AN INTRODUCTION
TO THE STUDY
OF DISEASE

WILLIAM BOYD, C.C., M.D.

DIPL. PSYCHIAT., M.R.C.P. (EDIN.), HON. F.R.C.P. (EDIN.), F.R.C.P.
(LOND.), F.R.C.S. (CAN.), F.R.S. (CAN.), LL.D. (SASK.), (QUEEN'S),
D.SC. (MAN.), M.D. (HON.) (OSLO).

*Professor Emeritus of Pathology, The University of Toronto; Visiting
Professor of Pathology, The University of Alabama; Formerly Professor
of Pathology, The University of Manitoba and the University of British
Columbia.*

SIXTH EDITION, Thoroughly Revised————————
200 Illustrations

LEA & FEBIGER   *Philadelphia*

First Edition, 1937
Reprinted, 1938
Reprinted, 1939

Second Edition, 1941
Reprinted, 1942
Reprinted, 1944

Third Edition, 1945
Reprinted, 1945
Reprinted, 1947
Reprinted, 1948
Reprinted, 1949
Reprinted, 1950
Reprinted, 1950

Fourth Edition, 1952
Reprinted, 1953
Reprinted, 1954
Reprinted, 1955
Reprinted, 1957
Reprinted, 1958
Reprinted, 1960

Fifth Edition, 1962
Reprinted, 1963
Reprinted, 1965
Reprinted, 1969

Sixth Edition, 1971
Reprinted, 1972
Reprinted, 1976

ISBN 0-8121-0333-5

Published in Great Britain by Henry Kimpton Publishers, London
Library of Congress Catalog Card Number 76-135679

Printed in the United States of America

To Enid

Preface

I⊤ is difficult for the author of a book on *An Introduction to the Study of Disease* to know what he should put into a new edition after the lapse of nine years, during which time spectacular advances have been made in so many fields involved in disease. The purpose of a Preface to a new edition is to indicate some of the more important changes which have been made in that edition. It should also include the outline of the main purpose of the book as indicated in the Preface to previous editions.

This book is, of course, merely an introduction to the study of disease, in which the important word is "introduction." It may be regarded as an airplane view of disease, its causes, and the bodily changes that accompany it. When we descend to earth again, it is easier to understand the details of the country over which we have flown. This introduction is merely a lifting of the dark veil, so that we may peep beneath and get some glimpse of the hidden mysteries. Emphasis is laid on disturbed function rather than disordered structure, although I, as a pathologist, should be more concerned with the latter. Such a survey must necessarily be brief, but this is no disadvantage provided the fact is recognized. A little knowledge may be a dangerous thing, but not if you know how little it is.

The book is designed principally for the assistants, or rather the partners, of the physician in his demanding task of caring for the sick, those members of the health team who are described nowadays as students of the allied disciplines. The relation may be that of nurse, laboratory technologist, x-ray therapist, physiotherapist, occupational therapist, medical secretary, medical librarian, or medical records librarian. Every doctor knows that he can practice medicine better with a good laboratory service, and it is not necessary even to mention that the same is true of a good nursing service. Those of us who have been ill know how true this is. It is obvious that for both of these groups of workers a sound knowledge and understanding of the nature of disease is essential. The pharmacist is, of course, an all-important member of the health team. To these groups we must add the premedical student, whose studies in the basic sciences have made

him aware of the vast field of disease awaiting him, as well as the
college student who may be toying with the idea of becoming a
physician.

In the process of acquiring new information, the student is confronted with two approaches to the subject represented by two very
different words, namely *what* and *why*. The question *What* connotes the
learning of facts, and represents the acquisition of new information;
it is a feat of memory. The question *Why* is far more penetrating and
difficult to answer; it is a leading out, that is to say an education
(which is the meaning of that word), and demands thinking rather than
memory. In the chapters that follow we must naturally be concerned
primarily with facts, but we would be stupid if we did not keep asking
the master word *Why*. Nor must we entirely neglect the third master
word *How*. The understanding of disease does not consist in learning
a vast number of scientific names, but in comprehending what is going
on in the body.

As is evident from the Table of Contents, the first part of the
book deals with the general principles of disease, while the second
part describes the individual organs and systems and their diseases.
Chapter 1 starts with the living cell and its functions. It is intended
for those who have had no previous contact with anatomy and physiology and can be skipped by those who have. So also may the chapters
on bacterial and viral infections by those who have had a course in
microbiology. Those with no interest in how we came to our present
knowledge of disease do not need to trouble themselves with Chapter 2.

Among the material that is either new or greatly amplified may be
mentioned: the thymus in relation to immunity; the intimate structure
of a cell, including sex chromatin, as revealed by modern technique;
the classification of viruses; interferon; bacteriophage and slow-acting
viruses; transplantation of the heart and kidney; the meaning of death
in relation to organ transplantation; cardiac catheterization and angiocardiography; drugs as a cause of disease; blood platelets and the
part they play in disease; the etiology of cancer; carcinoma-in-situ;
the resistance of the body to cancer; the malabsorption syndrome;
calcitonin and the regulation of the calcium content of the plasma;
surfactant, which allows the alveolar spaces of the lungs to remain
open; contraceptives; the treatment of Parkinson's disease with L-dopa;
memory; whiplash injury; and the hazards of prolonged rest in bed
for the elderly.

The increasingly important subject of emphysema is now discussed
in some detail early in the chapter on the Lungs, rather than briefly
at the end as formerly.

The final chapter on The Care of the Patient has been expanded with the allied personnel in mind, including occupational therapists and pharmacists. It may well be considered presumptuous for a mere pathologist to write a chapter on this subject, but the members of the allied health fields for whom the book is designed are all concerned in one way or another with the care of the sufferer from the diseases they have been studying. That is my excuse.

The reader may notice that there is no chapter on the eye or the ear. That is because I know next to nothing about diseases of these organs. Nor is there a chapter on diseases of the skin, which is so complicated a subject that it is better for the beginner, for whom this book is intended, to steer clear of it.

At the end of the book the reader will find a list of classic prefixes and suffixes, which provide a convenient type of shorthand in medical and other sciences. The classic derivation of many words is given in the text, as it serves to make these words more meaningful. I have indexed these words for ready reference. Words such as leukorrhea and thalassemia become less obscure when the derivations are made plain. With this in view, I have not felt it necessary to include a glossary.

Italics and bold face have been used to a greater extent than formerly, not only for words but also for sentences. This may be helpful to the reader who wishes to revise a subject.

At the end of each chapter there is for the first time a short list of articles for further reading. These are not references mentioned in the text, but papers giving further information if that is desired.

Many new illustrations have been introduced, some of which replace those that seemed somewhat worn and out-of-date.

I wish to express my appreciation to Dr. P. H. Pinkerton for help with revising the chapter on the blood, and in particular the blood platelets; to Dr. C. M. Godfrey for bringing the section on physio-therapy more up-to-date; and to Dr. Patoria of Nagpur, India, for donating such excellent pictures of malignant melanoma, aneurysm of the heart and of the aorta, and polycystic kidney.

I also wish to convey my very warm thanks to Miss Laura McKinnon for typing and helping me with the manuscript and index.

As with my other books, I have been extremely fortunate in having the skilful editorial assistance of Miss Mary E. Mansor.

WILLIAM BOYD

Toronto

Contents

Part One

GENERAL PRINCIPLES

Chapter 1

The Living Body

In order to study and understand disease, it is obvious that we must first know something of the structure and functions of the body in health, and in particular, the normal working of the basic units of which it is composed. The present chapter represents the merest outline or draft. A more detailed, although necessarily very incomplete, account will be found in the chapters of Part Two which deal with the various organs and their diseases.

The human body, that miracle of mechanical perfection, is composed of an infinite number of minute elements known as *cells,* which are collected to form definite structures or *tissues,* these again being grouped into *organs.* Thus certain cells with definite properties are set aside to form muscle tissue, and others with quite different properties to form nervous tissue; these and other tissues are combined to form organs such as the heart and stomach. *A tissue consists of cells of the same kind. An organ is composed of tissues of different kinds.* Cells and tissues must be studied under the microscope. This study is known as *histology,* from the Greek *histos,* tissue and *logos,* the study of. The word tissue itself comes from the French term *tissu,* which means weave or

3

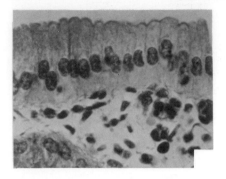

A

Fig. 1. Photomicrographs of types of epithelium. *A*, Simple columnar lining gallbladder. × 730; *B*, moist stratified squamous of oral cavity. × 365. (Finerty and Cowdry, *A Textbook of Histology.*)

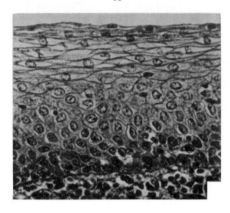

B

texture. There are four basic tissues: (1) epithelial, (2) connective, (3) muscular, and (4) nervous tissue. *Epithelial tissue* or epithelium serves to protect, absorb, and secrete. It is natural, therefore, that epithelial cells should be arranged in sheets or membranes, acting as *protective* coverings for external surfaces (skin) or *absorptive* linings for internal surfaces (intestine) (Fig. 1). For *secretion* there are groups of cells that have grown down from the surface epithelium to form *glands. Connective tissue* holds together, connects, and supports other tissues and cells. In addition to connective tissue cells it contains a large amount of *intercellular substance* (Fig. 2), which plays a prominent part in the reaction of inflammation. *Muscular tissue* consists of long muscle cells whose chief characteristic is contractility. *Nervous tissue* is highly specialized with the object of giving instant conductivity, which in turn is dependent on a high degree of irritability. It may be well to remember that a nervous system which is not irritable, *i.e.,* which does not respond to irritation, is completely valueless.

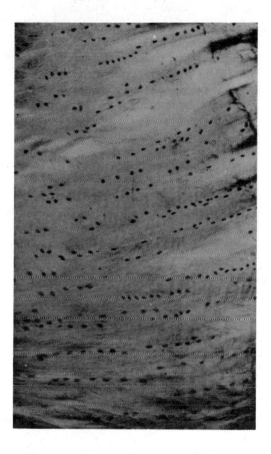

Fig. 2. Abundant intercellular substance in tendon. × 150. (Finerty and Cowdry, *A Textbook of Histology.*)

THE HEALTHY CELL

The word "cell" originally meant a small chamber, and it is still used in that sense in relation to a jail or a monastery. *But it is a chamber holding a living inmate, actually the smallest unit of living matter.* Some animals such as the ameba and the malaria parasite consist of a single cell, and are therefore called unicellular organisms or protozoa. Although these most primitive of animals are entirely undifferentiated, they breathe, digest, excrete, and move. Let us not forget that each of us started from a single cell, a fertilized ovum. This cell multiplies almost endlessly, and the resulting cells become differentiated to an incredible degree. All the cells of the body become specialized in form and function with the exception of the sex cells, which are set aside at a very early stage of development for the continuance of the race.

In the earliest stage of development the cells of the embryo are not notably different from one another. Later a finished muscle cell and a finished nerve cell and a finished liver cell are as far apart in visible structure as in what they do. Some of the cells will pour out cement which binds them together, as in cartilage and bone, some become fluid so as to flow along tubes too fine for the eye to see. Some become as clear as glass, as in the cornea of the eye, some as opaque as stone, some colorless, some red, some black. Some become factories of a furious chemistry, some develop into a system transmitting electrical signals. Each one of the 70,000 billion cells in each human body finally specializes into something helpful to the whole. The evolution of cells for different functions leaves us breathless—those functions we recognize in our own bodies as well as the incredible senses of "dumb animals," such as the vision of the eagle, the olfactory sense of the dog, the radar-like mechanism employed by the bat so that he can fly safely through a wood at night, and the sense of touch of the mollusc. This is the miracle of life and its development.

The human body has been likened by Rudolf Virchow, the father of modern pathology, to a "cell state" with a social organization and specialization of labor. This carries with it the hazard that one group of specialized cells becomes dependent on another group of specialists, and a strike on the part of a very small group may paralyze or reduce to chaos the entire community. Thus, the contractility of the heart depends on a very narrow bundle of conducting fibers. If this is put out of business the heart stops, every function of the body ceases due to lack of oxygen, and death results. The lowly ameba, consisting of only one cell, has no such hazards to fear. Specialization demands a price, in cells as well as in society.

We have seen that the body is composed of cells as a house is of bricks. But it is as if a house originated from one brick, a magic brick that would set about manufacturing other bricks. These bricks, without waiting for the architect's drawings or the coming of the bricklayers, assemble themselves into walls, and become changed into windowpanes, roofing-slates, coal for heating, and water for the kitchen and the bathroom.

There is a striking contrast between the durability of our body and the transitory character of its elements. Man is composed of a soft matter which can disintegrate in a few hours, and yet he lasts longer than if made of steel. Moreover, he accommodates himself marvelously to the changing conditions of his environment. The body seems to mold itself on events. Instead of wearing out like a machine, it changes.

Just as the atom is the unit in physics, so cells are the fundamental units of every living body, whether it be animal or vegetable, and in the last analysis it is they that eat the food, drink the water, and breathe the air, all of which are necessary for the life of the body. The marvelous arrangements of structure (*anatomy*) and function (*physiology*) are

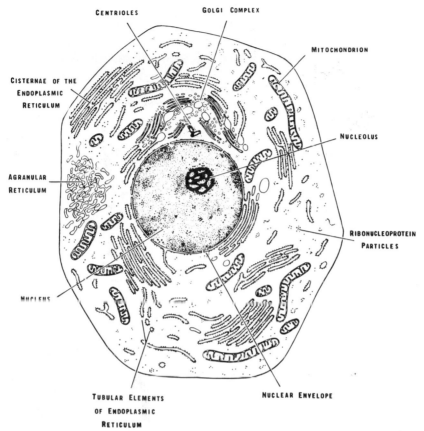

Fig. 3. Diagrammatic representation of the structure of a cell to indicate morphology and typical arrangement of its parts as seen with electron microscopy. (Courtesy of Dr. Don W. Fawcett; from Finerty and Cowdry, *A Textbook of Histology.*)

simply a complex mechanism to bring to the cells this food, water, and air, which are so far beyond their reach, as well as to perpetuate the species to which the organism belongs.

Every cell, whether of an animal or a plant, consists of *protoplasm,* a gelatinous substance composed of water (75 per cent) and protein (25 per cent) with the addition of various minerals. The protein molecules are made up of atoms of carbon, nitrogen, oxygen, and hydrogen. The three principal constituents of the cell are: (1) *cell membrane,* (2) *nucleus,* and (3) *cytoplasm.* The nucleus contains: (*a*) the *chromosomes,* which are the carriers of the genes, the transmitters of hereditary characteristics, and (*b*) the *nucleolus.* The cytoplasm contains a variety of structural constituents known as the *organelles* or little organs. The cell is indeed a *multum in parvo* (Fig. 4).

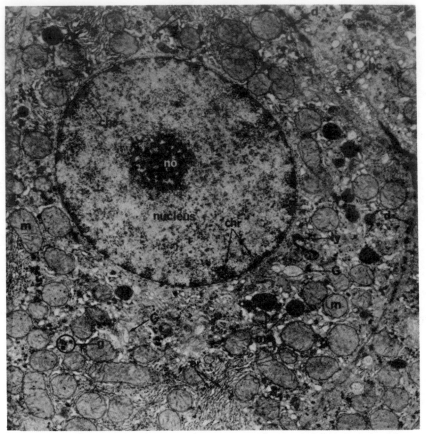

Fig. 4. Electron micrograph of a normal liver cell. Uranyl acetate and lead hydroxide stain. This shows the nucleus with its nucleolus (no) and chromatin (chr), and the cytoplasm with its mitochondria (m), endoplasmic reticulum (er), Golgi apparatus (G), desmosomes (d), microbodies (mb), and a bile canaliculus (bc). × 14,500. (Kindness of Dr. K. Miyai; Boyd's *Textbook of Pathology*.)

In recent years enormous advances have been made in our knowledge of the structure of the cell in health and to a lesser degree in disease. We owe these advances in the main to two new methods of technique: (1) The *electron microscope,* which gives us a magnification of 100,000 in place of one of 1,000, revealing a new wealth of structure, particularly the mitochondria, which could not be seen with the light microscope with ordinary stains. Electron microscopes are now being constructed at a cost of one or two million dollars which may make it possible for us actually to see the atom. (2) The development of *new methods of cytochemistry* by means of which chemical agents such as enzymes can be demonstrated not only in the intact cell, but also in particles such as mitochondria obtained by disrupting the cell by mechanical means and then separating the particles by means of the ultracentrifuge.

The stains usually employed in combination to show cellular detail in microscopic sections are *hematoxylin,* a basic stain which colors the nucleus a rather intense blue, and *eosin,* an acid stain which colors the cytoplasm a rather faint pink. It is the nucleus that stands out clearly, the outline of the cytoplasm being often vague and indistinct. The reason that the nucleus stains intensely is that it contains *chromatin granules,* which represent the chromosomes (*chroma,* color; *soma,* body) that are involved in mitotic division.

CELL MEMBRANE. The membrane or envelope of the cell is not evident with the light microscope, but it is well demonstrated by the electron microscope. Too little attention has been paid this membrane in the past, but it is now known to be a structure no less remarkable than the contents that it encloses. It is an all-important structure, for it regulates the internal environment of the cell, determining what goes in and what comes out. Thus it separates the high concentrations of potassium inside the cell from the high concentrations of sodium outside the cell, it can hold back red blood cells and plasma in the capillaries, but allow the passage of white cells, the leukocytes, and it can push out processes to engulf harmful bacteria which the cell then destroys, the process of phagocytosis. Water and all food particles must pass inward through the membrane freely, while metabolites must pass out. Virus particles are *adsorbed* to the surface of the cell before penetrating to the interior. It is to the surface structure that many dyes and effective drugs become attached, and antigens react at the surface of the cell with the formation of antibodies, which are then liberated to enter the blood stream. *From these facts it becomes apparent that the cell membrane is a structure of paramount importance.*

NUCLEUS. *The nucleus may be regarded as the heart of the cell.* When the nucleus dies, death of the cell will soon follow. There is one curious exception to this rule, for the erythrocyte or red blood cell loses its nucleus when it enters the blood stream from the bone marrow, yet its life span is about 120 days. Perhaps its passive role of carrying oxygen from the lungs to the tissues makes the presence of the nucleus superfluous. The nucleus contains 23 pairs (46 in all) of uncoiled *chromosomes* along which are strung 50,000 to 100,000 *genes,* which are the arbiters of hereditary characters. One of each pair of chromosomes, with all its tally of genes, comes from the father and the other from the mother. Actually it is only when the cell is dividing that the chromosomes become visible as separate units (p. 12). At other times they are in the form of a *chromatin network* of granules. The genes appear to be chemical particles of a nucleic acid known as DNA (deoxyribonucleic acid) (p. 11). Loss or abnormality of one of these genes may result in an *inborn error of metabolism,* which often manifests itself as a disease. It is hardly too much to say that a man's biochemistry is as individual as his fingerprints, and that both are determined by his genes. The nucleus is also concerned with cellular reproduction and multiplication, the development of separate chromosomal threads from the network being the first step in *mitosis* or cell division (*mitos,* a thread). We shall return to the subject of mitosis shortly (p. 12). In addition to the chromosomal network the nucleus contains a small darkly staining body, the *nucleolus,* of which at times there may be more than one. The function of the nucleolus is not certain at the present time, but it appears to be particularly concerned with the synthesis of protein by the cytoplasm. In this connection it may be remarked that the nucleic acid of both nucleolus and cytoplasm is RNA (ribonucleic acid), whereas that of the nucleus is DNA (see p. 11). Finally, the nucleus is believed to control the production of enzymes by the cytoplasm. These enzymes, which are discussed in connection with metabolism, are responsible for the chemical transformations associated with life.

CYTOPLASM.   If the nucleus is the heart of the cell, concerned with such major problems as genetic constitution and cellular reproduction, it is the cytoplasm that does most of the everyday work. As the cells are specialized to do different kinds of work, such as the contraction of muscle, the secretion of digestive juices, the production of hormones, and the sending out of nervous impulses, it is natural that the shape and appearance of cytoplasm should vary correspondingly. An examination of the nucleus will indicate whether the cell is living or dead, but the appearance of the cytoplasm will tell the pathologist looking down the microscope whether or not the cell has been sick and unable to work. A brief note on this appearance is given on page 14.

The cytoplasm contains a number of structural constituents known as *organelles.* These have been studied in detail by the modern methods already referred to, in particular *cell disruption, high speed centrifugation,* and photography with the *electron microscope.* Our knowledge of the functions of the various organelles is still very meager, so we shall limit our discussion to three, the mitochondria, the endoplasmic reticulum, and the lysosomes.

Mitochondria.   The mitochondria are thread-like bodies (*mitos,* thread; *chondros,* granule) when viewed with the light microscope and stained with appropriate stains, but as seen with the electron microscope they are rod-shaped or like a cucumber. Although they are not visible with hematoxylin and eosin staining, they are present in enormous numbers, with an average of 2500 per cell in the liver of the rat. They are surrounded with a double-layered membrane, so that each can be regarded as a separate chemical laboratory, and folds of the inner membrane project inward as shelves termed *cristae* (Fig. 5). It is on these shelves that the all-important enzymes are arranged, and it is these enzymes that are responsible for cell respiration, which uses oxygen and produces energy. *The mitochondria may therefore be regarded as the main power plants of the cell.* This activity, without which life would be impossible, is considered again in this chapter in connection with metabolism (p. 20).

Endoplasmic Reticulum. This is the skeleton of the cytoplasm, a series of vesicles and intercommunicating canals, whose primary function is the manufacture of protein. Many of the vesicles are dotted on their outer surface with fine dark granules which consist of ribonucleic acid or RNA, so that they are called *ribosomes.*

Lysosomes. The lysosomes are membrane-bound bodies containing powerful digestive enzymes, so that *they can be regarded as part of the* digestive system of the cell, just as the mitochondria represent the *power plants.* They may be called the stomach of the cell.

NUCLEIC ACIDS. The dominant constituents of both nucleus and cytoplasm are the nucleic acids, which are complexes of bases, sugars and phosphoric acid. They are divided into two groups, namely *ribonucleic acid* (RNA) and *deoxyribonucleic acid* (DNA), the two groups being distinguished by their sugar component, ribose. Both types stain with basic dyes, but they can be differentiated by means of the *Feulgen reaction,* which is based on a difference in the two sugars. DNA stains purple or magenta with the Feulgen method and is therefore said to be Feulgen-positive; RNA remains unstained and is Feulgen-negative. *DNA is confined to the nucleus and in particular the chromosomes, whereas RNA is present mainly in the mitochondria of the cytoplasm, but also in the nucleolus.* It is the DNA of the fertilized ovum that deter-

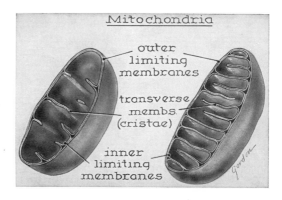

Fig. 5. Diagrammatic drawings to illustrate the structure of mitochondria in three dimensions. (Ham, *Histology;* J. B. Lippincott Co.)

mines the species of animal that will develop, as well as the individual characteristics of that animal. *The genes consist of DNA, and the chromosomes are assemblies of genes.* The RNA of the cytoplasm presides over protein synthesis, but it is the DNA that presides over the synthesis of RNA, and therefore dictates the formation of every kind of protein to be constructed from the choice of 20 amino acids, thus every possible enzyme and every sort of function. The RNA, however, is the real worker. It is believed by some to be related to memory, indeed it may be the very stuff that memory is made of. Unfortunately, with the passing of the years the code message stored in the nerve cells may become garbled. The giant molecule of DNA is pictured as a double spiral or helix. Each chain of the spiral consists of alternate deoxyribose and phosphoric acid groups. The two chains are cross connected by two pairs of four nitrogenous bases that follow each other in a nearly infinite number of possible arangements, and thus inscribe on the DNA molecule the *"four-letter code of life."*

Mitosis.   Reference has already been made to the varying life span of cells. Some are short-lived, while others enjoy a long life. In either case, when they die they are replaced by new cells. (An important and sad exception to this rule is the cells of the brain and spinal cord; once these are destroyed, as in cerebral hemorrhage or poliomyelitis, they cannot be replaced). In the lowliest unicellular organisms new cells are created simply by the division of the pre-existing cell. In all the higher forms the birth of new cells takes place through a complex and wonderful process known as mitosis or *mitotic division.* A nucleus in the process of mitosis is referred to as a *mitotic figure.* The meaning of the word will soon be evident. The process passes through a number of stages or phases, which have been given rather difficult names that the reader need not try to remember.

After the resting stage or *interphase* comes the *prophase,* in which the dispersed chromatin granules of the nucleus become organized into a darkly staining coiled thread (*mitos,* thread), which undergoes segmental division into chromosomes and longitudinal splitting into two longitudinal halves or *chromatids.* In this way the number of chromosomes is doubled, an equal number being destined for each of the two new daughter cells. It is to be presumed that each of the genes undergoes similar multiplication. A *spindle* of non-chromatin threads is now formed, stretching from one pole of the cell to the other, and in the *metaphase* (*meta,* after) the chromatids of each pair separate and line up in two parallel bands across the center of the cell and become attached to the threads of the spindle. This is called the *monaster,* because it suggests a star when viewed from the side. In the *anaphase* (*ana,* up) the two sets of new chromosomes separate and move to the op-

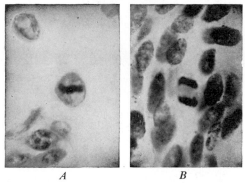

A   *B*

Fig. 6. Mitotic figures. *A* shows the monaster stage (metaphase) and *B* the diaster stage (anaphase). × 700.

posite poles forming a *diaster* (double star). In the end stage or *telophase* (*telos,* end) the cytoplasm becomes constricted in the middle of the cell until division is complete, while the chromosomes take on their original granular appearance, which probably represents the intact genes. The prophase is shown in Figure 3, and the metaphase (monaster) and anaphase (diaster) in Figure 6. The entire process is illustrated in diagrammatic fashion in Figure 7.

Mitoses (mitotic figures) are seldom seen in normal tissue, because very few cells are dying and being replaced. As might be expected, they are very common in the growing embryo. Cell division becomes very evident in the repair of wounds and in the replacement of excised tissue, especially so in the case of the liver. The study of mitosis is of particular importance in the case of cancer, where mitotic figures are not only numerous but often atypical in appearance. This fact may enable the pathologist to decide whether he is examining a benign (innocent) tumor or a malignant one.

THE SICK CELL

The infinitely complex and delicate structure of the cell may be damaged by a variety of influences, of which chemical poisons and bacterial toxins are the most obvious examples. The cell becomes sick, so that it does not function perfectly. This sickness is reflected in changes in the microscopic appearance of the cytoplasm and later of the nucleus. To these evidences of cellular damage the pathologist has given the name of *degenerations. They can be regarded as the fingerprints of disease,* but when the damage is slight the prints can be erased. Although these changes are of importance to the pathologist, they are of little interest to the reader of this book, and they will merely be mentioned so that the laboratory technologist will recognize the names when he

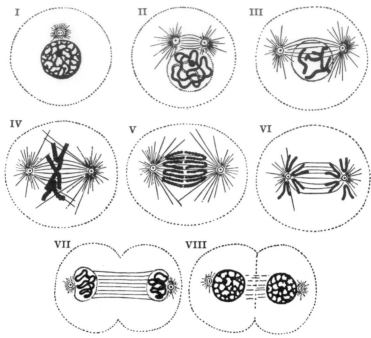

Fig. 7. Diagram of stages in mitotic cell division. I–III, prophase; IV, meta-phase; V and VI, anaphase; VII and VIII, telophase. (*Gray's Anatomy.*)

hears them discussed. It must be added that a cell may be sick without showing any microscopic evidence of that fact. We are coming to think of disease in terms of the molecule, and not merely in terms of the cell. The real work of the cell is done by enzymes (p. 21), and an enzyme may be poisoned without the pathologist being able to detect any evidence of damage. A person who dies in the terrible convulsions of tetanus (lockjaw) *appears* to have a normal nervous system, although we know that it must be profoundly, indeed fatally, abnormal functionally. *The same is true of mental disease.*

DEGENERATIONS. The commonest degeneration is called *cloudy swelling.* This is an old-fashioned and confusing name, for originally it was applied to the gross organ, which was swollen and had a cloudy surface, rather than to the cells of that organ. The cells, however, are also swollen and the cytoplasm has a granular appearance. The change seems to indicate *some disturbance in the protein metabolism of the cell.* The swelling is due to an accumulation of water in the cytoplasm. *Fatty degeneration* is an accumulation of fat in the cytoplasm in the sick cell. This accumulation may be caused by a *local breakdown of the mitochondrial metabolism of fat* produced by disruption of the en-

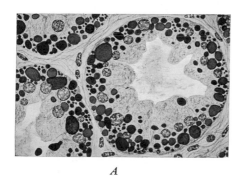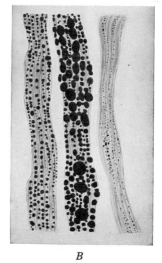

A   *B*

Fig. 8. *A*, Fatty degeneration of convoluted tubules of the kidney. Drawing. The rounded fat droplets are shown in a dark color. *B*, Fatty degeneration of cardiac muscle in chronic alcoholism. Drawing. The fat droplets are shown in a dark color. (Bell, *Textbook of Pathology,* Lea & Febiger.)

zymes concerned. Or it may be due to healthy cells being presented with an overload of fat as a result of some systemic metabolic derangement, a condition known as *fatty infiltration.* These fatty changes are of particular importance in cirrhosis of the liver, usually associated with nutritional deficiency, which may or may not be related to chronic alcoholism. The fat can be demonstrated with great ease in the sick cells by means of a variety of special stains, provided that precautions are taken to prevent the fat's being dissolved in the preparation of the microscopic section (Fig. 8). *Glycogen infiltration* is an *abnormal accumulation of glycogen in the cell,* which is the storage form of carbohydrates. It is best seen in diabetes mellitus, in which there is an excess of carbohydrate in the blood owing to a deficiency of the hormone insulin. In *von Gierke's* disease, a rare condition in children, there is an extreme accumulation of glycogen in the cells particularly of the liver, with great enlargement of that organ. The condition seems to be a congenital anomaly of metabolism. Other degenerations are described, but they need not detain us.

NECROSIS. Necrosis, as the name implies (*nekros,* corpse), is the local death of cells. The cellular changes characteristic of necrosis are changes that the cell undergoes *after* it has died while still remaining in the body, and are due to the action of enzymes. These turn their energies on the framework of the cell itself, a process known as *autolysis.* Death of the cell may be due to (1) chemical poisons, (2) bacterial toxins, (3) physical agents such as irradiation, and (4) loss of blood supply due to closure of an artery by thrombosis, a condition known as an *infarct,* cellular death in this last instance being caused by the sudden cutting off of the supply of oxygen to the cell, that is to say, *anoxia* (Fig. 9). The nucleus breaks up and disappears, and the cytoplasm becomes indistinct and fades away, with eventual liquefaction. In the case of some bacterial infections such as tuberculosis, the structural outlines of the part are wiped out. This process is known as *caseation,* because the gross appearance of the material is cheesy or caseous. In an infarct, on the other hand, the general outline of microscopic structure can still be recognized, such as the tubules and glomeruli in the kidney and the muscle fibers in the heart. The difference between the necrosis of an infarct and caseation is the difference between the site of ancient Pompeii in which the outline of the streets can still be recognized compared with that of the destruction of Hiroshima.

Somatic Death. This is death of the body as a whole. It occurs when respiration and the heart's action cease, although individual cells and even tissues may continue to live for short periods. Soon characteristic changes begin to make their appearance in the dead body. The most striking of these are: (1) a *fall in the temperature;* (2) *rigor mortis,*

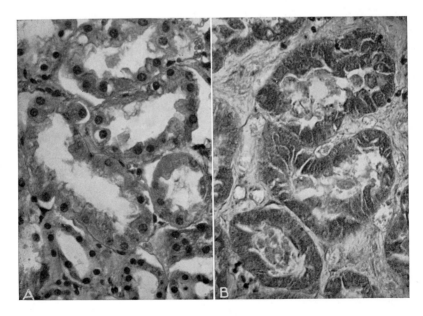

Fig. 9. *A*, Normal renal tubules. *B*, Tubules from an infarcted area showing coagulation necrosis. Note absence of nuclei and homogeneous cytoplasm. Photomicrograph. (Bell, *Textbook of Pathology,* Lea & Febiger.)

i.e., muscular rigidity due to chemical changes in the muscle, the stiffness beginning in four hours or more and passing off in about three days; (3) *postmortem lividity,* a reddish discoloration of the dependent parts of the body due to the sinking of the blood from gravity combined with a breaking down (hemolysis) of the red blood cells; (4) *postmortem clotting of the blood.* The doctor or the detective in the story book can tell to within a few minutes how long the body has been dead, but so many factors such as fever, high external temperature, and violent exercise at the time of death may influence the speed of the postmortem changes that anything approaching accuracy is out of the question. A note of these changes, however, may be useful in making a rough estimate of the time of death for medicolegal purposes.

BODY FLUIDS

The body fluids are of three kinds: tissue fluid, blood, and lymph. (1) The *tissue fluid* surrounds and bathes the cells; it is placid, a lake, not a stream (Fig. 10). (2) The *blood* is contained in the blood vessels, and nowhere comes in direct contact with the tissues except in the spleen. It is carried to an organ in arteries. These break up into a vast network of capillaries through whose infinitely thin walls the fluid of the blood (plasma or serum) is able to pass, mixing with the tissue fluid and carrying to it the nutriment and oxygen that the waiting cells absorb. The capillaries open into the veins by which the impoverished blood is carried away from the part. As the tissue fluid continually increases in amount, it is obvious that there must be some means of escape. This is provided by (3) the *lymph,* which, like the blood, is

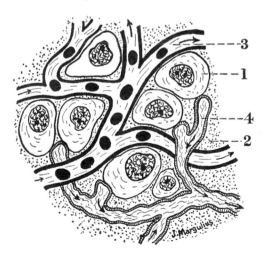

Fig. 10. Tissue fluid bathing body cells. 1, Tissue cell; 2, tissue fluid; 3, blood vessel; 4, lymphatic.

contained in a set of vessels, the lymphatics. The tissue fluid laden with waste products from the living cells passes through the thin walls of the lymphatics and is carried away as lymph. This is really a round-about way of getting back into the veins, for all the lymphatics eventually form one or two main ducts, which open into the large veins in the neck. The advantage of this method is that the lymph has to pass through a series of filters, known as the lymphatic glands or *lymph nodes,* in which bacteria and other injurious agents that may have gained access to the tissue fluid are strained out and usually destroyed. A small proportion of the tissue fluid passes directly back through the walls of the veins into the blood stream.

It is possible to estimate the rate of passage of water from the vessels into the tissue spaces by injecting some traceable substance, such as a radioactive isotope, into a vein and noting the rapidity with which it disappears from the blood. The rate of exchange shown by this method is incredibly fast, for *more than 70 per cent of the water of the blood is exchanged with extravascular water every minute.* The walls of the smaller blood vessels appear to be veritable sieves with regard to water.

WATER AND SALT. The most important single constituent of the body is water, for water is the fabric of everything that lives. Hunger can be endured for days or weeks, but thirst is unendurable; the cells of the whole body are crying out for water, not merely the parched mouth. Life started in the water in the very dim and distant past, for the sea is the original home of all life on the globe; even vertebrate life first appeared as a marine form. We still live in a watery environment, not, as we fondly imagine, in the air. For the surface of the body in contact with the air is either dead (the horny layers of the skin) or is separated from the air by a layer of water (eyes, nose, and mouth). After all, we are completely immersed in water during the first nine months of life before birth. The baby consists mostly of water, while the old man or woman shrivels up like a wilted plant. In the salt content of the blood plasma and the film of salt water through which we look upon the outside world, we carry the memory of the remotely ancient ocean in which we originated. Still more do we carry this modified salt water in the *interstitial fluid,* which constitutes what the great French physiologist, Claude Bernard, more than a hundred years ago called the *internal environment.*

The water of the body, together with the salts or *electrolytes* (substances decomposed in solution by electricity) that are dissolved in it, is contained in two major compartments: (1) intracellular and (2) extracellular. The *intracellular fluid* makes up nearly 50 per cent of the body weight, the bulk of it being contained in muscle. The *extracellular fluid* is mainly represented by the interstitial fluid, with a much smaller amount in the blood plasma. It is the fluid in the interstitial space that constitutes the real internal environment, and the freest communication exists through the cell membrane between the water in this compartment and the water inside the cells. The passage of fluids or solutions through a membrane is known as *osmosis;* this is the passage from the less concentrated to the more concentrated side of the membrane. *Osmolality* represents the osmotic concentration of a solute. Thus for each cell in the body the same conditions prevail as for the single-celled creatures fixed on the bed of a flowing stream which brings to them their food and oxygen and carries away their *waste* products. The cells are bathed in salty fluid; without that fluid they cannot live. They are indeed islands in the interstitial sea. In many diseases such as cholera this fluid is drained away from the body, the tissues become dehydrated, and they will die unless the water is replaced by intravenous injections of saline solution.

It is the delicate balance of electrolytes and water that serves to maintain the *constancy of the internal environment,* the importance of which Bernard was the first to emphasize. For the preservation of this constancy the mechanism of *homeostasis* has been evolved. The chief instrument in the homeostatic orchestra is the kidney, as we shall see when we come to that organ, but the posterior pituitary, the adrenal cortex, and the thyroid all play their part. *When the mechanism breaks down we see the clinical picture that we call disease, a breakdown which, if sufficiently profound and prolonged, results in death.*

The subject of the internal environment has become of much greater importance in the present day than in bygone years not only to the physician, but also to the nurse and the medical technologist, partly because of the strong likelihood of its being changed when the patient is placed in a hospital bed—especially on a surgical ward—and fluids begin to flow into his veins, partly because the physician, and still more the surgeon and the pediatrician, can do so much to correct disturbances of this environment, and to safeguard health and life itself in the process.

We have seen that an adequate and constant supply of tissue fluid is necessary for the health of the body cells. If this supply is insufficient or if the fluid is withdrawn too quickly, a condition of *dehydration* develops, which can be recognized by the sunken appearance of the face and the wrinkled condition of the skin. This may develop very quickly, as after a night of hard drinking, or in acute diseases associated with severe vomiting or profuse diarrhea. Dehydration and loss of salt may be the result of excessive sweating, as is seen in the tropics or the desert and in men working under conditions of great heat. When the heat of

Arabia comes out like a drawn sword and strikes you speechless, you realize that water comes before everything. In such cases it is important to drink large amounts of fluid to which salt has been added. On the other hand, tissue fluid may accumulate in excessive amount, so that the part becomes waterlogged, a condition known as *edema,* which can be recognized by the fact that when a finger is pressed into the swollen part, a temporary pit is formed owing to the fluid's being forced away into the surrounding tissues. Edema may be caused in many ways. (1) In *inflammation* the walls of the capillaries become unduly permeable and too much fluid passes from the blood into the tissue spaces. (2) In *heart and kidney disease* edema is an important symptom; its method of production will be considered in connection with these diseases. (3) *Pressure on the lymphatics* by a tumor will naturally be accompanied by edema.

Derangements of the body fluids are discussed further in Chapter 5.

METABOLISM

Metabolism is the sum total of the chemical reactions that proceed in that remarkable chemical laboratory, the living cell. There are many cellular laboratories that do different kinds of work, and each individual laboratory can do various kinds of work. *Intermediary metabolism* is the chemical transformation of foodstuffs in the body so that they can be used. The essence of metabolism is change (*metabole,* change), and the change may be a breaking down, known as catabolism, or a building up or anabolism. *Catabolism* involves the breaking down of foodstuffs as well as protoplasm into simpler materials; in the process there is an all-important *liberation of energy.* In *anabolism,* on the other hand, there is a *utilization of energy,* by means of which new substances, including protoplasm, are formed. The three main constituents of food are proteins, carbohydrates, and fats. All contain carbon, hydrogen, and oxygen, but proteins are also distinguished by their content of nitrogen, which has to be built into the cells to make up for the loss that occurs in the wear and tear of activity. Proteins are made up of a large number of small units differing from one another; these units are the *amino acids.* Speaking generally, proteins are used for body building, while carbohydrates and fats are used for the production of energy. Carbohydrates and fats have been compared with gasoline and oil in an automobile, but it is protein that replaces worn parts. We are apt to picture the protein of meat being built up into body protein, and so on with the other foodstuffs. It is now known that the derivatives of the ingested protein, carbohydrate, and fat of the diet pass into a common metabolic pool, in which one basic foodstuff can be converted into another according to need before being built into the tissues. The essential purpose of this disintegration is to provide energy, some of which is used to perform mechanical work, some to support metabolic processes, the remainder appearing as heat. *All living systems require an external source of energy for growth and activity.* Plants obtain their energy directly from the sun by virtue of the photosynthesis effected by their chlorophil. By means of photosynthesis plants build simple substances (carbon dioxide of the air and water) into more complex ones (starch, sugar, cellulose). In all other organisms energy originally comes from the sun by way of the plants. Thus it is that animals and plants must depend on each other. When we regard a plate of beefsteak with a liberal helping of vegetables we are really looking at a plateful of energy. *Pyruvic acid* is a key substance in intermediary metabolism, as it represents a stage reached by all the foodstuffs, not only carbohydrate but also protein and fat. The various complex steps by which pyruvic acid is broken down with the liberation of energy is known as the *Krebs cycle.* (For this work Krebs received the Nobel prize.) The energy is trapped or bound as "energy-rich phosphate bonds," more particularly *adenosine triphosphate,* for convenience known as ATP. This trapped energy can suddenly be released like the combustion of gunpowder when the call comes. What brings about these dramatic changes?

ENZYMES. The profound importance of the biological catalysts known as enzymes or ferments in every phase of metabolism has now come to be fully recognized. A *catalyst,* it may be remarked, is a substance that can enormously speed up a reaction without itself becoming altered or forming a part of the product of that reaction, so that it can be used over and over again for an almost infinite number of times. *Enzymes have been called the men and the machines of the body's assembly line; they seem, indeed, to be the very center of life.* They bring about reactions which, without them, would require great heat and strong chemicals. They are giant protein molecules, and over 600 of them have been isolated. They are remarkably specific for all kinds of proteins, carbohydrates, and fats, chemical specialists in the true sense of the word. Indeed the specificity is so precise that it may be likened to the fit of a key for a lock, as if to make sure that the right chemicals undergo the right reactions at the right time. The substance on which a specific enzyme acts is known as the *substrate.* Many enzymes are inactive unless united with a nonprotein organic molecule, known as a *coenzyme,* which is therefore of equal importance with the enzyme itself.

Enzymes may pass out of the cell and take part in the digestion of food, as is the case in the enzymes of the saliva, the gastric juice, and the secretion of the pancreas which is poured into the intestine. Or they may act inside the cell. It is customary to name enzymes by adding the suffix *-ase* to the name of the substrate, as in maltase and lipase, or to the task they perform. Some, however, retain their original names, such as ptyalin in the saliva, pepsin in gastric juice, and trypsin in pancreatic juice. *The cellular enzymes may spill over into the blood when produced in excess, and their detection in the blood stream is the work of the medical technologist.* The demonstration of such enzymes may be of great diagnostic value. Thus the presence of acid phosphatase may confirm a suspicion of cancer of the prostate, and the same is true of glutamic oxaloacetic transaminase in the case of myocardial infarction caused by coronary artery thrombosis.

Enzymes belong to two great groups as regards their action on the substrate; they may be (1) hydrolytic or (2) oxidizing. The *hydrolytic enzymes* are those concerned more particularly with the digestion of food, and are therefore found in the mouth, the stomach, and the intestine. Hydrolysis involves the decomposition (loosening) of a substance owing to the incorporation of water, followed by a splitting into simpler compounds with smaller molecules which are able to pass through the intestinal mucosa into the blood stream. Thus protein is split into amino acids (acids containing one or more amino or NH_2 groups), and the hydrolytic enzymes then recombine the products of digestion to build up complex tissue, proteins, carbohydrates, and fats. It is evident that this is an anabolic process.

The *oxidizing enzymes* are concerned more particularly with the metabolism of carbohydrates and the intracellular production of energy. All the activities of the cell require energy, and this energy is derived from the oxidation of carbohydrates and, a lesser degree, of fats and proteins. As a result of the oxidation of carbohydrate, the carbon is converted to carbon dioxide (CO_2) and the hydrogen to water (H_2O), while energy is released. The body may be compared to a gasoline engine, which also burns carbon and hydrogen. In the engine heat represents the source of energy, but in the body it is a waste product representing energy the cells have failed to use and expressed as calories.

It becomes evident that respiration is not basically a matter of breathing air into and out of the lungs, but rather an interchange of oxygen in the course of intermediate metabolism within the cell, which is known as *cellular respiration*. The oxidative enzymes of the Krebs cycle have been pictured as arranged in an orderly manner on the shelves of the cristae of the mitochondria, the ultimate purpose of the mechanism being the synthesis of *adenosine triphosphate* (ATP). With this picture in mind we can visualize how a poisonous compound such as carbon tetrachloride may play havoc with the physiology (functioning) of the liver cells by penetrating the cells, attacking the mitochondria, paralyzing their enzymes, and thus disrupting the Krebs cycle and the production of ATP. The cyanides and hydrocyanic acid (prussic acid) are deadly poisons because they damage the respiratory enzymes that normally transfer oxygen from the hemoglobin of the red blood cells to the cells of the tissue. Thus all the tissues immediately suffer from lack of oxygen (*anoxia*), although the blood cells remain oxygenated and therefore bright red. It may be noted in passing that cancer cells have fewer mitochondria than normal, because these cells are unfortunately more concerned with reproduction (mitotic division) than with functional activity.

We may conclude our necessarily brief study of that remarkable structure, the living cell, with the vivid words of Osgood in an address to the American Society of Medical Technologists: "In summary, can you imagine a mobile, self-reproducing factory, which selects its own raw materials, manufactures not one but many products, rebuilds and repairs itself constantly, provides its own power supply, has automatic local and remote controls, transports its fuels, products and waste products with great efficiency, which may be versatile or specialized, but is integrated by efficient communication systems with the needs of the community, and always provides reserves for emergencies? Such a factory is the cell."

We have considered the cell, together with the body fluids and metabolism, which make the life of the cell possible and give it meaning as the basic unit in the living body. Let us now turn our attention for a few moments to the systems that bring nutriment and oxygen to the cell, prepare the food for absorption, excrete waste products, make intercommunication between the cells and organs possible, and finally meet the supreme challenge of reproduction. All of these will be discussed in greater detail when we study the diseases of these systems in Part Two of this book.

CIRCULATION

The *circulatory system* is the mechanism by which fresh material is sent to the tissue fluid and waste material is removed from it. The fresh material is of two kinds, food and oxygen. The food is contained in the blood from the intestine, the oxygen in the blood from the lungs. Because the blood has to circulate from the intestine and lungs to the tissue fluid and back again, a pump is required. This pump is the heart, which is simply a hollow muscle. Contraction of the body muscles helps to force the lymph through the lymphatics, and when this is interfered with as the result of disease, massage may take its place. *The blood from the tissues is impure*. It contains waste products, in the form of solid material in solution, and gas (carbon dioxide), also in solution. The solid material in solution is excreted, mainly by the kidneys but also by the skin. If the kidneys go on strike, the skin may be stimulated to do at least part of the work through increased perspiration. The carbon dioxide in the blood is given off in the lungs and expired; in this way the blood is purified. At the same time oxygen is breathed in and taken up by the blood, as a result of which the color of the blood becomes a much brighter red. The system of blood vessels with the blood they contain (blood vascular system) is comparable to a system of roads and railways by means of which intercommunication between different parts of the cell state is maintained (Fig. 11).

The tissues contain abundant reserves of water, salts, proteins, carbohydrates, and fat. These reserves can be used when need arises. Unfortunately oxygen is not stored anywhere; it must be unceasingly supplied to the body by the lungs, for the blood contains only a three-minute supply at any given moment. That is why the absence of oxygen or *anoxia* can only be tolerated for the shortest time, and is rapidly fatal to a tissue such as heart muscle and to life itself.

An organ is like a pond completely filled with aquatic plants and fed by a small brook. The water in the pond is nearly stagnant, and is polluted by waste products of the plants. The degree of stagnation and pollution depends on the volume and rapidity of the stream. This is the reason why the health of every organ suffers in the condition of prolonged heart disease known as congestive heart failure.

The *impure blood* from the body is carried to the *heart* by veins. and is then sent by the pulmonary artery to the *lungs* to be purified. The *pure blood* from the lungs is also carried to the heart by another set of veins, the pulmonary veins. It is evident that if these two kinds of blood were allowed to mix in the heart, the whole object of the circulation would be defeated. The cavity of the heart is therefore divided by a longitudinal septum or partition into two sides, right and left. The right side receives the impure blood from the body and sends it to the lungs. The left side receives the pure blood from the lungs and sends it throughout the body in the arteries. Like any other pump the heart is provided with valves, so that the blood will always move in one direction. If these are diseased the blood may leak back through the valves with great disturbance to the circulation. The names and arrangement of the valves and of the various chambers of the heart will be considered in connection with diseases of that organ.

RESPIRATION

The *respiratory system* is designed to bring air, or rather oxygen, from the outside to the cells in the innermost recesses of the body. The air is inhaled through the trachea or windpipe into the lungs, where it is brought into intimate contact with a vast network of capillaries

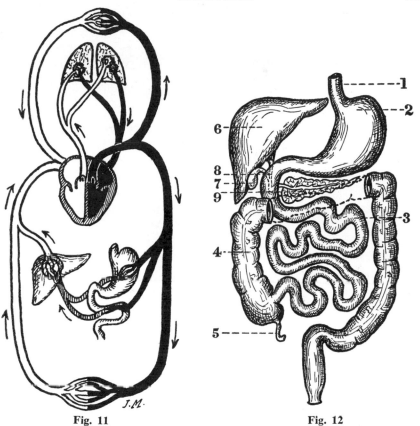

Fig. 11   **Fig. 12**

Fig. 11. Diagram of the circulation. The pure arterial blood is black, the portal blood is shaded and the impure venous blood is colorless.

Fig. 12. Alimentary canal. 1, Esophagus; 2, stomach; 3, small intestine; 4, large intestine; 5, appendix; 6, liver; 7, gallbladder; 8, bile duct; 9, pancreas.

through the thin walls of which the oxygen is able to pass. It is seized upon by the hemoglobin of the red blood corpuscles and carried throughout the body. When the capillaries of the tissues are reached the oxygen leaves the red blood cells, passes through the capillary walls, enters the tissue fluid, and is taken up by the cells. The energy of cells is obtained from burning food, particularly carbohydrates, with oxygen. At the same time the tissues give off one of their waste products in the form of the gas, carbon dioxide. The carbon dioxide passes into the venous blood, the plasma carrying three times as much as the red cells, and is taken up by the disengaged red blood corpuscles, carried back to the lungs, discharged into the air spaces of those organs, and exhaled into the outside air. *Tissue* or *cellular respiration is therefore*

*the real meaning and reason for the rising and falling of the chest which
we commonly call respiration.*

DIGESTION

The *digestive system* is concerned with preparing the food that is to
be carried by the blood to the tissue fluid for the nourishment of the
cells. The tissue fluid must receive its food in the simplest form,
for conversion into the *building stones* of the body and the *fuel* which
drives the engine. A beefsteak would be out of place in the tissue spaces;
the cells would not know what to do with it. The work of preparing
the food so that it may be utilized by the tissues is performed by the
alimentary canal and by certain *digestive glands,* which are derived from
the alimentary canal and pour their digestive juices into it. The
alimentary canal consists of the *mouth,* where the food is broken up
by the teeth and acted on by the saliva; the *esophagus* or gullet, which
is a mere passageway; the *stomach,* where the food is retained for some
hours and is acted on by the gastric juice; the *small intestine,* where
it is further digested and liquefied and from which it is absorbed; and
the *large intestine,* which conducts the indigestible part of the food to
the exterior. The food is converted into a soluble absorbable form by
digestive juices, which are produced by collections of cells to form
glands. The glands line the interior of the stomach and intestine and
are also collected to form a most important digestive organ, the *pancreas,* which pours its digestive juice into the very beginning of the intestine. *Bile* from the liver also enters the bowel at the same point and
assists in the digestion of fats (Fig. 12).

The *liver* plays a much more important role in the utilization of foodstuffs than merely by the production of bile, which in many respects
is simply a waste product. The three main constituents of food are
proteins, carbohydrates, and fats. We have already seen that all three
contain carbon, hydrogen, and oxygen, and that protein in addition
possesses nitrogen.

The complex *proteins* of the food are broken down in the intestine
into their simplest elements, the *amino acids* or building stones of the
body, still characterized by the possession of nitrogen. The amino acids
and carbohydrates are absorbed into capillaries in the wall of the small
intestine and carried to the liver by the *portal vein.* In the liver the portal
vein breaks up into fine capillaries, which come into intimate contact
with the liver cells, each of which is a little chemical factory filled with
hard working enzymes housed in the mitochondria. Some of the amino
acids pass on to the heart and are distributed to the tissues, where they
serve their important function of body building. The rest of the amino
acids lose their nitrogen in the liver, where it is converted into urea,

a waste product that reaches the kidneys by the blood stream and is excreted in the urine as nonprotein nitrogen. The valuable non-nitrogenous portion (carbon and hydrogen) of these amino acids reaches the tissue cells where it is utilized in the production of energy. This process of breaking down the protein of food into its constituents (catabolism) and rebuilding these into the tissues of the body (anabolism) is graphically portrayed by Best and Taylor (*The Living Body*) in the following passage: "The utilization of protein in the construction of body tissue may be compared to the building of a number of houses of different types from materials derived from the wrecking of other structures. Each brick and stone in the old buildings must be separated and then sorted and carted to the new sites. Some of this building material will be more suitable for one type of house, some more suitable for other types. Other materials again will not be utilizable at all, and will therefore be discarded as refuse. The new buildings, though constructed from materials taken from the old, will be quite different in structure and in general plan."

The *carbohydrates* of the food are converted in the intestine into *glucose* or sugar. From the intestine the glucose is absorbed into the capillaries and carried by the portal vein to the liver, where most of it is changed into a storage form known as *glycogen* and retained temporarily in the liver cells. Glucose is one of the important fuels of the body, necessary for muscular action and heat production. When fuel consumption is rapid the carbohydrate depot, the liver, is called upon to convert some of its glycogen into readily available glucose and give it back to the blood for transportation to the muscles.

Some of the *fats* are carried to the liver by the portal vein; here they are converted into a form more readily utilized. The rest of the fat is absorbed into lymphatic vessels known as *lacteals,* and is carried by the *thoracic duct* to the great veins of the neck, where it enters the general circulation and is stored in the fat depots of the body.

It will be seen that the journey of the blood stream from the intestine to the tissues is somewhat in the nature of a cafeteria, various additions to the tray being made on the way. Denatured amino acids, now freed from their nitrogen and therefore no longer deserving of their name, are added by the liver; glycogen is converted into glucose when the storehouse in the liver is called upon by the tissues; oxygen is added as the blood passes through the lungs; and fat is poured into the veins at the root of the neck.

EXCRETION

The *excretory system* is concerned with the removal of waste products from the body. This is brought about by the cooperation of a number of organs, *i.e.,* the intestine, kidneys, skin, and lungs. The *intestine* offers the simplest example of an excretory organ. Food contains elements that are indigestible and cannot be utilized. These are passed on into the lower part of the bowel, the large intestine, from which they are discharged periodically as feces or stools. The *kidney* is a complex structure, the details of which will be considered in a later chapter, but the essential arrangement is not unlike that of the lung, except that fluid instead of gas leaves the blood. The arteries to the kidneys break up into fine capillaries, through the walls of which pass fluid from the blood together with waste substances in solution. The fluid or urine passes into tubules that open into a duct, the ureter; this duct carries the urine to the bladder, from which it is periodically discharged. The excretory function of the *lungs* has already been indicated. Here the waste product is carbon dioxide which passes through the capillary walls into the air spaces or alveoli of the lungs and is breathed out through the trachea. The *skin* is an excretory organ by virtue of its sweat glands, which remove waste substances from the blood and pour them out on the surface in the fluid form of sweat. If the kidneys are not working properly the sweating function of the skin can be stimulated by heat, and thereby relieve the kidneys of part of their load. The skin is a remarkable structure. Despite its thinness it effectively protects the delicate internal structures and fluids against the unceasing variations of external conditions. It is moist, supple, elastic, and durable. Its durability is due to its being composed of several layers of cells that continually multiply. These cells die while remaining united to one another like slates on a roof, slates that are continually blown away by the wind and continually replaced by new ones. All the openings in the skin except the nostrils are closed by elastic and contractile rings known as sphincters. Thus it is the almost perfectly fortified frontier of a closed world.

COMMUNICATIONS

From what has already been said it is evident that the various highly specialized parts of the body are brought to work together for the common good. The runner breathes faster because his muscles need more oxygen; glycogen is converted into glucose when they need more sugar for energy; the rectum, the terminal portion of the large intestine, contracts (or should contract) so as to empty itself when it becomes full of feces; the eye is closed when threatened by a flying object; the foot is raised when its owner wishes to walk. What are the integrating influences that make the organs members one of another? They are of two kinds. The one is telephonic or telegraphic in type, urgent in character, demanding instantaneous response; the messengers are *nervous impulses,* electrical in nature, and they are transmitted by the nervous system. The other may be compared to a special delivery service, slower but more detailed in character; the messengers are the *hormones,* chemical instead of electrical in nature, produced by the endocrine or ductless glands, and carried by the blood stream.

NERVOUS SYSTEM. The nervous system is singularly like a gigantic telephone system, with a central exchange, an infinite number of wires, and receivers at the ends of these wires. The exchange is the brain and spinal cord, known collectively as the *central nervous system,* while the wires are represented by the nerves that form the *peripheral nervous system.* Some parts of the system act like automatic telephones without any conscious control; purely automatic messages are concerned in such functions as the beating of the heart, the contraction or dilatation of the blood vessels, the swallowing of food, the movement of food along the intestine, the process of childbirth. The automatic messages are carried for the most part by a special set of nerves known as *autonomic* or *sympathetic,* which form the *involuntary nervous system,* although *reflex action* also plays some part in automatic responses.

The greater part of the nervous system is operated on the principle of a nonautomatic telephone exchange. On the surface of the body as well as in its interior there are myriads of receivers which, when stimulated, transmit sensations of various kinds to the spinal cord and thence to the brain, or directly to the brain. These receivers are known as *receptors,* some of which are specialized for the reception of sensations of sight, sound, taste, etc. (the *special senses*), while others respond to stimulation by giving rise to sensations of touch, pain, heat, and cold. These varied sensations are carried to the central nervous system by *afferent* or *sensory nerves,* where they are sorted out and analyzed by the nerve cells of the brain. The sensory nerves form part of the *voluntary nervous system,* the other part of which is constituted by *efferent* or *motor nerves.* These nerves carry electrical messages from the nerve cells of the brain to the muscles, in response to which muscular contraction occurs. The actual stimulus that acts on the muscle fibers is apparently chemical in nature, for chemical substances of various kinds are liberated at the nerve endings when the nerves are stimulated. The structure of the nervous system is described in somewhat greater detail in Chapter 27.

ENDOCRINE GLANDS. The other means by which intercommunication between organs is established is through the agency of the chemical messengers, the *hormones.* These are produced by the *endocrine* or *ductless glands.* Ordinary glands such as the salivary glands and pancreas pour out their secretion into the mouth or intestine through ducts. The endocrine glands have no ducts, and so discharge their secretion directly into the blood vessels with which they are in contact. *These glands are among the most important structures in the body, for they control metabolism and regulate personality. In addition they influence growth and reproduction.* The effect that the ductless glands exert on the mind is equally striking, and the difference between endocrine health and disease may mean the difference between the finest mental power and imbecility. The principal endocrine glands are the pituitary at the base of the brain, the thyroid and parathyroids in the neck, the adrenals, the islets of Langerhans in the pancreas, and the sex glands.

It would be absurd to attempt even to outline the complex functions of the endocrine organs in this place, but it may be noted that not only do they regulate the behavior of many of the tissues (*e.g.,* the parathyroids determine the amount of lime salts in the bones), but they also influence one another so as to act in harmony. They are like the instruments of a string quartet noted for its perfect ensemble, and the leader of the glandular orchestra is the pituitary, the master gland of the body. The pituitary produces hormones that influence the activity of the thyroid, the parathyroids, the adrenals, and the ovaries, as well as other organs and glands.

The endocrines are stimulated to activity not only by hormones from other endocrine glands, but also by nervous stimuli. One simple example of this remarkable interrelationship must suffice. When a person is intensely activated by great rage or great fear he is impelled to immediate muscular activity for purposes of either attack or flight. The muscles are called on to contract to the utmost of their ability, and therefore require a maximum supply of carbohydrate fuel in the shape of glucose. This is lying stored in the liver in the form of glycogen. A nervous stimulus passes from the brain along the nerves to the adrenal glands, and causes them to pour out their hormone, adrenalin (epinephrine). This is carried by the blood to the liver, where it causes the conversion of inert glycogen into active glucose. The glucose is carried by the blood to the muscles, supplying them with the fuel necessary for intense and immediate activity.

REPRODUCTION

Reproduction is the most complex of the mechanisms of the body, but in its elements it is essentially simple. In the lowest forms of life, as in such a unicellular organism as the ameba, reproduction is *asexual.* A line of division is formed along the middle of the cell, and the cellular constituents, first the nucleus and then the cytoplasm, divide into two, one set passing to one half of the cell, the other set to the other half. Finally, the line of division becomes complete and two new individuals are formed. This is called *reproduction by fission.* As both cells go on living, indeed need never die, they seem to enjoy the fountain of youth and can be regarded as immortal.

In all the higher forms of life reproduction is sexual in type, and is brought about by the union of two cells specially set aside for the purpose. They are known as the male and female *gametes* or germ cells, as distinguished from the body or *somatic cells.* The sex cells are produced by the male and female sex glands or *gonads,* the *testicle* with its tubules lined by germinal epithelium in the male, the *ovary* in the female. The male sex cells are the *spermatozoa* or sperms, the female sex cells are the *ova.* The sperm is a highly specialized cell with an oval flattened head and a long tail-like process, which by violent lashing movements propels the cell with great speed. In the human female an ovum is liberated every month from the ovary, and passes along a duct, the *Fallopian tube,* to reach the *uterus* or womb, from which it is soon discharged in a flow of blood known as *menstruation (mensis,* month). If impregnation is to occur the male elements, the spermatozoa, ejected by the *penis* into the *vagina,* must pass through the uterus and enter the Fallopian tube. (We are apt to think that fertilization of the ovum depends on sexual intercourse, but this is not necessarily so. For instance, the female salmon lays her eggs in a quiet pool, after which the male salmon comes along and fertilizes the eggs with his sperms.) It is rather breathtaking to learn that not one but some 300,000,000 spermatozoa, more or less, start on their journey, perhaps because the secretion of the vagina is acid and only a few hundred thousand survive to pass into what is to them the huge cavern of the uterus. A further obstacle awaits them, for very many of the survivors enter the wrong tube, as only one tube contains the ovum. When the leading spermatozoon in the race encounters the ovum in the tube its head, carrying the paternal chromosomes and genes, penetrates the tough envelope of the ovum by means of an enzyme, *hyaluronidase,* its lashing tail is left behind because it is no longer needed, and *impregnation* has occurred. The sperm's remarkable journey has taken about 12 hours. A change at once occurs in the ovum's envelope, which renders it impermeable to any subsequent sperm that might wish to enter. When the male nucleus merges with that of the female, *fertilization* has taken place, and the result is *conception* and the creation of a new life. It is hard to believe, but the fertilized ovum, which is to produce all the mysteries of the human body in the course of a few months, is only the size of a grain of sand. The fertilized ovum continues on its way down the tube and enters the uterus. This time, however, it is not discharged, so that menstruation does not occur for the duration of the pregnancy. In the uterus it develops into an *embryo,* the original single fertilized cell at once beginning to divide and multiply, the resulting cells not separating from one another but becoming differentiated and arranged to form the infinitely varied tissues and organs, until in the fullness of time, nine months in the case of the human, a child is born.

There is one fundamental fallacy in the above account which the discerning reader will not fail to detect. We have seen previously that when a somatic cell divides, the chromosomes split longitudinally, one half passing to each of the new cells, which therefore possess the correct number. How is it that the fertilized ovum, which is a combination of two cells, male and female, does not come to have twice the number of chromosomes that it ought to? The reason is that the germ cells, while still in their respective gonads, have undergone a process of *maturation* in anticipation of the impending fertilization. This is effected by a *reduction division* or *meiosis*. In the mitosis of somatic cells each chromosome splits longitudinally and each pair separates into two, so that each daughter cell contains the original number of 46. Since these consist of 23 pairs, somatic cells are said to have a *diploid* (*diplous,* double) number of chromosomes. In the maturing germ cell there is no splitting of chromosomes, so that when division occurs each daughter cell contains only 23 chromosomes, which are said to be *haploid* (*haplous,* single) in number. *The new germ cells, both male and female, contain only half the number of chromosomes and genes.* Fusion of the two gametes after fertilization results in a restoration of the chromosomes to their original number, but now one half are maternal and one half paternal in origin.

DETERMINATION OF SEX. The wish is sometimes expressed that something could be done to determine or influence the sex of the unborn baby. This is particularly true in the case of farm animals. It also used to be true in the days when a king needed a male heir. It is felt that modern science, which can work such wonders, should be able to perform this miracle. The truth is that the sex of the newly created embryo has been determined at the moment of conception, and that nothing more can be done about it. To understand this, we must take a second look at the chromosomes. These are divided into 44 *autosomes,* which are the ordinary chromosomes, and two *sex chromosomes,* which determine the future sex. In the *immature female sex cell* both sex chromosomes, known as *X chromosomes,* are alike and equal in size, so that when the cell matures and undergoes reduction division, each daughter cell has one X chromosome, which can be regarded as the hallmark of femaleness. In the *immature male sex cell,* on the other hand, one of the sex chromosomes is similar to the X chromosome of the female, but the other, known as the *Y chromosome,* is very much smaller, and may be regarded as indicating maleness. It is evident that after reduction division of the male gamete, half of the sperm cells will receive an X chromosome and the other half a Y chromosome. If, now, the ovum containing one X chromosome should be fertilized by a sperm containing an X chromosome, a female (XX) will be produced, but if the sperm contains a Y chromosome, the result will be an XY individual, in other words a male. The result is pure chance and incapable of control.

Sex Chromatin. Unfortunately the matter is not always as simple as has just been suggested. When the gonads develop, the testicular or ovarian hormones which they produce profoundly influence what are called secondary sex characters, by which one is accustomed to distinguish a boy from a girl. Occasionally, owing to some defect in the genes, this development is not normal, and we are confronted with the tragic problem of *intersex,* when the child shares both male and female characteristics. In such cases a test for sex chromatin is of the greatest value. Thanks to the work of Murray Barr and his associates in 1949 at the University of Western Ontario, we now know that the cells of the body carry the fingerprints of their genetic sex, which may not correspond with the *apparent* somatic sex of the person. Barr has shown that a small mass of chromatin, the *sex chromatin,* lies against the nuclear membrane in about 85 per cent of cells of normal females, but in less than 10 per cent of cells of normal males (Fig. 13). This chromatin mass, now known as the **Barr body,** is quite easy to see if you know what you are looking for, but no one before Barr realized its significance. The female cells are said to be *chromatin-positive,* the male cells *chromatin-negative.* The most convenient source of cells is a smear made from the mucous membrane of the mouth. It would appear, as suggested by Mary Lyon, that in the somatic cells of the female one of the two chromosomes (one inherited from each parent) is genetically

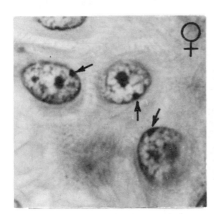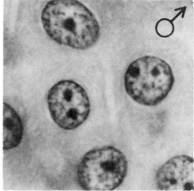

Fig. 13. Female and male cells showing presence or absence of sex chromatin. (Boyd's *Textbook of Pathology.*)

inactivated, becomes tightly coiled, and forms the sex chromatin or Barr body. There is at present no explanation for the occurrence of sex chromatin in a small proportion of male cells, unless it is related to the XY sex chromosome complex. With regard to the relation of sex to disease, nearly all the serious organic ailments are commoner in the male, with the notable exception of disease of the gallbladder and, to a lesser degree, mitral stenosis. There appears to be an inherent weakness in the male, a sex-linked inferiority, so that by comparison with the female he is a weakling at all periods of life from conception to death. In the investigation of sterility, if the sex chromatin test reveals a discrepancy between apparent sex and chromosomal sex, the chances of fertility are practically nil. The question of sex reversal and other sex anomalies will be discussed again in Chapter 14 on Heredity in Disease.

When we think of the incredible intricacy of structure and function which has been sketched in the briefest outline in this chapter, we can echo the words of Hamlet when he exclaimed: "What a piece of work is a man." But the inner mechanism of that piece of work, of which it is to be presumed he knew nothing, might have appeared to him even more "express and admirable." How we would have prized a soliloquy on the function of the pituitary, which used to be regarded as the seat of the soul.

FURTHER READING

ALLISON, A.: Scient. Amer., 1967, *217,* No. 5, 62. (Lysosomes and disease.)

BEST, C. H., and TAYLOR, N. B.: *The Human Body,* 4th ed., 1963, New York.

BOURNE, G. H.: *Division of Labour in Cells,* 1962, New York.

BRACHET, J.: Scient. Amer., 1961, *205,* No. 3, 50. (The living cell.)

CAMERON, G. R.: *New Pathways in Cellular Pathology,* 1952, London.

CANNON, W. B.: *The Wisdom of the Body,* 2nd ed., 1963, New York.

CHAMBERS, R. W. and PAYNE, A. S.: *From Cell to Test Tube. The Science of Biochemistry,* 1960, New York.

CRUICKSHANK, B., DODDS, T. C. and GARDNER, D. L.: *Human Histology,* 2nd ed., 1968, Edinburgh.

HAM, A. W.: *Histology,* 6th ed., 1969, Philadelphia.

LYON, MARY F.: Nature, London, 1961, *190,* 372. (The X chromosome.)

PORTER, K. R. and BONNEVILLE, M. A.: *An Introduction to the Fine Structures of Cells and Tissues,* 3rd ed., 1968.

Chapter 2

Historical Outline

Primitive Medicine	*Nursing*
Ancient Medicine	Florence Nightingale
Hippocrates	1860–70
Galen	*Bacteriology*
The Middle Ages	Pasteur
Arabian Medicine	1870–80
Avicenna	*Bacteriology*
Rhazes	Koch
Modern Medicine	1880–90
Sixteenth Century	*Preventive Inoculation*
Anatomy	*Protozoan Parasites*
Vesalius	Laveran
Seventeenth Century	1890–1900
Circulation of Blood	*Radiation*
Harvey	Roentgen
Eighteenth Century	The Curies
Pathological Anatomy	*Insect Carriers*
Morgagni	Manson
Nineteenth Century	Ross
1840–50	*Twentieth Century*
Anesthesia	*Chemotherapy*
Morton	*Organotherapy*
1850–60	*Deficiency Disease*
Pathology	*Genetics*
Virchow	*Mental Disease*
Physiology	
Bernard	

Medicine had its beginnings in mystery and superstition in "the dark backward and abysm of time." The three M's—mystery, magic, and medicine—were one and the same. Medicine was first a religion, then it became a science, but it is always an art. Unfortunately, as the science advances there is a danger of the art falling into the background. The regard with which medicine is held by the public at any one time has no relation to the benefits it bestows. Indeed it was regarded with the greatest veneration when it had nothing to offer. This is because regard depends on emotion. Religion and art appeal to the emotions; science, whether medical or otherwise, does not. It leaves us cold. Anyone, whether medical or not, who is occupied in the hospital or the laboratory is likely to encounter the names of some of the workers who have blazed the trail for us in time past. The prospective student of medicine who may happen to read these pages will get an inkling of some of the romance of the story of the slow and painful development of our present knowledge of disease and the struggle to control and prevent it.

As the practice of medicine is an art based on a science, let us briefly review the development of that science. It will simplify matters for us if we divide this outline roughly into four periods: (1) *primitive medicine,* (2) *ancient medicine,* with the supreme name of Hippocrates, (3) *the Middle Ages,* and (4) *modern medicine.* We may further subdivide modern medicine into the sixteenth century with Vesalius; the seventeenth century with Harvey, Sydenham, and Malpighi; the eighteenth century with Morgagni, Hunter, and Jenner (the last named rather out of his proper era); the nineteenth century, which we must divide into before and after 1840; and the twentieth century. Of these various periods the most significant and revolutionary was the latter part of the nineteenth century.

PRIMITIVE MEDICINE

When we look back into the dim and distant past we see primitive man terrified by the world around him and ascribing disease, as well as his other misfortunes, to supernatural malevolent forces, to the influence of spirits to be placated by sacrifice. It was the age of the witch doctor, the medicine man, the fetish and amulet, an age that has perhaps even yet not entirely passed away. As a matter of fact, the medicine man represents the oldest professional class of which we have record. Guthrie, in his admirable *History of Medicine,* remarks that primitive man at the present day, in whatever part of the world he is found, still does not admit the existence of disease from what we call natural causes. Death was and is a punishment for man's disobedience. The oldest surgical operation of which we have evidence is *trephining* or trepanning, which consisted in opening the skull with a sharp stone instrument for the purpose of letting out the evil spirit. If the patient died as the result of the operation, it could always be blamed on the invading demon, which refused to leave by the opening provided.

ANCIENT MEDICINE

The old civilizations of *Egypt* and *Babylon* had their medicine, and developed a knowledge of drugs and methods of embalming. The practice of medicine in Babylon must have demanded care, for we read that if a physician treats a severe wound successfully with a bronze lancet, or opens an abscess of the eye and cures the eye, "he shall take ten shekels of silver"; but if the patient dies of his wound or loses his eye, "one shall cut off his (the physician's) hands." Such a practice would at least encourage conservative methods of treatment.

Jewish medicine developed about the same time as that of Assyria. It was remarkable for its regulations for the prevention of disease and contagion, its hygiene of menstruation and the puerperium, and the establishment of social hygiene, details of which can be read in the Book of Leviticus.

Scientific medicine was born in Greece in the fifth century B.C.; it died in Rome 600 years later; it was resurrected after nearly 1500 years in the Renaissance or rebirth of learning. *Hippocrates,* born in 460 B.C., was its father, for he separated medicine from mystery and magic, relieved the gods of their responsibility for the prevention and treatment of disease, and laid that burden on the shoulders of man, its proper place. Hippocrates was the first and greatest physician, because he first threw aside all the demonology of the priests and looked upon disease as part of the order of nature, *having a natural cause.* The rise of natural medicine dates from Hippocrates. Dawson remarks with truth about Hippocrates that "probably no character in all history has through a single principle exerted so great an influence on civilization, upon the conditions of humans, as did he whom we revere as the father of modern medicine." He developed a system of thorough history taking. His methods of physical examination are still used. He advocated clean hands and nails and boiled water for operations! He preferred the "vis medicatrix naturae," the healing power of nature, to drugs. He was severely handicapped by a complete ignorance of anatomy and pathology, due to the fact that no dissections or autopsies were permitted, because the human body *after death* was regarded as sacred by the Greeks, an idea that was perpetuated later by the Church of Rome for many long centuries.

With the decline of Greece, due in part to the prevalence of malaria, the candle of learning continued to burn feebly in *Rome.* Here progress was marked by practical organization rather than by originality. The outstanding contribution of Roman medicine was sanitation: clean streets, pure water, public baths, sewage disposal—all necessary to public health. The only great figure to emerge from Roman medicine was *Galen,* who lived in the second century A.D. He was the real originator of experimental research methods in medicine, but he was dogmatic to a degree, and made facts fit his theories, instead of theories fitting the facts, which is the modern method. His dogmatism was fatal for a thousand years or more, because men soon lost the power of doubting, without which no progress is possible, and regarded his writings as those of an infallible medical Pope. His knowledge of anatomy was learned entirely from dissections on animals, and the brilliancy of his rhetoric prevented anyone from learning at first hand something about the structure of the human body.

MIDDLE AGES

Galen died in 200 A.D., and in 410 A.D. the German barbarians under Alaric entered Rome. Then the dark night of the Middle Ages fell upon Europe. Medicine ceased to be a science; it again became mystery and magic. Life itself was too precarious for mental development. Even when it became relatively safe, the authority of the Church did not encourage research in medicine, for it was far more interested in the immortal soul than in the frail and mortal body. When men become slaves to authority they lose the power of independent thought, in medicine as in other things. And so the clear stream of scientific medicine was lost in the morass of the Dark Ages. In Osler's moving words: "Following the glory that was Greece and the grandeur that was Rome, desolation came upon the civilized world in which the light of learning burnt low, flickering almost to extinction."

The flame was kept alight by *Arabian medicine,* many of the Greek and Roman texts being translated into Arabic, but it was not until the revival of learning and the founding of the universities that this knowledge became available to western Europe. Perhaps the overriding distinction between European and Arabian medicine at this period was that the early Christian church regarded disease largely as a punishment for sin rather than a result of natural causes, whereas the Arabians carried on the teachings of Hippocrates and the Greek school of thought, adding many drugs, such as laudanum, which have lasted to the present day. Perhaps the three greatest names were *Rhazes,* a Persian, who was the first to distinguish between measles and smallpox; *Avicenna,* another Persian, who was known as the Prince of Physicians; and *Maimonides,* a Jew, who has been called by a modern writer the William Osler of Medieval Arabic and Hebrew Medicine. Avicenna, the most famous physician of the Arab world, was not handicapped by undue modesty. In his autobiography, which covers only the first 21 years of his life, occurs this passage: "Medicine is not a difficult subject, and in a short space of time, of course, I excelled in it, so that the masters of physic came to read with me, and I began to visit the sick. I was then about sixteen years of age."

MODERN MEDICINE

It is not easy to know what period of time should be included under this heading. Taking the long view, I propose to review the advances made in the centuries that have elasped since the Dark Ages to the present day. It will be convenient to consider the advances in the separate centuries until 1840; after that date the advance becomes explosive.

SIXTEENTH CENTURY. The sixteenth century saw the dawn, for in 1543 *Vesalius,* a young Belgian who became professor of anatomy at Padua at the age of 22 years, published a textbook, "On the Fabric of the Human Body," in which he recorded what he saw and not what authority said he should see. Osler regarded this work as the greatest medical book ever written. Vesalius made his own dissections, begged all the doctors for their fatal cases, and even made friends with the judges, so that they would arrange executions to suit him, that is to say not too many at one time. No one represents the true spirit of the Revival of Learning in medicine better than Vesalius. To pass from the writings of Galen and his followers to those of Vesalius is like passing from darkness into sunlight, for he shattered the idol of authority in anatomical science and dared to show that Galen was often wrong. Without a knowledge of normal anatomy no hope of pathology, the study of diseased structure, was possible. *Ambroise Paré,* a great French military surgeon, whose life span covered the greater part of the sixteenth century, made surgery a practical art. Paré introduced the use of ligatures, the truss in hernia, massage, artificial eyes, and other innovations. His most famous aphorism: "I dressed the wound; God healed it."

SEVENTEENTH CENTURY. If the sixteenth century saw the birth of anatomy, the seventeenth witnessed the arrival of physiology in one of the greatest advances in the whole history of medical science, the discovery of the *circulation of the blood* by *William Harvey,* an English physician, in 1628. It is difficult to picture medical thought without this vital information. The function of respiration, diseases of the heart, hemorrhage, embolism, the spread of infection, the distribution of tumor metastases by the blood stream, and a host of other phenomena would be unintelligible without the magic words of Harvey: "I began to think whether there might not be a movement *as it were in a circle."* As usually happened in those days, the epoch-making discovery was greeted with ridicule and abuse. In reality it formed the beginning of modern medical science. There was one serious gap in Harvey's demonstration and argument. He had failed to show by what means the blood passed from the arteries to the corresponding veins. The gap was filled by the work of an Italian, *Marcello Malpighi,* who was born in the year that Harvey's book was published. Malpighi was the father of histology, the first man to apply the microscope to the minute structure of the body, although the instrument, which at that time was 1½ feet long, had been invented half a century earlier. The microscope was as essential to medical advance as the discovery of the wheel was to mechanical progress. Malpighi must be regarded as a great physiologist as well as the father of histology, for form and function are merely two aspects of the same truth. Soon after his appointment to the chair of medicine at Bologna he wrote a letter to a friend describing a minute vascular network joining the ending of the smallest arteries and the beginnings of the smallest veins. Thus he had found the missing link in the chain of Harvey's discovery, and made possible a sound view of the processes of nutrition. The great practitioner of this century was *Sydenham,* who has been called the English Hippocrates. He was not interested in theories or experiment, but if you fell sick in those days with one of the infectious fevers, you would do better with Sydenham than with Harvey as your doctor.

EIGHTEENTH CENTURY.   In the eighteenth century there was little of the stirring of spirit and uprush of new ideas that characterized the seventeenth. This was a period of consolidation, an age of criticism rather than discovery in medicine, of philosophers and philosophizing, culminating in the French Revolution. But it witnessed the birth of pathology in the limited sense of morbid anatomy, and the father was *Giambattista Morgagni* of Padua, who at the age of 79 in 1761 published a book entitled, "The Seats and Causes of Disease," which at once rendered obsolete all others dealing with the diseased body. Before Morgagni disease was considered as a general thing. Doctors speculated as to the nature of the process, built up a hypothesis no matter how fantastic, and gave it a name. Strangely enough they did not enquire as to the *seat* of the disease. It was Morgagni who was the first to correlate the symptoms of the patient during life with the changes in the organs found at autopsy. He showed that it was not true that dead men tell no tales. Dead men have for centuries been telling doctors the story of how they got sick and why they died. For the first time we could think of liver disease, kidney disease, and heart disease, and have a mental picture of the clinical condition in relation to the lesions in the organs responsible for that condition. Morgagni made few real discoveries, nor did he revolutionize pathology as did Virchow in the coming century; his great service to pathology was his emphasis on detail and thoroughness.

Many gifted clinical observers were born at the end of this century, *Laennec* in France, *Addison, Bright,* and *Hodgkin* in England. The first pathologists were merely medical men who performed autopsies as a sideline. But two men of this period stand out from the others as imbued with the true spirit of research. These are *John Hunter* and *Edward Jenner,* who was Hunter's pupil. We have seen that Paré, in the sixteenth century, made surgery an art. Two hundred years later Hunter,

an extraordinary and turbulent personality, made it a science. He cor-
related surgery for the first time with physiology and pathology, and
introduced a spirit of scientific enquiry which had been entirely lacking
in surgical practice. So great was his influence that it is no exaggeration
to say that surgery may be divided into two periods, before Hunter and
after Hunter; but the surgery was still only the surgery of the surface
of the body and the extremities. Jenner, by introducing vaccination
against smallpox, was the founder of preventive medicine, as well as
one of the greatest benefactors of mankind. Some idea of the ravages
and prevalence of the disease that he did so much to eradicate may
be gained from the old saying "mothers counted their children only after
they had had the smallpox."

NINETEENTH CENTURY. The nineteenth century dawned with no
indication of the stupendous and revolutionary discoveries that it had in
store. Until the nineteenth century the history of medicine is largely
a catalogue of the follies of medical mankind. As late as the end of
the eighteenth century the kings and queens of England and France still
"touched for the King's Evil," *i.e.,* laid their healing hands on those
suffering from scrofula (tuberculous glands in the neck)! In the
eighteenth century all doctors were general practitioners. The surgeon
could not open the abdomen, so he had plenty of time to practice medicine. In the first half of the nineteenth century hospitals were little more
than a refuge for sick poor, who died of mysterious infections. It was
only after the conquest of surgical infection that the teaching hospital
became a medical scientific center and the age of specialization began,
with the eventual development of intracranial, intrathoracic, and now
cardiovascular surgery. The first 40 years were quiet, but in the remaining years of the century medicine advanced further than in the entire
course of recorded history. It was a triumph for the application of experimental methods to medical problems. Time now has to be reckoned
not in centuries but in decades.

1840 to 1850. In 1846 *Morton* demonstrated to an audience of Boston doctors that *ether* would abolish the pain of a surgical operation.
In the following year *Sir James Young Simpson* of Edinburgh introduced *chloroform* to relieve the pain of childbirth as well as that of
general surgery. For the first time in the world's history it was possible
for a surgeon to operate without inflicting terrible anguish on his
patient.

1850 to 1860. *Nursing* is as old as the human race, but in this decade
Florence Nightingale organized it, made it a profession, and one for
trained gentlewomen. It is easy to forget that only 100 years ago
there were no nurses and no nursing as we know it today. In the
early Victorian period the level of nursing had sunk very low indeed.

The hospitals were dirty; the patients poorly cared for. How incredible a change to the modern nurse, that compound of science and sympathy! At the present day the nurse often means more to the patient than does the doctor, for she has the compassion of a woman, as well as being the computer arm of the doctor. In this same decade some of the most valued medical instruments of precision were invented; the *ophthalmoscope* by von Helmholtz, a German professor of physics, the *laryngoscope* by Manuel Garcia, a Spanish teacher of singing in London. Darwin's "Origin of Species" was published in 1859, and in 1858, Virchow's "Cellular Pathology."

Rudolf Virchow is the father of modern pathology as we know it, for he showed for the first time that the underlying structural changes in disease are to be found, not in the organ as a whole, but in the cellular elements of which the organ is composed; what the molecule is to the chemist and the electron to the physicist, the diseased cell has been to the pathologist since Virchow. He bestrode the world of pathology like a colossus, contributing to our knowledge in an endless variety of fields. Thus he was the first to demonstrate the occurrence of pulmonary embolism and the first to describe leukemia. But Virchow was much more than the supreme pathologist. He was also Germany's leading anthropologist, leading archeologist, and leading liberal statesman in opposition to Bismarck. We may ask how all this was possible? Perhaps an answer may be found in part in the title of his graduation thesis on leaving high school at the age of eighteen: "A Life full of Work and Toil is not a Burden but a Benediction."

We must not make the mistake of thinking that the structural changes connoted by the term morbid or pathological anatomy are the essence of disease, although they are certainly the easiest to recognize and to demonstrate. In the last analysis it is *function* that makes life possible, and *disordered function* that constitutes what we as patients regard as disease. Physiology constitutes the study of function, and in the middle of the nineteenth century the towering figure of *Claude Bernard,* the French physiologist, ranks equal with that of Virchow, the great German pathologist. It was Bernard who was the first to recognize that the pancreas was by far the most important digestive gland in the body, producing enzymes that act on proteins, carbohydrates, and fats. Of equal importance was his discovery of the glycogenic function of the liver. Before that time the only function of the liver was thought to be the production of bile. Bernard showed that the cane sugar of the food is changed by gastric juice to glucose, which is carried to the liver and there converted by an enzyme to a substance he called *glycogen.* This proved to be a storage form of sugar, which could be reconverted into glucose as the need arose and the metabolic fire demanded more

fuel. Another great achievement was his demonstration of the existence
of the *vasomotor nerves,* which control both the constriction and dilatation of blood vessels. In the realm of pure thought his supreme contribution was his concept of *the constancy of the internal environment* as
the condition of free and independent life, to which reference has been
made in the preceding chapter. His character and moral worth were
so outstanding that at his death all Paris wept, and he was the first man
of science to be laid to rest with a state funeral in the cathedral of Notre
Dame.

1860 to 1870. The greatest discovery in the long history of medical
science, namely the role that bacteria play in the causation of disease,
was made in this and the following decades. The existence of bacteria
was well known. They had been guessed at by Kircher in the seventeenth century, and seen and accurately described by the Dutchman
Leeuwenhoek later in the same century. For our knowledge of the overwhelming importance of bacteria as agents of disease we are indebted
to three men—Pasteur, a Frenchman; Lister, an Englishman; and Koch,
a German. *Louis Pasteur* was a chemist, not a physician, but he became
interested in the problem of why wine spoils, and he came to the conclusion that the fermentation of wine and beer was due to the action of
living bacterial agents. From this he was led to the study of putrefaction,
i.e., the decomposition of meat and other dead organic material. This
was again found to be due to the same living agents, and the process
could be prevented by heating organic fluids, such as milk, to a temperature below the boiling point, the procedure now known as *pasteurization.* At this time the surgeon, *Joseph Lister,* afterwards Lord Lister,
was pondering on the problem of wound infection following surgical
operations, which rendered the most brilliant operation worse than useless, and gave origin to the popular gibe "the operation was successful
but the patient died," when he came across Pasteur's work. At this
time the mortality from operations, now frequent owing to the use of
anesthetics, was appalling. *At least 45 per cent of amputations resulted
in death from septicemia, pyemia, and gangrene.* Lister had previously
realized that putrefaction of dead organic material and infection of
wounds were intimately related, and now he saw in one lightning flash
that if putrefaction was bacterial in origin, so also was wound infection.
Destruction of bacteria in infected wounds (antisepsis), and later exclusion of bacteria from the field of operation (asepsis), wrought a revolution in surgery so far-reaching, so overwhelming, that surgery as we
know it today is essentially the gift of Lister to humanity. His work
alone made possible the surgery of the abdomen, chest, brain, and
joints, as well as rendering a hundredfold more safe operations on the
limbs and the practice of obstetrics.

In this same wonderful decade there is evidence of an awakening social conscience in medical matters in the founding of the *International Red Cross* by a Swiss, *Henri Dunant,* an organization designed to help sufferers in war and great natural disasters.

1870 to 1880.   This is the decade of bacteriological advance. Pasteur and Koch are the two supreme figures. *Robert Koch,* at first a German country practitioner, must share with Pasteur the title of the founder of modern bacteriology, for he introduced the methods of bacteriological investigation, such as the use of pure cultures and special stains and reproduction of the disease by animal inoculation, which are employed at the present day. In addition he demonstrated the bacterial cause of many infections such as anthrax, cholera, and above all tuberculosis. In this decade a large number of infectious diseases (as opposed to wound infections) were shown to be due to specific bacteria. Pasteur also introduced the idea of *ultramicroscopic filterable viruses,* agents of disease so small that they could not be seen with the microscope and were able to pass through the finest filter, although ordinary bacteria were held back by such a filter. It should be added that at the present day the electron microscope, with its enormously increased power of magnification, has brought even the smallest viruses into view, so that they no longer deserve the term ultramicroscopic.

1880 to 1890.   The two outstanding discoveries of this period were *preventive inoculation* against disease, and the fact that the microscopic *animal parasites known as protozoa* may cause widespread epidemics. Jenner's discovery in 1798 of the value of vaccination against smallpox (now known to be a viral disease) was an isolated miracle that led to further advances. Pasteur now introduced the principle of preventive inoculation by means of "vaccines" against bacterial and virus disease. The modern development of protection against poliomyelitis by virus inoculation need only be mentioned here. The discovery of protozoa as agents of disease was of special importance in the case of malaria, the most widespread disabling and killing disease in the world. It was *Laveran,* a French Army doctor, who first discovered the malaria parasite.

1890 to 1900.   The nineteenth century ends with a tremendous burst of activity in scientific medicine, but only three outstanding achievements can be mentioned here. These are: (1) the discovery of *x-rays* (Roentgen) and *radium* (Marie and Pierre Curie) and their application to medicine; (2) the treatment of infectious disease by *antitoxins;* and (3) the discovery of the *insect transmission of disease.* The use of x-rays has revolutionized diagnosis in every region of the body, and radiations either of this type or those of radium constitute the greatest recent advance in the treatment of many forms of cancer. The first and the most successful of the antitoxins was against diphtheria, but the other antitoxins have been replaced by antibiotics. The demonstration that infection can be carried by insects was one of the most important contributions ever made to preventive medicine. It was *Sir Patrick Manson* who was the first to show in 1877 that the embryos of the minute worm filaria, the cause of elephantiasis, were present in the blood at night and transmitted by the culex mosquito, and *Sir Ronald Ross* who proved in 1897 that malaria was spread in the same way. We know now that the anopheles mosquito carries malaria and yellow fever, the flea bubonic plague, the louse typhus, the tsetse fly sleeping sickness, and so on. Haggard, in his delightful little book, "Mystery, Magic, and Medicine," sums up the effect of these discovers as follows: "Six hundred years ago men believed that disease was due to the wrath of the gods; they prayed—and died. Three hundred years ago they believed it due to meteorological disturbances and contaminated air; they closed their windows at night and burned coal and powder in the streets—and died. Today we turn from such omniscient powers as the gods and the weather to prosaic matters such as the exterminating of the mosquito, the killing of the rat and its fleas, and the delousing of the traveller— and we live free from plague, malaria, and yellow fever."

TWENTIETH CENTURY. In the twentieth century the emphasis is directed to disturbed function rather than to the description of structural changes, so that physiology and biochemistry have come to assume front rank, especially with regard to enzymes and hormones, and to water and electrolyte balance. *It is for this reason that the work of the medical technologist in the laboratory has come to be of such commanding importance.* The most striking achievements of medical science so far may be grouped under the three headings of chemotherapy, organotherapy, and the discovery of the importance of dietary factors in the causation of disease. To these must be added medical genetics and the tentative beginnings of a biochemical approach to mental disease. The great advances in what may be called social medicine lie outside the scope of this review.

Chemotherapy made its real debut in the first decade of the new century in the treatment of syphilis. At that time the cause of the disease was unknown, accurate diagnosis was difficult and often impossible, and treatment was unsatisfactory and inefficient. Incredible though it may appear, these three problems were solved in the space of five years. In 1905 *Schaudinn* discovered the cause of syphilis (Treponema pallidum, formerly called Spirocheta pallida); in 1906 *Wassermann* introduced his famous blood test; and in 1910 *Ehrlich* demonstrated that *arsenical preparations* provide a specific treatment against the disease. Seeing that these preparations have a direct action on the treponema of syphilis, it was hoped that other chemicals would soon be found which would have a similar action on other bacteria. No major success attended repeated efforts until 1935, when the sulfonamide group of agents, the so-called sulfa drugs, were introduced. This produced a revolution in the treatment of bacterial infections. An even more remarkable discovery was that of the dramatic effectiveness of penicillin in 1940. The *sulfonamides* are synthetic chemicals invented and manufactured in the chemist's laboratory. *Penicillin,* on the other hand, is a substance naturally produced by one of the common green molds growing in nature, called Penicillium notatum. As it prevents the growth of certain bacteria it is known as an antibiotic. Penicillin was followed by streptomycin, which acts on another group of bacteria, and later by aureomycin, terramycin, chloromycetin, and many others. All of these antibiotics have their particular use, which will be described later. Some are bacteriostatic rather than bactericidal, that is to say they inhibit the growth of the bacteria, thus leaving them an easy prey to the defensive forces of the body. These dramatic and epoch-making therapeutic advances are due to the entry of chemistry into medicine, one of the most important features of twentieth century progress.

Organotherapy, i.e., treatment by the administration of organs or extracts of organs, has also made great advances, particularly in the field of endocrine diseases. In the days when medicine was compounded of mystery and magic primitive man ate the heart of a lion to make him brave. Now, with considerably more satisfactory results, he eats liver so that he may recover from pernicious anemia, that previously invariably fatal disease, or receives injections of extract of the thyroid gland for myxedema, or insulin (the extract of the pancreas first prepared by Banting) for diabetes. Hormones from the sex glands, especially those of the female, are extensively used in the practice of gynecology. Among the more recent and exciting of the hormones are those obtained from the cortex of the adrenal gland (cortisone), and the hormone of the pituitary (ACTH) which stimulates the production of the adrenal cortical hormones.

Dietetics is largely a twentieth century product, although scurvy, that scourge of armies and navies, had already been conquered by fruit juice. Knowledge of vitamins and the mineral requirements of food is extremely modern. It is of importance in the prevention rather than the cure of disease, and will go far to the future physical betterment of the race. *Medical genetics* really originated with the studies of *Gregor Mendel* in 1866 on the inheritance of color in sweet peas, the transmission of characteristics from one generation to another, but the ability to separate and study the chromosomes carrying their cargo of genes composed of DNA is very recent, and has thrown a flood of light on such mysteries as sex anomalies and sex reversal as well as the complex problems of inherited disease (see Chapter 14). The *biochemical approach to mental disease* may prove the next and most important breakthrough, for at last it is becoming apparent that so-called diseases of the mind may be in essence a disturbance of the biochemistry of the brain, a disturbance that can be remedied by chemical means. This matter is discussed further in Chapter 27. It is worth noting that although there are more inmates of mental hospitals than of general hospitals, far less money is available for research in mental disease than in any other branch of medical science.

In this lightning review of the development of medical science far, far more has been omitted than has been mentioned. Only a few men and a few supreme achievements have been selected. The aim has been to show the different position of the sick person now compared with that in bygone days. What once seemed impossible and then miraculous is now almost commonplace. Perhaps the three biggest steps in the past have been: (1) *the development of dissection* of the human body, (2) *the use of the microscope* in the examination of pathological tissue, and (3) *the introduction of chemistry and biochemistry* in the investigation and treatment of disease. The healing art from the humblest beginnings has developed into the greatest benefactor of mankind: the leaves of its tree are for the healing of the nations.

FURTHER READING

DAWSON, BERNARD: *The History of Medicine: A Short Synopsis,* 1931, London.

GUTHRIE, DOUGLAS: *A History of Medicine,* 1958, revised edit., London.

HAGGARD, H. W.: *Mystery, Magic, and Medicine,* 1933, New York.

LONG, E. R.: *A History of American Pathology,* 1962, Springfield, Ill.

OSLER, SIR WILLIAM: *The Evolution of Modern Medicine,* 1921, London.

Chapter 3

Causes of Disease

WHAT IS DISEASE?

Before entering on a discussion of the possible causes of disease, it may be well to ask, "What is disease?" This is a question that is a good deal easier to ask than to answer. To the patient it means discomfort, dis-ease, dis-harmony with his environment, to the physician or surgeon it means a variety of symptoms and signs, and to the pathologist it means one or more structural changes or *lesions,* which may be *gross, i.e.,* seen with the naked eye, or *microscopic,* only made visible with the light or the electron microscope. The study of lesions forms part of the science of *pathology.* Pathology itself may be defined as *that branch of medicine that deals with the essential nature of disease* (*pathos,* disease).

Pathology was originally simply an investigation in the autopsy room known as morbid anatomy, at first gross (naked eye) and later microscopic. From the very beginning the aim was to throw light on, or explain, the clinical picture. In 1483 the amazing Leonardo da Vinci dissected an old man in Florence "to see the cause of such a quiet death." (We do not need to ask if the cause became evident to Leonardo.) When after very many years the investigation of disease moved from the autopsy room or "dead house," as it was unpleasantly called, to the bedside of the living patient, the study was called *clinical pathology,* or in recent years, because so much of this work is done in the laboratories, the term *laboratory medicine* has gained in popularity. Our knowledge of the processes of disease and the techniques for investigating them has continued to grow with ever-increasing and sometimes terrifying speed. It is now obvious to everyone that the practice of good medicine without adequate laboratory facilities is impossible. The diagnostic laboratory is no longer a matter of a single outstanding pathologist, but rather a team of experts in the various fields—medical, scientific, and technical. The tremendous increase in the amount of work required from clinical laboratories has led to the introduction of automation, which in turn has resulted in an enormous increase in the volume of work that can be done. This is the age of the computer. But we must never forget that the whole complex structure has one and only one objective, namely the care of the patient, a matter to which we shall return in the final chapter.

The lesions laid bare by the pathologist may bear an obvious relation to the symptoms, as in the case of the gross lesions of acute appendicitis or the microscopic lesions of poliomyelitis. But there may be lesions without symptoms, as in early cancer or pulmonary tuberculosis. Finally there may be symptoms without obvious lesions, as in the so-called psychosomatic (*psyche,* spirit and *soma,* body) diseases and the various psychoses. As we have already seen, it is possible, if not probable, that future research may reveal hitherto unsuspected *biochemical lesions* in these cases also. For disease itself is merely life under abnormal conditions. The presence of lesions distinguishes *organic disease,* in which there are definite observable gross or microscopic changes in an organ from so-called *functional disease,* in which there is some temporary disturbance of function without any corresponding organic change. Although it is true that at the present time diagnosis consists largely in the naming of lesions (cancer of the lung, coronary thrombosis, etc.), *disease should be considered as disordered function rather than changed structure.* By our forebears disease was regarded as an evil thing or devil, which inhabited the body and had to be expelled or exorcised. Now it has changed from a thing to a concept involving in the last analysis the chemistry of the cells and tissues.

We must also recognize that in addition to disease entities, each with its specific cause, there are syndromes. A *syndrome* (from the Greek meaning running together) is an aggregate of symptoms not due to a specific disease factor, but to interference at any point with a chain of physiological processes and as a result some impairment of bodily function. There is no constant lesion.

Fortunately there is a natural tendency to recovery from disease, more especially in acute illnesses. This was attributed by the ancient writers to *vis medicatrix naturae,* the healing power of nature, a phrase that even at the present day we cannot improve upon. Perhaps the very best example is the spontaneous healing of a clean wound, which we all take so for granted. This healing power, however, presents us with great difficulties in assessing the value of new therapeutic measures, especially new drugs. Is the happy outcome *post hoc* or *propter hoc,* that is to say, is it merely a natural event thanks to mother nature or is it the result of the therapy? This illustrates the importance of controls in our work, but naturally such controls are very much more difficult in human material than in the laboratory animal. The outcome of disease will vary between the extremes of complete recovery and death. This outcome is *prognosis;* it is a forecast of what may be expected to happen. *Diagnosis* is the art of determining not only the character of the lesion but also its etiology. Diagnosis is often difficult, but accurate prognosis is much more difficult and calls forth the very highest powers of the physician. It is largely the result of experience and judgment.

ETIOLOGY

The causation of a pathological process is known as the *etiology. Pathogenesis,* a term easily confused with etiology, is the method of production and development of the lesion. It might be supposed that the relation of etiological agent to disease, of cause to effect, was a relatively simple matter. The reverse is the case. Perhaps we are misled into imagining that only one cause is responsible. We say that the cause of tuberculosis is the tubercle bacillus, but we know that many people may inhale these bacilli yet only one may develop the disease, and that the bacilli may lurk in the body for years and only become active as the result of an intercurrent infection, prolonged strain, or starvation. The pathologist who investigates the causation of a disease must consider such elements as heredity, sex, environment, immunity, allergy, and many others. From this it becomes evident that there is no simple answer to such questions as: Does cigarette smoking cause cancer of the lung, or what is the cause of cancer or of arteriosclerosis? Even such an apparently simple matter as the relation of a blow to fracture of a bone may not be simple at all, for the real cause may be a softening of the bone or the presence in the bone of an unsuspected tumor which weakens the bone to such a degree that a very slight injury may result in what is known as a *pathological fracture.* Moreover internal and personal factors may come into conflict with external and environmental ones with resulting *stress,* a word that has become very popular. Finally, it must be admitted that the cause of a great number of diseases is completely unknown, for instance, multiple sclerosis and the various psychoses.

TRAUMA

Trauma or mechanical injury may damage a part to such an extent that the tissues may be killed. It may take the form of a blow, a wound, a fracture of bone, or a sprain to a joint. Lesser degrees of trauma cause inflammation. Mechanical injury may act as a predisposing cause of a nontraumatic disease. One of the best examples is acute osteomyelitis, an acute inflammation of bone and bone marrow caused by circulating microorganisms, usually staphylococci, which settle in the bone often at the site of a traumatic injury. It is the possibility that the disease may be predisposed or precipitated by trauma that makes workmen's compensation cases so difficult to decide. Trauma may injure a bone, causing a fracture, or it may injure the soft parts, with a resulting wound or bruise. In the condition known as *whiplash injury* of the neck, the head is thrown forward suddenly and violently, then backward, as a result of a thrust on the body from behind; the common cause is a car being rammed from the rear. The soft brain moves more slowly than the solid skull that contains it, with resulting concussion and perhaps hemorrhage on the surface, or injury to the nerve roots in the neck and even the vertebrae.

FRACTURES. A fracture may occur without the skin's being torn; this is a *simple fracture.* If the broken ends of the bone project through the skin the condition is a *compound fracture.* The great difference between the two types of fracture is that in the compound fracture there is danger of infection from the skin or air, which in the days before antisepsis and antibiotics often proved fatal. Compound fractures and battlefield wounds in general before the middle of the nineteenth century were full of hazard. A *greenstick fracture* in children is a crack rather than a frank break of the pliable bone, which has been likened to the injury caused by bending a green twig. The relation of a *pathological fracture* to some unrelated cause of weakening of the bone has already been mentioned. *Fractures of the skull* are of particular importance, because even a minor crack may tear one of the numerous meningeal arteries that run in relation to the inner surface of the skull, with the possible development of a dangerous or even fatal meningeal hemorrhage.

WOUNDS. An injury of the soft parts associated with rupture of the skin is known as a wound. It is obvious that there can be a great variety of wounds. The wound may be clean or infected, incised, punctured, penetrating, and so on. Trauma may injure the soft tissues even though the skin is not broken. The finer vessels, especially the capillaries, are ruptured, so that there is bleeding into the tissue spaces. The result is a *bruise* or *contusion,* which is at first red, then greenish or yellow before it fades. This is the basis of the so-called "black eye." The changes in color are caused by changes that the hemoglobin undergoes after the blood has been shed. The damaged area loses its normal capacity for resistance to infection, so that bacteria that may have been carried into the tissue by the foreign body causing the injury can multiply rapidly. Even if the surface has not been broken, bacteria circulating in the blood may enter the damaged area because of the increased permeability of the dilated capillaries, and they find the fluid medium to their liking.

INFECTIONS

By far the commonest cause of disease is *bacteria.* These, together with *molds* or *fungi,* properly belong to the vegetable kingdom, but certain lowly forms of animal life known as the *animal parasites* may also live in the body and produce disease. Finally there are *filterable viruses,* forms of living matter so minute that they pass through the pores of filters fine enough to hold back bacteria, so tiny that they cannot be seen with the most powerful light microscope, and are therefore said to be ultramicroscopic, although, as pointed out previously, they can now be made visible with the electron microscope. This last group has attracted a great deal of attention in recent years.

Bacteria, microorganisms or germs can be divided into three main groups: (1) *cocci,* which are round; (2) *bacilli,* which are rod-shaped; and (3) *spirilla,* or spirochetes, which are spiral like a corkscrew. They cause disease either by their presence in the tissues or by producing toxins (poisons), which either act on the surrounding structures or are carried by the blood stream to distant organs; in both instances they cause inflammation and degeneration.

It would be useless to give in this place a list of the bacteria that cause disease, for it would be merely a list of names with little meaning. Many of these are considered in Chapter 8, and others in connection with the organs that they are most prone to attack.

PHYSICAL AGENTS

Trauma is the most obvious physical agent causing injury, but it has already been considered. Other physical agents that may prove dangerous are unusually high or low temperatures, irradiation, and increased or decreased atmospheric pressure.

TEMPERATURE. A *high temperature* may produce local or general damage. *Local damage* takes the form of *burns.* The burn may be *first degree* (slight reddening of skin), *second degree* (blistering), or *third degree* (destruction of whole thickness of skin). The threat to life depends as much on the size of the area burnt as on the severity of the burn. If death occurs in a day or two it is due to shock, if delayed it is due to absorption of toxins from dead tissue.

General damage or *heat stroke* may be caused by direct exposure to the sun (*sunstroke*), or to a very high temperature. The heat-regulating mechanism of the body seems to be paralyzed, so that the temperature shoots up to an alarming height, collapse and unconsciousness develop, and death may result.

A *low temperature* may cause *frostbite,* which usually involves exposed parts such as the ears, tip of nose, hands, and feet. The fluid in the cells becomes converted into ice crystals, a change that tears the cells apart. The result varies, as in the case of burns, from mild blistering to necrosis and gangrene.

RADIATION.   One of the most destructive of physical agents is radiation, which is likely to be the result of the injudicious use of x-rays or radium. It must be borne in mind that radiation, so valuable for destroying cancer cells, can also destroy normal tissue more certainly and extensively than any other known agent. *What is powerful for good can also be potent for evil.* The subject of radiation damage is discussed more fully in Chapter 13.

ATMOSPHERIC PRESSURE.   As in the case of temperature, the pressure of the atmosphere may be too high or too low.

Increased Pressure.   This is involved in building piers under water when water-tight boxes called caissons are used, in constructing tunnels under rivers, and in deep-sea diving. Additional pressure of two or three atmospheres may be used, and this results in additional air becoming dissolved in the blood plasma. When the person involved passes too rapidly from a high to a normal atmospheric pressure the air is released as bubbles in the blood. The oxygen is absorbed, but the nitrogen may form bubbles of air emboli in the small arteries to the brain with resulting damage. Pains develop in various parts of the body ("the bends"), and there may be temporary or even permanent paralysis. The condition in general is known as *caisson disease.*

Decreased Pressure.   This may be experienced by aviators flying at altitudes over 30,000 feet unless the plane is pressurized. The gases in the body cavities such as the intestine expand, causing marked discomfort, and gas bubbles are released in the blood and cause air embolism, with results similar to those of caisson disease.

CHEMICAL POISONS

The subject of poisoning or toxicology is a large and specialized one which need not detain us. Poisonous chemicals may be introduced into the body under four very different circumstances: (1) *by accident,* especially in the case of young children, (2) *for suicide,* (3) *for homicide,* (4) *as an industrial hazard.* In these days when every industry seems to use a new and different chemical, the last-named has become of particular importance. Strong acids and alkalis burn and kill the skin or the mucous membrane of the mouth and stomach if taken internally. *Lead poisoning* (*plumbism*) deserves special mention, because it belongs to both the first and fourth groups. Children are apt to put painted objects in their mouths and repeatedly swallow small amounts of the lead in the paint. Lead is used in a large number of industries—painting, glass making, lacquering, and many others. In these occupations it is particularly important to wash the hands well before eating. Poisons such as lead, mercury, arsenic, and phosphorus interfere with the working of some of the cell enzymes, thus producing sickness and even death.

ANOXIA

Loss of blood supply to a part is called *ischemia.* This is a local loss of blood, in contrast to anemia, which is a general condition of bloodlessness affecting the entire body. The result is *anoxia* or loss of oxygen to the part. As the food and oxygen are carried by the blood it is evident that if the supply of blood is diminished by narrowing of the lumen of an artery, the part of the body deprived of its blood supply will suffer and become diseased. An example of this is seen in arteriosclerosis (hardening of the arteries) of the vessels supplying the leg; the tissues of the foot will finally die, a condition known as *gangrene.* An even more important example of ischemia is blockage of the coronary arteries to the heart muscle, either by arteriosclerosis or thrombosis, resulting either in sudden death or in permanent damage to the heart. Thrombosis of one or more of the cerebral arteries is the most common cause of a stroke, by reason of the resulting cerebral anoxia.

STRESS

Overwork or *overstrain* is an occasional cause of disease. It is best seen in the heart, which may be permanently damaged by the chronic strain thrown upon it by prolonged high blood pressure.

The concept of *stress,* although an old one, has reasserted itself through the work of Selye. This will be discussed in connection with the endocrine glands. Here it may be said that stress of various kinds, both physical and mental, may upset the normal hormonal balance, especially that between the pituitary and adrenal, with resultant disturbance of health. This far-reaching concept has aroused widespread interest. *Health indeed may be regarded as the result of success in the ceaseless struggle between man and his environment,* and much of this struggle is with stress. The outcome of the struggle depends largely on the adrenal cortex, itself controlled by the pituitary. When the stress is continued over too long a period, the adrenals become exhausted.

DEFICIENCY DISEASES

The idea that disease may be due to something lacking, rather than to some positive hostile factor such as bacteria, injury, or poison, is a comparatively new one, but enormously important and far-reaching. It has, of course, always been recognized that starvation will affect the health of the body and will eventually result in death. But there may be an insufficient supply of some particular element in the food, such as proteins, carbohydrates, and fats. Even more important as a cause of disease is an inadequate supply of *minerals* and of the essential food factors known as *vitamins.* Even though actual disease may not be present, *perfect* health is impossible if there are deficiencies in the food. This is particularly true of the growing period of life.

With every year that passes the importance of nutritional deficiencies is becoming more apparent. It is the quality rather than the quantity of the food that is essential. During starvation the demands of the body are so much lowered that true deficiency disease may not become apparent. But if the food is abundant, particularly in carbohydrates, but deficient in minerals or vitamins, the health of the cells is impaired and evidence of disease becomes manifest.

The most obvious method of production of nutritional deficiency is lack in certain elements in the diet. But the same result may be brought about in a number of other ways. If a patient suffers from persistent vomiting he cannot assimilate his food, no matter how excellent it may be. Such conditions as gastric ulcer and diabetes may necessitate the long-continued use of diets that may be deficient in particular food elements. Widespread disease of the intestine, commonly associated with diarrhea, may interfere so seriously with the absorption of food that deficiency must result. Even when satisfactory absorption has occurred, such an important digestive organ as the liver may be unable to deal with the food elements owing to cirrhosis, etc., and once again symptoms of deficiency may appear. This list, which could be extended considerably, will indicate how readily a condition of dietary deficiency may arise.

Resistance to infection appears to depend to some extent on the food supply, and particularly on the proteins, for it is from proteins that antibodies to bacteria are manufactured. It is for this reason that a state of chronic starvation is associated with a greatly lowered resistance to such infections as tuberculosis. A tragic demonstration of this fact is provided by the high incidence of tuberculosis and other serious infections among the peoples of Europe impoverished by a great war.

The earlier work on food deficiency, particularly vitamin deficiency, was concerned with what may be termed full-blown diseases such as scurvy, rickets, and beriberi. It is now realized that minor manifestations of deficiency are much more common, though they have been overlooked in the past. In certain localities where, for geographic or economic reasons, there is a grave lack of such essential foods as milk and fresh vegetables, a large proportion of the population may exhibit symptoms and signs of deficiency disease, though they may be quite unconscious of that fact.

The minerals and vitamins have been called the *"protective elements"* of the diet, and they are really more important than proteins, carbohydrates, and fats, which are energy foods necessary for running the engine. Without the protective foods a child cannot enjoy buoyant as compared with merely satisfactory health.

MINERAL DEFICIENCY. The three important minerals that may be deficient in the food are calcium, iron, and iodine. *Calcium* is necessary both for the formation and the continued health of bone. If it is deficient in the diet during early childhood there is danger that *rickets* may develop; the bones that are deficient in calcium are soft and easily bent, so that bowlegs and other deformities develop. In adult life calcium deficiency may also lead to softening of the bones or *osteomalacia* (the same thing in Greek). *Iron* is absolutely necessary for the health of the red blood corpuscles, and when it is deficient in the diet *anemia* inevitably develops. As will be seen when diseases of the blood are studied, anemias are now divided into iron-deficiency anemias and other forms of anemia. It is of interest to note that the most important member of the latter group, pernicious anemia, is also a deficiency disease. *Iodine* is essential to the proper functioning of the thyroid gland, and when it is deficient one form of *goiter* develops. Although minerals are so essential for the health of the body, the actual amounts needed are extraordinarily minute. For instance, the amount of iodine needed to prevent the development of goiter is only 10 to 20 mg. *a year.*

Potassium deficiency has come to assume a position of special importance. The deficiency of the mineral is due to loss from the body, not to an insufficient supply in the food. We owe the realization of the importance of potassium in the body's economy to an advance in medical technology, for the use of the flame photometer has made it possible to estimate the potassium content of body fluids and tissues. At least

98 per cent of the potassium of the body is located in the intracellular fluid, mainly in the muscle cells, in contrast with sodium, which is mainly in the extracellular fluid. Potassium deficiency (*hypopotassemia*) may develop from a variety of causes, of which the most important are: (1) *stress,* usually the result of surgical trauma, the cells of the postoperative patient leaking potassium into the extracellular fluid and thence at once into the urine, the leak being activated by aldosterone liberated as part of the reaction of the adrenal cortex to stress; (2) *vomiting and diarrhea* when severe and prolonged; (3) *deficiency caused by therapy,* especially the continued intravenous administration of salt and glucose solutions, which may lower the serum potassium level to a dangerous degree. The muscles suffer most, with lack of tone, weakness, and finally paralysis. The abdominal distention so common in the postoperative patient is caused by lack of tone of the muscular wall of the intestine due to potassium depletion caused by stress. Cardiac dilatation and myocardial failure with marked changes in the electrocardiogram are among the most serious of the sequelae.

There is a curious relationship between mineral metabolism and the ductless glands, which will be discussed in more detail when diseases of those organs are considered. Iodine metabolism is regulated by the thyroid gland, and as we have just seen, lack of iodine will cause disease of the thyroid, just as disease of the gland will cause disturbed iodine metabolism. The parathyroid glands bear the same relation to calcium metabolism, and the adrenals govern the metabolism of sodium chloride.

VITAMIN DEFICIENCY. An adequate supply of protein, carbohydrate, fat, and mineral salts is not sufficient for the needs of the living body. Certain *"accessory food factors"* are also necessary for life. These are therefore called vitamins. *They are formed or synthesized by plants, not by animals.* Man's supply therefore comes directly from plants, or from animals (including fish) that have eaten the plants and stored up the vitamins—unless these happen to be bought at the corner drugstore. They need only be present in minute amounts, but their absence (*avitaminosis*) leads to profound pathological changes. Some of these deficiency diseases such as rickets and scurvy have been known for centuries. Although it was not recognized that they were due to a simple deficiency in diet, empirical methods of treatment were successfully employed. The old explorers recognized the value of fresh fruit in the prevention of scurvy, and cod liver oil has been used in the treatment of rickets for more than a hundred years.

The original list of four vitamins (A, B, C, D) has been greatly extended, and the end is not in sight. Moreover vitamin B, a complex, has been separated into a number of distinct chemicals. With such complexity, the alphabetical system of names has broken down, and the chemical names have come into general use. An exception to this rule are vitamins A and D, which are not manufactured chemically, but are sold as concentrates from fish liver oils. Vitamins are organic catalysts of exogenous origin, which are intimately related to the enzyme systems. They play the part of coenzymes in the chemical mechanism of the cell by which the true foodstuffs are metabolized. In many respects they resemble the hormones, which also act through the enzymes, the chief distinction being that hormones are endogenous in origin, whereas vitamins are exogenous, the body being unable to synthesize them.

It is customary to divide the vitamins into two groups, the fat-soluble and the water-soluble. The *fat-soluble vitamins* are A, D, E, and K, the *water-soluble* being B and C. The fat-soluble members are naturally less easily absorbed than the water-soluble, so that they are more readily affected by conditioning factors (see below), but the advantage possessed by the water-soluble group in this respect is offset by the fact that they are more readily lost as the result of cooking or the modern processing of food.

Avitaminosis or vitamin deficiency may be due to two very different conditions. (1) The supply of the food factor may be inadequate. This is known as *primary deficiency,* and is exogenous in origin. This is no longer of great importance in developed countries, except among food faddists and other health cranks, but it is widely prevalent in undeveloped countries, particularly Africa and the Orient. (2) The supply is adequate, but for various reasons it cannot be used properly. This is *secondary conditioned deficiency.* Conditioning factors may be: (1) *reduced intake,* as may occur in prolonged vomiting, esophageal obstruction, and loss of appetite; (2) *malabsorption,* such as occurs in chronic inflammation of the pancreas and small intestine; (3)*excessive demand,* seen especially in infancy and puberty, but also during pregnancy and lactation; (4) *reduced storage facilities,* the best example being cirrhosis of the liver in the chronic alcoholic. Before proceeding to a consideration of the various vitamin deficiencies it should be pointed out that man seldom shows the picture of pure vitamin deficiency seen in the experimental animal, and that the administration of a single vitamin in a chemically pure state may not serve to correct the condition. We now know enough, however, to prevent the *five major vitamin-deficiency diseases,* namely *beriberi* (vitamin B complex—thiamin), *pellagra* (vitamin B complex—niacin), *scurvy* (vitamin C), *rickets* (vitamin D), and *keratomalacia* (vitamin A).

Vitamin A.   This is a fat-soluble vitamin, so that it is found in butter, cream, egg yolk, and fish liver oils, as well as in yellow and green vegetables such as carrots, spinach, peas, and beans. The plants do not really contain vitamin A, but a yellow pigment called *carotene* which is converted by the liver into the vitamin. The vitamin A content of milk and butter depends on the carotene content of the plants the animal eats. Even the vitamin in fish liver oil comes from marine plants (plankton). Minute invertebrates feed on the plants; they are devoured later by small fish; these in turn serve as food to large fish in whose livers the vitamin is stored.

Lack of vitamin A in the diet leads to degeneration of the epithelium lining mucous membranes in the respiratory and digestive tracts as well as in certain glands such as the lachrymal and salivary. Such mucous surfaces are especially susceptible to infection. In children, in whom the deficiency is most likely to develop, drying of the cornea, known as *xerophthalmia* (*xeros,* dry) may occur, owing to lack of secretion of the lachrymal glands. This may lead to softening of the cornea (*keratomalacia*), with ulceration and subsequent blindness. Bronchopneumonia in children may be caused by the changes in the mucous membrane of the bronchial tree. A peculiar symptom is *night blindness,* or inability to see in a dim light. This is due to deficiency in the visual purple of the retina, a substance necessary for vision in poor light.

Under ordinary conditions of life vitamin A deficiency is seldom seen in Europe and North America, although quite common in India, China, and other countries where the diet is often of low quality. Where war brings restrictions in diet, however, night blindness and xerophthalmia may become common, the former being particularly dangerous during blackouts. Governments have recognized this to such an extent that they have added vitamin A to bread when necessary.

Vitamin B Complex. One of the earliest discoveries regarding vitamins was that beriberi, a disease of the Orient, was due to eating "polished" rice, *i.e.,* rice from which the outer covering and the germ had been removed in the milling process. The vitamin responsible was called vitamin B. It is now known that what was thought to be a single vitamin is really a complex, from which a number of components have been separated. The three best known of these are thiamin, niacin, and riboflavin. This group of vitamins is one of the most widely distributed, being present in all natural foodstuffs. The various members of the group are water-soluble, so that they are readily absorbed, but they pay a penalty, because much is lost in the process of refining and of converting natural into artificial foods, as in the case of white bread and polished rice. Fortunately most of the B complex vitamins utilized by the body are produced by the bacteria in the intestine.

Thiamin (formerly vitamin B_1) is the antiberiberi factor. The principal features of *beriberi* are peripheral neuritis (marked by weakness of the limbs), widespread edema, and myocardial weakness. When rice is polished the skin and the germ, which contain the vitamin, are removed, so that in rice-eating countries such as China beriberi is a common disease. Thiamin is now added to enriched white flour, to restore what is lost from the whole wheat in milling.

Riboflavin (formerly vitamin B₂) is also desirable for the enrichment of bread, but the supply is still small. Mild symptoms of its absence (ariboflavinosis) are not uncommon among the undernourished and those women who subsist on absurdly inadequate diets with the object of improving their figure. Severe manifestations are seen principally in the southern states of America and in Newfoundland. There may be fissured lesions at the corners of the mouth (*cheilosis*) and erosions around the eyes and the sides of the nose. The tongue may acquire a characteristic magenta color. The most serious disturbances are those involving the eye. In persons whose occupation exposes them to bright light, including workers with the microscope, there may be eyestrain and redness of the conjunctiva and the lower lids. In advanced cases there is invasion of the cornea by capillaries. In the past these ocular symptoms were never attributed to the real cause, namely, vitamin deficiency. The principal source of riboflavin is milk.

Niacin (formerly nicotinic acid) is the pellagra-preventing vitamin. *Pellagra* is a disease common in Italy and the southern United States, but not confined to these regions. It is characterized by reddening and scaling of the skin on the exposed parts of the body, as well as gastrointestinal, nervous, and mental disorders. The tongue may become smooth and fiery red. Although a deficiency disease, it is also in some way connected with eating diseased maize.

Vitamin B₁₂ is a growth factor in the maturation of red blood cells in the bone marrow. It is derived from the food, but it is absorbed from the intestine only in the presence of an "intrinsic factor" secreted by the stomach. Absence of this factor leads to the development of pernicious anemia, in which the progenitors of the red blood cells in the marrow do not develop into adult erythrocytes, but enter the blood stream as abnormally large red cells (macrocytes), which have a shortened life span, even though the bowel is full of vitamin. *Vitamin B₁₂ deficiency is therefore an excellent example of a conditioned deficiency, depending on absence of the gastric intrinsic factor.*

Vitamin C (Ascorbic Acid). This is the *antiscorbutic vitamin,* which prevents scurvy or scorbutus. It occurs in fruits and fresh vegetables rather than in fats. It is particularly abundant in tomato, orange, lemon, and grapefruit. It is destroyed by heat and drying, so that preserved foods and fruits are lacking in it. In vitamin C deficiency the level of ascorbic acid is low in the urine and very low in the blood. By estimation of this level, deficiency of the vitamin can be readily detected. Linus

Pauling, Nobel Prize winner, believes that taking large doses of vitamin C in the form of powdered ascorbic acid leads to increased vigor, increased protection against infections, and increased rate of healing of wounds.

When ascorbic acid is lacking, the cement substance, which holds together the endothelial cells lining the capillaries, becomes deficient. The vessels thus develop leaks through which bleeding occurs into the tissues. The health of the ground substance of the connective tissue in general also suffers.

Scurvy or *scorbutus* is the great manifestation of vitamin C deficiency. It used to be a common disease among sailors, soldiers, arctic explorers, and others deprived of fresh fruit and vegetables. The old Elizabethan seaman, Captain Hawkins, called it "the plague of the sea and the spoil of mariners," adding that "the sea is natural for fishes and the land for men." That was all changed by Captain Cook's discovery that limes and lime juice would prevent the disease, and now even that is not necessary, for the vitamin can be put up as tablets of ascorbic acid.

Hemorrhage occurs owing to lack of cement substance in the capillaries. The gums are soft, spongy, bleed readily and are heavily invaded by bacteria, while the teeth fall out, so that the condition of the mouth becomes foul and very distressing. The skin presents numerous small hemorrhages (petechiae). There is hemorrhage into the joints and the internal organs. Owing to the deficient ground substance of connective tissue there is *delayed healing of wounds,* and after healing they tend to break down under strain. If the scorbutic condition is not relieved it may end fatally, and in the past it frequently did so.

Infants who are artificially fed may develop *infantile scurvy* (*Barlow's disease*), of which the chief symptom is extreme tenderness of the legs due to hemorrhage under the periosteum of the tibia. The disease should never occur, as it can so readily be prevented by including tomato or orange juice in the feedings.

Vitamin D. Much of the romance of the vitamins centers around this member of the group. Several factors are concerned in the action of this vitamin, and the unraveling of these might easily have taken half a century, but the whole problem was cleared up in little more than half a dozen years by workers in many widely separate countries.

Vitamin D is the *antirachitic vitamin;* it *prevents rickets* or rachitis. It does this by controlling calcium metabolism. It is a *fat-soluble vitamin,* so, as might be expected, it is found in milk, butter, egg yolk, and other fats, but by far the most abundant supply is in cod liver oil.

One of the most remarkable discoveries was that the vitamin is formed by the *action of ultraviolet light* on certain waxy compounds known as sterols, particularly ergosterol, found in yeast, and cholesterol, present in the skin. When the skin is exposed to abundant sunlight, a sufficient amount of the vitamin is formed from the cholesterol. In dark and gloomy climates, however, and in the slums of cities, there is not enough light to form the vitamin. It is prepared commercially by irradiating yeast, which is rich in ergosterol, by the mercury vapor lamp, and is then called *viosterol*. The vitamin has been synthetized in the laboratory; it is a yellow crystalline substance, which has been named *calciferol* because of its influence on calcification.

Without a sufficient supply of vitamin D the proper calcification of bone in the child cannot take place, and rickets is the result. It is also required for the formation of normal teeth in the growing child. Marked deficiency of the vitamin is rare in adults, but when present it may produce *osteomalacia* or softening of the bones. This disease is more likely to be seen in such countries as India and China, where the diet is deficient, and commonest in women who are little exposed to sunlight in those countries.

Rickets or rachitis is a disease of young children. The bones are not properly formed, owing to insufficient deposition both of calcium and phosphorus. The bones are therefore soft and bend easily, so that deformities (bowlegs, etc.) result. These are described in more detail in connection with disease of bones. The disease occurs usually in bottle-fed babies, and in young children brought up in the slums of smoky cities in northern latitudes. It is unknown in the tropics. As we have seen, it may be due to one of two factors, or often to a combination of the two: (1) *insufficient vitamin D in the diet;* (2) *insufficient sunlight (ultraviolet) which could produce the vitamin by activating the cholesterol in the skin.*

The disease is easily arrested by the administration of cod liver or halibut liver oil or viosterol, or by exposing the child to ultraviolet radiation from sunlight or the mercury vapor lamp or carbon arc.

Vitamin E. This vitamin is necessary for normal reproduction, so it has been called the antisterility vitamin. The chief sources are the germ of various cereals and green vegetable foods. Wheat germ oil contains a large amount of the vitamin. Knowledge as to its action is limited to animals. Deficiency in female rats causes the embryo to die early, and in males spermatozoa are not produced because of degenerative changes in the testes. This has not been established for humans.

Vitamin K. The story of vitamin K is quite as remarkable as that of vitamin D. In 1930 a Danish observer, Dam, noticed that chicks fed on a deficient diet developed hemorrhage and that this was prevented when they were given alfalfa. There was evidently some factor in the alfalfa which was necessary for the coagulation of the blood and without which hemorrhage would occur. Soon this factor was extracted and crystallized. It was called Koagulationsvitamin, being German for the vitamin which promotes coagulation; this became shortened to vitamin K.

The *prothrombin of the blood* must be at a normal level if the coagulation of blood, which is necessary to stop hemorrhage, is to occur in a normal way. It was soon found that animals deficient in vitamin K were also deficient in prothrombin, and so it became apparent that vitamin K is necessary for the formation of prothrombin. The mere presence of a sufficient amount of vitamin K in the food is not enough; it has to be absorbed before it can be used for the manufacture of prothrombin.

The next discovery was that *the vitamin is not absorbed unless bile is present in the intestine.* It had long been known that operations on jaundiced patients were apt to be followed by hemorrhage, often fatal, at the site of operation. In jaundice the bile is unable to reach the intestine. Now it was clear that the reason for the bleeding tendency in jaundice was lack of vitamin K, that lack being due to failure in absorption, which in turn was due to absence of bile in the bowel. The prothrombin in the blood was found to be very low in cases of jaundice, as was to be expected.

This was a discovery of great practical importance, because now it is possible to raise the prothrombin in the blood of jaundiced patients before operation. This is done by administering bile, or rather bile salts, combined with vitamin K. The vitamin is absorbed, the prothrombin rises to normal, and the operation can be performed without danger of hemorrhage.

Another condition in which the prothrombin is low is *hemorrhagic disease of the newborn.* Shortly after birth the baby may show a tendency to bleeding, and if there has been any birth injury to the head there may be fatal intracranial hemorrhage. This is due to vitamin K deficiency in the baby, and can readily be prevented by administering the vitamin to the mother before delivery.

Table 1 is a summary of some of the principal clinical features of the vitamin deficiencies in man.

The various vitamins are necessary for perfect health. Deficiency in any one of them may lead to disease. It is important, however, to remember the following facts, which are apt to be overlooked in view of the flood of articles on vitamins in the press and periodicals, not to mention the persuasive pamphlets from the pharmaceutical houses. (1) Under modern conditions outspoken deficiency disease is uncommon except in a few less favored localities, in Oriental countries, or as the result of war, although minor degrees are far from rare. (2) An average mixed diet including fresh fruit and green vegetables contains

Table 1. *Vitamin Deficiency Diseases*

Vitamin A	Night blindness, xerophthalmia, keratomalacia
Thiamin (B₁)	Beriberi
Riboflavin (B₂)	Cheilosis, eye lesions
Niacin (nicotinic acid)	Pellagra (skin, alimentary canal, central nervous system)
Vitamin B₁₂	Pernicious anemia
Vitamin C	Scurvy
Vitamin D	Rickets, osteomalacia
Vitamin K	Hypoprothrombinemia, tendency to bleeding

an ample supply of vitamins. (3) Whereas pure vitamin deficiency can be produced in the experimental animal, in human cases an inadequate diet is likely to be lacking in more than one vitamin, so that the clinical picture will tend to be a mixed one. (4) More than $100,000,000 are spent by the United States public in buying vitamins. (5) It is better and infinitely cheaper to get your vitamins from the grocery store, where they have been manufactured by Nature, than from the drugstore, where they have been manufactured by man. Although this is true for healthy persons, it may not be true for those suffering from avitaminosis. When the condition is of long duration it may be necessary to administer artificially prepared vitamins for a correspondingly long period before the needs of the tissues are fully satisfied and the normal balance of vitamins is restored. *Finally, it must be borne in mind that vitamins, although essential to life, are no substitute for food. They provide no energy, calories, or body-building materials, and are merely accessory to diet.*

DRUGS

The causes of disease are endless, and it is sad to have to finish with a reference to drugs. There is nothing better both for the prevention and cure of disease than drugs. But, as we have already seen, what is powerful for good may also be potent for evil. The picture of disease is changing before our very eyes, and while old diseases are passing away as the result of modern therapy, new diseases are taking their place, and many of these new diseases are due to drugs, which are a two-edged sword. These are usually drugs used by the general public, but they may be drugs prescribed by the doctor. In these days when tranquilizers take the place of baby-sitters, blood transfusions are given indiscriminately and often needlessly, antibiotics are regarded as the cure-all for the most minor infections, and steroid therapy is the refuge of the destitute, it is small wonder that old maladies are replaced by new man-made ones.

There never has been a period in human history when such a deluge of new drugs has been poured forth. The public press daily reports a quota of miracle drugs, which the public demands. No drug is completely safe. One person may have an allergy to such a harmless drug as aspirin. If the reader will consult the table of contents of Spain's "The Complications of Modern Medical Practices," he will see the truth of this statement. The most tragic example is, of course, thalidomide given to pregnant women with results which we all know. The use of "The Pill" involves a distinct danger of thromboembolism.

HEREDITY AND CONSTITUTION

HEREDITY. Heredity is a factor in the causation of disease and its importance is recognized by life insurance companies. If one has the misfortune to inherit poor materials from one's ancestors the machines constructed from those materials can never be first class, and "causes of disease" may wreck that machine, whereas they might have little effect on one of high grade. In most diseases, certainly in all bacterial infections, there are two factors to be considered, an extrinsic or external factor, such as the bacillus of tuberculosis, and an intrinsic or internal factor, which we may call the constitution of the patient, the body's power of defense, and the like. *It is a question of the seed and the soil.* If the soil is suitable, even a minute quantity of seed will grow abundantly and bring forth a rich harvest of disease. Some people get every infection that is going around, while others never seem to be ill. Much of this is a question of heredity. The subject of genetic factors in the causation of disease is discussed in Chapter 14.

CONSTITUTION. The constitution comprises those features of the mind and body that a man derives from heredity and upbringing. It is the sum total of his being. There can be little doubt that nutrition is a factor of great importance, especially in the early formative years of life. Every day and every hour the cells of the body are taking up elements from the food, including vitamins, and if these are deficient in quantity or quality the constitution as a whole cannot fail to suffer. It has been said, with what truth I am unable to tell, that if all the diseases now described in the textbooks could be removed by the wave of a wand, doctors would still be left with 80 per cent of their patients. There ill health would be due not so much to any known disease as to the failure of the constitution to adapt itself to the life led. *A good constitution is not to be confused with a good physique; it is something more and something more valuable.* Those who have it seem able to do whatever they wish without impairing it in any way. When it is poor, small causes may impair health or even endanger life. The athlete with the most perfect physique may be attacked by every infection that he encounters, and may early develop arteriosclerosis and other degenerative conditions. Constitution can be divided into the hypersthenic, the hyposthenic, and the normal. The *hypersthenic* individual is bubbling over with energy; he is the man of action. The *hyposthenic* may be the very reverse of this, but it is this group that supplies the great thinkers. It is obvious that a doctor must distinguish between these groups if he is going to give advice of value as to the way of life that a patient should follow.

It is sometimes said that the nature of disease is changing, that we hear much more about people dying of heart failure and cancer than used to be the case. This does not mean that these diseases have become actually more common, although more people do die from them. Long ago Addison, in the *Vision of Myrza,* drew a picture of the great masses of mankind walking over the bridge of life which spans the dark river of death. In the bridge there were many hidden trapdoors through which the unwary travellers dropped into the flood below. Their numbers became ever fewer as they approached the far side, but none succeeded in completing the journey. The trapdoors represent diseases. At the near end of the bridge there are many trapdoors—infantile mortality, typhoid, malaria, smallpox—which have been so securely closed by medical science that they seldom open now. But at the far end there is a small number of wide trapdoors—cancer, heart failure, apoplexy—and great numbers must fall through these into the dark flood of oblivion.

MAKING THE DIAGNOSIS

The detection of disease and the determination of its precise nature are as elaborate and sometimes as difficult a matter as the detection of crime. *The methods employed fall into two main groups, the clinical and the laboratory.*

CLINICAL METHODS.   The *clinical* group consists of an analysis of symptoms and physical signs. *Symptoms* include the complaints of the patient, either voluntary or elicited by careful cross-examination. It is often possible to make a correct diagnosis from the symptoms alone. Thus the agonizing pain over the heart in coronary thrombosis, or the digestive distress and pain relieved by taking food so characteristic of ulcer of the stomach, may tell the doctor in clear and unmistakable language the disease from which the patient is suffering. In the majority of diseases there is a close relationship between the symptoms of the patient and the lesions that the pathologist may be able to demonstrate. Thus if the air spaces of the lung are filled with inflammatory material in pneumonia it is only natural that the patient should be severely short of breath. This close relationship of lesions to symptoms is one of the chief reasons why a knowledge of pathology is of value to the doctor. One of the peculiar effects of cortisone, a hormone of the cortex of the adrenal, is that it may break this relationship without having actually altered the lesions and therefore without having benefitted the patient, no matter how much better he may feel. Unfortunately the number of symptoms of which a patient can complain are limited, and pain, shortness of breath, fever, and loss of strength can be caused by many very different diseases. On this account the doctor has to turn to physical signs for further help.

Physical signs are elicited by physical examination of the patient. By listening to the heart a murmur may be heard, palpation of the kidney may show it to be enlarged, and pressure over the appendix may elicit tenderness even though the patient has not complained of pain. These signs are of the greatest help in diagnosis.

Simple visual inspection of the patient may tell the doctor or the nurse all that needs to be known. The patient with pneumonia can be recognized by reason of the rapid respiration, cough, and flushed feverish appearance. In chronic heart failure there is shortness of breath (dyspnea), swelling of the legs, and the bluish tinge of cyanosis. In an acute heart attack, such as that of coronary thrombosis, the face is clammy and ashen in color, the expression that of deep anxiety, and there is a strange immobility as if the patient feared to move a muscle. In nephritis the face and eyelids are swollen and the skin presents a typical pallor. Acute intestinal obstruction can be suspected from the sunken appearance of the eyes due to extreme loss of fluid (dehydration), the leaden skin, and the board-like rigidity of the abdomen. The wasted and emaciated appearance (cachexia) of the cancer patient is only too readily recognized. Among the most characteristic of clinical pictures are those of certain diseases of the endocrine glands, as illustrated by the pigmentation of the skin in Addison's disease associated with destruction of the cortex of the adrenals, and the striking contrasts presented by Graves' disease due to hyperactivity of the thyroid and myxedema due to hypoactivity of the same gland.

What may be called the *scopes* can be included in a discussion of physical signs. They are instruments that enable the doctor at the bedside to see what would otherwise remain hidden from him. They consist of a tiny electric light bulb at the end of a metal tube. When this is introduced into one of the hollow organs of the body, the walls of the organ can be studied by means of an ingenious system of mirrors. The *laryngoscope* reveals the interior of the larynx, the *bronchoscope* the interior of the bronchial tree, the *gastroscope* the interior of the stomach, the *sigmoidoscope* the interior of the colon (sigmoid), the *cysto-*

scope the interior of the bladder, and so on. In the case of the *ophthalmoscope* a beam of light is directed into the eye, the interior of which is illuminated and can be studied.

LABORATORY METHODS. These comprise tests that cannot be done at the bedside, but require the use of laboratory apparatus such as the microscope and the test tube with all its complicated extensions. It must be emphasized that laboratory tests, with which must be included x-ray pictures, do not provide the doctor with a ready-made diagnosis; they merely give him additional information which, taken in conjunction with the clinical evidence (history of the illness, symptoms, and signs), enable him to arrive at a correct conclusion—we hope.

These tests constitute what has now become the specialty of *clinical pathology,* and comprise the examination of fluids (including blood) and cells taken from the patient during life. When I was a junior resident in Edinburgh I used to carry out these tests myself, for they were simple and easy, consisting chiefly of examining the urine for albumin, sugar and abnormal cells, counting the red and white cells of the blood, testing the sputum for tubercle bacilli, and similar elementary procedures. Now all that has changed, and the change has been vast in scope and unbelievable in degree. This is largely due to the development of chemistry and biochemistry in relation to their application to the examination of the blood and other fluids, to the introduction of methods for estimating the enzyme activity of liver and heart muscle cells in diseases of those organs, and so on. The material is collected and the tests performed mainly by the medical technologist, the laboratory technician, a highly trained individual whose work has become as valuable and essential to the clinician in the diagnosis of disease as is that of the trained nurse in the treatment and care of the patient. This is the nurse-technologist-doctor team.

Laboratory tests are numerous and complex. Indeed entire books are devoted to them. Only a few of the more important will be mentioned here. In what follows I have confined myself to the barest outline, to be skipped by even the embryo technologist, but intended for the uninitiated as a preview of some more detailed accounts in the second part of this book.

Urinalysis is the commonest of all laboratory tests. Examination of the urine serves not only to indicate the condition of the kidneys, but may also reveal disease of the bladder and urethra. Other diseases not connected with the urinary tract may be detected by urinalysis, *e.g.,* the presence of sugar in the urine in diabetes. As a matter of fact, the urine represents the main route by which abnormal substances are eliminated from the blood. It is obvious how many of these substances, such as minerals and hormones, may be revealed by skillful urinalysis.

Examination of *stomach contents* and *feces* gives valuable information as to the presence of disease in the stomach and intestine.

A *blood count* shows the number and the condition of both the red blood cells and the leukocytes. The red cells are diminished in various forms of anemia. The number of the leukocytes is increased in acute infections (appendicitis, pneumonia), and in the blood disease leukemia.

Blood chemistry is becoming of ever-increasing importance. Thus the blood sugar is increased in diabetes, the urea and nonprotein nitrogen are increased in renal failure, the phosphorus is lowered in rickets, and various enzymes may be increased in amount, while others not normally present may make their appearance.

The *cerebrospinal fluid* shows changes in many diseases of the nervous system. Thus the diagnosis of acute meningitis is made by finding large numbers of leukocytes in this fluid, together with the bacteria causing the infection. The fluid, which is obtained by means of lumbar puncture, is a mirror in which is reflected disease of the brain and spinal cord.

Bacteriological examination is of the greatest importance in the diagnosis of many of the infectious diseases such as diphtheria, pneumonia, and tuberculosis A blood culture may show the presence of streptococci and other organisms in the circulating blood.

Serology, which is a branch of bacteriology, consists in the examination of the blood serum for substances that indicate the presence of bacterial infection. Examples of such tests are the Widal test for typhoid fever and the Wassermann test for syphilis. It must be understood that these are not tests for the bacteria, but for substances produced by the body in response to the infection.

Tissue diagnosis is the microscopic examination of pieces of tissue. When such a piece is removed during life for the purpose of diagnosis the procedure is called a *biopsy,* in contrast to the examination of tissues at autopsy. It is usually done to determine whether a tumor is malignant.

The *electrocardiogram* is an electrical record of the contractions of the heart. All contracting muscles produce an electric current, and such a current is produced by the contractions of the auricles and ventricles. The current is made to write a permanent tracing (electrocardiogram), which is of one pattern when the heart muscle is healthy, but of a different pattern when the muscle is diseased. These fingerprints of the heart's action are of great value to the heart specialist.

Basal metabolism or the *basal metabolic rate* (B.M.R.) is the heat production of the body. It is determined from the amount of carbon dioxide eliminated or the amount of oxygen consumed over a given period of time. The two important conditions that raise the basal metabolic rate are fever and overactivity of the thyroid gland (hyperthyroidism, exophthalmic goiter). The chief value of the test is to estimate the functional activity of the thyroid in cases of goiter.

Radiography. The radiologist provides invaluable asistance to the clinician in search of a diagnosis. X-rays have the power of passing through solid objects and affecting a photographic film on the other side of that object. But their use is limited by the fact that they can only show differences in density. An opaque object like a bullet will stand out clearly; large solid organs can be seen on the film, but the outlines of hollow structures, such as the stomach, intestine, gallbladder, and bronchi, are indistinguishable. It is these outlines, however, that are most likely to be altered in disease.

This serious limitation to the usefulness of x-ray examination has been largely overcome by the ingenuity of the radiologist. He has found it possible to introduce into the cavities of the body substances such as barium and iodine which are opaque to x-rays and thus provide the contrast necessary for the making of a picture. The method has its greatest use in examination of the gastrointestinal tract, which when filled with a barium meal becomes opaque to the rays, so that an exact outline of the stomach or intestine appears on the film. An ulcer stands out on the edge of the stomach as a crater, while a tumor shows as a dent (filling defect) which the barium cannot fill out. A *cholecystogram* is a picture of the outline of the gallbladder; an opaque substance is administered which is excreted by the liver in the bile and thus enters the gallbladder where it becomes sufficiently concentrated to throw a shadow on the film. Similarly in *urography* an opaque substance is injected into the ureters through the bladder and thus shows an outline of the renal pelvis. Or similar material (*Uroselectan*) can be injected intravenously; this is excreted by the kidneys, and the outline of the renal pelvis again becomes visible. *Lipiodol* is an oil containing iodine which can be injected into the bronchi or the spinal canal, so that an outline of these spaces is seen. A *ventriculogram* is a picture of the ventricles of the brain obtained by injecting air into these cavities through an opening made in the skull. As air is less dense than the surrounding brain, an outline of the ventricles is obtained. Of particular value has been the introduction of *angiography,* by means of which a radiopaque substance injected into an artery can show narrowing of that vessel, the presence of an aneurysm, etc. This technique has acquired particular importance by reason of the surgeon's ability to operate on diseased arteries and replace them with artificial tubing. Angiography has proved particularly useful in the investigation of cases in which disease of the intracranial arteries is suspected.

In all of these cases a photograph is made on a film by the rays that have passed through the body. An equally valuable method of examination is by means of the *fluoroscope*. This is a sensitive screen on which a faint outline of opaque structures becomes visible when x-rays pass through the body. The value of the fluoroscope is that it shows movement; an aneurysm of the aorta can be seen to pulsate, the movements of the diaphragm can be studied, the ability of the stomach to empty itself is noted, and the peristaltic movements of the intestine can be observed. The fluoroscopic screen shows the observer what is happening in the body from moment to moment, but the x-ray film gives a permanent record of any structural changes that may be present.

DEATH

We have discussed the various causes of disease and how to circumvent them, but there remains the fact that the end of life is death. This raises a question that has only recently aroused acute interest and concern: What is death, and when is a person dead? At first sight the answer would seem to be simple: when the heart has stopped beating, when the patient no longer breathes, when the brain has ceased to function. But from the biologist's point of view death is a process, not just a moment in time. There is a major difference between the life of a person and life of tissue within that person. After the patient is pronounced dead the cells of the body, those of the skin, the kidneys or the heart, can continue to function if placed in the right environment. The individual dies by degrees, and he may be maintained "alive" by the heart-lung machine and other wonders of modern physics and chemistry. Finally, an organ from another person, alive or very recently dead, may be used to replace one that has failed because of disease. The whole subject of *organ transplantation,* particularly that of the heart, has been brought before the public eye and ear to an embarrassing degree. There are two major questions to be faced: (1) When is a person sufficiently "dead" to justify removal of his heart? (2) To what extent is it justifiable to keep the moribund person "alive" by means of artificial or transposed heart, lungs, or kidneys, even though the brain has ceased to function normally? It was the author of the book of Ecclesiastes who said: "There is a time to be born, and a time to die." Fortunately it is the clinician, not the pathologist, who has to make this difficult decision.

To me it is sad that we regard death with such horror. Only too often it is a welcome relief to the sufferer. After all, it is a natural end. Robert Louis Stevenson, himself a sufferer from tuberculosis, wrote:

> Glad did I live and gladly die,
> And I lay me down with a will.

> This be the verse you grave o'er me:
> Here he lies where he longed to be;
> Home is the sailor, home from the sea,
> And the hunter home from the hill.

We may conclude this chapter on the causes of disease with the thought that when all the natural frailties of our bodies are considered, it seems

> Strange that a harp with so many strings
> Should stay in tune so long.

FURTHER READING

BOYD, W.: A Textbook of Pathology. (Chapter 1 Disease and its Causes), 8th ed., 1970, Philadelphia.

BOYD, W.: Can. Med. Ass. J., 1965, *92*, 868. (Cause and effect.)

BRUNSON, J. G. and GALL, E. A. (Eds.): *Concepts of Disease,* 1971, New York.

BURKITT, D. C.: Lancet, 1970, *2*, 1237. (Relationship as a clue to causation.)

BURNET, SIR F. M.: Lancet, 1968, *1*, 1383. (A modern basis for pathology.)

SPAIN, D. M.: *The Complications of Modern Medical Practices,* 1963, New York.

WILENS, S. L.: *My Friends the Doctors,* 1961, New York.

Chapter *4*

Disturbances of the Blood Flow

Hemorrhage	*Effects*
Thrombosis	Infarction
Fibrinolysis	**Ischemia**
Embolism	*Gangrene*

Through every organ and tissue of the body the life blood flows cease-
lessly night and day. Health is dependent on the maintenance of that
flow which is governed partly by the heart, the pump of the circulation,
and partly by the intact conditions of the blood vessels. Heart disease
will be considered in a later chapter. In this place we shall concern ourselves with three topics: (1) The intactness of the vessel walls and the
possibility of hemorrhage; (2) clotting of blood circulating in the vessels, a process known as thrombosis; (3) narrowing of the lumen of
the vessel with the production of ischemia.

HEMORRHAGE

When a vessel is ruptured blood will naturally escape into the surrounding tissue or onto a free surface. The hemorrhage may be large
and form a tumor-like swelling known as a *hematoma.* Or the hemorrhages may be as small as a pin's head and are then called *petechiae.*
The effect depends on the *size* and the *site* of the hemorrhage. If it
occurs into a muscle it does little damage, but if it takes place into the
brain or onto a free surface such as the interior of the stomach where
it cannot be arrested, it may cause death. *Rupture of a vessel* may be
produced in several ways: (1) The commonest cause is *trauma* in the
shape of a wound or bruise. (2) A *destructive process* in the neighborhood of a large vessel may finally perforate the wall and give rise to
profuse hemorrhage; this may happen in ulcer of the stomach or in a
tuberculous cavity in the lung. (3) The wall of the vessel may be weakened by a degenerative condition such as *atherosclerosis,* and finally
give way under the pressure of the blood; this is what happens in

apoplexy or cerebral hemorrhage. Often this is preceded by a localized bulging of the vessel wall, known as an *aneurysm*.

But the remarkable thing about hemorrhage is not that it should occur, but that it should ever stop. If a hole is made in a pipe through which water is passing, the water will flow out until the pipe is empty. It is true that if we fill the pipe with a glue-like material too thick to pass through a small hole none will escape, but such a material would never be able to flow through the small arteries and the minute capillaries. The problem to be solved in the case of hemorrhage is how a fluid thin enough to pass through the finest channels ceases after a short time to flow through a comparatively large opening in the vessel wall.

The *arrest of hemorrhage* is brought about by the *coagulation* or *clotting of the blood*. As long as the blood is inside the vessel it does not clot, but when it escapes into the surrounding tissue or onto the surface of the skin, it begins at once to coagulate, and soon the clot thus formed is able to plug the hole in the vessel unless that hole be too large. The clotting of blood is due to the interaction of two substances in the plasma called *fibrinogen* and *thrombin*. The thrombin is formed by the interaction of *prothrombin* with *calcium salts*. Prothrombin has recently become a substance of great importance; it appears to be formed from vitamin K, and when a person suffers from vitamin K deficiency his blood prothrombin is low and the blood has lost the power of clotting. What prevents this mechanism from making the blood clot in the vessels of a normal person is the presence of *heparin* (*antithrombin*), which prevents the prothrombin and calcium from uniting to form thrombin. Heparin is present in extremely minute quantities in the blood. It was first obtained from the liver, hence its name (*hepar,* liver), but is also present in large amount in the lung and intestine, from which it can be extracted. When blood is shed the blood platelets disintegrate and liberate *thromboplastin;* this neutralizes the heparin, and when it is eliminated the whole complex machinery of clotting is set in motion.

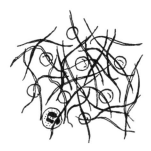

Fig. 14. Network of fibrin containing red blood cells and one leukocyte in its meshes.

The clot is formed of interlacing threads of *fibrin* (Fig. 14), and these threads seal over the opening in the vessel in much the same way as the threads of a spider's web might do. This plug is greatly reinforced by the *blood platelets,* tiny particles that float in the plasma and form a sticky mass which effectually seals up the hole in the vessel wall. In time this emergency plug is converted into fibrous or scar tissue, just as an inflammatory exudate becomes changed into scar tissue, and the opening is closed safely and permanently. In actual fact coagulation is infinitely more complex than what has been outlined above, but nothing would be gained by detailing its minutiae in this *Introduction.*

When a surgeon ties a ligature around a bleeding vessel during the course of an operation, he does not intend it to remain in place permanently. In the course of a few weeks the ligature will be absorbed, but its place will be taken by a firm, permanent clot. In studying inflammation we shall see that healing will not take place properly as long as infection is present. The same is true of the formation of the permanent clot. In an infected wound there is always the danger that the temporary plugs may become weakened by the action of bacteria, and that severe hemorrhage may occur a week or two after the operation. This is called *secondary hemorrha*ge.

Occasionally, though fortunately rarely, it happens that the mechanism for the temporary arrest of hemorrhage is defective, so that the blood continues to flow out. This is most marked in the hereditary disease called *hemophilia,* sufferers from which are known as bleeders and may die of hemorrhage from a trivial wound, cut, or tooth extraction. It appears that the essential defect is a lack in the globulin fraction of the plasma. This is known as the *antihemophilic factor* (AHF). When this is added to hemophilic blood it causes coagulation to occur, and when it is injected into the patient clotting time is reduced. The prothrombin seems not to be utilized properly in the hemophiliac. *Hemophilia is a striking example of sex-linked heredity; only the males of a family suffer from the disease, and only the females transmit it.* Everyone is familiar with the fateful part that hemophilia has played in the misfortunes of the house of the Romanoffs and in the matter of the Spanish succession. Excessive bleeding may also occur to a lesser degree in patients suffering from jaundice and in a number of blood diseases, known as the bleeding diseases.

THROMBOSIS

Clotting of the blood should occur when the blood escapes from the vessel, but not when it is flowing through the lumen of the vessel. Should this occur the process is called *thrombosis* and the clot within the vessel is known as a *thrombus. This consists mainly of platelets, which adhere to the vessel wall on account of their stickiness and gradually form a mass that may finally close the lumen of the vessel and stop the flow of blood through it.* In addition to the platelets a large amount of fibrin may be formed, as is found in an ordinary blood clot. It has been said with truth that throughout his entire existence man is almost constantly hemorrhaging or thrombosing.

The *causes* of thrombosis are threefold, as Virchow stated over a hundred years ago (*Virchow's triad*). They are: (1) *slowing of the blood stream,* (2) *changes in the vessel wall,* and (3) *changes in the blood itself.* Of the three the last is perhaps the most important and the one of which we know the least. As the first of these factors is commoner in veins than in arteries it is natural that thrombosis should usually occur in veins. The normal vessel has an exquisitely smooth lining known as the endothelium. When this is destroyed by injury or inflammation the platelets adhere to the rough spot and gradually build up a thrombus from the blood as it flows past. The slower the flow the more likely are the platelets to fall out of the stream and adhere to the vessel wall, so that thrombosis is associated with varicose (dilated and tortuous) veins and failing heart. A very important form of thrombosis is that which follows abdominal operations, particularly on the pelvic organs. Closely related to this is the thrombosis that may occur in the puerperium, the period following childbirth.

The principal *sites of thrombosis* are the *veins* and the *heart.* Thrombosis may occur in the *arteries,* particularly the coronary arteries, the cerebral arteries, and the arteries to the leg in old persons. In all of these cases there is preliminary narrowing of the lumen by arteriosclerosis. The veins of the leg are frequently affected because of the tendency for postoperative and puerperal thrombosis to involve these veins. Thrombosis of the veins of the leg is also common in chronic heart failure owing to the sluggish circulation, particularly when a patient is confined to bed for some time. A number of cases of thrombosis in the legs followed by fatal pulmonary embolism occurred during World War II in London air raid shelters in elderly persons who sat all night in deck chairs, the wooden supports of which pressed continuously on the thighs. The leg is swollen owing to interference with the return of blood and the thrombosed vein may be felt as a hard tender cord. In the heart a common site of thrombus formation is an inflamed valve, on which the platelets are deposited as the blood flows past, until they form a large thrombus which, in this situation, is known as a *vegetation.* Even more common is thrombus formation in one of the atria, particularly in the part called the atrial appendix, which is a kind of cul-de-sac in which the blood is apt to stagnate.

Thrombosis may be a serious complication in surgical operations, particularly in operations on large blood vessels such as arteries. This can now be prevented by the use of *heparin,* which prevents the platelets from sticking together and to the vessel wall, so that a thrombus is not formed. Heparin has also been used to prevent thrombosis in the veins of the leg after an operation. The substance *Dicoumarol* resembles heparin in prolonging the coagulation time, and it has the advantage that the action is much more prolonged and that it can be taken by mouth instead of being injected intravenously.

The *subsequent history of a thrombus* varies: (1) The thrombus may become converted into fibrous tissue with permanent closure of the vessel. (2) It may contract or become canalized so that blood can flow through the lumen once again (Fig. 15). (3) Finally, the thrombus may become detached from the vessel wall and enter the blood stream as a floating body known as an *embolus,* a catastrophic occurrence, as we shall see in the next section. This detachment of the thrombus is particularly likely to occur when there is sepsis at the site of thrombosis, as the infection causes the thrombus to break down and become loosened. Another factor is rough handling of the part. It is evident that a thrombosed leg has to be treated with the greatest care and anything in the nature of massage must be avoided.

FIBRINOLYSIS. Blood clots are not necessarily permanent structures, and Nature tries to remove an obstructing thrombus by means of a fibrinolytic enzyme in the blood. This enzyme, called *plasmin,* or *fibrinolysin,* is carried in the globulin fraction of the plasma in the form

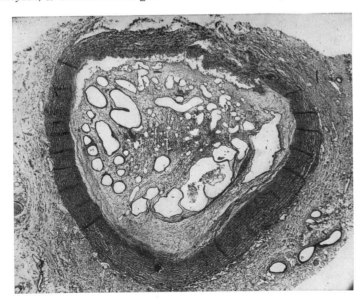

Fig. 15. An arterial thrombus showing canalization. Photomicrograph. (Bell, *Textbook of Pathology,* Lea & Febiger.)

of a precursor, plasminogen, and digests the fibrin of the thrombus. Unfortunately, Nature is often far from successful in its efforts, although it must be admitted that cardiac infarction associated with thrombotic occlusion of the coronary arteries is accompanied by the production of fibrinolysin. In view of the profound damage that a thrombus can do in obstructing such arteries as the coronaries and cerebrals, not to mention the veins, great efforts have been made to find some substance that would dissolve the fibrin of the thrombus. These efforts have been much more successful in the test tube than in the living body, and the work is still in the experimental stage. *Streptokinase,* a bacterial filtrate, activates plasminogen with the formation of fibrinolysin. Use of this substance appears to have a beneficial effect on the clinical condition, although there is little evidence that the clot has been dissolved.

EMBOLISM

An embolus is a thrombus that has become detached and has entered the blood stream. As it is usually a vein that is the site of the thrombus and as the veins become larger as the heart is approached, it follows that the embolus will meet with no obstruction in its voyage to the heart. But no sooner has it passed through the right side of the heart and entered the pulmonary artery that carries the blood to the lungs than the chances of arrest of the embolus increase with every inch the embolus travels, for the arteries become narrower the farther they pass from the heart. Finally, the embolus will lodge in one of the arteries of the lung, the size of the vessel blocked depending entirely on the size of the embolus. Indeed, the main pulmonary artery may be blocked if the embolus is sufficiently large.

An embolus may *originate* from the *heart* instead of in a vein, usually on the left side of the heart. The original thrombus may have been a *vegetation on a valve,* as has already been described, or it may be formed in *one of the chambers of the heart,* usually the left atrium. In either case the destination of the embolus is now quite different, for it *enters the aorta,* the great vessel that leaves the left side of the heart, and passes not to the lungs but to the brain, kidneys, and other organs.

There are other types of emboli besides those that originate as a thrombus. The most important of these are fat emboli, air emboli, and tumor emboli. *Fat embolism* occurs as the result of crushing injuries to bones, which allows the fat in the bone marrow to enter the veins in that substance in the form of globules. *Air embolism* is due to the entrance of air into the veins either during a surgical operation or because of the injection of air into the uterus in an attempt at the production of criminal abortion. *Tumor emboli* are groups of cancer cells that have invaded the vein, become detached, and are then carried to the lungs or other organs. It is by this means that cancer is disseminated throughout the body with the formation of secondary growths known as *metastases.*

EFFECTS OF EMBOLISM.   When an embolus sticks in an artery it blocks the lumen and cuts off the blood supply to the organ or part supplied by that artery. The effect will depend on the size of the embolus and on the circulatory arrangements of the part. It is obvious that if an embolus is large enough to block the main artery to an organ or a limb the effect will be as disastrous as the cutting off of the main water supply to a city. In the case of a smaller embolus the question of the vascular arrangements is all-important (Fig. 16). In most parts of the body there is what is called a *collateral circulation,* a communication between two sets of arteries. The blood to the hand is carried by two main arteries, one on each side of the wrist, and between the branches of these there pass numerous small communicating vessels. Should one of the main arteries be blocked by an embolus or ligatured by the surgeon, the communications from the remaining artery become greatly dilated so that sufficient blood can still reach the area supplied by the blocked vessel. *Under these circumstances an embolus does little or no harm.*

Infarction.   It is a different matter, however, if the main artery to a limb, such as the femoral artery in the thigh, is blocked. Here there can be no efficient collateral circulation, and the tissues are completely deprived of their blood supply and die. A similar state of affairs is met with in a number of organs such as the brain, heart, kidney, and spleen. Here there is no very efficient collateral circulation between the small arteries in the organ, so that if one is blocked no great help need be expected from its neighbors, and the area deprived of blood soon dies. The dead area is pale, sharply demarcated from the surrounding tissue, and is known as an *infarct* (Fig. 17). It is evident that an infarct is the result of a *sudden* cutting off of the blood supply to part of an organ with an insufficient collateral circulation. An *infarct may be produced by thrombosis as well as embolism.* Thus an infarct of cardiac muscle is nearly always caused by thrombosis of one of the coronary arteries; an infarct of the brain may be caused either by thrombosis or embolism of the cerebral arteries. *The most important sites of infarction are the heart, lung, brain, spleen, kidney, and intestine.*

Before leaving the general subject, reference must be made to *pulmonary embolism* and *infarction.* As the blood from the veins passes to the right side of the heart, and as the pulmonary artery to the lungs arises from that side, it is evident that emboli from the veins will lodge in the lungs. The effect on the patient depends entirely on the size of the embolus. If it is small it will not be arrested until it reaches a cor-

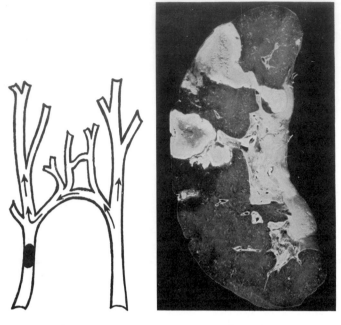

Fig. 16   **Fig. 17**

Fig. 16.   Embolus blocking an artery. In this instance the collateral circulation prevents serious damage to the part supplied.
Fig. 17.   Infarct of spleen. The large white areas are infarcts. (Bell, *Textbook of Pathology,* Lea & Febiger.)

respondingly small arterial branch, and the area of the infarct produced will be equally small. The patient will experience a sharp pain in the chest, and may cough up a little blood during the next few days, after which recovery will be complete. *Tragically different is the course of events when the embolus is large enough to block the main pulmonary artery or one of its principal branches* (Fig. 18). The operation is usually abdominal, and the more serene the events during and following the operation, the more likelihood there is of venous thrombosis and pulmonary embolism. After an uneventful convalescence, suddenly, almost out of a clear sky, there is strange restlessness, rapidly ensuing shock, air hunger, and collapse, and death usually in two to fifteen minutes. The exact explanation of sudden death is not easy. We have suggested that the cause is the shock of the abrupt pulmonary ischemia. But when the surgeon ties off the main pulmonary artery before removing a lung for cancer he does not expect the patient to die. Perhaps a more probable explanation is the release of *serotonin* from the blood platelets at the site of embolism. Serotonin is a vasoconstrictor substance that was obtained from clotted blood as long ago as 1884, is stored in the platelets, is readily released, and stimulates plain muscle, including that of the bronchial tubes. The full tragedy of this accident is evident in those cases in which the embolism occurs about a week after an abdominal operation or after childbirth when the patient is convalescing splendidly, but after sitting up in bed suddenly feels faint, drops back on the pillow panting for breath, and is dead in the course of a few minutes. Often, however, embolism is a complication of medical rather than surgical cases, and it is particularly likely to complicate heart failure.

In all these cases the patient is confined to bed, and the condition (failing heart, childbirth, abdominal operation, immobility) tends to interfere with the flow of blood from the veins of the leg to the heart. It is in these veins that thrombosis occurs, the thrombus becomes dislodged by some sudden movement, and pulmonary embolism is the result. *Nursing precautions* can be of real value in preventing the stagnation of circulation that leads to thrombosis. Voluntary movements of the legs, frequent change of position, and elevation of the foot of the bed all contribute to this end. Circulation is assisted by stimulating the respiration, and this may be done most conveniently by getting the patient to breathe into a rubber bag, the carbon dioxide which he is thus forced to inhale being the most powerful of known respiratory stimulants. In order to counteract the tendency to thrombosis, which is associated with prolonged rest in bed after pelvic operations and childbirth,

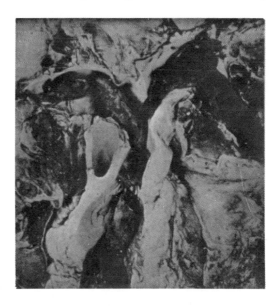

Fig. 18. Pulmonary embolism. A twisted embolus occludes the pulmonary artery and its two main branches. The patient died in the course of a few minutes. (Boyd's *Textbook of Pathology*.)

it is becoming the fashion to make the patient get up, if only for a short time, at a much earlier date.

ISCHEMIA—ITS CAUSES AND EFFECTS

Ischemia is a condition in which the blood supply to a part is diminished or stopped. It is a local rather than a general bloodlessness. As the blood is carried to the part by an artery, it is evident that ischemia will be caused by anything that narrows or closes the lumen of an artery, provided the collateral circulation is not sufficiently abundant to compensate fully for the primary loss of blood supply.

The closure of the artery may be sudden or slow, and the effect varies accordingly. We have already studied the effect of *sudden closure* of an artery, whether by the formation of a thrombus or by the lodgment of an embolus. If the collateral circulation is inadequate the result will be an infarct. *Slow closure* is due to the degenerative disease of arteries known as *arteriosclerosis* or *atherosclerosis,* commonly called hardening of the arteries (Fig. 19). The exact cause of this condition is not known, a matter that is discussed in Chapter 16, but it is a degenerative condition of advancing years, just as is graying of the hair. The blood vessels begin to feel the effect of the sharp tooth of time. Occasionally, however, it may begin before the age of 30, and a person of advanced years may be singularly free from the disease, so that the saying that "a man is as old as his arteries" is profoundly true. The essential change is a nodular thickening of the intima or inner coat of the artery, as a result of which the lumen slowly becomes narrowed, until finally a mere chink may be left through which the blood can only trickle with difficulty. The smooth endothelium lining the vessel in time becomes lost over the atherosclerotic nodules, so that the inner surface is now roughened, and as the platelets tend to stick to the rough surface a thrombus may form which suddenly completes the closure of the already narrowed vessel. This is what happens in *coronary artery thrombosis,* one of the commonest causes of sudden death in persons over 50 years of age. The coronary arteries are the vessels that supply blood to the

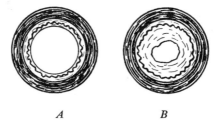

A   *B*

Fig. 19. Atherosclerosis. *A,* Normal artery; *B,* atherosclerotic artery showing great thickening of inner coat (pale part) and narrowing of lumen.

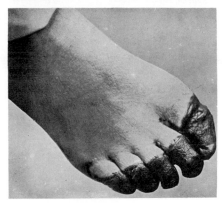

Fig. 20. Gangrene of the toes. (Bell, *Textbook of Pathology*, Lea & Febiger.)

heart muscle, the most essential muscle in the body, and if that supply is suddenly cut off the heart will stop beating.

For some reason not understood at present arteriosclerosis is not a general process affecting all the arteries in the body, but a selective process that picks out an artery here and there. *The three principal sufferers are the heart, kidneys, and brain,* to which must be added the arteries of the leg. Not all of these are attacked in the same person, so that one person may have symptoms pointing to injury to the heart, another to the kidneys, and a third to the brain. Strokes and "little strokes" are usually due to thrombosis, not to hemorrhage as used to be believed. It is probable that a hereditary or inherited weakness plays a part in the selection, for several members of one family may die of coronary thrombosis at about the same age.

The effect of ischemia is gradual death of the specialized cells of the part, *i.e.,* nerve cells in the brain, heart muscle cells, and so on, and their replacement by scar tissue, so that the organ loses the power to do its proper work. In the brain there is failure of memory and of the power of accurate thinking, and there may be actual softening of the part of the brain affected owing to degenerative processes.

Closure of the arteries in the leg and rarely in the arm may lead to death of the parts farthest from the heart, the toes or fingers, as in them the circulation is likely to be most sluggish. Here another change becomes evident, for bacteria invade the dead tissue through the skin and cause decomposition and putrefaction of the dead tissue, a process known as *gangrene* (Fig. 20). The gangrenous part undergoes a series of color changes, becoming first green and finally black. The gangrene tends to spread slowly up the limb as the narrowing of the arteries becomes more extreme and widespread. Diabetes often leads to the occurrence of marked atheroma in the arteries of the leg, so that *diabetic gangrene* is a common complication in elderly patients.

When a patient shows evidence of marked interference with the circulation in the leg, special care is necessary to prevent the onset of gangrene. Any injury, however trivial, may start the process in the devitalized tissues, a process that may eventually require amputation of the affected foot. Special care must be taken in cutting the nails lest the toe be injured. Bandages must not be too tight, and the limb must be kept warm to encourage any circulation that may still remain in the collateral vessels, yet too much heat in the form of an electric foot warmer or a hot-water bottle is a particular source of danger.

FURTHER READING

ASHFORTH, F. P., and FREIMAN, D. C.: Am. J. Path., 1967, *50,* 257. (Role of endothelium in initial phases of thrombosis.)

BIGELOW, W. G.: Can. J. Surg., 1964, *7,* 237. (The microcirculation.)

BIGGS, R., and MACFARLANE, R. G.: *Human Blood Coagulation and its Disorders,* 3rd ed., 1962, Oxford.

DORAN, F. S. A., and WHITE, H. M.: Brit. J. Surg., 1967, *54,* 686. (Prevention of deep-vein thrombosis in legs by stimulating calf muscles.)

HARDISTY, R. M., and INGRAM, G. I. C.: *Bleeding Disorders,* 1965, Oxford.

LINTON, R. R.: Ann. Surg., 1953, *138,* 415. (Results of thrombosis.)

MACFARLANE, R. G.: Nature, 1964, *202,* 498. (Blood clotting.)

SEVITT, S.: Am. J. Med., 1962, *33,* 703. (Venous thrombosis in pulmonary embolism.)

Derangements of Body Fluids

Water Balance
Electrolyte Balance
Acid-Base Balance
  Buffer Systems
  Respiratory Control
  Renal Control
  Acidosis
    Metabolic
    Respiratory

Alkalosis
  Metabolic
  Respiratory
Dehydration
Edema
Shock
Burns

WATER BALANCE

The supreme importance of water has already been discussed in Chapter 1. Water, which comprises about 70 per cent of the weight of the body, is present in the vessels (in the form of plasma), in the interstitial tissue, and in the cells. These may be regarded as three compartments between which a continual exchange of fluid is going on (Fig. 21). Water lost from one compartment can be supplied from another compartment. Thus plasma that is lost may be replaced by fluid from the interstitial compartment. There is 12 times as much water in the cells as in the blood, and 4 times as much in the interstitial tissue. *Water balance* is the remarkably constant balance between the fluid in the vessels and the fluid in the tissues, both cellular and interstitial. It is in the cells themselves that the correct content of water is so important. The balance will be influenced by both the intake and the output of water. Water balance is for the most part regulated by *water loss,* which averages about 2500 cc. a day in the adult, although much more proportionately in children, whose surface area is large in proportion to their weight. The loss takes place by four routes: (1) from the intestine, (2) from the lungs in expired air, (3) from the skin, and (4) from the kidneys. It is the kidneys that are mainly responsible for removing excess fluid in health, although the large amount that may be lost in severe and continued diarrhea or in the profuse sweating of natural or artificial

Relationships between Plasma, Interstitial Fluid, and Intracellular Fluid

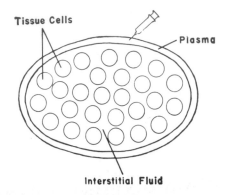

Fig. 21. *Relationships between plasma, interstitial fluid, and intracellular fluid.* The cells are islands in the interstitial sea. Oxygen, electrolytes, and nutrients must traverse the capillary membrane, the interstitial fluid, and the cell membrane to maintain normal cellular activity and composition. (Hardy, *Fluid Therapy;* Lea & Febiger.)

heat is obvious. The renal glomeruli excrete water and sodium chloride, but these are reabsorbed by the renal tubules in the right quantities to maintain the correct balance. The entire mechanism, known as *homeostasis,* is designed to maintain the constancy of the internal environment to which reference has already been made in Chapter 1.

It is this mechanism that serves to maintain the constancy of the acid-base balance, the osmotic pressure, the concentration of the different solutes or of ions, the blood sugar no matter how much glucose is consumed, the body temperature despite changes in the outside temperature, and the blood volume even after severe hemorrhage or copious intravenous fluid infusion. It is on the internal environment that the multiplicity of laboratory tests are now performed to determine the state of health of a person. The relation of water balance to electrolytes is discussed in the next section.

ELECTROLYTE BALANCE

The various substances that are present in solution in the body fluids are not in the form of salts, such as sodium chloride or calcium phosphate, for these salts are *electrolytes,* that is to say those substances which when placed in water become dissociated into electrically charged particles called *ions.* This dissociation was first observed 150 years ago when an electric current was passed through a solution of inorganic compounds with the result that some elements passed to the negative pole and the adjacent fluid became alkaline, while others went to the positive pole and the fluid became acid. Ion is derived from the Greek word meaning to pass or go. The ions may be *positively charged cations,* so-called because they collect at the negative or cathode pole, the more important being sodium (Na^+), potassium (K^+), and calcium (Ca^{++}). The *negatively charged* ions are *anions*, which pass to the positive pole or anode, the chief being chlorine (Cl^-), carbonates, and phosphates. The fact that the positively charged cations pass to the negative pole is merely an illustration of the generally recognized truth that opposites attract one another. Substances are not electrolyte unless they become dissociated into charged particles. All the sodium and potassium of the body is ionized and much of the calcium. The cations include all the metals and hydrogen. The anions include the nonmetals, the acid radicals, and the hydroxyl (OH^-) ion. It is the ions of the electrolytes with their positive and negative charges and their consequent chemical combining power which determine the constancy of the acid-base balance (see below).

Electrolytes exert an important effect on the amount of water in the various compartments (water balance) because of the *osmotic pressure* that they produce. *Osmosis* is the passage of a fluid through a semipermeable membrane to that side that has the higher concentration of molecules. A semipermeable membrane offers no obstacle to the passage of electrolytes, but does not permit the passage of large molecules such as those of protein. The salt content in the cellular compartment is quite different from that of the interstitial and vascular compartments. *Potassium* is the chief constituent in the *cellular compartment; sodium* and *chlorine* are present in the *two extracellular compartments.* A main function of the sodium and chlorine is, by means of their osmotic pressure, to maintain the delicate water balance that is controlled by the kidneys.

The normal figures for the principal electrolytes in the plasma, which vary within fairly narrow limits, are given below, together with round or average figures, which are easier to remember:

Sodium	135–155	mEq./liter	150
Chloride	97–105	" "	100
Potassium	3.6–5.0	" "	4
Bicarbonate	25–32	" "	30

The *equivalent weight* of an electrolyte is the weight in grams that combines with or displaces 1 gram of hydrogen. Because the concentrations of electrolytes in body fluids are so low, we express them as milliequivalents per liter (mEq./L). This is in place of milligrams per 100 cc. as has been used in the past, and which must still be used for nonelectrolytes that cannot be dissociated into ions. The use of milliequivalents facilitates the expression of the total amounts of cations and anions in body fluids. Thus plasma contains about 155 mEq./L of cations and an equal number of anions.

The total amount of electrolytes may determine the amount of body fluid and its osmotic tension. Their relative proportions determine the reaction of that fluid and influence the action of nerve on muscle. The *total* electrolyte concentration is essentially the same in all three phases of body fluid, but the *relative* amounts of the different electrolytes vary widely. *In the extracellular fluid* (plasma and interstitial fluid) the important ions are *sodium, chloride,* and *bicarbonate,* of which sodium is the principal basic ion (cation), and chloride and bicarbonate are the chief acidic ions (anions). *In the intracellular fluid potassium* is the great cation, and *organic phosphate* the corresponding anion.

ACID-BASE BALANCE

In addition to changes in the volume of the fluids in the various compartments, we must consider changes in the ionic equilibrium that affect the reaction of the acid-base balance of the fluid. The *concentration of hydrogen ions* in the body fluids indicates their reaction, and this is expressed as the *negative* logarithm of this concentration. In practice this is abbreviated to pH. Thus 10^{-7} becomes pH 7.0, which is the hydrogen ion concentration of pure water, representing electroneutrality, and is taken as the reference point for expressing the ionic concentration of other solutions. The pH of serum is 7.4, and the normal limits of variation are very narrow, between 7.35 and 7.45. An increased concentration of hydrogen ions, giving a shift of pH toward 7 (on account of the *negative* logarithm), indicates acidosis, while a decreased concentration, giving a higher pH, signifies alkalosis.

It is of extreme importance that the H^+ ion concentration be maintained within normal limits. The *regulation of the acid-base balance* depends on three principal factors: (1) buffer systems; (2) excretion of acid or alkali by the kidneys; (3) excretion of carbon dioxide by the lungs.

BUFFER SYSTEMS. Body fluids contain substances known as buffers, which "soak-up" excess acid or alkali and thus minimize changes in hydrogen ion concentration. They convert strong acids and bases into weaker ones, so that the narrow limits of hydrogen ion concentration are not transgressed. Hydrochloric acid is a "strong" (strongly ionized) acid because in solution it is highly ionized, and as a result nearly all its hydrogen is present in the ionized form, whereas carbonic acid is a "weak" acid, because only a small number of dissociated ions are in solution. The chief buffers of the blood are carbonic acid (H_2CO_3), its bicarbonate salt ($NaHCO_3$), and hemoglobin, which is weakly acid. *Sodium bicarbonate buffers strong acids, whereas carbonic acid buffers strong bases such as sodium hydroxide, converting it into sodium bicarbonate and water,* with only a few OH⁻ ions. Both plasma protein and hemoglobin are buffer systems. Hemoglobin is the buffer for carbonic acid derived from carbon dioxide and changed into carbonate in the red cells as part of the respiratory mechanism.

RESPIRATORY CONTROL OF pH. The respiratory center in the brain is extremely sensitive to changes in the H⁺ concentration of the plasma. The amount of sodium bicarbonate present in the extracellular fluid available for the neutralization of acids stronger than carbonic acid is known as the *alkali reserve.* It is a measure of the degree of disturbance of the acid-base balance. The plasma bicarbonate is expressed as the *carbon dioxide combining power. The simplest measurement for the demonstration of acidosis or alkalosis is the estimation of this combining power,* which is done by a gas analysis test. The quantity of carbon dioxide normally present as bicarbonate is from 55 to 75 volumes per cent. In moderate acidosis the carbon dioxide combining power is less than 40 volumes, in alkalosis it is above 80 volumes. As bicarbonate is continually being formed by tissue metabolism and as carbonic acid is readily eliminated as carbon dioxide it is easy to appreciate the paramount importance of respiration in conjunction with bicarbonate in maintaining the acid-base balance.

RENAL CONTROL. *Although carbonic acid is regulated by the respiratory mechanism, all the other electrolyte components of the plasma structure are under the control of the kidneys.* There is a constant production of acid products such as sulfuric and phosphoric acids from protein metabolism, lactic acid from muscle activity, and ketone acids in high fat diet when the carbohydrates are low. These acids must be eliminated without a loss of base, so that the alkali reserve will not be depleted. Urea is formed from the blood by the cells of the renal tubules; ammonia is formed in turn from the urea; and the ammonia thus formed combines with the acid phosphate and sulfate radicles to be excreated in the urine. Another renal device for conserving fixed base is the ability of the kidney to separate sodium from fixed acid salts in the tubules and return it to the blood, where it combines with bicarbonate, while the acid radical is excreted in the urine in the form of free acid.

ACIDOSIS. We have already seen that the alkali reserve of the blood is represented by bicarbonate. Any change in this reserve is reflected in the plasma carbon dioxide level. The buffer system $\dfrac{H_2CO_3}{NaHCO_3}$ has a normal ratio of 1/20. Four things may happen to upset this ratio. Acid may be increased if the numerator, carbonic acid, is increased, or if the denominator, sodium bicarbonate, is decreased; the reverse is true of alkali. A primary alkali deficit with resulting acidosis is the most important disturbance of the acid-base balance. The mechanism for the change may be metabolic or respiratory.

Metabolic Acidosis. This condition develops whenever the available alkali is diminished. Such a state of affairs may arrive in one of three ways: (1) An *excess of acid ions* may develop as the result of disease that uses up the bicarbonate. This may occur in diabetic acidosis or the ketosis of starvation. (2) An *inadequate excretion of acids* due to renal failure. This is retention acidosis. (3) *Loss of sodium bicarbonate,* as in chronic diarrhea, the secretions of the bowel being quite alkaline. The ratio of carbonic acid to carbonate may fall from a normal of 1/20 to 1/10, with a fall in pH to as low as 7.1.

Respiratory Acidosis. When there is interference with the exchange of gases in the pulmonary alveoli an insufficient amount of carbon dioxide is blown off. The retention of carbon dioxide leads to an increased carbonic acid concentration in the blood and acidosis. The carbonic acid-bicarbonate ratio may be only 1/15. The exchanges of gases may be depressed by advanced chronic pulmonary disease such as fibrosis or emphysema, or by impairment of the respiratory muscles due to diseases such as poliomyelitis.

ALKALOSIS. It is only natural that alkalosis is not nearly so common as acidosis, nor does it have the same clinical significance. Again it may be metabolic or respiratory in character.

Metabolic Alkalosis. Here there is a primary bicarbonate excess. Occasionally this is due to an increased intake of alkalies as in overdone sodium bicarbonate therapy for duodenal ulcer. Much more important is loss of fixed acids, as in the depletion of free hydrochloric acid in the vomiting of duodenal ulcer. When chloride is lost, its place is taken by bicarbonate.

Respiratory Alkalosis. This is the result of a primary carbon dioxide deficit. The usual cause is the deep and rapid breathing that may accompany hysteria or fear. It may also result from the anoxia of heart disease or of high altitudes. The increased ventilation blows off such large volumes of carbon dioxide that the concentration of carbonic acid in the blood falls in relation to the bicarbonate, so that a relative alkalosis results. If the pH is above 7.6, the spasmodic attacks known as *tetany* may occur, owing to increased neuromuscular irritability.

DEHYDRATION

Under normal conditions more water is taken in than is needed, and the excess is excreted in the urine by the kidneys. If the *intake* is *insufficient,* the output due to evaporation from the skin and the lungs and the excretion in urine and feces results in a negative water balance and a state of *dehydration*. The same result will be produced by *excessive loss* of water via the skin, lungs, kidneys, or gastrointestinal tract. A patient suffering from Asiatic cholera may become completely dehydrated in the space of 24 hours. Death occurs when the loss reaches 15 per cent of the body weight. As this percentage is reached twice as quickly in an infant as in an adult, it is evident that the water in the tissues will be exhausted at twice the rate of an adult, and that the infant will die in half the time. *Dehydration is therefore a much more acute problem in infants and young children than in adults.*

From what has been said it is obvious that *fluid balance depends not only on water but also on salt.* If both water and salt are lost, as in vomiting and diarrhea, or even in profuse and continued sweating, as occurs in the tropics or in men working at blast furnaces, salt must be replenished as well as water. One of the hormones of the adrenal cortex, aldosterone, controls the excretion of sodium chloride by the kidneys. If this hormone is insufficient excessive salt is lost in the urine, the salt content of the plasma falls, water is not retained in the tissues, and dehydration results. This is seen in marked degree in Addison's disease, which is due to destruction of the adrenal cortex.

Decrease of body water from whatever cause is naturally first seen in the intravascular compartment with a reduction in blood volume, carrying with it the possibility of shock. The regulating mechanism at once comes into play, withdrawing fluid from the interstitial compartment, and finally the intracellular fluid. *This is significant, for cellular dehydration creates thirst that may become so intense as to be unendurable,* and *it interferes with cellular enzymes to a degree that may be fatal.*

Disturbance in the water (and salt) balance may occur in a number of diseases, some of which will be discussed in this book. Examples are *shock, acute intestinal obstruction, renal failure,* and *Addison's disease.*

EDEMA

Edema is an abnormal collection of fluid in the tissue spaces. This accumulation may be local or general. The fluid can be moved from one place to another, so that when the edematous part is pressed on, a pit is left; this is known clinically as *"pitting on pressure."* The accumulation of fluid is most marked and most readily recognized in the subcutaneous tissue of the skin. An edematous tissue has a pale watery appearance. Subcutaneous tissue may come to resemble jelly. In the lung, where edema of the alveolar spaces is very common, the affected part may feel solid, but fluid pours from the cut surface.

CAUSES OF EDEMA. There are three main causes of general edema. The *first* of these is *increased permeability of the capillary wall.* All edema fluid comes from the blood and passes into the tissues. It is evident that if the permeability of the smallest blood vessels is increased, fluid passes from the blood into the tissues. It must be remembered that this passage of fluid through the wall of the small vessels is a normal one, for it is the process by which nourishment is carried to a part and reaches the individual tissues. *The most important cause of increased permeability of capillaries is inflammation.* This is the explanation for the large amount of edema fluid that collects during the inflammatory process, and is mainly responsible for the swelling of inflammation. The *second* cause is a *decrease of the osmotic pressure of the plasma proteins.* These proteins exert an osmotic influence on the fluid in the blood which holds it in the vessels and prevents it from escaping. It is evident that in the event of a reduction in the amount of proteins there will be a corresponding loss of this "pool," which normally keeps the fluid from escaping. If proteins such as albumin are lost in the urine as a result of disease of the kidneys, a development of edema may be expected. The *third* cause is an *increase in the pressure in the small veins and capillaries.* This has nothing to do with high blood pressure, but is the result of chronic heart failure in which the blood is prevented from reaching the heart rapidly and accumulates in the veins. As a result, the fluid tends to pass from the inside of the vessel to the tissues outside.

From what has been said it will be apparent that there are three principal types of edema encountered by the physician. These are (1) inflammatory edema, (2) renal edema, and (3) cardiac edema. *Inflammatory edema* is localized. *Renal edema* is general, but appears first in the face and the lower eyelids, giving a puffy appearance. *Cardiac edema* is also general, but usually makes its first appearance in the dependent parts of the body, particularly the ankles and feet. The *fourth* cause of edema, local rather than general, is *lymphatic obstruction.* If the lymphatics are obstructed by inflammation or by the pressure of a tumor, the lymph within the lumen passes outward and accumulates in the tissues. A striking example of lymphatic edema is sometimes seen after extensive operations for the removal of cancer of the breast or radiation to the part for the treatment of that disease. The subsequent swelling of the arm is not due to a recurrence of the cancer, but to an accumulation of lymph fluid that is unable to escape from the tissues.

The subject of edema is very involved and the accumulation of tissue fluid is dependent on many complex disturbances of chemical processes. A detailed account of the subject would be out of place here.

SHOCK

In a state of health not all the capillaries of an organ are open at the same time, for some parts of the organ are working and some are resting. If all the capillaries and venules in the body were filled with blood at the same time, the entire supply would be contained in these vessels, the heart would have insufficient blood on which to contract, the stimulus to work would be lost, and the heart would fail. This is essentially the state of shock, in which there is an enormous dilatation of the capillary bed in which the blood collects, and the effect on the heart is disastrous.

Shock may be produced in a variety of ways. *Very severe injury* or *prolonged surgical operations* may cause so severe a nervous disturbance that the capillaries are allowed to dilate to a dangerous degree. The blood disappears into the vast capillary bed as if sucked up by a sponge, so that the patient may be said to bleed into his own capillaries. *Great loss of fluid* from the body, either loss of blood itself, as in severe hemorrhage, or loss of fluid from the stomach, as in continuous vomiting, or from the bowel, as in continuous diarrhea, may deplete the blood volume so much that the heart has not sufficient to work upon, even though the capillaries are not unduly dilated. Many other pathological conditions may lead to shock.

The *appearance of a person in shock* is characteristic. He lies quite still, his face is pale and gray, drawn and anxious, and the skin is cold and clammy. The temperature is subnormal, the pulse feeble, the respirations shallow and sighing, and the blood pressure alarmingly low. Shock is usually a temporary condition, a step toward death which the patient can retrace, but sometimes the step is final and return impossible.

It is obvious that the most important point in the *treatment* of shock is to refill the empty vessels and give the heart fluid to work on. Saline solution is of no value, because it pours through the permeable walls of the vessels into the interstitial tissue as fast as it is administered. Blood plasma when given intravenously remains in the vessels, because its large protein molecules cannot pass through the walls of the capillaries, and the protein in turn holds back the fluid by virtue of the osmotic pressure that it exerts. Still more valuable is whole blood.

BURNS

Burns are coming to assume an ever-increasing importance by reason of the industrial age in which we live with its great furnaces, domestic heating with highly inflammable agents, automobile and airplane accidents, and last but not least, atomic and hydrogen bombs. Over 80 per cent of the casualties at Nagasaki and Hiroshima suffered from burns. Burns present two very different features: (1) the *local lesions,* which have already been mentioned (p. 53), and (2) the *physiological disturbances,* which are essentially those of shock and may result in a fatal outcome. In the burned area *capillary permeability* is greatly increased, and through the injured walls plasma rich in protein pours in large amount and continually. It is the extent of the burned area rather than its depth which determines the amount of loss of this vital fluid. The local outpouring of fluid results in a remarkable concentration of the blood as shown by hemoglobin estimation, and this leads in turn to circulatory failure and oxygen starvation of the tissues, a condition that has been called *burn shock.*

It is evident that this chapter has been concerned with *disturbances of the internal environment,* on the integrity of which health and life itself depend. We have examined the incredibly intricate and ingenious mechanisms by which that integrity is maintained, and we have watched what happens when the mechanisms break down. In this brief discussion of the physiology and pathology of the internal environment no reference has been made to methods by which its disturbances can be corrected. As I am ignorant regarding the details of this all-important subject, I shall remain silent. The real authorities, however, say that it is probable that the proper use of water and salt has saved the lives of more persons seriously ill than any other therapeutic measure. These two substances can be so used that they achieve seeming miracles, but they can be so misused as to lead to a fatal issue. What is powerful for good, is potent for evil.

FURTHER READING

CANNON, W. B.: *The Wisdom of the Body,* 1932, New York.

GAMBLE, J. L.: *Chemical Anatomy, Physiology and Pathology of Extracellular Fluid.* (The bible of the subject.) 1954, Cambridge, Mass.

GOLDBERGER, E.: *A Primer of Water, Electrolyte, and Acid-Base Syndromes,* 4th ed., 1970, Philadelphia.

MOORE, F. D., et al.: *The Body Cell Mass and its Supporting Environment,* 1963, Philadelphia.

MOYER, C. A.: *Fluid Balance,* 1952, Chicago.

ROBINSON, J. R.: *Fundamentals of Acid-Base Regulation,* 1962, Oxford.

STATLAND, H.: *Fluid and Electrolytes in Practice,* 3rd ed., 1963, Philadelphia.

Inflammation and Repair

INFLAMMATION

Of all the forms of disease that the doctor is called upon to treat, inflammation is the commonest, the most important, and the most amenable to treatment. Every disease whose name ends in *itis* is a form of inflammation, so that appendicitis is inflammation of the appendix, tonsillitis is inflammation of the tonsil, and so on. Some important examples of inflammation, such as pneumonia and pleurisy, were given their names long ago, so that they do not follow the usual rule regarding nomenclature.

Inflammation is the *local reaction of living tissue to injury*. It is important to realize that although inflammation may be unpleasant and painful to the patient it is a defense reaction, a beneficial one, for without inflammation life would be impossible. It is true that the ancients gave the condition its name to indicate a flaming or burning, but in the course of evolution only those animals survived who were capable of this response.

CAUSES. The cause of the local reaction is said to be an *irritant,* a conveniently vague term which merely means something that excites inflammation—whether physical or mental.

Inflammation is the *local reaction of the body to an irritant.* Now there are many kinds of irritants, but they can all be placed in one or other of three great classes, *physical, chemical,* and *bacterial.* The simplest example of a *physical irritant* is a *foreign body,* that is to say some solid substance introduced into the tissues from outside, like a

95

splinter in the finger. The foreign body injures and irritates the tissues, and the attempt that the body makes to remove the irritant is the process of inflammation. Sometimes the attempt is crowned with success, sometimes it is a miserable failure, and occasionally a truce is established between the invader and the defense forces of the body. *For inflammation is like life: it is a continuous struggle between two opposite forces, the one friendly, the other hostile. Trauma* or injury may cause inflammation even though no bacteria are present, as every footballer knows who has wrenched his knee. When tissue is traumatized a substance known as *histamine* is liberated, and this causes the local changes of inflammation. Other physical irritants that may produce intense inflammation are great *heat* (burns) and *cold* (frostbite), *light* (sunburn), *roentgen rays,* and *radium*. It is true that here there is no question of expelling the irritant, but the changes in the tissues are similar to those produced by a foreign body. Examples of *chemical irritants* are strong acids and alkalis, and poisons of every description.

The *bacterial irritants* are by far the most important, because bacteria are universally present, and are continually gaining access to the tissues. They are destroyed by the process of inflammation, but the fight is usually so short and so localized that the patient is not aware of its existence; it is only when it becomes more severe that symptoms develop that demand medical attention. The great majority of acute infections are caused by staphylococci (which are always present in the skin) and streptococci (which are similarly present in the throat), but pneumococci cause the inflammation of pneumonia, meningococci the inflammation of meningitis, and so on. Of less importance as a cause of inflammation are the animal parasites.

SYMPTOMS.   The symptoms of inflammation have been known since the beginning of medical history; they are *heat, redness, swelling,* and *pain.* The infected finger or the finger containing a sliver is hot, red, swollen, and painful. If the injury is mild, the symptoms are correspondingly mild. Some *loss of function* is common. The meaning of these symptoms has only become apparent in recent times, and in order to understand them we must ask what we mean by saying that inflammation is the local reaction to an irritant, or an attempt to remove the irritant from the body.

The main defense of the body against bacteria, which we shall take as the standard type of irritant, is contained in the leukocytes of the blood. These blood cells have the power of engulfing the bacteria and finally digesting them, an operation known as *phagocytosis* (*phago,* to eat; *cytos,* cell). Bacteria damage the tissues not merely by their physical presence in enormous numbers, but by the poisons or toxins that they produce. Antagonizing substances called *antitoxins* are produced in the blood which neutralize the bacterial toxins. It is evident, then, that the most important defense forces against bacterial infection lie in the blood. But unfortunately the invaders against which these forces are to operate are not in the blood stream but in the tissues outside the blood vessels. Something has to be done to bring the defenders out to meet the invaders, and it is this something that is largely responsible for the heat, redness, swelling, and pain which constitute the clinical picture of inflammation.

There are two great phases of the inflammatory process: (1) *the vascular or blood vessel changes,* and (2) *the formation of the inflammatory exudate.* It will be evident in what follows that these two cannot be sharply separated from one another, but it is of help to keep them in mind.

VASCULAR CHANGES. In the inflamed finger or appendix we can only guess what is going on, although microscopic examination of the tissue will show us the state of affairs at the particular moment the tissue is removed. But the whole process can be watched under the microscope in the living animal if we use a transparent tissue such as the web of a frog's foot. When an irritant such as a drop of weak acid is applied to the frog's foot, the small blood vessels and capillaries are seen to dilate, so that very much more blood comes to the part, bringing with it great numbers of leukocytes. An increased blood supply means that the part becomes red and hot, and this is the basis for the heat and redness of the inflamed finger. If we continue to look down the microscope it will be seen that the blood flow becomes slower in the dilated vessels, and that the leukocytes collect along the walls of the vessels to which they become adherent. The vessel wall becomes looser in texture, and through this loosened wall the leukocytes, which are of

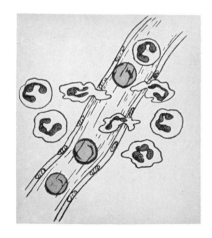

Fig. 22. Leukocytes passing through vessel wall and collecting outside. No emigration of red cells. (Best and Taylor, *The Human Body;* Henry Holt & Co.)

jelly-like consistency, can be seen to make their way, much as a soap bubble might pass through a closed door by flowing through the keyhole (Fig. 22). In this way great numbers of leukocytes accumulate in the tissues immediately outside the vessels where they have the desired opportunity of attacking the bacterial irritant (Fig. 23).

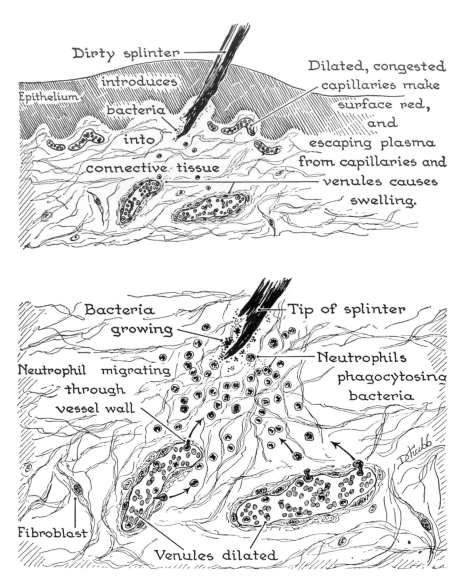

Fig. 23. Diagrams to show how neutrophils migrate from congested, dilated small blood vessels to combat bacteria introduced into tissues by means of an injury. (Ham, *Histology;* courtesy of J. B. Lippincott Co.)

Still further assisting the local accumulation of leukocytes is the fact that the bone marrow, which is the storehouse and factory of the leukocytes, pours out vast numbers into the blood, so that the total number of leukocytes is greatly increased. This increase is known as *leukocytosis,* and is an indication that inflammation is going on in some part of the body. A blood examination (*leukocyte count*) is therefore an invaluable test for determining whether a pain in the right side of the abdomen is due to appendicitis or a pain in the chest is due to pneumonia. The normal leukocyte count is about 6000 (6000 leukocytes in each cubic millimeter of blood), but in severe inflammation the count may be 30,000 or even higher.

INFLAMMATORY EXUDATE.   Let us now consider more in detail the elements of the blood that pass through the vessel walls whose permeability has become so greatly increased (Fig. 24). The white cells of the blood are of various kinds, but the two important ones in acute inflammation are the polymorphonuclear leukocytes and monocytes. The *polymorphonuclears* are the first to collect outside the vessels; they are the first line of defense. Later they are followed by the *monocytes,* which perform a very different function. Finally there is the fluid part of the blood, the *plasma.* This also passes through the permeable vessel walls and collects in the tissues around the irritant. The plasma that passes

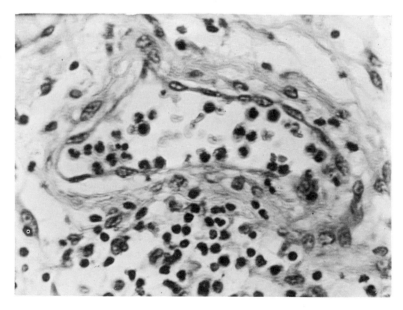

Fig. 24. Acute inflammation. The exudate is formed by the inflammatory cells passing through the vessel wall. × 500.

out is changed in character and is called *serum* or inflammatory lymph. The various leukocytes and the serum together form what is known as the *inflammatory exudate*. It is this exudate that is responsible for the swelling that is such a striking clinical feature of inflammation. The swelling causes tension and pressure on the nerves of the part, and this is the cause of the pain, the fourth and most important of the symptoms. It is obvious that the more dense the tissue, the more severe is the pain, so that the pain is worse in inflammation of bone (mastoid disease, toothache) than in inflammation of a loose structure such as the skin. The throbbing of an inflamed finger is caused by the increase of pressure in the dense tissues each time the heartbeat forces more blood into the part.

Now that the defense forces have passed from the inside of the vessels to the outside it is time to ask what part the various elements of the inflammatory exudate play in disposing of the irritant, which we shall presume to be invading bacteria. The first line of defense, the polymorphonuclear leukocytes, approach the bacteria, and when they meet them they throw out arms of protoplasm (the jelly of which they are composed), arms that surround the germ with a deadly embrace, and draw it into the interior of the leukocyte, where it is slowly digested (Fig. 25). The process is known as *phagocytosis* or swallowing by a cell, just as the esophagus is the structure that swallows food. Inflammation is essentially a fight between the defenders and invaders of the body, and the result depends largely on the shock troops, the polymorphonuclears. But the fight is not entirely one-sided. The bacteria discharge their poisonous toxins, which kill great numbers not only of the polymorphonuclears but also of the tissue cells. The battlefield therefore becomes strewn with the dead bodies of cells. At this stage, if the defense forces are in the ascendant, the *monocytes* begin to arrive. They also are actively phagocytic and on that account, and also because of their large size, they are called *macrophages* (*macro,* large; *phago,* devour). *These macrophages are the scavengers of the body, for they remove the debris of the battle by the simple process of engulfing the*

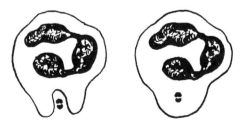

Fig. 25. Phagocytosis by polymorphonuclear leukocyte.

dead cells. In more chronic inflammations, such as tuberculosis, they also devour the bacteria.

In addition to the polymorphonuclears and the macrophages, other cells may play an important part in the inflammatory process. The chief of these are the lymphocyte, the plasma cell, and the eosinophil. The *lymphocyte* is a small round cell which is present in enormous numbers in the lymphoid tissue and lymph nodes of the body. It may put in an appearance in the acute stage of inflammation, but is more characteristic of the later stages. For many years its function was completely unknown, but *it is now known to be an important source of the immune bodies that are so essential for the neutralization of bacterial toxins and for damaging the bacteria themselves.* The *plasma cell* is probably derived from the lymphocyte. It is somewhat larger, and is characterized by the fact that its nucleus is at one side of the cell rather than in the center. It also is concerned perhaps to an even more important degree with the production of immune bodies. The *eosinophil* is similar to the polymorphonuclear leukocyte, but contains granules that stain intensely with the red stain eosin. Its function is not certain, but it appears in large numbers in those types of inflammation in which allergy plays a part. It is of interest to note that the eosinophils of the blood disappear almost entirely when cortisone is administered.

HUMORAL DEFENSE. So far the conflict has been prehistoric in type, a hand-to-hand encounter. But more subtle methods are also employed by both sides, suggestive rather of modern warfare. Reference has already been made to the toxins of the bacteria. Against these the phagocytes are of no avail, but the value of the serum in the inflammatory exudate now becomes apparent. The serum contains antibacterial and antitoxic substances, which increase steadily in amount as the infection progresses, and which are, of course, present not only in the circulating blood but also in the serum that pours through the vessel walls into the inflammatory exudate. The *antitoxins* neutralize and destroy the toxins of the bacteria, and the *antibacterial substances* paralyze the bacteria so that they readily fall prey to the phagocytic leukocytes. To prepare an antitoxin, small doses of toxin are injected into an animal repeatedly until the animal becomes immunized. When the serum of such an immunized animal is injected into a patient suffering from a bacterial infection, the antitoxin it contains destroys not only any toxins that may be in the patient's blood, but also those that are being produced in the tissues. One of the best examples of this method of treatment is afforded by diphtheria antitoxin.

FIBRIN FORMATION. When the serum is poured out on the surface of a serous membrane such as the pleura or peritoneum, it tends to clot with the formation of *fibrin*. This takes the form of fine interlacing

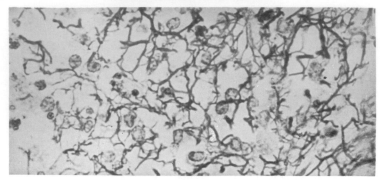

Fig. 26. Exudate consisting mainly of fibrin. × 600. (Boyd, *Textbook of Pathology;* Lea & Febiger.)

threads (Fig. 26), and a surface covered with fibrin becomes sticky so that it tends to adhere to a neighboring surface. In this way *adhesions* are formed between adjacent coils of bowel, between the pleura covering the lung and that lining the chest wall, and between other surfaces. These adhesions usually disappear when the inflammation subsides, but sometimes they persist and may cause serious subsequent trouble in the abdominal cavity. By and large, however, fibrin formation must be included in the defense mechanisms, for it has a distinctly limiting effect on the spread of infection throughout and beyond the inflamed area.

VARIETIES OF INFLAMMATION. Inflammation has been divided into a number of varieties, although the essence of the process is always the same. The principal types are acute inflammation, chronic inflammation, and granulomatous inflammation. In *acute inflammation* the process is of rapid onset and of comparatively short duration. The characteristic cell is the polymorphonuclear leukocyte. *Chronic inflammation* is a more long-drawn-out process, and is sometimes described as a low grade type of inflammation. The characteristic cells are the lymphocyte and plasma cell. *Granulomatous inflammation* is really a subvariety of chronic inflammation. *Whereas acute inflammation is characterized by the formation of an exudate from the blood vessels into the tissues, granulomatous inflammation is characterized by a proliferation of cells at the site of inflammation.* It is spoken of as proliferative or productive in type. The result is that a mass of new tissue is formed which is called a *granuloma*, because of a somewhat fancied resemblance to the microscopic picture of granulation tissue, which will be described in connection with the healing of inflammatory lesions. The best known examples of infective granulomas, as they are called, are tuberculosis and syphilis. Diseases caused by fungi, which are becoming more and more common and important, are granulomatous in character. The bacteria have been displaced to such an extent by antibiotic therapy that they have made room for the fungi to enter.

LOCALIZATION OF INFECTION. Once infection has occurred, its localization depends on a number of factors, many of which have already been considered. When the organisms have entered the body, as through a wound in the skin, they may be held more or less *in situ* or they may drift through the ground substance with amazing rapidity. It is evident that the consequences to the patient are entirely different in the two cases. *The inflammatory reaction tends to prevent the dissemination of infection.* Speaking generally, the more intense the reaction, the more likely is the infection to be localized. The main battleground is the ground substance of the connective tissue which separates the cells and fibers. It consists mainly of hyaluronic acid, a markedly viscid substance which constitutes a barrier to the spread of infection. The microorganisms of highly invasive infections, such as erysipelas or gas gangrene, produce an enzyme, *hyaluronidase*, which breaks down this barrier.

RESULTS OF INFLAMMATION. The outcome of the conflict depends on two factors, the virulence or destructive power of the bacteria and the resistance of the patient. In most cases the former is weak and the latter is strong. When a needle infected with germs is run into the finger of a healthy person a mild degree of inflammation ensues, but there is every chance that the defenders will overpower the invaders before the latter have time to multiply, and the resulting heat, redness, swelling, and pain may be so trivial as hardly to attract the notice of the patient. Sometimes, however, the bacteria are of such overpowering virulence, as in the case of a pathologist who receives a prick in the finger when performing an autopsy on a patient who has died of streptococcal septicemia, that they paralyze the leukocytes with their toxins, invade the blood stream, set up *septicemia* (blood poisoning), and spread throughout the body with fatal results. This was particularly likely to happen with streptococcal infections before the advent of antibiotics.

More frequently the infection is kept within bounds or localized, although there may be extensive damage to the tissues. *Infections caused by staphylococci generally remain localized.* A digestive ferment is liberated from the bodies of the dead polymorphonuclear leukocytes, and this ferment digests and liquefies the tissue cells that have been killed by the bacterial toxins. *Pus* or matter is a thick yellow fluid consisting of liquefied tissue and the fluid of the inflammatory exudate, and containing polymorphonuclear leukocytes, known here as pus cells, and living and dead bacteria. Inflammation accompanied by the formation of pus is called *suppuration*, and the bacteria responsible are known as *pyo-*

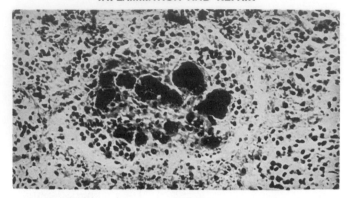

Fig. 27.   Abscess of kidney showing dark masses of bacteria and destruction of tissue. × 275. (Boyd, *Textbook of Pathology;* Lea & Febiger.)

genic or pus-producing (*pyon,* pus). A cavity is produced in the tissues as the result of the destruction, and this cavity is called an *abscess,* and is filled with pus (Fig. 27). The cavity is surrounded by a wide barrier of leukocytes, which prevent the infecting bacteria from spreading further into the tissues. If the abscess extends and reaches the surface it is said to *point;* finally it bursts, and pus is discharged on the surface. This may be regarded as a method that the body has of ridding itself of infection and the bursting of the abscess is likely to be followed by healing. When suppuration spreads diffusely through the tissues, usually owing to streptococcal infection, the condition is known as *cellulitis,* only too common before the advent of antibiotics.

If the abscess is some distance from the surface, the track leading from the abscess to the surface is called a *sinus* (Fig. 28). A sinus may remain open for a considerable time. If the abscess should discharge onto both skin and a mucous surface the track is known as a *fistula* (Fig. 28). Thus if an abscess of the appendix should open onto the skin,

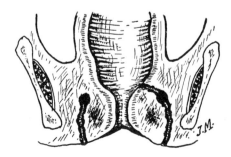

Fig. 28.   Sinus (left) opening on to skin. Fistula (right) connecting rectum and skin surface.

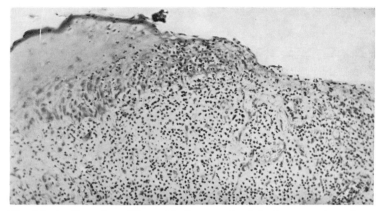

Fig 29. Nonhealing ulcer. The epithelium on the left shows no sign of growing over the inflamed floor of the ulcer. × 125. (Boyd's *Textbook of Pathology*.)

a fistula is formed between the skin surface and the interior of the bowel. An *ulcer* is a superficial lesion caused by destruction of the skin (Fig. 29) or of a mucous membrane (*e.g.*, ulcer of the stomach). The cause of the destruction may be a focus of inflammation a short distance below the surface leading to disintegration of the overlying skin or mucous membrane. Or it may be in the nature of a shallow wound, which subsequently becomes infected. A *boil* is an abscess of the root of a hair and is caused by bacteria that have penetrated from the skin, often owing to friction, so that it is commonest on the buttocks and the back of the neck. The root of the hair is a dense fibrous structure, so that an inflammatory swelling within it causes much tension and pain until softening occurs and the hard "core" of the boil is liquefied and extruded. Spontaneous softening may fail to occur owing to lack of the liquefying ferments of the polymorphonuclears, *but the local application of heat will cause an outpouring of leukocytes and greatly hasten the process.* A *carbuncle* is a group of boils connected by underground channels. It is a much more serious lesion, with extensive destruction of tissue and great absorption of septic material.

HEALING OR REPAIR

In the living body destruction of tissue is followed by healing or repair. The process is the same whether destruction has been due to inflammation or to a wound, surgical or otherwise. The first requisite for healing is complete destruction of bacteria. *Neither an inflammatory lesion nor a wound can heal if it is infected.* The next step is removal of dead fragments of tissue by macrophages. When this has been done, healing can commence. In the case of a surgical incision, the edges

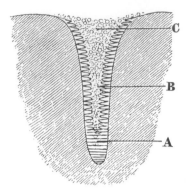

Fig. 30. A healing wound. *A,* Wound closed by connective tissue cells; *B,* gap filled by exudate; *C,* discharging surface of wound. (Bowlby and Andrewes', *Surgical Pathology;* J. & A. Churchill, Ltd.)

of which can be brought together, the *fibroblasts* or connective tissue cells in the sides of the wound proliferate and bridge across the narrow gap (Fig. 30). At the same time they form fibers of connective tissue which sew together the edges of the wound much more securely than can the surgeon; the sewing is completed in about five days. The thin connective tissue fibers are then converted into strong, dense *scar tissue,* a process that takes about three weeks.

When the edges of a wound cannot be united or when healing of an abscess takes place, young vascular connective tissue fills up the cavity from below. This gives the surface of the wound or cavity a granular appearance, so that it is known as a granulating surface and the new connective tissue is called *granulation tissue.* The granulating surface is slowly covered by epithelium, which grows inward from the edges. At first this is a very thin blue layer, like ice forming on a pond in the fall of the year, but after a few weeks it becomes thick and white. At the same time the underlying granulation tissue is becoming converted into dense *scar* tissue (Fig. 31). This has an unfortunate tendency to contract as it gets older, and marked deformities may result in this way. The adhesions of fibrin to which reference has already been made also become converted into scar tissue, and if these adhesions are between loops of bowel, the subsequent contraction may lead to kinking of the bowel and serious intestinal obstruction.

It will be noted that although the word repair has been used, the repair is but a makeshift. The human machine has no replacement parts. If the greater part of a kidney is destroyed by inflammation, it is not replaced by new kidney tissue but only by scar tissue. This is useful for plugging a hole, but it has no other use. With advancing years many tissues wear out, but they can only be replaced by scar tissue, a poor substitute. Any house runs down in the wear and tear of seventy years' continuous occupancy by the same tenant. Unfortunately with the

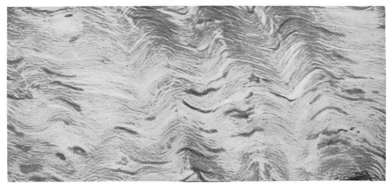

Fig. 31. Scar tissue. Bundles of collagen fibers, between which are flattened fibroblasts. × 400. (Boyd, *Textbook of Pathology;* Lea & Febiger.)

human body, as with the automobile, the older the model is the more repairs are required, and the harder it is to make them.

The process of *healing* is a complex one. Suffice it to say here that newly formed connective tissue grows inward from the walls and fills up the abscess cavity, and this is followed by an ingrowth of the skin epithelium, which covers the new connective tissue. The process is exactly the same as the *healing of a wound* (Fig. 31).

In this discussion of inflammation we have taken for convenience the example of a finger infected with staphylococci or streptococci. But it will be realized that inflammation may occur in any organ and that it may be caused by many different agents. Pyogenic bacteria cause acute inflammation with suppuration and the production of pus. Other bacteria produce a slow or chronic form of inflammation without the formation of pus. Tuberculosis, syphilis, and other important diseases are examples of chronic inflammation, but in these cases the defense forces are the cells of the tissues rather than those of the blood. Here again healing takes place by the formation of scar tissue, so that a former tuberculous lesion in the lung or the glands of the neck can be recognized by the scar that it leaves.

PRINCIPLES OF TREATMENT. In the treatment of any infectious disease the doctor may adopt one or both of two methods; he may assist the healing powers of Nature, what the old writers used to call *vis medicatrix naturae,* or he may directly attack the infecting bacteria. *Rest* of the inflamed part is the most important of all therapeutic measures. Exercise not only acts as an additional irritant, but serves to disperse the bacteria through the tissues and thus increase the area of inflammation. It tends to break down the barrier that the leukocytes try to build up around the bacteria. Thus the inflamed finger is splinted, the inflamed arm is placed in a sling, the inflamed eye is shaded so that it cannot be used, and purgatives are avoided as if they were poison in the treatment of the inflamed appendix.

The second principle is *free drainage*. The quickest way to get an abscess to heal is open it and let out the pus. This not only allows the infecting bacteria to escape, but also relieves the tension in the inflamed area, and thus encourages the further flow of healing substances from the blood vessels in addition to relieving the pain. But if pus has not yet formed and a barrier of leukocytes has been built around the bacteria, the knife may do more harm than good, for it may open fresh channels for spread of the infection.

Heat in the form of fomentations, poultices, and so on is one of the oldest and most efficient methods of treating inflammation. The warmth sends messages up the sensory nerves of the part to the spinal cord; these pass down the nerves to the blood vessels and cause the latter to dilate, so that additional blood is brought to the part, thus adding to the supply of leukocytes and antitoxins. *Cold* in the form of an ice-bag or cold compresses will relieve the pain by causing the vessels to contract and thus diminish the swelling of the tissues, which is responsible for the pain, but it will not increase the local resistance.

The *direct attack* on the invading bacteria, first by the sulfa drugs and later by the antibiotics, has come to occupy so dominant a place in the treatment of inflammation due to infection that we are apt to lose sight of the healing powers that used to be our only hope, powers that proved to be sufficient in the great majority of cases. It is well to remember, however, that the wonder drugs do not actually kill the bacteria, but rather inhibit their growth, so that the *vis medicatrix naturae* still remains man's best friend.

FURTHER READING

Inflammation

ARCHER, R. K.: *The Endothelial Leucocytes,* 1963, Oxford.

CAMERON, R., and SPECTOR, W. G.: *Chemistry of the Injured Cell,* 1961, Springfield, Ill.

DIBLE, J. H.: Ann. Roy. Coll. Surg. England, 1950, *6,* 120. (Inflammation and repair.)

DUBOS, R. J.: Lancet, 1958, *2,* 1. (The microenvironment of inflammation.)

EHRICH, W. E., DRABKIN, D. L., and FORMAN, C.: J. Exper. Med., 1949, *20,* 157. (Plasma cells and antibody formation.)

FLOREY, H. W., and GRANT, L. H.: J. Path. and Bact., 1961, *82,* 13. (Leukocytic emigration in inflammation.)

MOVAT, H. Z., and FERNANDO, N. V. P.: Am. J. Path., 1963, *42,* 41. (Allergic inflammation.)

MOVAT, H. Z. (Edit.): *Inflammation, Immunity and Hypersensitivity,* Chapter 1, The Acute Inflammatory Reaction, New York, 1971.

PAGE, A. B., and GOOD, R. A.: Am. J. Path., 1958, *34,* 645. (The neutrophils in the inflammatory response.)

REBUCK, J. W., and MELLINGER, R. C.: Am. J. Path., 1953, *29,* 599. (Cortisone and inflammation.)

SPENCER, W. G., and LYKKE, A. W. J.: Path. and Bact., 1966, *92,* 163. (The cellular evolution of inflammatory granulomata.)

ZWEIFACH, B. W., GRANT, L., and McCLUSKEY, R. T. (Eds.): *The Inflammatory Process,* Academic Press, New York and London, 1965.

Repair

DUNPHY, J. E.: New Eng. J. Med., 1963, *268,* 1367. (The fibroblast—a ubiquitous ally for the surgeon.)

DUNPHY, J. E., and UDUPA, K. N.: New Eng. J. Med., 1955, *253,* 847. (Wound healing.)

HARTWELL, S. W.: *The Mechanisms of Healing in Human Wounds,* 1955, Springfield, Ill.

Chapter 7

Immunity and Hypersensitivity

Immunity
  Natural Immunity
    Species Immunity
  Passive Immunity
  Acquired Immunity
  Antibodies
  Thymus
Hypersensitivity
  Acquired
  Immediate
    Anaphylactic shock
    Serum sickness

Delayed
  Tuberculin reaction
Natural: Allergy
  Hay Fever
  Bronchial Asthma
  Food Allergy
  Drug Allergy
  Plant Poisons
Autoimmunity
  Diffuse Collagen Diseases
  Tissue Transplantation

IMMUNITY

Immunity is a difficult subject—difficult to understand and difficult to write about. The first difficulty for the thoughtful reader (and 99 per cent of the readers of this book are presumed to be thoughtful) is presented by the double title of this chapter, for we are apt to think of immunity and hypersensitivity as two unrelated opposites, like virtue and vice. We shall find that this is not necessarily the case. Considering immunity merely as a defense against infection, our thinking can be summarized in the words of Sir Macfarlane Burnet: *"In the broadest terms the development of immunity is a process by which the body learns from experience of past infections to deal more efficiently with subsequent ones."* Unfortunately the immune system is a two-edged sword which, as we shall see, can be turned against the body in that biological paradox nicknamed *autoimmunity,* in which the same forces that normally reject foreign material act in reverse and reject the cells and tissues of the body itself, with very unpleasant consequences.

Early in the course of evolution animals learned to protect themselves against external enemies by developing armor, spines, or poison. But some of the enemies gained entrance to the interior of the body in order to adopt the easy life of a parasite. Resistance to these invaders evolved as a result of the development of the mechanism of immunity. It was first necessary for the cells of the body to recognize the invader in order that protective substances called *antibodies* could be produced against it. Burnet has introduced the concept of the *self-marker*, perhaps a molecular pattern of the body proteins marked "self" in contrast to organic material from outside which is marked "not-self." The latter is thus at once recognized as an alien enemy, against which antibodies are produced with rejection or destruction of the invader. The not-self foreign material, nearly always a protein, responsible for the production of antibodies, is known as an *antigen* (*gen,* to form).

Basically we may say that the development of immunity depends on the recognition of differences in the chemical structure of substances, just as friend and foe may be distinguished by the different uniforms they wear. Antibodies to the invading antigen can be detected in the circulating blood, and the antibody-producing cells are so modified that they can rapidly produce fresh supplies of antibody on contact with the *same* antigen in the future. *This is the key to the whole process.* The antibodies are formed by cells of the *reticuloendothelial system* (reticular or supportive cells and lining endothelial cells, more particularly in the spleen, lymph nodes and bone marrow), the chief of these being *immature plasma cells.* Lymphocytes are also involved, but more as carriers than producers of antibody.

Several different varieties of immunity have acquired names and thus crept into the books, so that they must be learned by the student, although the differences are not necessarily fundamental.

NATURAL IMMUNITY. This is a condition that is said to exist in persons who can pass through a virulent epidemic without acquiring the disease. It would seem that they have inherited a constitution (? molecular pattern) different from that of their less fortunate fellows. But before jumping to this conclusion we must realize that a person may have one or more attacks of an infection so mild as to be undetected and therefore known as *subclinical,* yet sufficient to stimulate the antibody-forming cells and thus render the subject immune to a future more severe infection. *This is really an acquired immunity, although unrecognized as such.* We must also recognize that a person may develop a complete immunity owing to previous subclinical or clinical attacks, and yet continue to harbor the infecting organism. Such a person is a *carrier.* Typhoid infection is one of the best examples of the carrier state. Antibodies circulate in the blood, but the typhoid bacilli continue to live quietly in the lumen of the intestine and gallbladder. They are beyond the reach of immune bodies, but they can infect people with whom the carrier comes in contact. In some infections a transient natural immunity is due to the transmission of antibodies (acquired) from the mother to child via the placental circulation. The best example is diphtheria, 80 per cent of newborn children having diphtheria antitoxin in their blood, which disappears by the end of the first year.

Species immunity provides an excellent example of a true natural immunity. Some diseases such as gonorrhea and typhoid fever are peculiar to man, and have not been reproduced in animals by inoculation with the specific microorganisms. The rat is peculiarly resistant to tuberculosis and several other human infections. Other diseases are limited to certain animals. It is a matter of chemical relationship between the tissues and the microorganisms. If there is no affinity between the infective agent and the cells of the body, the animal will possess perfect immunity against that infection.

The *properdin system* appears to be an important element in natural immunity. Properdin is a globulin of large molecular weight, and acts only in conjunction with complement and magnesium, hence the term properdin system. It is intimately involved in the destruction of bacteria, the neutralization of viruses, and the hemolysis of red blood cells. The importance of the properdin system lies in its lack of specificity and therefore wide range of defense. Among laboratory animals the rat has the highest titer of properdin, whereas the guinea pig, notoriously susceptible to infection, has the lowest.

PASSIVE IMMUNITY.   This is that form of immunity in which a person receives his antibodies from a previously immunized animal or human. As the cells of the body have undergone no change, the immunity is only temporary, passing off in a few weeks. Its great value in practice depends on the fact that the immunity is immediate, and therefore becomes operative when the patient shows evidence of disease but has not had time to manufacture his own antibodies. The best example is diphtheria, in which blood serum containing large amounts of antitoxin manufactured by a horse inoculated repeatedly with diphtheria bacilli is injected into a child suffering from the disease. This used to be one of the most valuable measures in the treatment of infectious disease, but it is no longer required if the child has been actively immunized by inoculation with diphtheria toxoid (denatured toxin).

ACQUIRED IMMUNITY.   Immunity may be acquired as: 1. *The result of disease*. The immunity develops during an attack of the disease, it is the main reason for recovery, and it may persist for years or even a lifetime. Long-lasting immunity is the rule in many viral diseases such as smallpox and in the common childhood fevers, which therefore occur once and once only. In contrast to these viral diseases, the majority of bacterial infections produce only temporary immunity to a second infection, and some, such as gonorrhea, produce none at all. Other infections produce little or no immunity; we all know how true that is of the common cold. 2. *The result of artificial immunization,* which may be passive or active. The *passive type* induced by the injection of immune serum has already been considered.

The *active type* of acquired immunity is induced by inoculation with a suspension of dead or attenuated living bacteria or viruses, or their toxic products, or of a related organism. The inoculum is called a *vaccine,* a term taken from the first example of successful active acquired immunity, namely protection against smallpox by the use of the infective material from cowpox (*vacca,* a cow). The specific organism in the vaccine is usually in the form of a killed culture, as in typhoid vaccine, but sometimes it is more effective to use living organisms of attenuated virulence, as in the B.C.G. vaccine (Bacille Calmette-Guérin) against tuberculosis, which is a culture of a living bovine strain of tubercle bacilli attenuated by years of artificial culture. Immunization against poliomyelitis illustrates the two techniques: the Salk method using killed virus inoculated into the skin, and the Sabin method using attenuated living virus given orally. For some diseases the antigen of the vaccine is a bacterial toxin rather than the bacteria themselves, the toxicity having been removed by chemical means without diminishing the immunizing power. The denatured toxin is called a *toxoid.* Toxoids are used particularly in protection against diphtheria and tetanus, both diphtheria and tetanus bacilli forming powerful exotoxins.

ANTIBODIES. Passing reference has already been made to antibodies, but they merit closer attention. They are *immune bodies* produced in response to antigens that attach themselves to the surface of cells of the reticuloendothelial system, *in particular immature plasma cells,* and these penetrate to the interior of these cells. Like antigens, the antibodies are protein in nature, and belong to the gamma globulins of the blood plasma. The *plasma proteins* are: (1) *fibrinogen,* from which fibrin is formed in the clotting of blood, (2) *albumin,* on which depends the all-important osmotic pressure that holds the fluid of the blood inside the vessels, and (3) *globulin,* which consists of alpha, beta, and gamma types. Fractionation (separation) of the plasma proteins can be done by highly accurate but complicated and time-consuming chemical analysis or by the much simpler and more rapid method of *electrophoresis.* **When plasma proteins are subjected to an electric field, the different protein components move at different speeds, so that they can be separated.** The speeds can be recorded on paper in an electrophoresis cell. The fastest moving is albumin, followed by alpha globulin, beta globulin, and fibrinogen, with the large molecules of gamma globulin bringing up the rear. Alpha globulin is made in the liver, gamma globulin in the plasma cells.

In *agammaglobulinemia,* as the name indicates, there is *a deficiency of the gamma globulin fraction of the plasma proteins, with a corresponding very low resistance to infection.* The condition is usually *congenital,* familial, and sex-linked, being confined to males. These children are apt to die of infections which in normal people are quite trivial. It is noteworthy that there is atrophy of lymphoid tissue and failure of the plasma cells to differentiate on antigenic stimulation. The *acquired form* may occur in either sex, comes on in later life, and is not familial. It may be added that the newborn infant synthesizes little gamma globulin or antibodies until three to twelve weeks of age, depending on the original supply from its mother.

Antibodies are of varied character. Some are *agglutinins,* so-called because they cause agglutination or clumping of bacilli in suspension seen under the microscope by imparting a stickiness to the surface of the bacteria. The presence of agglutinins in the blood is of great advantage in defense against bacteria, because it causes them to stick together and to the surrounding tissues, so that they are unable to spread to a distance before the leukocytes arrive on the scene and devour them. The presence of agglutinins in the blood as shown by agglutination of the bacteria in a fluid culture is the basis of the Widal test for typhoid fever. Other antibodies are *bacteriolysins,* which cause lysis or solution of the invading bacteria. *Opsonins* (from the Greek for a sauce or appetizer) are antibodies that make bacteria or other antigens attractive to the leukocytes. Leukocytes washed free from blood serum do not phagocytose bacteria, but when a trace of serum is added they commence to do so.

Antibodies are produced in excess in the cytoplasm of the plasma cells, and are then liberated into the blood stream, where they unite with and neutralize the circulating corresponding antigen. For this union a substance named *complement* is necessary, and it is believed to be responsible for the actual destruction of the antigen after it has united with the antibody. When complement, which is a normal constituent of blood plasma, has united with antigen and antibody it is said to be fixed or bound, for it is unable to enter into combination with another antigen-antibody pair. *Complement fixation* can therefore be used as an indicator of the presence of an antigen and its corresponding antibody. If antigen and complement are placed in a test tube and the blood serum of a patient is added, the complement will be fixed if the serum contains the corresponding antibody, but it will remain free if the antibody is absent. This is the basis of the *Wassermann reaction* for syphilis, which is a test for the presence of specific syphilitic antibody in the suspected serum.

Complement is therefore an indicator. Unfortunately, in the Wassermann reaction and in other complement-fixation tests it is an invisible indicator, for the reagents, namely antigen, immune body (antibody), and complement are all colorless. A colored indicator must therefore be added. This takes the form of *sensitized* red blood cells. The red cells of a sheep are injected a number of times into a rabbit until an immune body in the form of a hemolysin is produced. Like other immune bodies, it is unable to act on its antigen without the presence of complement, but when complement is present union occurs, and the red cells are hemolyzed, a change that can be seen in the test tube at a glance. The Wassermann reaction is considered again on page 154.

Dye molecules can be chemically linked with antibody globulin molecules without impairing the capacity of the latter to react with antigen. This has been a most important advance, for the antibody can be now seen, photographed, and located in a particular tissue. The most useful method is the *fluorescent-labeled antibody technique of Coons,* in which the antibody is conjugated with fluorescein isocyanate. The antigen-antibody reaction can now be seen and photographed because of the fluorescence of the dye. It is obvious that such a method is equally valuable for demonstrating the site of the antigen with which the labeled antibody reacts.

THYMUS.   In previous editions of this book no mention was made of the thymus gland in relation to disease. That is because nothing was known of the subject, or even of the function of the thymus. The breakthrough came with the observation that removal of the thymus (thymectomy) in the newborn laboratory animal, more particularly the mouse, resulted in loss of power of rejecting a skin graft from other mice, and even a graft from another species, such as the rat, was accepted. The golden age of thymology had begun. Nor can the animal respond to antigens by producing appropriate antibodies. *It would now appear that during the first few weeks of life the thymus produces immunologically competent cells which are distributed to other factories of lymphocytes in the lymph nodes and spleen,* their function being to protect the body against foreign invaders. In addition the thymus is believed to produce a hormone that has the power to endow cells having immunological potential with immunological competence.

HYPERSENSITIVITY

We have seen that the body protects itself against foreign protein invasion by the mechanism of immunity. But during the development of immunity there may appear a very different and indeed opposite type of reaction, namely *hypersensitivity* or *allergy*. This reaction is a hypersensitivity to bacterial protein as well as to any foreign protein that may be injected or enter the body. **Hypersensitivity is essentially an altered state of reactivity of the body.** Indeed this is what the word allergy means (*allos,* other, *ergon,* energy). The first injection may produce no evident effect, but a second injection is followed by striking and often dramatic phenomena, which may be local or general. Immunity is a manifestation of what has been termed **the wisdom of the body,** but hypersensitivity might well be called the stupidity of the body. The conditions of life in modern "civilization" have vastly multiplied the chances of a person's developing hypersensitivity. This is due partly to our industrial development, but even more to the unbelievable number and variety of chemicals and drugs that it has become fashionable to swallow, to inhale, to apply to the skin, or to have injected.

There are several types of hypersensitivity, and almost as many ways in which they can be classified. Much depends on whether allergy is regarded as synonymous with hypersensitivity or as a special variety of that condition. Either course is fully justifiable, but the latter will be followed here (see page 118). We may then recognize two main types of hypersensitivity: (1) *acquired* by exposure to an antigen or induced experimentally, (2) *natural* and synonymous with allergy. The acquired group may be subdivided into (*a*) *immediate* or early, also known as *anaphylactic,* and (*b*) *delayed* or late, also known as the *cellular* or *tuberculin* type. Details of the classification can be seen in the outline of contents at the beginning of this chapter.

IMMEDIATE HYPERSENSITIVITY.   The immediate or anaphylactic reaction develops with dramatic suddenness, shows circulating antibodies in the serum, is of short duration, is induced by artificial means, and is not heritable, and the symptoms are mainly due to smooth muscle spasm. In this group we may include anaphylactic shock and serum sickness.

Anaphylactic Shock.   The word anaphylaxis (*ana,* backward, and *phylaxis,* protection) means the opposite of protection. The reaction is much more readily induced in the experimental animal, particularly the guinea pig, than in man. The animal is sensitized by the subcutaneous injection of a minute amount of foreign protein such as horse serum. After an interval of at least ten days a second, somewhat larger, dose of the *same serum* is injected intravenously. The reaction is rapid or immediate, the animal passing into a state of acute shock, with severe respiratory embarrassment, terminating in death. In man fatal anaphylactic shock is fortunately rare, but it may occur as the result of the intravenous injection of therapeutic serum, particularly antidiphtheritic serum. One of the first persons to receive a prophylactic dose of diphtheria antitoxin was the young son of Professor Langerhans, who described the islets in the pancreas. The boy was all right for five minutes, but ten minutes later he was dead from anaphylactic shock. It must be remembered that most therapeutic sera are manufactured by the horse. For this reason, if it is known that the patient has previously (over ten days) received an injection of serum, it is wise to test for possible hypersensitivity by the intracutaneous inoculation of a small amount of the serum before giving an intravenous therapeutic injection.

In rare cases fatal anaphylactic shock may be produced in man by the *sting of bees or wasps.* Most bee keepers become immunized to the poison as the result of frequent stings, but occasionally the effect is hypersensitivity rather than immunity, and a single sting may have fatal results.

The *mechanism* responsible for the anaphylactic reaction appears to be a combination of the injected antigen with already circulating antibodies to form an *antigen-antibody complex,* which then acts on sensitized cells with the release of histamine. It is of interest to learn that shock may be induced by the use of preformed antigen-antibody complexes acting on sensitized cells. The histamine released causes a spasmodic contraction of smooth muscle in the walls of the bronchioles, the pulmonary arteries, and the gastrointestinal tract, as well as increased capillary permeability leading to edema, particularly of the lungs. *All the major manifestations of anaphylactic shock can be reproduced by the intravenous injection of histamine.*

Serum Sickness. In man anaphylactic shock is fortunately rare, but a much milder reaction known as serum sickness is not uncommon following the subcutaneous injection of serum. This is marked by an urticarial rash, fever, pains in the joints, and swelling of the lymph nodes. The symptoms are attributed to a reaction of the foreign antigen with *sessile* rather than circulating antibodies resulting from a previous injection. Occasionally the clinical picture develops after a single injection. In such a case we must presume the presence of already existing antibodies.

DELAYED HYPERSENSITIVITY. This form is also known as the *bacterial* or *tuberculin* type of hypersensitivity, although an even better term would be *cellular hypersensitivity.* The delayed reaction is seen in many diseases caused by bacteria, viruses, fungi, spirochetes, and parasites. The maximum inflammatory response does not develop for 24 hours or more after the application of the test antigen. How different in this respect from the dramatic immediate response! Perhaps explaining this difference is the fact that **circulating antibodies produced by plasma cells play no part in the reaction, which takes place on the surface or in the interior of tissue cells sensitized by the primary bacterial infection, hence the term cellular hypersensitivity.** The reaction is most readily shown in the case of tuberculosis. When tuberculin, a sterile extract of tubercle bacilli, is injected into the skin of a normal animal or person there is no reaction, but if the animal or person is already tuberculous a small dose will cause redness and swelling of the skin. This is the *tuberculin reaction,* and constitutes the *von Pirquet test* for the presence of tuberculosis in man. If the dose of antigen is larger there will be extensive necrosis and sloughing, which constitutes the *Koch phenomenon.* In the natural disease as it occurs in man there is the same sequence of events. The initial lesion produced in the lung by inhaled tubercle bacilli may be insignificant and remain so, but the primary infection has led to sensitization of all the cells of the body, so that a subsequent reinfection with the same antigen causes a violent intracellular reaction in the enzyme systems resulting in degeneration and death of the cell. From this account it will be seen that such terms as delayed, cellular, and bacterial type are all well justified in describing this form of hypersensitivity. It will also be evident that this form is of much greater importance in relation to common bacterial diseases than the anaphylactic or immediate type.

ALLERGY.   Reference has already been made to the difficulty of deciding on a suitable nomenclature for the hypersensitivity states and reactions. Hypersensitivity and allergy both mean the same thing, so that many writers very properly use the terms interchangeably. On the other hand the public, for whom allergy has become an everyday and household word, uses the term to indicate an individual hypersensitivity or idiosyncrasy to pollens, some kinds of foods, plant poisons, and the emanations of animals. To this group the immunologist applies the name *atopy* (*atopia,* a strange disease), but I prefer to use the common name, allergy. The respect in which it differs most from other forms of hypersensitivity is that it is a natural rather than an acquired condition. An excellent though rather an awkward name would be *natural hypersensitivity.* The idiosyncrasy is a quantitative rather than a qualitative difference from the normal. The greater the concentration of the substance, the more people are found to be allergic. Idiosyncrasy has been described as individuality run wild. **The condition is an inherited predisposition,** and this hereditary tendency forms one of its most striking characteristics, following the laws of mendelian inheritance. The hypersensitivity is not present at birth, and takes some years to develop. Cases are on record of identical twins who have become allergic to the same protein at the same age. The person with pronounced allergy is likely to show an increase in the number of eosinophil leukocytes in the blood.

The manifestations vary in different people, depending on which particular tissue happens to be hypersensitive. If that tissue is the lining of the nose and eyelids the result is hay fever, if it is the musculature of the bronchi the result is asthma, if it is the wall of the bowel the result is abdominal cramps and diarrhea, if it is the skin the result is urticaria or nettle rash. The same protein may produce effects on different tissues. Thus plant pollen may cause both hay fever and asthma in the same individual, and certain foods such as shellfish (shrimp, oysters) and strawberries may cause eczema and urticaria as well as gastrointestinal disturbance.

Hay Fever. **Hay fever is one of the most clear-cut of the allergic diseases.** The attacks are strictly seasonal, occurring in spring, summer or autumn, depending on whether the patient is hypersensitive to the pollens of trees, grasses, or such a fall plant as ragweed. The symptoms are itching and congestion of the eyes, violent paroxysms of sneezing, and a profuse watery discharge from the nose. The particular protein responsible can usually be determined by means of skin tests, *i.e.,* scratching the arm and rubbing in the suspected protein; if an inflamed area or wheal is produced, the patient is hypersensitive to that protein. When the protein is known, the patient may be desensitized against it by means of repeated small injections of the protein before the onset of the hay fever period. In about two thirds of the cases this is followed by marked improvement.

Many sufferers from hay fever obtain marked benefit from the use of antihistamine drugs. There are many of these materials now available. They counteract the effect of histamine, which is liberated in the tissues following exposure to the offending protein material. In some people, these drugs have a marked sedative action producing drowsiness, which must be watched for if these drugs are taken while the patient is carrying on his usual activities.

Bronchial Asthma. Asthma is an allergic condition in which there is hypersensitiveness of the walls of the bronchi, either to foreign proteins of external origin or to bacteria that have their habitat in the respiratory passages. The foreign proteins (*i.e.,* foreign to the body) may be the pollens of plants, the dander and emanations of animals (especially horses), vegetable dusts such as face powders containing orris root, and certain foods such as egg white, especially in children. Bronchial asthma is often associated with infection by intestinal parasites. The walls of the bronchi consist mainly of a lining of mucous membrane and layers of plain muscle. **In an allergic attack the muscle contracts and the mucous membrane becomes swollen.** The patient therefore suffers great difficulty in breathing, even more in expiration than inspiration, and wheezing is a marked feature of the respiratory distress. The treatment of an acute attack of asthma is best carried out by the use of epinephrine by hypodermic injection, or by inhalation of epinephrine spray. Aminophylline and ephedrine are also valuable drugs in the alleviation of an attack of asthma. In severe attacks ACTH has been of value in many instances. The general principles of treatment of asthma from the standpoint of prevention of attacks should be concerned with the removal of any materials to which the patient may be sensitive, but only too often all attempts in this direction end in failure. In addition, **many attacks of asthma are precipitated by emotional disturbances,** and assistance to prevent this factor may be of great help in this disease. The continued use of drugs such as aminophylline and ephedrine are frequently of value in preventing attacks. The use of the antihistamine drugs in the treatment of asthma is generally disappointing.

Food Allergy.   Many persons are hypersensitive to such articles of diet as oysters, fish, strawberries, pork, cereals, eggs, and milk. In these persons a very small amount of the food in question may produce an immediate attack of vomiting and diarrhea accompanied by collapse, of urticaria and other skin eruptions, or of asthma. The fault lies in the person, not in the food, clearly illustrating the old adage that "what is one man's meat is another man's poison." The search for the article at fault may tax the detective powers of the physician to the utmost. It may be accomplished by means of skin tests, or even more reliably by elimination of one article after another from the diet.

Drug Allergy.   A wide variety of medicinal substances may cause drug allergy which is in a rather different category, for these substances are not in themselves antigenic, but by becoming *conjugated with serum proteins* they acquire antigenic properties and cause serious and sometimes fatal disturbances. Sulfonamide allergy deserves special mention, as, in addition to fever, chills, and a skin eruption, there may be renal failure with anuria about a week after the administration of the drug.

Plant Poisons.   Hypersensitivity to plant poisons is a rather common affliction. Such plants as poison ivy, poison oak, and the primula family may set up a severe inflammation of the skin (*dermatitis venenata*) when the sensitive person touches the leaves. Even the smoke of burning poison ivy can produce the same result. It often happens that florists only develop hypersensitivity after they have been handling primulas for many years, a fact that we must admit is suggestive of induced rather than natural hypersensitivity.

AUTOIMMUNITY

The immunity mechanism is a reaction against substances of foreign origin. We have already seen that this reaction can be either beneficial or harmful to the host. Both are due to the response of the antibody-producing apparatus in contact with an exogenous antigen, that is to say one with foreign protein. It used to be thought that the body would never make the grave mistake of responding immunologically to its own protein antigens by the formation of antibodies. Thus horse serum injected into human beings acts as a powerful antigen, but it does not elicit antibody formation when injected into a horse. A skin graft from a child to its mother is rejected because it is a *homograft,* not an *autograft,* on account of the presence of paternal antigens in the cells of the graft, but of course it is accepted by the child itself, for whom it is an autograft.

Reference has already been made to the self-marker concept of Burnet, according to which the molecular pattern of the body proteins seems to be marked "self," thus providing them with a passport for identification. Organic material from outside is marked "not-self," so that if it gains entrance to the body, antibodies are formed against it.

It has now come to be recognized that under certain conditions not at present clearly understood **antigenic substances formed in the body (***autoantigens***) may excite the formation of antibodies, with a resulting antigen-antibody reaction.** That is to say, certain body proteins are now regarded as not-self or foreign by the body itself. Possibly the entry of a *foreign nonantigenic substance* such as a drug may combine with an *endogenous body protein* and modify it enough to make it antigenic, so that antibodies are formed to this complex. A foreign substance with this ability to combine with a body protein is known as a *hapten,* from the Greek meaning to seize.

The concept of autoimmunity, which might more appropriately be termed *autosensitivity,* is one of far-reaching importance, and at present we only stand on its threshold. It is possible that a number of diseases which in the past have been labeled as idiopathic, that is to say of unknown etiology, may prove to be caused by an autoimmune or, to use a better although less popular term, an autoallergic mechanism. Indeed there is a danger that this easy diagnosis may become a refuge for the destitute when the real problem case is encountered. It is much easier to establish evidence in support of this concept in the experimental animal than in man. In the animal the inoculation of brain, thyroid, adrenal, kidney, and other organs will produce a reaction of delayed type hypersensitivity, with the same fundamental lesions as are seen in hypersensitivity to exogenous antigens. In man the evidence is much less convincing, although still suggestive. The best example is *Hashimoto's disease of the thyroid,* and others that may be mentioned are the *idiopathic form of Addison's disease* of the adrenals, *acquired hemolytic anemia* in which circulating autoantibodies to erythrocytes can be demonstrated, and the increasingly important group of the *collagen diseases, including rheumatoid arthritis.* It is now believed that it is the *antigen-antibody complexes* that may do the damage. Thus when these become attached to the basement membrane of the renal glomeruli they may set up the condition known as glomerulonephritis. The antigens may be either autogenous or exogenous (bacterial) in origin.

DIFFUSE COLLAGEN DISEASES.   This is a convenient place in which to refer to a group of diseases that have several features in common, although they are not necessarily of allergic or autoimmunological origin. From the days of Morgagni we have been accustomed to think of disease in terms of organ pathology; we speak of tuberculosis of the lung or cancer of the breast. The diseases to be considered here do not involve any one *organ* or even one system but rather a *diffusely distributed tissue,* namely fibrous connective tissue or collagen. Thus rheumatic fever is a disease of this tissue, whether it occurs in the heart, arteries, joints, skin, serous membranes, or internal organs. The principal members of the group are *polyarteritis nodosa* and *disseminated lupus erythematosus,* which are considered in connection with diseases of arteries (Chapter 16), *rheumatic fever,* discussed in relation to diseases of the heart (Chapter 15), *rheumatoid arthritis,* described with diseases of joints (Chapter 28), together with the rarer diseases, *scleroderma* and *dermatomyositis,* the names of which indicate the chief site of involvement.

The diseases, with the exception of scleroderma, are characterized by an inflammatory reaction which is at first acute, yet no bacteria or other irritant can be found in the lesions. The acute lesion is in the nature of an allergic inflammation with rapid and massive exudation of protein-rich fluid. The nature of the antigen is unknown, but in the absence of any evidence of an external agent it is natural to suspect an autoimmune mechanism. There is no reason to suppose that there is one single causal agent for the various members of the group, but throughout the variations there seems to run a fairly constant theme of hypersensitivity, an antigen-antibody reaction in the connective tissue and the walls of the arteries. The evidence in favor of an allergic basis is a good deal more convincing in the experimental animal than in man.

The most characteristic lesion is so-called *fibrinoid degeneration* or *necrosis,* best seen in the walls of arteries. This consists of loosening and separation of the collagen bundles with swelling of the ground substance and disintegration into granular necrotic material which stains bright red with eosin. This material reacts with special stains for fibrin, hence the name fibrinoid degeneration. For long it was believed that fibrinoid was the result of an allergic reaction on the part of the ground substance of collagen fibers, but now it appears even more possible that it represents a local conversion of plasma fibrinogen into fibrin, the basis being a local increase in vascular permeability so that plasma oozes through the vessel wall, together with an abnormal release of thromboplastic substances in the area as a result of local necrosis. After the acute reaction has subsided there is a tendency to fibrosis and sclerosis. In general terms it may be said that in *polyarteritis nodosa* the *inflammatory reaction* is a striking feature, in *disseminated lupus erythermatosus fibrinoid formation* is the dominant lesion, in *diffuse scleroderma,* as the name suggests, *collagenous sclerosis* overshadows the other components, and in *rheumatic fever all three* are well represented.

Biochemical changes are a feature of the various collagen diseases. The most characteristic change is *increase in gamma globulins,* probably due to proliferation of plasma cells, which are the cellular source of antibodies and other gamma globulins. *Cortisone* and *hydrocortisone* are of great value in several of the collagen diseases, apparently acting by destroying plasma cells with rapid degradation of antibodies. They also suppress the permeability of membranes and thus interfere with the outpouring of plasma rich in fibrinogen, which would otherwise give rise to the formation of fibrinoid. It is particularly in acute diseases of relatively short duration, such as rheumatic fever, that these hormones arc of benefit.

TISSUE TRANSPLANTATION. In the general subject of autoimmunity, of self and not-self, one question of particular importance is that of tissue transplantation. Each of us is so individual that we can recognize and reject the tissues of another person when they are introduced into ourselves. We refuse integration, produce antibodies, and reject the intruder. This is even true of the erythrocytes in a blood transfusion. If the antigens of the donor do not belong to the same blood group as those of the recipient, antibodies are produced and the red cells are destroyed.

The same holds true for tissue transplants. These transplants may be (1) *autogenous* (*auto,* self), in which the transplant is made from one part of an individual's own body to another part, (2) *homologous* (*homo,* same), in which the transplant is from another member of the same species (from man to man), and (3) *heterologous* (*heteros,* another), in which transplants are made between different species. It is obvious from what we have just said that an autogenous graft will be accepted and a heterologous will be rejected. It is unfortunate that the homologous graft is also regarded as not-self, and is therefore rejected, but this obstacle can now be overcome in part by a number of devices. Of these the most important are (1) *total body radiation* of sufficient strength to interfere with antibody formation to such a degree that homologous and even heterologous transplants are accepted, and (2) *cortisone* and particularly *hydrocortisone,* the use of which can allow human tissue, even cancer, to be transplanted into rats.

The matter of the transplantation of tissues and organs is vitally important to the surgeon. Thus if both kidneys of a patient have been destroyed by disease, the obvious thing to do would be to transplant a kidney from a healthy donor or even a dead body. This procedure will work and save the patient from certain death in the case of identical twins (self and self), but not under other circumstances (self and not-self). Success, however, has attended kidney transplantation between *nonidentical* twins by inducing at least partial tolerance by means of subtotal whole body irradiation combined later with cortisone therapy.

It may be that one of these days we shall learn how to break down the barrier so that healthy organs can be transplanted to replace diseased ones in persons other than twins. It is now known that the self-marker stamp is not placed on cells until late in embryonic life. Before a certain point of embryonic development the entry of foreign cells provokes a specific *acquired tolerance* in later life, so that tissue transplants can be made. This acquired tolerance may be related to the absence of plasma cells in the fetus, so that antibodies are not formed. Possibly in the future our knowledge of acquired or induced tolerance may have developed to such a degree that the surgeon may be able to transplant organs with impunity from one body to another.

It must not be supposed from what has just been said that tissue transplants in the past have been of no value. Autogenous transplants in man are of course most desirable, and these are used in skin grafts. Heterologous transplants, however, have also proved of great use, particularly in the case of bone, fascia, nerves, blood vessels, and the cornea of the eye. In these instances we are really using not the cells but the *intercellular substance* of the transplant, and even though antibodies may destroy the cells, the intercellular substance acts as a scaffold on which the cells of the host can build a new structure. This is particularly well illustrated in arterial transplants, which provide a temporary skeleton on which a new vessel can be constructed, the skeleton itself being later discarded.

FURTHER READING

BOYD, W. C.: *Fundamentals of Immunology,* 4th ed., 1967, New York.

BURNET, F. M.: *The Integrity of the Body,* Harvard University Press, 1962, Cambridge, Mass.

COOMBS, R. R. A.: Brit. Med. J., 1968, *1,* 597. (Immunopathology.)

DIXON, F. J., and HUMPHREY, J. H.: *Advances in Immunology,* vol. IV, 1965, New York and London.

GAIDUSEK, D. C.: Arch. Int. Med., 1958, *101,* 9. (Auto-immunity in disease production.)

GARDNER, D. L.: *Pathology of the Connective Tissue Diseases.* Ed. Arnold, Ltd., London, 1965.

GLYNN, L. E., and HOLBOROW, E. J.: *Autoimmunity and Disease,* Blackwell Scientific Publications, 1965, Oxford.

GOOD, R. A.: in *The Thymus in Immunobiology;* edit. R. A. Good and A. E. Gabrielsen, 1964, New York.

MACKAY, L. R., and BURNET, F. M.: *Autoimmune Diseases,* 1963, Springfield, Ill.

MILLER, J. F. A. P.: Lancet, 1967, *2,* 1299. (The thymus: yesterday, today and tomorrow.)

NOSSAL, G. J. V.: Scient. Amer. Dec. 1964, p. 106. (How cells make antibodies.)

PILLEMER, L., *et al.*: Science, 1954, *120,* 279. (Properdin system immunity.)

WEISER, R. S., MYRVIK, Q. N., and PEARSALL, N. N.: *Fundamentals of Immunology,* 1969, Philadelphia, Pa.

Bacterial Infections

GENERAL CONSIDERATIONS

BACTERIA AND DISEASE. Bacteria are the greatest single cause of disease. Fortunately for man it is only a small number of bacteria and fungi that have acquired the power of existing in the living body and thus producing disease. The vast majority of bacteria live only on dead matter and are therefore called *saprophytes* (*sapros,* decayed), in contradistinction to *parasites* which exist on living matter, although the term parasite is often wrongly restricted to those animal forms as opposed to plant forms which invade and live in the body. Parasitism is a remarkable phenomenon, for in its essence it is a breaking down of that vital resistance which, as we have seen in the preceding chapter, every living thing presents to invasion by another living entity. A microorganism may be both a parasite and a saprophyte, for it may exist for a time in the living body and for a time outside the body, drawing its sustenance from dead matter. An example of such an organism is the typhoid bacillus. Other parasites have become so dependent on the support of the living body that they have lost the power to exist on dead matter; such is the spirochete (treponema) which causes syphilis. It is evident that the problem of infection will be different in the two cases; in the former it is not necessary for the infecting agent to be conveyed directly from person to person, while in the latter this is an essential requisite.

Some bacteria can produce disease in practically every organ of the body; such are the staphylococcus, streptococcus, and tubercle bacillus. Others have a special predilection for one organ and are rarely found elsewhere; examples of this group are the gonococcus (genital tract), meningococcus (meninges covering the brain and spinal cord), pneumococcus (lungs and upper respiratory passages), and typhoid bacillus (intestine). The latter group will be considered more fully in connection with the organs that they usually attack. Some members of the former group will be considered in this chapter, together with such questions as how pathogenic bacteria enter the body, how they leave it, how they spread from person to person, and how they produce disease. No attempt will be made to give bacteriological detail, as that would merely usurp the function of a text on bacteriology. It may be added that the term *microbiology* has become popular in place of bacteriology, because it includes the study not only of bacteria, but also of fungi, viruses, rickettsiae, and even unicellular protozoan animal parasites. Bacteria and fungi belong to the vegetable kingdom, protozoa to the animal kingdom.

Bacteria are the lowest forms of life, and therefore have the highest power of reproduction, so that one bacterium can give rise to hundreds of millions in the course of twenty-four hours provided the conditions are suitable, *i.e.,* food supply, moisture, and suitable temperature. This enormous increase is possible under laboratory conditions (not necessarily in the body) because reproduction is not the complicated process that it is in the higher animals, nor does sex enter into it. One bacterium gives rise to two by the simple process of fission or splitting down the middle.

Bacteria are so small that they can only be seen with the higher powers of the microscope, but, although minute, they vary much in size. When stained with chemical dyes in the laboratory they are seen to vary also in shape, and on this basis they can be divided into three groups: *cocci* which are rounded, *bacilli* which are rod-shaped, and *spirilla* which have the form of a spiral (Fig. 32).

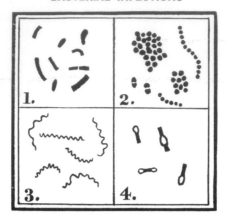

Fig. 32. Various bacteria. 1, Bacilli; 2, staphylococci and streptococci; 3, spirilla, small spirals—spirillum of syphilis; 4, spore-forming bacilli.

Pneumonia is caused by a coccus, tuberculosis by a bacillus, and syphilis by a spirillum. Diplococci grow in pairs, staphylococci in clusters like a bunch of grapes, streptococci in long or short chains. Bacteria are named according to the disease that they produce, but a new and much more complex nomenclature has been developed in recent years, and the old group of bacilli (bacillus tuberculosis, bacillus typhosus) has disappeared. The new names are derived from the discoverer, *e.g.,* Pasteurella pestis (plague), Eberthella typhosa (typhoid); or from the cultural requirements, *e.g.,* Hemophilus pertussis (whooping cough), which requires hemoglobin for its growth in culture; or from the appearance of the cultures, *e.g.,* Mycobacterium tuberculosis (*mykes,* a fungus), Clostridium tetani (*kloster,* a spindle). A few bacteria (staphylococci, streptococci) have fortunately escaped this renaming process. The new names have not entirely replaced the older ones even in textbooks of bacteriology, and on that account the old names more or less fixed by common usage are used in this book, although the new names sometimes are given in parentheses.

Physicians, as well as the paramedical workers for whom this book is intended, are so much concerned with disease-producing (pathogenic) bacteria that they are apt to forget that the great majority of bacteria are harmless. Indeed we can go farther than this and say that *without bacteria life would long ago have ceased on this planet, for they are the agents that keep the supply of food in constant motion.* They prepare food materials for plants, which are eaten by animals, which are eaten by man, and finally the dead bodies of animals and man are broken down by bacteria into their original elements, which are then returned to the soil. Bacteria close the gap between the form in which nitrogen is excreted by animals (urea and uric acid) and that in which it becomes serviceable to plants (nitrates), and thus prevent a continuous deterioration of the soil which would lead to the disappearance of all vegetation. *Without bacteria the nitrogen cycle would come to a full stop, and the continued existence of all higher forms of life would be impossible.* It used to be thought that individual life in animals and man was impossible without the presence of bacteria, particularly those in the bowel. This is now known not to be true, for first birds (from eggs) and now mammals (delivered by cesarean section) have been raised in a germ-free environment. It is interesting in the light of our studies on natural immunity in the previous chapter to observe what happens to animals brought from a germ-free to a normal germ-laden environment. All of the guinea pigs die of overwhelming infection within forty-eight hours, only 50 per cent of the mice die, and rats or chickens show no ill-effects.

It is easy enough to kill bacteria outside the body by means of antiseptics. It is very much more difficult to do so in the living body, because poisons that are injurious to the bacteria are even more harmful to the cells of the body. Treatment is *specific* when it attacks the bacteria without injuring the cells. In the past specific forms of therapy have been only too rare. Antibiotic therapy has changed that picture. The modern antibiotics such as penicillin and streptomycin, which are prepared from fungi in the soil, can kill bacteria *in vitro* with startling rapidity. In the living body they may not do this directly, but they prevent the bacteria from multiplying, and thus give the defense forces of the body time to mobilize and attack the invaders. That is to say they are *bacteriostatic* in their action, but some are also directly *bactericidal.* **We have now come to realize, however, that the antibiotics may also kill off the useful bacteria in the intestine and leave a vacuum, which is soon occupied by pathogenic organisms.** Moreover, it is the antibiotic-sensitive strains that are killed. The antibiotic-resistant strains, if there are any, survive, and may come to dominate the situation. This is particularly true for staphylococcal hospital infections, and this has now come to assume alarming proportions.

BIOLOGICAL ACTIVITY. When a microorganism invades the tissues of a host, one of three things may happen. (1) The invader may die; this is the most likely thing to happen. (2) It may survive without giving rise to what we call disease, but often causing a host immune reaction which may prevent reinfection. (3) Only exceptionally it may survive and produce clinical disease, which in rare cases may prove fatal, not only to the host but probably also to the invader.

The *biological effects* are produced in the main by *bacterial enzymes,* which are remarkably like those produced by the cells of higher animals.

They break down complex food materials, whether protein, carbohydrate, or fat, into simpler substances which can be assimilated by the bacteria. In the intestine this enzymatic activity results in the decomposition of dead organic material, with a resulting return to the soil of elements needed for the growth of plants. Indeed **these helpful intestinal bacteria have been called Nature's garbage disposal plant and fertilizer factory.** They also serve to purify sewage and make it inoffensive. Many of the essential vitamins, such as the B complex, are formed by bacteria in the large intestine. It is for this reason that over-use of antibiotics may lead to vitamin deficiency. When given before a surgical operation they may interfere with the formation of vitamin K, with resulting dangerous hemorrhage. What is powerful for good can be potent for evil.

Bacterial activity is manifested in various ways. (1) *Fermentation of carbohydrates,* as a result of which acid and gas are produced, a fact utilized by the bacteriologist for identifying certain bacteria, and by the industrialist for the manufacture of alcohol, vinegar, cheese, and other good things. Indeed Pasteur was first drawn to the study of bacteria through working at the fermentation of wines. (2) *Proteolysis,* a breaking down of proteins into simpler substances, some of which are very foul-smelling, mainly by the enzymes of anaerobic bacteria. *Putrefaction, i.e.,* the decomposition of *dead tissue,* is an example of proteolytic change. (3) *Toxin production* varies with different bacteria. Comparatively few produce exotoxins, that is to say poisons that are excreted by the living bacteria. Good examples are the diphtheria bacillus and the *Clostridia* group of gram-positive spore-bearing bacilli. The three members of the latter group, namely the organisms of tetanus, gas gangrene, and botulism, provide an interesting example of variation in exotoxin production and action. Tetanus bacilli grow under anaerobic conditions (without air) in dead tissue and there produce an exotoxin, which causes no local inflammatory reaction, but passes along the course of the peripheral nerves to the central nervous system where it causes catastrophic clinical results but still without *apparent* tissue damage. The organisms of gas gangrene, on the other hand, produce profound and widespread local damage in wounds by means of their enzymes. Finally, the bacilli of botulism do not need to live in the tissues of the host, but proliferate in insufficiently sterilized canned goods, where they elaborate one of the most deadly poisons known, which when ingested swiftly kills. When an exotoxin is treated with formaldehyde, it no longer causes disease when injected, but confers immunity. Such a modified toxin is called a *toxoid.* Toxoids are used more particularly for protection against diphtheria and tetanus. Practically all bacteria contain *endotoxins,* which are only liberated when the bacteria die and disintegrate. Examples are the gram-negative intestinal bacilli.

SPREAD OF INFECTION. Different pathogenic or disease-producing bacteria have different portals of entry to the body. Some may be introduced through the skin, but the great majority enter through the natural passages. Some prefer the respiratory passages, others the alimentary or the genitourinary tracts. Some are discharged from the body in the feces and urine, others by the mouth, nose, respiratory tract, saliva, and even the blood by means of insect bites. **Knowledge and appreciation of these routes are necessary if the spread of infection is to be prevented.** When an infection is transmitted intentionally through a series of laboratory animals, the *virulence* is likely to be *increased,* probably because the bacteria adapt themselves to their environment. The same thing is seen in human epidemics, in which virulence increases until a peak is reached, followed by a decline, perhaps because only the resistant members of the community remain to be infected. There are four principal methods of spread: (1) physical contact, (2) air, (3) food, and (4) insects.

Physical Contact. The contact may be *direct,* the infecting bacteria not surviving outside the body; of this the classic example is the venereal diseases. Or the contact may be *indirect* through *fomites,* that is to say clothing, utensils, and other possessions of the patient, the bacteria surviving for some time outside the body. The water of swimming pools deserves special mention.

Air-borne Infection. Bacterial and viral infections of the respiratory tract are transmitted through the air by dust or droplets. *Dust infection* comes from bacteria in dried sputum which become attached to dust particles; this is particularly true of tuberculosis. The danger comes from sweeping the dust. *Droplet infection* is the basis of epidemics of upper respiratory disease. It is estimated that 20,000 droplets containing possible pathogens may be expelled by one sneeze, and that droplets 1 mm. in diameter may pass over a distance of 15 feet. Were it not for immunity we would all be ill.

Food-borne Infection. This constitutes an important public health problem. The possibility of infection by food or water must be considered in every major epidemic of intestinal disease. The method of transmission does not have to be direct, for the feet of fecal-feeding flies may foul the food. Epidemics of typhoid, dysentery, and cholera are due to infection of food or water.

Insect-borne Infection. Insects are potent conveyers of infection, not only bacterial, but also viral and protozoal. Thus plague is spread from the rat to man by the rat-flea, typhus by lice, and the yellow fever virus and the malaria parasite by mosquitoes. *It is obvious how necessary is a knowledge of the spread of infection by insects if some of the great scourges of the tropics are to be controlled.*

DIAGNOSTIC METHODS.   It might be thought that it would be a simple matter to determine the bacterial agent causing a given disease. In some cases this is really quite easy, but in other cases it may be extremely difficult. It was Robert Koch who in 1881 first established the criteria necessary to justify the assumption of an etiological relationship. These criteria, which are four in number, have long been known as *Koch's postulates.* They are as follows: **(1) The suspected organism must always be present in the lesion. (2) It must be grown in pure culture on laboratory media. (3) It must cause the same disease when injected into a susceptible animal. (4) It must be recovered from the experimental animal.** The most notable of the many contributions that Koch made to bacteriology was his demonstration of the true cause of tuberculosis, for in the space of one year he (1) demonstrated the tubercle bacillus in the lesions by special staining, (2) grew the bacilli on a medium which he invented, (3) reproduced the disease by injecting the culture into suitable laboratory animals, and (4) recovered tubercle bacilli from these animals. But such conclusive proof is not always possible. Thus in leprosy the human lesions are simply swarming with bacilli very similar in appearance to the tubercle bacillus, but these will not reproduce the disease in any of the ordinary laboratory animals, nor can they be grown in artificial culture on the commonly used media.

Special stains are of value in recognizing and classifying certain bacteria. The aniline dye, methylene blue, will stain the vast majority satisfactorily, but two special methods are invaluable. The first of these is *Gram's stain,* in which the film is stained with gentian violet followed by iodine, and then decolorized with alcohol and counterstained. Bacteria which resist the decolorization and so remain stained blue are said to be *gram-positive;* those that are decolorized by the alcohol, but are shown up by a counterstain of a different color, are said to be *gram-negative.* This method is indispensable in routine laboratory work, for it separates bacteria, both cocci and bacilli, into two great groups. The second method is *acid-fast staining.* The term "fast" is taken from a German word meaning resistant. Bacilli that resist decoloration with acid after being stained red with hot carbol fuchsin are said to be acid-fast. The reader will appreciate that acid-fast corresponds to gram-positive; in the former acid is used as the decolorizing agent, in the latter alcohol. The only two important members of the acid-fast group are the bacilli of tuberculosis and leprosy. There are many other special stains, but these two have been chosen for mention, because we shall have to keep referring to acid-fast bacilli and gram-positive and -negative organisms in the course of this chapter.

Cultural characteristics also play an important part in determining the nature of an infection. The four requirements for successful culture are food, temperature, moisture, and oxygen. *Food* is represented by the culture medium. Some media suit some types of bacteria, while other media, such as those containing hemoglobin, are better for other types. *Moisture* is essential, because water is as vital to bacteria as to all other forms of life. It is for this reason that a swab of infective material must never be allowed to dry out in its passage from the bedside to the laboratory by being left lying around. *Temperature* best suited for pathogenic bacteria is usually that of the body to which they are accustomed, so that the incubator in which the media are placed is kept at 37° C. (98.4° F.). *Oxygen,* represented by air, is required for growth by most bacteria; they are said to be *aerobic.* Some can live with or without air. An important group are peculiar enough to demand absence of air for continued growth; they are therefore called *anaerobic* bacteria or *anaerobes,* and the laboratory technique must be regulated accordingly. To this group belong the spore-bearing bacilli which live in soil that has been fertilized by manure and which infect wounds contaminated with such soil, the most important being the bacillus of tetanus and the bacilli that cause gas gangrene.

Serological Tests. Reference has already been made to tests for antibodies in the circulating blood by means of which the nature of the infecting bacteria can be determined. The most familiar of these are the agglutination Widal test for typhoid and the complement fixation Wasserman test for syphilis. The serological tests for syphilis present a special problem which will be discussed when that disease is considered.

In *summary* of the diagnostic aspects of bacterial infections we may say that **an immediate laboratory diagnosis of the nature of the infective agent has become of prime importance, so that appropriate antibiotic therapy may be started at the earliest possible moment.** The first step is gram-staining of the smears, which allows a preliminary classification before the final culture and sensitivity tests become available. An *exact* bacteriological diagnosis is far more necessary than formerly, because of the fact that microorganisms respond so differently to different chemotherapeutic agents.

TISSUE CHANGES. Different bacterial pathogens produce widely differing lesions. Some are focal, others diffuse, some are suppurative, others granulomatous, and so on. A general idea of the types of the infecting agent may be gathered from a consideration of the character and histological appearance of the lesions, but absolute certainty can only come from such bacteriological techniques as staining the organisms in smears or tissue, growing them in culture, reproducing the disease in an animal, or demonstrating the presence of immune bodies by appropriate serological methods.

Suppurative lesions are produced in the great majority of cases by one or other of the pyogenic cocci. When the suppuration remains *localized,* as so often happens with Staphylococcus aureus, the lesion takes the form of an abscess, with necrosis of tissue and collections of polymorphonuclear leukocytes (see Fig. 27, p. 104). *Diffuse* suppuration spreading through the interstitial tissue without abscess formation (cellulitis) is more likely to be caused by hemolytic streptococci (see Fig. 23, p. 98). *Granulomatous inflammation* is characterized by a histiocytic reaction without the participation of cells from the blood, the lesions often terminating in healing with fibrosis. This is the antithesis of pyogenic inflammation. The classic example is, of course, tuberculosis.

CHANGING PICTURE OF INFECTION.   Even under normal conditions life in the bacterial world is a constant intense competition for survival. The main function of the enzymes in the bacterial cell is to produce the protein needed for growth of the bacteria. *If the local environment becomes unfavorable, the power to mutate or to bring latent enzyme systems into play becomes apparent.* Modern conditions, and particularly the widespread *and often unnecessary use of antibiotics,* have greatly exaggerated this tendency. Resistance to the antibiotics is seen in most striking degree in the case of Staphylococcus aureus in relation to penicillin. In the Toronto General Hospital resistant strains of Staphylococcus aureus rose from 6 per cent in 1947 to 60 per cent four years later. We are now faced with the situation that our hospitals are filled with carriers of antibiotic-resistant strains of staphylococci ("hospital staph") in the nose and throat of both patients and staff, and the distance between the nose of a surgeon and an operation wound is very short. The incidence of penicillin-resistant staphylococci is much higher in hospital in-patients than out-patients, and it is still lower in the general population. Nature likes to maintain a biological balance, and this is true of the bacteriological field. A chemotherapeutic agent can displace the normal harmless flora of the throat, which are soon replaced by intestinal bacteria, also harmless in their proper habitat. In the new environment, however, they may cause serious local infections and even invasion of the blood stream. It is indeed a tragic paradox that the more an antibiotic is used (or abused) in a hospital community, the less valuable does it become. As we have already seen so frequently, what is potent for good can be powerful for evil, and *the wonder drugs may become harbingers of death.*

We must not suppose that this changing picture of bacterial infection is a new thing. **The incidence, character, and severity of microbic diseases may change from one generation to another.** This may be due to change in environmental conditions, to development of immunity in the population, or to the introduction of prophylactic measures such as vaccination against smallpox and toxoid inoculation against diphtheria. In many instances no good reason can be given. In such cases we may turn for an explanation to the natural tendency to mutation in the rapidly recurring generations of bacteria. Leprosy practically disappeared in England during the sixteenth century. Long before the modern era of chemotherapy syphilis had changed its character profoundly, and the mortality from tuberculosis had fallen steadily. It would appear that the changing picture of infection, although partly man-made, is also partly natural. We must admit, however, that the majority of fatal infections used to be produced by streptococci, staphylococci, and tubercle bacilli, originating in apparently healthy persons outside a hospital. Now the common culprits are gram-negative bacilli, staphylococci, viruses, and fungi.

Lest the picture presented above may be too depressing, we may recall that of the children born in London between 1762 and 1771, two-thirds died before the age of five years. This was in the century called the Age of Reason. There was certainly no danger of an exploding population. At the same period and in the same country Queen Anne had twelve pregnancies, but not one child survived—an example of effort unrewarded. Modern antibacterial therapy is one of the greatest benefits medicine has given to man.

STAPHYLOCOCCAL INFECTIONS

The staphylococcus is a gram-positive organism which grows in small clusters like a bunch of grapes (Fig. 32). There are two principal forms, Staphylococcus aureus (golden) and Staphylococcus albus (white), depending on the color of the colonies on solid media. The white form is always present on the skin, and is usually, though by no means always, harmless. It is the cause of the stitch abscesses of the skin which sometimes follow a surgical operation.

The staphylococcus is a pyogenic organism, a pus-producer, and is a common cause of acute inflammation. It enters the body through cracks in the skin often as the result of local irritation, such as the rubbing of a hard collar-stud on the neck. The mere pricking of a pimple may start the infection. *In contrast to streptococci, the staphylococcus usually produces inflammation which remains localized.* Some staphylococci produce an enzyme, *coagulase,* which causes a marked formation of fibrin from the fibrinogen of the plasma. *The coagulase-positive organisms are more dangerous, because the film of fibrin protects them from the action of antibodies and antibiotics.* The presence of this enzyme is the most reliable criterion of virulence. It must be admitted that the fibrin tends to limit the spread by blocking paths of dissemination. Some strains of staphylococci produce a "spreading factor" which markedly increases the permeability of the tissues. Certain strains have the power of forming an extremely powerful *exotoxin in culture.* The toxin can be detoxicated by the addition of formalin; the resulting product is a toxoid, which still retains its antigenic property and can be used to build up immunity to the infection. Staphylococci can survive dried in dust for many months. We have already seen that resistance to antibiotics is readily acquired, more especially in hospitals. *Penicillin-resistant strains always produce the enzyme, penicillinase, which destroys penicillin.* We must always remember that staphylococci are normal inhabitants of the body. They have been called the jackals of the microbial parasitic world, usually unable to mount an attack against the healthy body, but ready to invade the tissues when resistance is lowered by other disease states.

The chief lesions may be external or internal. **External lesions** occur in the following places: (1) *Skin pimples* are staphylococcal infections in the surface layer of the skin; *boils* are in the deeper layer; and a *carbuncle* is a large collection of pus in the subcutaneous tissue which communicates with the surface by several openings. *Infected wounds and stitch abscesses* are caused by staphylococci. (2) Boils on the *upper lip and nose* are of especial importance, as the infection is apt to pass back along the facial vein (which has no valves) into the cavernous venous sinus in the base of the skull, with a resulting *thrombophlebitis,* a condition of grave danger. (3) On the *eyelid* staphylococci may cause a *stye.* **Internal lesions** take the form of abscesses principally in the bones (osteomyelitis) and kidneys. Some persons, especially when young, are subject to repeated staphylococcal infections, particularly boils.

STREPTOCOCCAL INFECTIONS

The streptococcus is a gram-positive spherical organism identical in appearance with the staphylococcus except that it grows in chains of varying length instead of in clusters. (Fig. 32). It is more difficult to grow than the staphylococcus, and flourishes best on media enriched with blood (blood agar). Streptococci can be divided into two groups, depending on the reaction on blood agar. In the first group, *hemolytic streptococci,* the bacteria cause hemolysis or breaking down of blood in the medium, so that the colonies are surrounded by a pale colorless halo. In the second group the bacteria produce a green color on the blood agar, so that the group is called *Streptococcus viridans.* The hemolytic group causes much more acute and virulent infections than the viridans group. Streptococcus viridans is of low virulence and does not cause a sharp, acute reaction. Nevertheless it is an important cause of disease. It gives rise to focal or limited infection in the tonsils, at the roots of teeth, in the sinuses of the nose and face, and in the valves of the heart, where it causes subacute bacterial endocarditis, a condition that used to be uniformly fatal.

The habitat or natural home of the streptococcus is the mucous membrane of the respiratory and intestinal tracts. It is found less often on the skin. It tends to produce spreading inflammation which extends widely throughout the tissues in comparison with the circumscribed lesions caused by the staphylococcus. *This power of infiltration seems to depend largely on the power to produce fibrinolysin and hyaluronidase. Fibrinolysin* prevents the formation of fibrin and tends to dissolve any that has formed, thus eliminating the fibrin barrier to the spread of infection. *Hyaluronidase* is the enzyme which digests hyaluronic acid, the mucopolysaccharide of the ground substance that forms a natural obstacle in the interstitial compartment.

Some of the most widespread infections, such as septicemia and peritonitis, are caused by streptococci. It is the commonest cause of puerperal sepsis, the frequently fatal infection which used to follow childbirth. Most cases of septic throat, tonsillitis, and ear infections are due to streptococci.

Streptococcal infections may start in two different ways: (1) Cocci already present on the mucous membrane may invade the underlying tissue owing to some lowering of resistance. It is in this way that tonsillitis, streptococcal pneumonia, and appendicitis may be produced. (2) Virulent streptococci may be introduced from outside the body through the skin or mucous membrane. It is in this way that a surgeon's hand may be infected while operating on a septic case, or that the uterus may be infected owing to lack of care during or after labor.

Two manifestations of streptococcal infection are of so special a character that they merit separate descriptions; they are erysipelas and scarlet fever. Two others, namely rheumatic fever and glomerulonephritis, are sequelae not caused by the streptococcus pyogenes directly, but representing an immunological response to hypersensitivity byproducts. The former will be described here, the latter in connection with diseases of the kidney.

ERYSIPELAS. This is an acute spreading *inflammation of the lymphatics of the skin* caused by hemolytic streptococci with marked erythrogenic (rash-producing) power. The usual site is the face or scalp, the bacteria probably entering from the nose. The inflamed skin is of a bright red color and curiously firm. Like other streptococcal and staphylococcal infections it is accompanied by fever and an increase in the leukocytes of the blood (leukocytosis).

SCARLET FEVER.   Scarlet fever is an acute streptococcal fever characterized by *a high temperature, sore throat, and a widespread rash, often followed by complications in the ear, kidneys, and lymph nodes of the neck*. The throat is always actively inflamed, and this is probably the starting point of the infection, which may spread along the eustachian tube (the communication between the throat and ear) and cause acute inflammation of the ear. The lymph nodes of the neck are swollen, and sometimes abscesses are formed in them. The tongue shows a rash like that of the skin, so that it has a strawberry appearance (*strawberry tongue*).

The symptoms are caused by the erythrogenic toxin of the streptococcus. This toxin is used in the *Dick test* for susceptibility to scarlet fever. The diluted toxin is injected into the skin, and the appearance of a red area in the course of a few hours shows that the patient has no natural antitoxin in his blood, *i.e.,* he is susceptible to scarlet fever. In early childhood nearly everyone shows a positive reaction, but with increasing years the number of susceptible individuals steadily decreases, owing to the fact that most persons are exposed to infection too slight in degree to cause the disease but sufficient to stimulate the formation of antitoxin.

RHEUMATIC FEVER.   Rheumatic fever is an acute infection affecting principally the joints and the heart, and accompanied by sore throat. It is difficult to speak with certainty as to its cause, but it may be regarded as a manifestation of infection with group A hemolytic streptococci, which are located in the throat or tonsils. These bacteria are not found, at least in any numbers, in the organs attacked by rheumatic fever, such as the joints and the heart. It is assumed, therefore, that *these organs have become hypersensitive or allergic to the streptococci, a chemical group in the organisms uniting with connective tissue protein to create an antigen. This in turn excites the formation of specific antibodies, the reaction of the two resulting in a focal allergic necrosis accompanied by a characteristic cellular response.* This is the type of interaction that we have already studied in relation to autoimmunity in the preceding chapter.

We must not rest satisfied with the above account, for we have not explained why only a few individuals show the rheumatic response to streptococcal infection, and why 75 per cent of the cases occur in children or at least before the age of twenty years. There appear to be one or more unknown factors. The incidence of rheumatic fever parallels in a striking manner the incidence of hemolytic streptococci in the throat. Both are common in cold, damp climates, but rare in many parts of the tropics. Both are common in the children of the poor, but rare in the children of the wealthy. The elusive factor may be a vitamin or other food deficiency.

The invariable presence of *C-reactive protein* in the serum in acute rheumatic fever, while the reaction is completely negative in normal persons, provides a valuable laboratory test, but it is of course in no way specific for rheumatic disease. The name comes from the fact that the blood of patients with pneumococcal pneumonia contains a protein which reacts with the carbohydrate (hence the *C*) of the pneumococcus to form a precipitate.

The most striking and obvious *clinical feature* is acute inflammation of the *joints,* which become so exquisitely tender that the slightest movement of the joint produces excruciating pain. Nevertheless the inflammation is not a suppurative one, there is little destruction of tissue, and when the infection subsides the joints return to their normal condition. The acute joint symptoms such as swelling and pain are greatly relieved by the use of sodium salicylate, which is practically a specific remedy for this infection.

The same is not true, however, of the *heart.* During the acute illness there may be no evidence of any cardiac lesion, but months or years later symptoms of these lesions may make their appearance. Rheumatic fever is the commonest cause of heart disease. Both the heart valves and the heart muscle are attacked, but the lesions need not be described here, as they will be considered in connection with diseases of the heart. The characteristic microscopic lesion is the *Aschoff body,* marked by fibrinoid necrosis (p. 122) and collections of large chronic inflammatory cells. It is evident that the heart lesions of rheumatic fever are much more serious than the joint lesions, although it is the latter that first claim the attention of the patient and the doctor. For this reason one of the important elements in the treatment of rheumatic fever is prolonged rest in bed, so that the affected heart may have every chance of recovering to the greatest extent possible. Moreover in some persons, particularly in children, the inflammation in the joints may be so slight that the disease is not diagnosed as rheumatic fever, yet the heart may be seriously affected. Patients with rheumatic heart disease may therefore give a history of repeated sore throats, but not of acute joint pains. From all this the truth of the saying becomes apparent that *"rheumatic fever licks the joints, but bites the heart."*

Rheumatic fever may belong to the group known as the *collagen diseases,* other members of the group being disseminated lupus erythematosus, polyarteritis nodosa, and rheumatoid arthritis. Collagen is another name for the connective tissue of the body, and the chief characteristic of the collagen diseases is degeneration and necrosis of connective tissue fibers and of the ground substance or cement which binds them together. The lesions are found chiefly in the vascular system (heart and arteries), the joints, the serous membranes, and the skin. The lesions are controlled to a remarkable degree by cortisone, one of the hormones of the adrenal cortex, or by ACTH, the pituitary hormone which stimulates the production of cortisone.

The *treatment* of rheumatic fever consists of a combination of skilled nursing and drug therapy. During an attack of acute rheumatic fever damage may occur to the heart valves and to the heart muscle, and may progress unrecognized at first. During the period in which any activity of the rheumatic process is suspected the patient should be kept at rest in bed until the signs of the acute stage are past. This may require many weeks or months. The use of salicylates, and more recently of cortisone, during this acute phase relieves the symptoms and may prevent some of the progress of the disease. The great value of rest lies in the fact that the greater the strain on the heart the longer will the inflammation take to subside and the greater will be the subsequent damage to the valves and heart muscle. But this does not mean that rest must be prolonged indefinitely; as the heart muscle recovers from exhaustion and resumes its tone, graduated exercise can be resumed and soon the patient may be able to live a normal life again.

PNEUMOCOCCAL INFECTIONS

The pneumococcus is a gram-positive diplococcus surrounded by a polysaccharide capsule. It is a pyogenic organism, with a marked ability to excite the formation of fibrin. The chief lesion produced is lobar pneumonia, and the pulmonary alveoli are filled with an exudate composed mainly of pus cells and fibrin. Other lesions caused by pneumococci are endocarditis, pericarditis, peritonitis in children, meningitis, and middle-ear suppuration.

MENINGOCOCCAL INFECTION

We now turn from the gram-positive to the gram-negative cocci, that is to say, the Neisseria. The two members of the group which concern us are *Neisseria meningitidis* and *Neisseria gonorrhoeae*. They resemble one another morphologically as closely as the proverbial two peas. In addition to being gram-negative, they are bean-shaped diplococci with the convex surfaces opposed. Both the meningococcus and the gonococcus are found in large numbers within the polymorphonuclears of the pus, an environment in which unfortunately they seem to flourish (Fig. 33).

The *meningococcus* is a normal inhabitant (commensal) of the nasopharynx, and in times of epidemic as many as 90 per cent of persons in a crowded army camp may carry the germ. It does not grow at all readily on culture media. The meningococcus is extremely sensitive to sulfonamides and a wide range of antibiotics, and it is pleasant to learn

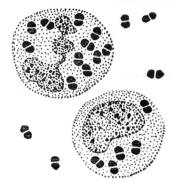

Fig. 33. Meningococci, mostly intracellular.

that, unlike the case of the staphylococcus, acquired resistance is unknown. If infection reaches the meninges from the nasopharynx by passing along the sheath of the olfactory nerves, an *acute meningococcal meningitis* is set up. **The bacteriological diagnosis is made by examining the cerebrospinal fluid, obtained by lumbar puncture, for the tell-tale gram-negative intracellular diplococci. The disease used to be frequently fatal, but modern chemotherapy has entirely altered the prognosis.** The lesions and clinical features of meningococcal meningitis are described in the chapter on the nervous system.

GONOCOCCAL INFECTION

In physical appearance and staining characters the gonococcus is the split image of the meningococcus, but we could not get a better example of the truth that *things are not always what they seem.* It is still harder to grow in culture than the meningococcus; when allowed to dry it dies immediately when removed from the body; *it is a complete parasite living on a human host;* and it does not live in the body as a harmless commensal. With these facts in mind it is perhaps surprising that the gonococcus manages to hold its place in the natural world, but that it does succeed is only too evident.

With two exceptions to be mentioned below, gonococcal infection is essentially a venereal disease, being transmitted through sexual intercourse. The initial site of infection is the mucous membrane of the anterior urethra in the male, and the urethra, vaginal glands, and cervix in the female. Once the gonococcus reaches the male or female genital tract, it makes itself at home. The initial process is an acute suppuration developing in a few days after infection, with a copious discharge of pus loaded with intracellular gonococci. *If prompt and effective treatment is given, the discharge disappears like magic and the infection clears up.*

The *untreated* case is quite a different matter. The inflammation becomes chronic, spreading upward and followed by fibrosis. This leads to stricture of the urethra and stenosis of the vas deferens in the male causing sterility, whereas in the female the Fallopian tubes are closed and converted into bags of pus, with sterility again an inevitable result.

As already mentioned, the infection may be nonvenereal in two instances. (1) *Ophthalmia neonatorum* is a gonorrheal conjunctivitis of the newborn, the infection being conveyed from a gonorrheal mother to her child at the time of delivery. This used to be an important cause of blindness in children before the days of the local application of penicillin and silver compounds to the eyes of the newborn. (2) *Epidemic vulvovaginitis* spreads by nonvenereal contact in girls' institutions, because the gonococcus can gain a ready hold in the vagina before it becomes lined by dense epithelium at the age of puberty.

The *treatment* of gonorrhea is still an important public health problem. When the sulfonamides were first introduced the gonococcus proved to be so susceptible that it seemed as if the disease might be completely eliminated, especially in view of the fact that the organism is unable to live outside the body. Soon, however, most strains became resistant. Penicillin took the place of the sulfonamides with complete success, but again the sad story of resistant strains was repeated. Then came streptomycin, but the gonococci proved as resourceful as ever. Yet they had now again become sensitive to the sulfonamides. And so the battle of attack and defense continues with varying fortune.

DIPHTHERIA

The diphtheria or Klebs-Loeffler bacillus (*Corynebacterium diphtheriae*) is a thin gram-positive bacillus, often slightly curved. It stains irregularly with methylene blue, some parts appearing dark while others remain light; for this reason the bacilli may have a granular appearance. There is apt to be pleomorphism, *i.e.,* variation in structure, and some of the bacilli may have an expanded end, giving an Indian-club appearance (Fig. 34). The bacilli are easily stained and easily grown in culture within 24 hours. Loeffler's blood serum (solid) is the standard medium for this purpose. Under the microscope the bacilli present an arrangement that suggests a box of spilt matches.

Unlike many of the other pathogenic bacteria the diphtheria bacillus does not invade the tissues of the patient. *It remains on the surface of the mucous membrane of the throat and produces a powerful exotoxin which kills the cells with which it comes in contact.* It also excites a plentiful production of fibrin. The dead or necrosed cells are not shed off, but are bound together by the threads of fibrin to form a tough leathery layer known as the *false membrane,* so-called because

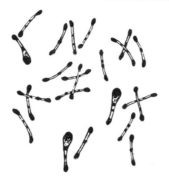

Fig. 34. Diphtheria bacilli showing granules and Indian clubs.

it is not one of the natural or true membranes of the body. The name diphtheria is from the Greek meaning leather. Sometimes the nose and rarely the ear, conjunctiva of the eye, and even wounds may be affected. In each of these instances a diphtheritic (false) membrane is formed, which is swarming with bacilli. The incubation period is two to seven days.

The danger to the patient is twofold: (1) he may die of suffocation owing to the false membrane obstructing the air-passages, especially the glottis; (2) the toxin may be absorbed into the blood and cause paralysis either of the heart or of the peripheral nerves.

Infection may be *spread* directly, *i.e.,* from person to person, or indirectly by infected articles such as cups, handkerchiefs, and even books. Direct infection may be from a patient, but often it is from a healthy carrier, *i.e.,* a person carrying diphtheria bacilli in his throat but not suffering from the disease; often, indeed, he has never had a previous clinical attack, but he has established a complete immunity, presumably from a subclinical infection.

Immunity against diphtheria may be natural or artificial. About 85 per cent of nursing babies have natural immunity which comes from the mother. This disappears after eight months. Most children are therefore susceptible, and 80 per cent of the deaths occur under five years of age. Susceptibility can be shown by means of the *Schick test.* A minute quantity of diphtheria toxin is injected into the skin. If a red area develops, the person is susceptible to diphtheria. If it does not, he is immune, because his blood contains antitoxin which neutralizes toxins. Susceptible children can be immunized by means of diphtheria *toxoid.* This is diphtheria toxin which has been rendered harmless by the addition of formalin. The immunity is of variable duration, but usually lasts for several years. These procedures are of value both for persons who have been exposed to infection and for children during an outbreak of diphtheria. *It can be stated with confidence that the use of toxoid in conjunction with the Schick test has placed in the hands of the physician a weapon with which diphtheria can be finally eradicated, and has been in many communities.*

WHOOPING COUGH

Whooping cough or *pertussis* is caused by a minute gram-negative bacillus, which is found in great masses entangled in the cilia of the bronchial mucosa. It is known as *Hemophilus pertussis,* because it belongs to the group of hemophilic bacilli, so-named because they require hemoglobin for growth in the culture medium. Another member of the group is *H. influenzae,* poorly named for the reason that it was thought at one time to be the cause of influenza, but is now known to be a common inhabitant of the nasopharynx, which invades the lung when resistance is lowered by virus infections such as influenza and measles. The laboratory diagnosis of *H. pertussis* is made by means of a "cough plate"; the patient coughs onto a plate of blood agar, and this is examined next day for colonies of bacilli.

Whooping cough is a far more dangerous and widespread disease than is generally recognized. The mortality rate for whooping cough is higher than for measles, scarlet fever, and even typhoid fever. It is the pulmonary complications that follow on the initial infection which are responsible for the deaths, and it is the subacute and chronic inflammations of the lung that lead to prolonged illness and pave the way for tuberculosis.

As with diphtheria, it is children who are in danger. About 33 per cent of the cases and 90 per cent of the deaths occur in children under three years of age.

The disease tends to come in periodic epidemics, especially in early spring and late summer. Susceptibility seems to be almost universal. Transmission is either direct, from a sick person to a healthy one, or by the common use of freshly contaminated utensils.

TUBERCULOSIS

Tuberculosis is a chronic inflammation caused by Bacillus tuberculosis (*Mycobacterium tuberculosis*), and is one of the most widespread of all diseases. Among the poorer classes of the large cities it is hardly too much to say that after middle life nearly everyone shows evidence of having had tuberculous infection. This is not the same as saying that they are suffering from the disease. The lesions may be extremely small and quiescent, and the presence of the infection may only be demonstrable by means of laboratory tests, but it is there nonetheless, and the sword of Damocles hangs over the unsuspecting victim's head, occasionally falling where living conditions are unfavorable. *It is evident that the natural defensive power of the body against tuberculous infection is sufficiently great to hold it in check in the majority of cases,* This defense may be broken down on the one hand by an infection such as influenza which undermines the health, by overwork, poor hygienic conditions, insufficient food, etc., and on the other hand by a fresh overwhelming dose of tubercle bacilli. The long-continued use of cortisone, as in rheumatoid arthritis, may not only disguise the symptoms, but depress resistance and activate the disease.

The *tubercle bacillus* is a thin curved rod which does not grow on the ordinary culture media. It can be stained in a specific way, being colored red by carbol fuchsin and retaining the color after treatment by acid which removes the color from other bacteria. Bacteria with this property are called *acid-fast,* a rather misleading term which really means acid-resisting. They are coated with a sheath of waxy material, and it is this sheath that prevents the acid removing the red fuchsin, whereas other bacteria not so protected lose their color. Another example of an acid-fast organism is the bacillus of leprosy. *On account of its waxy sheath the tubercle bacillus is an exceptionally hardy germ. It may live outside the body for six months if not exposed to sunlight.* Direct sunlight, however, will kill it in a few hours, a fact of obvious importance in the prevention of spread of the disease.

The laboratory diagnosis is made by direct microscopic examination of the infected material (sputum, urine, etc.) rather than by culture as is done with most bacteria, because the bacilli do not grow readily on culture media and several weeks may need to elapse before the colonies can be seen. Inoculation of a susceptible animal such as a guinea pig is also of great value, but again several weeks must pass before the animal develops evidence of the disease. There are two forms of tubercle bacilli, the human and bovine, the latter causing disease in cows as well as in man. They are identical under the microscope, but can be differentiated by special culture methods and by the inoculation of animals.

Tuberculosis used to head the list of the killing diseases, so that Osler called it the "Captain of the Men of Death." During the nineteenth century, man slew on the battlefield 19 million persons, but during the same period the tubercle bacillus slew 34 millions. The disease is steadily becoming less common as well as less dangerous, and in some communities tuberculosis sanatoria are being closed for lack of patients. These facts must not breed a spirit of false complacency, for it is estimated that at the present time there are 30,000,000 infected persons in the United States, and that 2,000,000 of these will develop active tuberculosis in their lifetime. It used to kill the young adult; now it is often seen in the aged. The reduction in the tuberculosis rate is due to the following factors: (1) improved social living conditions with better nutrition, fresh air, and sunlight; (2) education in hygiene, so that people lead more healthful lives as regards exercise and fresh air; (3) segregation of the sick in sanatoria and destruction of tuberculous sputum; (4) people seek medical advice earlier; and (5) improved methods of treatment.

METHODS OF INFECTION. In trying to prevent a disease it is essential to know the method of infection. In the case of tuberculosis infection may occur in a number of ways:

1. *By Inhalation.* The only likely source of infection from man is the sputum of a patient with tuberculosis of the lungs. There is practically no danger of infection from tuberculosis of any other organ. The bacilli may be inhaled from sputum which has dried and been changed into dust. They are soon killed by sunlight, but may survive a long time in the dark. When a patient with pulmonary tuberculosis coughs he infects the air in the immediate neighborhood with millions of tubercle bacilli contained in tiny drops of moisture. It has been estimated that a moderately advanced case may expel from 2 to 4 billion bacilli in twenty-four hours. This gives some idea of the infectivity of such a patient. This is probably the most important method of infection in the adult, for the "dose" of bacilli will be much larger than in the case of inhaled dust, and a large dose has much to do with breaking down the resistance of the exposed person. It is evident how vitally important it is to instruct the patient with pulmonary tuberculosis how to conduct himself so that he will not be a source of danger to those with whom he comes in contact. Attention to certain rules of hygiene, which are also rules of polite behavior, such as coughing into a handkerchief and never expectorating on the floor, remove practically all the danger from living in close contact with a patient suffering from active tuberculosis. *The technique of prevention, however, must be as unremitting and relentless as the similar technique in an operating room.* Bacilli may also be inhaled from the mouth into the lungs in minute droplets of fluid. It is probable that many children become infected through the introduction of bacilli into the mouth by contaminated hands followed by inhalation into the lungs. The danger to a child crawling about the floor on which tuberculous sputum has been expectorated is self-evident. There are thus three principal methods of infection by inhalation, *e.g.,* dust infection, droplet infection, and mouth infection.

2. *By Swallowing.* Children may readily acquire tuberculosis by drinking infected cow's milk. Here, of course, the bacillus is of the bovine type, and the lesions are naturally abdominal, either in the bowel or in the abdominal lymph nodes. But the nodes in the neck may also

be infected by bacilli passing through the tonsils. The amount of infection with the bovine tubercle bacillus in a community depends on the strictness of the milk inspection. The danger of milk infection is greatest in the first five years of life, and remains marked to the age of sixteen. It is comparatively slight in adults, who are relatively insusceptible to bovine infection. The importance of the rigid sanitary control of milk supplies to children is self-evident.

3. *Through the Skin.* Although this method is rare it is of importance to the laboratory technician and the nurse, because the disease may be acquired through the handling of infected material. A warty lesion develops on the hand, and the infection may spread up the arm to the lymph nodes in the axilla, but there is little danger of general infection or infection of the lungs.

METHODS OF SPREAD. The tubercle bacillus is like the streptococcus, as it causes a spreading infection and may invade the blood stream. The infection may spread in three ways: (1) *Through the tissues.* In the organ infected, unless the defense forces gain the mastery, the disease gradually spreads until the greater part of that organ is destroyed. (2) *By the lymphatics.* The bacilli tend to spread from the site of infection along the lymphatic vessels to the lymph nodes that drain the part, where they set up tuberculous disease. Thus the nodes in the neck are infected from the tonsil, the nodes in the chest from the lung, the abdominal nodes from the bowel. (3) *By the blood stream.* A breaking-down tuberculous lesion may perforate the wall of a vessel and discharge millions of bacilli into the blood stream. These are arrested in every organ in the body, where they cause the formation of numberless minute lesions the size of a pin's head; these are called miliary tubercles and the condition is known as generalized *miliary tuberculosis.* In addition to this massive infection, occasional bacilli may enter the blood stream and set up a single tuberculous focus in one organ such as kidney or bone.

LESIONS. Tuberculosis is a chronic inflammation. *The characteristic cell of the inflammatory exudate is the macrophage, which becomes changed in character so that it has a swollen pale body and indefinite outlines.* These characteristics are due to the fact that the fatty envelope of the bacilli is dissolved and taken up by the cells, which in their new form are called *epithelioid cells* (epithelial-like) and are the most characteristic single feature of the tuberculous reaction. The bacilli are surrounded by a mass of these cells, which are actively phagocytic. Sometimes a number of epithelioid cells fuse together to form a large *giant cell,* with as many nuclei as there are cells concerned with its formation. Further out there is a zone of *lymphocytes,* also called small round cells. The lymphocytes are one of the principal sources of the gamma globu-

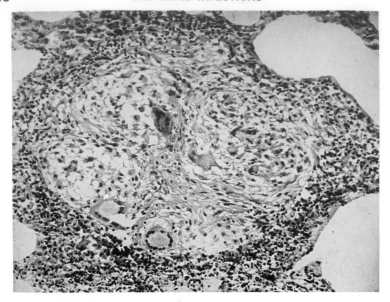

Fig. 35. A miliary tubercle in the lung, showing epithelioid cells, giant cells, and peripheral lymphocytes. × 150. (Boyd, *Textbook of Pathology;* Lea & Febiger.)

lins, which constitute the immune bodies. *There is none of the dilatation of blood vessels nor exudation of serum that is so characteristic of acute inflammation, and for this reason the heat and redness of acute inflammation are also absent.*

The collection of inflammatory cells around the clump of tubercle bacilli forms a little mass which becomes visible to the naked eye and is called a *tubercle* or *miliary tubercle* (*milium,* a millet seed) (Fig. 35). This is the standard lesion of tuberculosis, and is found in whichever organ the disease occurs, be it lung, kidney, or brain. Indeed, it is the tubercle that originally gave the disease its name. As the bacilli spread throughout the organ large numbers of tubercles are formed, and these grow ever larger, fuse together, and thus come to form extensive tuberculous areas.

Meanwhile a further change takes place in the center of the tubercle. The cells are killed by the bacilli, undergo necrosis, and finally lose all vestige of structure and fuse together to form a cheesy mass which is called caseous (cheesy) material, the process being known as *caseation.* In the course of time the caseous material may become liquefied, so that a cavity or cavities are formed in the organ.

Practically every organ of the body may be involved by tuberculosis. It is exceptional, however, for more than one or two organs to be attacked at the same time, except in general miliary tuberculosis. Although such a bone as the femur must necessarily be infected from the blood stream, it is nevertheless unusual for other bones to be involved in the same case. It is difficult to give a satisfactory explanation for this behavior.

The *lungs* and *pleura* are most frequently attacked, and pulmonary disease accounts for 85 to 90 per cent of all deaths from tuberculosis. *Lymph nodes* come next, most often those in the neck, less frequently the abdominal nodes. Tuberculosis of the *larynx* is a serious form, secondary to pulmonary tuberculosis. The *intestine* may be the seat of tuberculous ulcers, due in children to the drinking of infected milk, in adults to the swallowing of tuberculous sputum. The bacilli may spread from these ulcers to the *peritoneum* and cause tuberculous peritonitis. Tuberculosis of the *kidney* is not uncommon, and it tends to spread down to the *bladder,* and in the male may infect the *prostate* and *testes.* In the female the *Fallopian tubes* are often infected, a condition known as tuberculous salpingitis. The *bones* and *joints* are often involved, especially in children; in the *spine* the condition is called Pott's disease. Tuberculous *meningitis* is the most fatal form, although chemotherapy has now greatly changed the former gloomy picture. Other organs may also be attacked, but the above-named are the commonest.

The microscopic picture in tuberculosis is characteristic and readily recognized, but it must be borne in mind that a histological diagnosis of the disease is only presumptive. *Other conditions may present a similar or even identical microscopic picture, for example sarcoidosis, syphilis, and other conditions we shall study.*

POSSIBLE OUTCOME.   Tuberculosis is a fight in which the forces of attack and defense, of destruction and conservation, are usually fairly evenly balanced. *The outcome depends on two main factors, the resistance of the tissues and the size of dose of the bacilli.* If the resistance is good and the dose small there is a proliferation of fibrous tissue around the tubercle which limits the spread of the infection and eventually invades the tubercle and converts it into a mass of scar tissue known as a *healed tubercle.* This process of encapsulation and scarring is seen particularly well in the lung, and may occur even when the tuberculous area is of considerable size. Tuberculous scars are commonly found at the apex of the lung, and these scars often contain calcium which is deposited in the caseous material as healing occurs, and which can be detected in the roentgenogram. Healing of the tuberculous lesion is by far the most common outcome.

When the dose of bacilli is larger or the resistance of the patient is lowered by overwork and other causes, the disease tends to progress slowly, but fibrous tissue formation is continually going on, so that the destruction of tissue is gradual, and the process may be halted after it has lasted for a long time. Halting, however, is not synonymous with recovery, and unless the patient pays strict attention to the rules of hygiene the process may light up again, with recurrence of the severe symptoms. He is metaphorically sitting on a barrel of gunpowder and he must not forget that fact.

Finally, the infection may be overwhelming and resistance at a minimum. In these cases there is almost pure destruction with practically no attempt at limitation; the disease rages like a fire throughout the lung, huge cavities are formed, and the patient dies in the course of a few weeks or months. These are the cases which used to be popularly and justifiably known as galloping consumption.

Though particular mention has been made of the lung, because it is the organ most commonly attacked by tuberculosis, it will be understood that the same variations of the disease may occur in any organ with the same caseation, cavity formation, fibrosis, calcification, and so on. When we think about these varied possibilities it becomes obvious that nothing could be more different from the story in, say, infection by the pyogenic cocci, thus illustrating the difference between an essentially acute and an essentially chronic type of infection.

Many years ago Osler illustrated the possible outcome in tuberculosis by reference to the parable of the sower. "Some seeds fell by the way-side, and the fowls of the air came and destroyed them"; these are the bacilli that are scattered broadcast from an infectious case, but few are inhaled by other persons, and the majority of these bacilli die. "Some fell on stony places"; these bacilli fail to grow in immune persons, or form only small lesions that wither away "because they have no root." "Some fell among thorns"; these seeds grow, but the protecting forces serve to choke them. "But others fell on good ground and sprang up and bore fruit a hundredfold"; these are the cases in which the dose is overwhelming and resistance at a minimum.

TREATMENT AND PREVENTION. The *treatment* of tuberculosis, whether of the lung or elsewhere, has been revolutionized by a combination of streptomycin, isoniazid, and para-aminosalicylic acid. The great value of *isoniazid* is that it penetrates the large phagocytes within which the bacilli lurk, and it crosses the barrier that separates the blood from the brain (blood-brain barrier), so that *it is invaluable in the treatment of tuberculous meningitis, which used to be so extremely fatal. The bacilli easily acquire resistance to the individual drugs, but combinations of the drugs are remarkably effective.*

Prevention rather than treatment is of course the ideal method of controlling a disease that used to be such a scourge. Nothing could be done before Koch first showed that tuberculosis was a bacterial disease and therefore infective. There are two sources of infection: the human patient with pulmonary tuberculosis and infected cows' milk (bovine infection). The latter, which used to be of special importance in children, can be combated by the testing of dairy cows with tuberculin, by pasteurization of milk, and by other public health measures. Spread of infection from the patient can be prevented by careful disposal of the sputum, and education in the dangers of unguarded coughing and spitting. Tubercle bacilli can live outside the body as long as they have food and moisture and are protected from direct sunlight. Under these conditions they may survive for months. Sputum cups that can be burned are preferable. If these are not available, the regular cups and their contents should be boiled for ten minutes. Gauze used for the collection of sputum can be burned. If the patient does not go to a sanatorium, the other members of the household should undergo a periodic check-up by the tuberculin test and roentgenographic examination for the development of infection.

With such an insidious disease as pulmonary tuberculosis it is not possible to be certain that all danger of infection has been eliminated. Now we have a method of immunizing those most likely to be exposed to infection, such as children, nurses, and hospital employees, by inoculation with *B.C.G.* This is short for the Bacille-Calmette-Guérin vaccine, which is a *bovine strain* of tubercle bacillus rendered avirulent by prolonged culture on special media. The bacilli, which are living, have lost all power of producing disease, but when injected they still have an immunizing power against infection with a virulent strain. It is a remarkable fact that the method was introduced as long ago as 1922 by the French bacteriologist Calmette as a means of protecting infants born into tuberculous families, but the method did not gain general favor by reason of the fear of injecting a live culture. This fear has proved to be groundless. The reader will recognize that the principle is similar to that of the oral (Sabin) vaccine for protection against poliomyelitis (p. 182), and that it is related to toxoid immunization against diphtheria. Isoniazid has also proved of great value in protecting persons who live in household contact with an open case of tuberculosis.

LEPROSY

The reader of this book will almost certainly never see a case of leprosy. So why include it here? Because of the fascinating bacteriological problems it presents. The disease is caused by *Mycobacterium leprae,* an acid-fast bacillus almost identical in appearance with the tubercle bacillus. It is remarkable to learn that it was discovered by Hansen as long ago as 1874, or eight years before Koch discovered the tubercle bacillus, yet proof of a causal relationship between the organism and the disease was never really

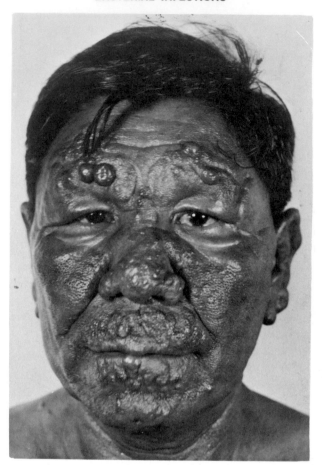

Fig. 36. Leprosy. A striking example of the nodular form, with multiple nodules in the skin. (Kindness of Dr. George L. Fite, Carville, La.; Boyd's *Textbook of Pathology.*)

established, because the disease could not be reproduced in the usual laboratory animals nor grown on culture media. Now at last a breakthrough has been achieved, and the lesions have been reproduced in the golden hamster and the organisms grown slowly on special media.

The reason that the lepra bacillus is assumed to be the cause of leprosy is that the skin lesions are simply teeming with these organisms. This would agree with the dread reputation that the disease enjoyed in the Middle Ages and in still earlier times. The leper was provided with a large bell, which he had to ring when passing through a village so that the inhabitants could shun him, nor was he allowed to enter a church to partake of mass. All this suggests a marked infectivity and a high virulence. The opposite is the case. A tissue may be swarming with bacilli, yet show no obvious change, the disease may remain latent for twenty years, and nurses and doctors in charge of leper colonies are seldom infected. The explanation may be that over the centuries the bacilli have slowly lost their virulence, although not their power of spreading slowly through the body and producing marked deformities. Leprosy is now largely confined to hot moist climates, more than 1 per cent of the population of Central Africa and of the west coast of India suffering from the disease.

Two main forms of the disease are recognized, the one characterized by skin nodules, the other by anesthetic patches, although the two are often combined. The *nodular form* is marked by the development of nodules and larger masses in the skin of the fingers, face (Fig. 36), and elsewhere, as well as in the liver, spleen, and other organs. The nodules ulcerate, and it is the ulceration and subsequent scarring that is responsible for the horrible deformities, with loss, it may be, of fingers, nose or ear, which has given the disease its fearsome reputation. In the *anesthetic form* the infection involves the peripheral nerves, which become greatly thickened and finally destroyed, thus producing areas of anesthesia in the skin. Sulfones and thiosemicarbazones make the open ulcerating cases noninfective in the course of two years.

SYPHILIS

Syphilis, like tuberculosis, is a chronic inflammatory disease of long duration, but differs in being one of the venereal diseases. It is acquired by contact with a syphilitic lesion in a patient suffering from the disease, usually but by no means invariably during sexual intercourse, so that the first lesions to appear are on the genital organs. Sometimes, however, the primary lesion may appear on the fingers as in the case of a doctor examining a syphilitic patient, or on the lip from kissing an infected mouth.

BACTERIOLOGY. Although syphilis has been the subject of study for hundreds of years, our modern knowledge of the disease is based on three great discoveries that were made in the course of five years at the beginning of the twentieth century, for its cause was discovered in 1905 by Schaudinn, an invaluable test for its presence was introduced by Wassermann in 1906, and a specific treatment in the form of arsenic ("606") was given to the world by Ehrlich in 1910.

The *cause* of syphilis is a delicate spiral-shaped organism, *Treponema pallidum,* formerly called Spirochaeta pallida. It cannot be grown on any of the ordinary culture media nor stained by ordinary staining methods. It is best demonstrated by the dark-field method, in which a special attachment to the microscope enables the organisms to be seen as bright white threads against a dark background (Fig. 37). The early lesions, both on the genital organs and in the mouth, contain enormous numbers of treponemata (still commonly referred to as spirochetes), so that

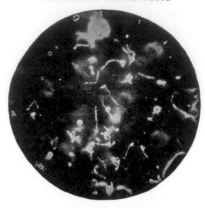

Fig. 37. Treponema pallidum as they appear under the dark-field microscope.
× 600.

these lesions are highly infectious. The pale spirochete resembles the gonococcus in being unable to survive outside the body.

Immunology.   A patient suffering from syphilis is immune to reinfection. This immunity, which becomes established as soon as the primary lesion develops, is associated with the appearance of two distinct antibodies in the serum, namely syphilitic reagin and treponema-immobilizing antibody. *Reagin* is a substance normally present in the plasma in small amount associated with gamma globulin. It reacts like antibody with certain extracts of normal tissues. In syphilis reagin is very greatly increased in amount, as a result of the interaction of the treponema with tissue, and this forms the basis of the complement fixation (Wassermann) and the precipitin (Kahn) reactions. The *complement fixation test* is a method for demonstrating a pathological increase of reagin, using an antigen-like lipid substance present in bovine heart muscle and other tissues. There are now various modifications of the Wassermann such as the Kolmer, Kline, and Eagle, but they are often still referred to as the Wassermann reaction (WR). The technique, by means of which "fixation" of complement is recognized to have taken place, is outlined in the previous chapter (p. 114). It will be seen that the Wassermann is in no sense a specific test for syphilis, because a syphilitic antigen is not used, but fortunately it works in practice. The *Kahn* and the *VDRL (Venereal Disease Research Laboratory) precipitation* or *flocculation tests* are also nonspecific, depending on the production of a precipitate by the interaction of an increased amount of reagin (antibody) with a tissue antigen containing lipid. Precipitation tests are more sensitive in treated cases, so that the VDRL test may be positive when the WR has become negative.

The *treponema-immobilization (TPI) test,* unlike the complement fixation and precipitation methods, is a specific test for a true syphilitic antibody. Living spirochetes from the testis of a rabbit are immobilized and finally killed by serum from a patient with syphilis as shown by dark-field microscopy. The test is considerably more reliable than the ordinary reagin reactions, but unfortunately at the present time it is too highly specialized a procedure to be a practicable routine method like the VDRL test with its rapid slide flocculation technique.

Finally it must be emphasized that in all laboratory tests for syphilis the results of a wrong report are so far-reaching and disastrous that the most meticulous care is needed not only in the performance of the test, but also in the collection and labeling of the sample of blood.

NATURAL HISTORY OF THE DISEASE. Syphilis seems to have lost much of its virulence since it was first introduced into Europe by the sailors of Christopher Columbus returning from the New World. At that time it swept through Italy like a pestilence, so that it came to be called *lues* (a plague), the name by which it is still known at the present day. This is another example of the natural changing picture of disease, such as we have already seen in the case of leprosy. Until recently, however, syphilis has still remained one of the most common and important diseases in the world. It has now fallen from its high estate because of treatment with penicillin, and the late manifestations, particularly those due to involvement of the central nervous system, are rapidly becoming a thing of the past. *At the same time it must not be thought that syphilis is no longer to be feared, and it is already beginning to raise its ugly head.*

What may be called the natural history of the disease is peculiar and highly interesting, and can be divided into three stages known as primary, secondary, and tertiary. For three or four weeks after infection the person feels perfectly well and shows no evidence of the disease. Then a lesion known as the **primary sore** or **chancre** appears at the site of infection. It takes the form of a curiously hard nodule, quite painless, which may become ulcerated, enormous numbers of spirochetes being discharged from the raw surface. The lesion consists of masses of chronic inflammatory cells, with no sign of acute inflammation. In the course of a few weeks it heals and may or may not leave a tell-tale scar. The regional lymph nodes, *i.e.,* those that drain the part, are enlarged and hard in the primary stage. Usually these are the nodes in the groin, but if the primary lesion is on the lip the nodes below the jaw will be involved. At the end of the primary stage the patient appears to have recovered, but the reaction to a serological test on the blood has now become positive, and shows that although he seems to be so well he is really suffering from active syphilis.

The **secondary lesions** appear after two or three months, and are due to the spirochetes having been carried far and wide throughout the body by the blood stream from the primary lesion. The skin, mucous membranes, and lymph nodes are principally affected. A great variety of *skin rashes* may appear, which may easily be mistaken for some other skin disease. White patches develop on the mucous membrane lining the mouth, tongue, and tonsils; they are called *mucous patches,* and as they discharge countless spirochetes they are highly infective. The *lymph nodes* all over the body become slightly enlarged. All of these secondary lesions finally disappear without leaving any trace, and the patient again appears to be well, although results of serological tests are still positive.

The **tertiary lesions** appear after an interval of one or many years, with something of the inevitability of a Greek tragedy. Two main types of tertiary lesion may occur. The one is gross and localized (the gumma), the other is microscopic and diffuse. The *gumma* is a necrotic, localized mass composed of the usual mononuclear cells. *It used to be so common that it had to be considered in the differential diagnosis of any mass of obscure character. Now it is hardly ever seen.* The *diffuse lesions* frequently involve the arteries. They are essentially destructive, and even if they do heal they leave the organ damaged and badly scarred. Ulcers followed by *scarring in the upper third of the leg* below the knee in the past were often syphilitic. *Syphilis frequently attacks the arteries;* in the brain the small arteries become thickened and narrowed so that thrombosis is apt to develop; in the main arteries such as the aorta the wall becomes so weakened that the diseased part of the vessel dilates and forms a bulging known as an *aneurysm. The most serious of all the tertiary lesions are those in the nervous system, which may develop many years after the original infection.* The spinal cord may be involved with the production of *tabes dorsalis,* also known as *locomotor ataxia,* or the chief lesions may be in the brain causing *general paresis,* also known as *general paralysis of the insane.*

CONGENITAL SYPHILIS. Syphilis may be either acquired or congenital. In congenital syphilis the child is infected with the disease from the mother before birth, although it does not necessarily show signs of the disease at birth. Indeed there are three possibilities: (1) The child may be born dead, usually showing well-marked evidence of syphilis. Syphilis is an important cause of stillbirth. (2) The child may be born alive with external evidence of syphilis. The skin shows inflammatory patches on the buttocks, the spleen is enlarged, and the mucous membrane of the nose is ulcerated with subsequent destruction of the bridge of the nose (saddle-nose of congenital syphilis). (3) The child may appear healthy at birth, but lesions appear later. These lesions are on the whole similar to those of acquired syphilis, but in addition the teeth may be small and peg-shaped, and the cornea of the eye may become hazy and opaque.

COLIFORM BACTERIA

The intestine is the natural home of myriads of gram-negative, motile bacilli, most of which are not only harmless but serve a useful purpose, such as synthesizing vitamin K and members of the B complex, so that *we must beware of banishing them too completely by overenthusiastic antibiotic therapy.* In addition to the harmless and even helpful saprophytes there are some, such as the *Coliform* group, which cause disease when implanted in tissue with diminished resistance (this is the jackal group); others, such as the *Salmonella* (typhoid) and *Shigella* (dysentery) groups, are dangerous pathogens, which invade the intestine in contaminated food and water, and set up violent inflammation in the wall of the bowel. These various gram-negative bacilli are indistinguishable from one another morphologically, but the coliform organisms are *lactose-fermenters,* producing acid and gas from this sugar, whereas the majority of the pathogens are not, a simple means of differentiation.

E. Coli. *Escherichia coli,* which used to be better known as *B. coli* or the colon bacillus, is a gram-negative, motile bacillus producing acid and gas in lactose. It is generally a harmless inhabitant of the bowel, but it is a common cause of acute and chronic inflammation elsewhere, especially when supported by other organisms. It can cause acute inflammation in the appendix and gallbladder, as well as in the pelvis of the kidney and the urinary bladder in cases of obstruction to the outflow of urine. It is in children and the aged that infection with *E. coli* is most to be feared.

Proteus and Pseudomonas. These two groups of motile gram-negative intestinal bacilli have come to assume increased importance because of their extreme resistance to antibiotics, so that they tend to supplant other bacteria when such therapy is long-continued. The proteus group ferments carbohydrates; the pseudomonas group does not, but produces a distinctive blue-green pigment (*Bacillus pyocyaneus*). Both groups belong to the jackal tribe, only becoming dangerous invaders when general resistance is lowered or local tissues damaged. The urinary tract is most frequently involved. Pseudomonas infections are now common in burns.

BACTEROIDES. This group of organisms perhaps does not deserve to be included with the coliform bacteria because, although they are gram-negative and easily confused with *E. coli,* they are strictly anaerobic and difficult to grow. This is the reason they have been overlooked and unrecognized in the past. They are resistant to penicillin, streptomycin, bacitracin, and neomycin, although quite sensitive to tetra-

cyclines and chloramphenicol. They are normal saprophytes but faculta-
tive jackals, and become pyogenic in tissues with depressed resistance
and in association with other invaders. The pus, in whichever organ,
is thick and foul-smelling with a characteristic odor like that of over-
ripe Camembert cheese.

TYPHOID FEVER

The gram-negative, motile bacillus that causes typhoid fever belongs
to the Salmonella group, and its official name is *Salmonella typhosa,*
but we shall refer to it as the typhoid bacillus. The group differs from
E. coli in being *non-lactose-fermenters, and although powerful pathogens, they are nonpyogenic in action,* indeed suppressing the polymorphonuclear leukocytes, which are the hallmark of suppuration. The
motility of the organisms is due to the presence of numerous flagella
(Fig. 38).

The *infection is spread* from some person with typhoid bacilli in his
digestive tract. This person may be a patient suffering from the disease,
or he may be a *carrier.* A carrier is one who has had an attack of the
disease, sometimes so mild that it fails to be diagnosed, but who continues to harbor the bacilli after he has recovered. The bacilli live in
the gallbladder of the carrier, from which they pass into the intestine
and are excreted in the feces. A carrier is only dangerous to others if
he is a food-handler (*e.g.,* a cook or a dairyman), or if the infection
can be carried from his excreta to food or water, as in the case of troops
on active service or contamination of wells from cesspools in the
country. The patient suffering from an attack of typhoid fever is an active source of infection, but knowledge and care on the part of those
nursing him should prevent spread of the infection to others.

The infecting agent has to be swallowed to produce the disease, and
*the bacilli may be conveyed by infected water, milk, or food, or by direct
contagion.* Epidemics usually can be traced to either water or milk infec-

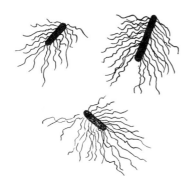

Fig. 38.   Salmonella typhosa with flagella.

tion. Water infection is generally due to fecal contamination. Food and milk infection may be caused by the contaminated fingers of a nurse who has been looking after a typhoid patient, a cook or dairyman (usually a carrier), or by flies. One of the most famous examples of the danger of a cook being a carrier is that of Typhoid Mary, a cook in New York, who was responsible for at least 50 cases of typhoid fever, many of whom died, before she was finally tracked down. Oysters grown in shallow water at the mouths of infected streams occasionally have been responsible for outbreaks. *Apart from the water- and milk-borne epidemics, the important causes of infection are the fouling of food by fingers and by the feet of fecal-feeding flies.*

Typhoid fever used to be a very common disease. Now it has vanished from our cities. In 1910 there were 4637 deaths from typhoid in 78 United States cities with a total population of 22 million; in 1936 there were only 342 deaths from this disease in 78 cities with a population of 36 million, and the majority of these cases were infected in the country. This is a triumph of sanitation in the prevention of disease.

LESIONS. *The lesions of typhoid are in the lymphoid tissue of the intestine, the spleen, abdominal lymph nodes, and bone marrow.* The *intestinal lesions* are most marked at the lower end of the small intestine. Here the lymphoid tissue is collected into small masses in the deeper part of the mucous membrane called Peyer's patches. The bacilli, which have been swallowed, lodge in these masses and cause an inflammatory reaction with accompanying swelling of the patches. By the end of a week the mucous membrane covering the patches is shed and the underlying lymphoid tissue becomes necrotic, disintegrates, and is lost so that many ulcers of varying depth are formed (Figs. 39 and 40). As a rule the ulcers heal by the end of the third week, but one or more of the ulcers may extend deeply, just as in the case of a gastric ulcer, until finally *perforation* may occur into the abdominal cavity. The *gallbladder* is always infected, although the lesions may be negligible. The bacilli live in the bile and pass down into the bowel. *Most of the bacilli in the stools come from the gallbladder, not from the ulcers in the bowel.* The bacilli in the typhoid carrier come from the gallbladder. The bacilli are carried by lymphatics to the *abdominal lymph nodes,* and these are markedly enlarged. The organisms also enter the blood stream, by which they are conveyed to all parts of the body. The *spleen* is considerably enlarged, so that it often can be felt by the physician. *Microscopic examination* of the *bone marrow* shows the presence of masses of the characteristic mononuclear inflammatory cells (typhoid cells) which are found in all the lesions.

BASIS OF SYMPTOMS. The symptoms are partly general, partly intestinal, and partly related to the blood and blood-forming organs.

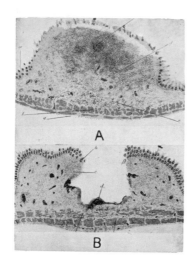

Fig. 39

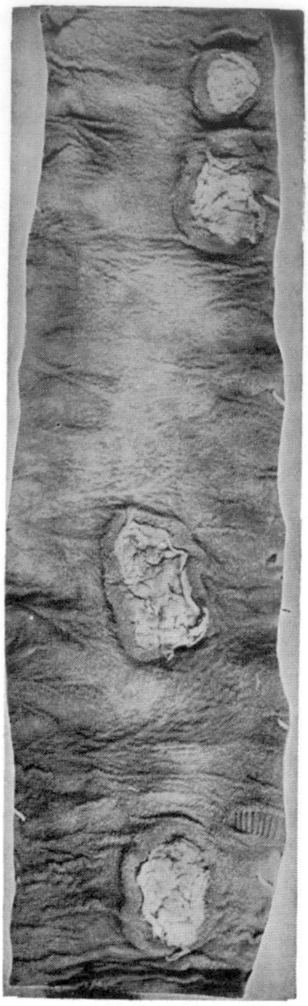

Fig. 40

Fig. 39. Formation of a typhoid ulcer (microscopic picture). *A*, Swelling and necrosis of Peyer's patch. *B*, Discharge of soft Peyer's patch leaving a deep cavity (ulcer).

Fig. 40. Typhoid ulcers of the bowel.

1. The *general symptoms* are fever, headache, malaise, lethargy, and a clouding of the mind, which gives the name to the disease (*typhos*, a cloud). The *fever* usually lasts about three weeks, but sometimes considerably longer. The temperature chart is characteristic; the temperature rises gradually for a week, remains elevated (103° to 105° F.) for a week, and gradually returns to normal during the third week. There is none of the sudden rise and sudden fall (crisis) so characteristic of lobar pneumonia. About the end of the first week small red patches appear on the abdominal wall; these are known as *rose spots*. Bronchitis and *nosebleeds* are early symptoms. The center of the *tongue* is heavily furred. *The fever, headache, and lethargy are due to the toxins of the bacilli in the blood stream. The rose spots are caused by clumps of bacilli lodging in the capillaries of the skin.*

2. The *intestinal symptoms* are abdominal discomfort, and constipation or diarrhea. With diarrhea the feces may have an appearance described by the rather unpleasantly vivid term "pea-soup stools." *Hemorrhage* from the bowel may take place owing to an ulcer having opened into a blood vessel. The hemorrhage may be very severe and may prove fatal. It usually occurs late in the disease, about the third week, and is accompanied by a sudden drop in the temperature. An even more serious complication is *perforation* of the bowel, owing to an ulcer having penetrated the entire thickness of the intestinal wall. This also usually occurs in the third week. The intestinal contents are poured into the abdominal cavity, and cause a fatal peritonitis unless an immediate operation is performed. *As the patient may have a deep ulcer and yet be only slightly ill, it follows that every case of typhoid fever must be treated with the greatest of care.* **The recognition of the symptoms of perforation is the nurse's duty, and it is no exaggeration to say that the patient's life is literally in her hands.** Perforation causes a sudden, sharp, intense abdominal pain quite different from any he may have experienced hitherto, but it only lasts a few seconds, and is quickly followed by a feeling of complete relief. This remarkable relief causes the ignorant observer to fall into grave error, but to the instructed mind it is a clear indication of the intense gravity of the situation. The subsequent peritonitis produces very few symptoms, because of the dulled condition of the patient's mind.

3. The *blood* and blood-forming organs show important changes. There is *enlargement of the spleen.* In most acute infections the number of leukocytes in the blood is markedly increased, a condition of leukocytosis. The opposite, however, is the case in typhoid fever, for not only are the leukocytes not increased in number, they are actually diminished, so that there may be less than 3000 instead of the usual 6000 or more. This condition of *leukopenia* is of great value in making the diagnosis. It is probably due to the fact that the bone marrow, the factory of the leukocytes, is damaged by the bacilli.

LABORATORY AIDS IN DIAGNOSIS. The four most valuable laboratory tests are: (1) blood culture, (2) the Widal agglutination test, (3) the demonstration of the bacilli in the feces, and (4) the leukocyte count. *Blood culture* is positive at the beginning of the disease (the period of bacteremia) and during the first week. The *Widal test* indicates whether agglutinins against typhoid bacilli in broth culture are present in the blood. A few drops of blood are taken from the finger or the ear and allowed to clot; a drop of the serum is then added to a drop of a broth culture of typhoid bacilli and examined under the microscope. If the result is positive the bacilli are seen to become agglutinated into small clumps; if it is negative they remain separate (Fig. 41). The test

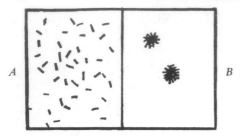

Fig. 41. Widal test. *A*, Negative; *B*, positive.

has a great reputation, but in many cases of typhoid it does not give a positive reaction until late in the disease, by which time the diagnosis is self-evident. After recovery the agglutinins persist for months and sometimes for years, and the test is frequently negative in carriers. *Bacilli in the stools* are most numerous in the third week, and they are found even more readily in carriers. Culture of the *bile* obtained by duodenal drainage is one of the best methods of detecting a carrier. The *leukocyte count* shows leukopenia from the beginning of the illness. **In the first week blood culture, in the second the agglutination test, and in the third week culture of the stool may be expected to yield positive findings.**

A clinical picture resembling typhoid fever but milder in type may be caused by other members of the Salmonella group, more particularly *S. paratyphi A* and *B*. Paratyphoid A infection is more common in Asia: paratyphoid B, usually due to dairy products, occurs in Britain and North America. The vaccine used for protection against typhoid is known as TAB; it indicates that it contains all three types of organism.

Food Poisoning.   This term denotes acute gastroenteritis (with the exception of botulism) caused by bacterial contamination of food or drink. The condition is a toxemia rather than a bacterial invasion. **There are two distinct forms of different origin but with a similar clinical picture:** (1) the *infection type,* in which bacteria in the contaminated food multiply and produce their toxins in the bowel, and (2) the *toxin type,* in which toxins are produced in the food before ingestion. Both forms are marked by violent vomiting and diarrhea accompanied by severe prostration. The symptoms usually come on from six to twelve hours after eating the infected food, being naturally earlier in the toxin type, and perhaps delayed for 24 hours in the infection type.

The *infection type* is usually caused by one of the Salmonella group (although not by the typhoid bacillus itself), sometimes by one of the Shigella (dysentery) group. The food (animals or game birds) usually has stood for two or three days, but it does not smell nor does it look bad. The outbreak is likely to involve all the members of a family or the guests at a large social gathering or picnic where there is a common food supply, probably imperfectly cooked or shielded from infection. In the *toxin type* the poison is formed in the food before it is eaten, so that the onset is early, sometimes within an hour. The bacteriology is obscure. It is known that some strains of *Staphylococcus aureus* and some *Proteus* strains can produce a powerful enterotoxin in decomposing meat. The very different problem of botulism must be mentioned here, although it is discussed in relation to the anaerobic spore-bearing Clostridia on page 169. The spores of *Cl. botulinum* can resist boiling for hours, and if they develop in canned goods they produce one of the most powerful poisons known. The symptoms are due to the action of the toxin on autonomic nerve endings.

BACILLARY DYSENTERY

Dysentery is an acute colitis characterized by *diarrhea.* Two entirely different diseases go by this name as the result of ancient usage; they are *bacillary dysentery and amebic dysentery,* only the first of which will be considered here. The bacillus belongs to the *Shigella group*, of which there are several types, only a few being pathogenic. These gram-negative bacilli differ from the coliform and typhoid organisms in two respects: (1) they are *nonmotile*, and (2) they damage the bowel *not* by invading it at first, but by secreting a powerful *exotoxin* which produces necrosis of patches of the wall of the colon and lower part of the ileum, followed by ulceration.

Infection is acquired through the ingestion of contaminated food and water, just as in the case of typhoid. The infection may come from a patient suffering from the disease or from a carrier. Like amebic dysentery the disease is very prevalent in the tropics, but also may occur in a temperate zone, especially when men are crowded together under poor hygienic conditions. In the past it has been a great destroyer of armies in the field. It is prevalent in large mental hospitals, and it is an important cause of acute diarrhea associated with the passage of pus and blood in children, especially in hot weather.

CHOLERA

Asiatic cholera, like leprosy, is a disease which I trust the reader will never encounter, but he ought to know something about it. It is caused by a motile, gram-negative bacillus shaped like a comma, and therefore easily distinguished from the ordinary gram-negative bacilli seen in the stools. It is called *Vibrio cholerae,* and the disease is known as Asiatic cholera because the lower basin of the Ganges is the one area where the disease is endemic and from which fearful epidemics would spread across the world before it was known that infection was due to drinking water polluted by fecal discharge. The vibrios release a powerful endo-toxin on dying, which causes intense dilatation of the capillaries along the length of the small and large intestine. Huge quantities of watery fluid pour into the lumen from the dilated capillaries, and the result is a *dehydration* so profound that it kills the patient in 75 per cent of untreated cases. The vibrios proliferate in the watery fluid as in a culture, so that the *"rice-water stools"* are intensely infective and can con-taminate wells, streams, and other sources of drinking water. Before this was known, 50,000 persons died of cholera in England in 1831. Treatment consists in restoring fluid and electrolytes to the blood at the earliest possible moment. Prophylactic inoculation is of value, but ensuring a pure water supply is infinitely more important.

PLAGUE

The disease is caused by Bacillus pestis (*Pasteurella pestis*), a small, gram-negative, extremely virulent organism. There is no more terrifying chapter in the story of disease than that of plague. The great plagues of the Middle Ages were worse than any wars. The Black Death came the nearest to exterminating the human race, for it killed 25 million people in Europe at a time when the population of that continent was very small. Zinsser, in his delightfully written *Rats, Lice and History,* refers to plague and typhus as "those two calamities sharing with human ferocity the greatest responsibility of wholesale sorrow, suffering, and death throughout the ages."

The bacillus usually enters the body through the skin by means of the bite of a flea which carries the infection from the rat to man. Indeed **plague is primarily a disease of rats.** A human epidemic is ac-companied or preceded by a rat epidemic. When a rat dies the infected fleas leave it and go in search of a new and preferably a human victim. **A patient with plague is not infective unless fleas carry the infection from him to others.**

There is no inflammation at the site of the flea bite, but the nearest lymph nodes become swollen and acutely inflamed, forming masses called *buboes.* It is these that give the disease its name of *bubonic plague.* The bacilli then invade the blood stream and are found in enormous numbers in the internal organs. The patient dies of over-whelming septicemia before there is time for marked lesions to develop. The mortality is extremely high, and the patient may be dead in less than 24 hours.

Sometimes an epidemic takes a pneumonic form, in which the infec-tion is spread by droplets of sputum. *Pneumonic plague* is one of the most deadly and rapidly fatal of all infections.

The *control of plague consists in the extermination of rats and in preventing them from leaving a ship coming from a country in which plague is prevalent.* This is done by placing large discs on the ship's cables, which prevent the rats running down the ropes. The problem of the flea is met with insecticides. The deadly triangle of the rat, the flea, and man must be broken.

TULAREMIA

Tularemia is a plague-like disease which *affects animals principally,* but which may be spread from them to man. It is caused by another member of the Pasteurella group, *Pasteurella tularensis. Ground squirrels* and *jack rabbits* are the animals most often affected. The name comes from Tulare County in California, where an epidemic of the disease killed large numbers of ground squirrels, the causal organism being named *Bacterium tularense.* Infection is carried from animals to man (1) by biting flies, (2) by ticks, and (3) most often by contact with skins of infected rabbits. It is seen, therefore, in farmers, hunters, butchers, housewives, and others who are likely to skin rabbits. In man the disease is fortunately not nearly so fatal as in animals.

The bacteria enter through cuts and cracks in the skin, and an ulcer develops at the site of infection. In this respect the disease differs from plague. The regional lymph nodes are swollen and tender, as in plague. There is prolonged fever and prostration. Recovery is the rule, but convalescence may take some months. In fatal cases areas of necrosis are found in the internal organs.

UNDULANT FEVER

This disease is caused by a very small organism midway in form between a coccus and bacillus. For this reason it is called neither, but is given the name of its discoverer, Sir David Bruce, and is known as *Brucella.* Infection with Brucella (*brucellosis*) is essentially an animal disease, attacking particularly cattle and goats. The germs infecting these two kinds of animals are of slightly different strains, although indistinguishable under the microscope. That infecting goats is known as *Brucella melitensis,* because it was first discovered by Bruce in the goats on the island of Malta. The strain infecting cattle is called *Brucella abortus,* because it produces contagious abortion in these animals. Infection in swine is caused by *Brucella suis.* Man acquires the infection by drinking cows' milk or goats' milk. Brucellosis is said to be the most common illness conveyed to humans from animals. In North America the only infecting agent that need be considered is Brucella abortus.

The disease is extraordinarily prevalent in cattle. In some parts of the eastern states 90 per cent of the herds are infected. Fortunately the abortus infection is not so pathogenic for man as the melitensis form. Most of the persons who drink infected cows' milk show no sign of the disease, though they may have agglutinins in the blood, indicating that they have been infected. But the disease is undoubtedly very much commoner than is usually thought. Its great importance lies in the fact that it is apt to be confused with such long-continued fevers as typhoid, miliary tuberculosis, and subacute bacterial endocarditis. These are all serious diseases, whereas in undulant fever the mortality is less than 2 per cent.

The disease begins insidiously with an evening rise of temperature, and the patient may be ill for some time without knowing that he has any fever. *The fever may come in waves, hence the name undulant fever, although this feature is often absent.* Its most striking characteristic is its remarkable persistence; three months is an average duration, but it may last for years. Persistent weakness, muscle pains, joint pains, and marked perspiration with a peculiar sweet sickly odor to the sweat are some of the common features of a disease which may easily pass unrecognized. The patient may feel extraordinarily miserable, and one doctor remarked on recovering from the disease: "If the cows felt as miserable as I did, I do not blame them for aborting." Strange to say, there are no characteristic lesions, merely those of any septicemia.

The most reliable means of diagnosis is the test for agglutinins in the blood against *Brucella abortus,* a test identical with the Widal test for typhoid. Agglutination in a dilution of over 1 in 300 indicates active disease; agglutination in a dilution of 1 in 80 in the absence of clinical symptoms indicates latent infection. *The most satisfactory antibiotic treatment is with cathomycin, which seems to be specific for undulant fever, preventing relapses.*

ANTHRAX

The anthrax bacillus is a large square-ended gram-positive bacillus, which outside the body forms spores. *The spores are extremely resistant to chemical disinfectants and also to heat. They may remain alive in the soil for many years,* and when they finally get a chance to enter the body again develop into bacilli. This is a fact of profound importance. The organisms grow readily in culture. They are aerobic, in marked contrast to the anaerobic spore-bearers about to be considered.

Anthrax is a disease of animals, principally cattle and sheep. It is very prevalent in European animals, but is much less common in North America, so that in this country the human disease is correspondingly uncommon. Cattle and sheep are usually infected by feeding on pasture contaminated by spores from other victims of the disease, a fact originally discovered by Pasteur. It is indeed remarkable that more than

100 years ago the father of bacteriology immunized sheep against anthrax by means of a vaccine consisting of the bacilli attenuated by culture at a raised temperature.

Man is infected from animal material, not from other persons; usually from the hides of cattle or the wool of sheep. The skin is the common site of infection, and the disease may be acquired by those using infected shaving brushes, or working with the hides of diseased cattle. The spores may be inhaled into the lungs, usually in the process of the "carding" of wool; the pulmonary form is known as "woolsorters' disease."

The skin lesion is called a *malignant pustule* and is easily recognized. A pimple appears on the surface of the hand, forearm, or face, which develops into a boil and then a pustule containing blood-stained fluid swarming with anthrax bacilli. The surface turns black, and then presents a highly characteristic appearance. *If it is recognized and promptly excised, recovery follows.* If not, the blood stream is invaded, the bacilli multiply with frightful rapidity, filling the capillaries of all the organs, and death soon results. A specific antiserum gives good results when used in conjunction with early excision of the lesion. The pulmonary form is always fatal. Penicillin and aureomycin have been used with beneficial results in anthrax infections in recent years.

ANAEROBIC SPORE-BEARERS

All the bacteria that have been considered so far are able to live and multiply in air, or rather in oxygen. They are aerobes. We now come to a group that cannot do so, and in particular the genus *Clostridium*, composed of many members which live in the soil, where they take part in the process of putrefaction, so that they are readily ingested in vegetables and establish themselves in the colon. Being strict anaerobes, they are unable to multiply in living tissue which is supplied with oxygen, confining themselves to dead tissue in which they can manufacture very lethal toxins. All the Clostridia are large gram-positive bacilli that produce spores that can survive in dry earth for years and are extremely resistant to heat and antiseptics. The three important pathogens of the group are: (1) *Cl. welchii,* causing gas gangrene, (2) *Cl. tetani,* causing tetanus, and (3) *Cl. botulinum,* causing botulism.

GAS GANGRENE. The common cause of gas gangrene is *Cl. welchii,* although other members of the Clostridia group are sometimes responsible. This anaerobic bacillus was discovered by the great American pathologist William Welch in 1891. It occurs in the intestinal tract of men and animals where it does no harm, but wounds may become infected either by soil containing animal manure or from contaminated clothing. It is in war wounds that *Cl. welchii* infection is of the greatest

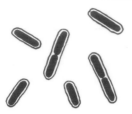

Fig. 42. *Cl. welchii* showing capsules.

importance. The bacillus is short, plump, gram-positive, produces spores, and is surrounded by a capsule that gives it a characteristic appearance (Fig. 42).

Unlike ordinary disease-producing bacteria it does not invade living tissue, growing only in dead or injured tissue in which there is a sufficiently low supply of oxygen to meet its requirements. It is therefore a saprophyte. It flourishes in muscles that have been torn up by bullets or fragments of shrapnel, have been deprived of their blood supply, and are thus anaerobic.

The chief characteristic of *Cl. welchii* is that it *produces gas from the muscle sugars,* so that it is commonly called the "gas bacillus," and the disease itself is known as gas gangrene. The gas is the result of fermentation, which may be defined as the splitting of a complex organic compound (in this case muscle sugar) into simpler elements. The gas spreads along the muscle sheaths, separating these from the muscles, and bubbles of foul-smelling gas and blood-stained fluid can be pressed up and down the length of the muscle. This fluid is highly toxic, so that it kills the muscle fibers which are then invaded by the bacteria. The process is one of putrefaction or breaking down of muscle, and is marked by a terrible odor. A toxin is also produced, which poisons the patient. Against this toxin an antitoxin has been prepared.

The most important part of the *treatment* of gas gangrene is to reduce the likelihood of anaerobic environment for the organisms by adequate surgical treatment to remove dead tissue and blood clots. The use of antiserums and large doses of penicillin have also been effective in controlling this type of infection in wounds.

TETANUS. *Clostridium tetani,* the tetanus bacillus, is a slender anaerobic organism with a spore at one end, giving it an appearance like a drumstick which is highly characteristic (Fig. 43). It lives in the intestine of horses, and occurs in about 15 per cent of horses' feces, so that it is found in soil that has been fertilized with manure.

It is the cause of a highly dangerous wound infection, which results when infected soil or the dirt of streets gains entrance to a wound. The spores can live in dust for long periods. Another source of infection

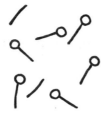

Fig. 43. *Cl. tetani* showing terminal spores.

in surgical wounds is catgut, which is prepared from the intestine of the horse, not the cat. If this is imperfectly sterilized, the spores may persist, and later cause infection in the wound.

The organism remains localized in the wound and does not invade the tissues. In this respect it is the exact opposite to the clostridia causing gas gangrene. As it is anaerobic, it grows best when other bacteria are present which kill the tissue so that the supply of oxygen diminishes.

The tetanus bacillus is dangerous because it produces one of the most powerful toxins known, far more virulent than the most deadly snake venom. The toxin gradually passes along the nerves from the wound to the spinal cord. There it becomes anchored to the motor nerve cells which it stimulates. so that the muscles become rigid and the patient is thrown into terrible convulsions. The jaw muscles are early involved by stiffness and the mouth cannot be opened, so that the common name of the disease is *lockjaw.*

The incubation period, *i.e.,* the time between infection and the first appearance of symptoms, is considerable, for the toxin travels along the nerves only slowly. The average time is seven to ten days. In wounds of the face it is shorter, as there is less distance for the toxin to travel. In other cases it may be several weeks. *This long incubation period is fortunate, because it makes preventive inoculation possible.* When the possibility of tetanus is suspected, and this should be the case in all street accidents or contaminated wounds, a prophylatic injection of tetanus antitoxin is given. This neutralizes the toxin before it has time to reach the nerve cells in the spinal cord. After that it is usually too late to do much good, as the toxin is firmly anchored to the nerve cells. In war time every wounded man received a dose of antitetanic serum on the chance that the wound might have become infected with tetanus.

BOTULISM. *Cl. botulinum* is essentially a soil bacterium, but it is also found in the intestine of domestic animals. This anaerobic bacillus is entirely different in its action to anything so far considered. We are really not concerned with the organism itself, for it does not grow in the human body. But it does grow in spoiled sausage (*botulus,* a sausage), preserved meat, canned vegetables, and ripe olives. Its spores are very resistant, and if the temperature employed in home canning is insufficient, the bacilli will produce a very potent toxin, which if taken in even very small amounts, may cause death. The condition is called botulism. The toxin does not produce any inflammation in the stomach or intestine, but is absorbed and acts on the brain, producing eye disturbances such as double vision and squint, and finally coma and death. The symptoms are apt to be mistaken for those of encephalitis, so that the correct diagnosis of food poisoning may be missed. Prevention is the best treatment, and this means proper attention to detail in the matter of home canning.

FURTHER READING

BURNET, F. M.: *Natural History of Infectious Disease,* 2nd ed., 1953. (A fascinating account of infection and parasitism.) Cambridge.

COLEBROOK, L.: Lancet, 1955, *2,* 885. (Hospital infections.)

DUBOS, R. J.: Can. Med. Assn. J., 1958, *79,* 445. (Historical evolution of infectious diseases.)

FINLAND, M.: New Eng. J. Med., 1955, *253,* 909. (Antibiotic-resistant bacteria.)

JESSON, O., et al.: New Eng. J. Med., 1969, *281,* 627. (Changing staphylococci and staphylococcal infections.)

KING, A.: Lancet, 1958, *1,* 651. (The varying incidence of venereal diseases.)

WHITBY, SIR L., and HYNES, M.: *Medical Bacteriology,* 6th ed., 1956, London.

Viruses and Rickettsiae

VIRAL DISEASES

General Considerations

NATURE. We now come to the most exciting division of the infectious diseases, namely those caused by viruses. Since 1950 some 200 new viruses have been described. But as we shall see presently, we must distinguish sharply between infection and disease. Many viruses, perhaps most, exist as inapparent or latent infections. It is true that they live at the expense of the cell, but without injuring their host. The pathogenic virus devours the cell, or at least deviates the metabolism to make more virus instead of more cell. This is really suicidal behavior, because when the cell dies the virus can no longer exist unless it succeeds in entering another cell. Viruses come not only in many sizes, but in a variety of shapes, some with elegant geometrical patterns in their substance as shown by the electron microscope.

A virus represents the most minute and primitive form of life. It is

171

a submicroscopic unit consisting of a core of nucleic acid with a coating of protein. The nucleic acid may be the ribose (RNA) or deoxyribose (DNA) type. Unlike bacteria, viruses are not capable of supporting life on their own because they lack enzymes. **In order to exist and multiply they must occupy living cells, which provide them with the necessary material and energy.** It is evident that a virus is a perfect example of a parasite, never a saprophyte. No wonder it cannot be grown on ordinary culture media, but only on tissue culture in *living* cells. When the nucleic acid component enters a cell it leaves its protein overcoat outside, and breaks into smaller units which are replicated a hundred times or more, each acquiring a new protein overcoat from the cell before leaving its shelter. Small wonder, then, that the multiplication of a virus is explosive in suddenness and rapidity. Their intracellular position makes viruses singularly difficult to attack, for the sulfonamides and antibiotics, which are so effective against extracellular invading bacteria, are unable to penetrate the cell and reach the virus.

Some viruses have a *host-specificity,* attacking only man, as in the case of measles and mumps, or only other animals or birds. When we use the word "attack," we are of course speaking from the point of view of the host, not of the virus. The latter is merely seeking food and shelter best adapted to its needs. Many also show a striking *tissue-specificity,* some being *dermatotropic,* as in smallpox, some *neurotropic,* as in poliomyelitis, and some *viscerotropic,* as in hepatitis. The introduction of the electron microscope has shown that viruses differ not only in shape but also in size to remarkable degree, the largest approaching the dimensions of the smallest bacteria, the smallest little larger than the largest molecules.

A *bacteriophage* is a virus that has a bacterium as a host. It is a bacterial virus. For a description of the method by which the nucleic acid component of the virus enters a bacterial cell, see above. Bacteriophage particles are now known to resemble tiny sperms with both a head and a tail-like structure. The tail penetrates the bacterial wall, and serves for the introduction of nucleic acid from the head, but the shell of the head and part of the tail are left outside. It is evident that the bacterial virus, the bacteriophage, toils not, neither does it spin, for it has learned the art of living at someone else's expense. In participating in this remarkable union, however, the bacterium commits suicide.

The *history of viruses* and viral diseases is quite remarkable. More than 100 years ago Pasteur showed that disease could be produced by agents too small to be seen with the microscope (ultramicroscopic), so minute that they are not held back by the finest filter (filter-passing), and refusing to grow on culture media. These unknown agents were called viruses. It is amazing to learn that he was able to immunize persons suspected of being exposed to one of these viral infections, namely rabies. Equally remarkable was Jenner's success in 1796, when he immunized persons against smallpox, which we now know to be a viral disease. The first virus to be actually demonstrated was in a plant disease, *tobacco mosaic*. The first demonstration of an animal viral disease in 1898 was *foot-and-mouth* disease of cattle. In 1901 came the proof of the first viral disease in man, namely *yellow fever*. But it is in the last twenty-five years that the most startling progress has been made. This has been largely due to the discovery that viruses can be grown outside the body in tissue culture. This was done first in the yolk sac of a hen's egg (the living embryo), and more recently in a tissue culture of the epithelial cells of monkey kidney. For this work Enders and his associates in Boston were awarded the Nobel prize. The virus not only grows luxuriantly in these epithelial cells, but is also present in large quantity in the supernatant fluid. The tissue culture technique is also used for the development of vaccines, especially for poliomyelitis. Not so long ago the public had never heard of viruses, but now everyone diagnoses his own complaints as being due to a virus.

CELLULAR CHANGES. A virus may enter a cell and produce no change in structure or disturbance of function. This is seen in the enteroviruses, (cultured from the stools of infected persons who therefore act as carriers), the Coxsackie viruses being an example. At the other extreme we have the explosive effects of the yellow fever virus on the liver cells and the poliomyelitis virus on the anterior horn (motor) cells of the spinal cord. **There is thus a world of difference between viral infection and viral disease.** In *viral infection,* which is very much commoner than viral disease, the virus may sojourn indefinitely in the comfortable surroundings of the cell. It is more than a boarder, for it has become one of the family, and multiplication of the virus proceeds without damage to the cell. *Various circumstances such as age, stress, or nutritional or hormonal imbalance may upset the harmony and convert the latent virus into a virulent one.* So may bacterial infection, one of the best examples being the well-known relations between herpex simplex ("cold sore") and pneumococcal infection. In *viral disease* the cell may be blown to pieces by the explosive proliferation of the virus, but evidence of *cellular degeneration,* what is called the *cytopathic effect of the virus,* is much commoner. In some diseases there are *intracellular inclusion bodies,* which are so characteristic that they can be regarded as the finger-prints of the invader. More bodies may be in the cytoplasm or in the nucleus. Two of the best-known examples are the *Guarnieri bodies* of smallpox and the *Negri bodies* of rabies (Fig. 44). When a dog suspected of rabies has bitten a person, the dog's brain must be examined for Negri

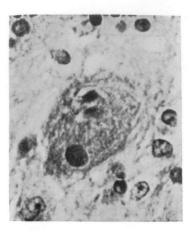

Fig. 44. Rabies, showing Negri body in a nerve cell. Photomicrograph. (Bell, *Textbook of Pathology*.)

bodies, so that if these are found preventive inoculation can be commenced immediately.

Slow-acting viruses have recently been recognized. The ordinary viruses with which we are familiar spend a few days or even weeks incubating in the recipient's body, but the slow-acting group may take two or three years in small animals and decades in humans to produce their effects. These infections seem to result in progressive degenerations in the central nervous system. The best example is *kuru,* an extraordinary disease confined to the Fore people of New Guinea, but many diseases of the muscular and nervous systems may be due to slow-acting viruses. Of these the most important are multiple sclerosis and Parkinson's disease.

IMMUNITY.   Immunity to viral infections is remarkably variable. Thus in smallpox, measles and chickenpox immunity is permanent or prolonged, whereas in the common cold, influenza and herpes simplex the immunity is transitory, and the patient is liable to recurring attacks. Can we explain this profound difference? *The duration of the immunity probably depends on the behavior of the virus within the cells.* If it produces rapid destruction of the cells, as in smallpox, the virus is liberated into the blood stream in enormous numbers, and there is every opportunity for abundant antibody formation. If on the other hand growth in the cell extends over a prolonged period, antibody formation is inadequate and no prolonged or permanent immunity is established.

It is now known that a protein is produced by virus-treated cells in tissue culture which is capable of inhibiting or interfering with the growth of many viruses. This material has been named **interferon,** and it seems to have many of the properties of a viral antibiotic. Immune antibodies are specific, differing for each disease, but interferon is the same, no matter what the infecting virus. Antibodies only begin to make their appearance relatively late in the disease, whereas interferon is found in the tissue in large quantities often during the early stages of the infection. Perhaps the most important difference from antibodies is that *interferon changes the invaded cell, so that it will no longer support the multiplication of a virus.* The therapeutic possibilities of such a substance are obvious.

SPREAD OF INFECTION.   We have already seen how disappointing the chemotherapy of virus disease has proved to be, largely because of the intracellular location of the virus. We therefore turn to prevention, which is always better than cure. Some knowledge of how the infection spreads from one person to another is obviously desirable if we are going to prevent that spread, especially in time of epidemics. The method of spread depends on the virus involved. Spread may be by *direct contact,* as in molluscum contagiosum, or due to *inhalation of droplets,* as in the common cold, influenza, and measles, or to *dust* from clothing or scabs, as in smallpox, or to *bites of animals,* as in rabies, or of *insects,* as in yellow fever. Some of this knowledge has proved invaluable, as in the case of yellow fever; some has been of little use, as in the case of influenza and the common cold. The other method of prevention is by immunization, which has proved of very great value in smallpox and poliomyelitis.

LABORATORY DIAGNOSIS.   It is obvious that the study of viruses is much more difficult than ordinary bacteriological studies, for neither the light microscope nor the culture tube can be used. But just as the presence of electricity can be recognized by the effect it produces on a light bulb, so the presence of an invisible virus is recognized by the effect it produces on the living body (man or the experimental animal) or on the living cells of a tissue culture. The *cytopathic effect* produced by a virus in these cells is of great diagnostic value. Reference has already been made to the presence of *inclusion bodies,* but these are more likely to be observed post mortem.

CLASSIFICATION OF VIRUSES.   Bacteria are classified according to their shape, staining character, and need of oxygen. The classification of viruses is much more difficult. The grouping may depend on the target organ or tissue (*e.g.,* neurotropic), the effect produced (herpes, smallpox), and so on. The morphology as well as the size varies to a remarkable degree, as will be evident from Figure 45. For the sake of simplicity we shall group according to the target organ, and therefore consider viruses of the skin, respiratory tract, nervous system, liver, and finally a miscellaneous group.

MORPHOLOGY	VIRUS GROUP	VIRION SIZE (mμ)

	Picornavirus
	    rhino
	    polio, Coxsackie, echo
	Reovirus
	Papovavirus
		18 - 30
		
		70 - 75
		40 - 55

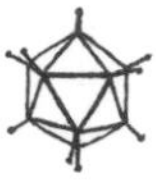	Adenovirus	70 - 80

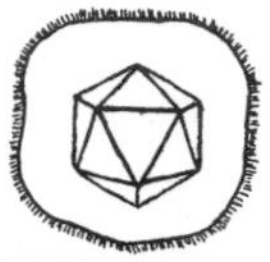	Herpesvirus
	    herpes simplex
	    herpes zoster
	    varicella
		180

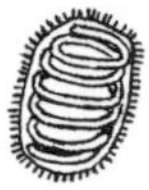	Myxovirus influenza	80 - 120

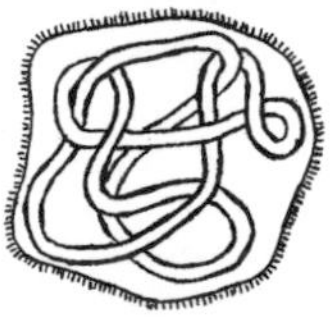	Paramyxovirus
	    parainfluenza
	    measles
	    mumps
		150 - 300

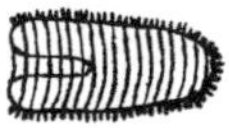	Rhabdovirus
	    rabies
		60 x 160
		    - 225

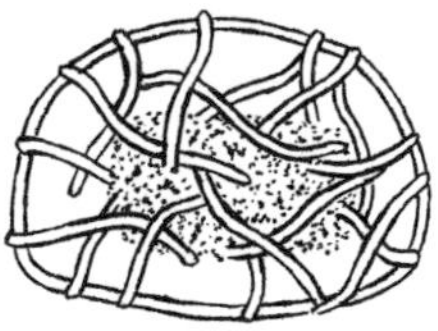	Poxvirus
	    smallpox
	    vaccinia
	    molluscum contagiosum
		230 x 300

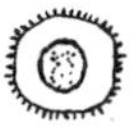	Togavirus
	    some arboviruses
	    rubella
		40 - 100

Fig. 45. Basic morphology of major human viruses. (Kindness of Nancy Jean Alfred.)

Skin

The *pox group* of viruses have a primary affinity for the skin, in which they produce a vesicopustular eruption. In the Middle Ages, when diseases began to be named, there were four types of pox or pocks. These were known as the Great Pox (syphilis), the Small Pox (variola), Cow Pox (vaccinia—from *vacca,* a cow), and Chicken Pox (varicella), so-called because the chicken typified something gentle and mild. Only the last three are now known as poxes; syphilis, of course, is not due to a virus.

SMALLPOX (VARIOLA). This is one of the most virulent of infectious diseases. All races of men are susceptible, and no one from childhood to old age is exempt. Actual contact, direct or indirect, with a patient is not necessary for transmission. It will sweep through a country with the speed of a prairie fire. (Other virus diseases, such as influenza, may travel with the same terrifying speed.) Small wonder, then, that in bygone years nearly everyone, high or low, rich or poor, bore the marks of "the pox" on his or her face. The picture in seventeenth-century England is drawn thus by the vivid pen of Macaulay: "The smallpox was always present, filling the churchyards with corpses, tormenting with constant fears all whom it had not stricken, leaving on those whose lives it spared the hideous traces of its power, turning the babe into a changeling at which the mother shuddered, and making the eyes and cheeks of a betrothed maiden objects of horror to the lover." Now almost no doctor living in countries where this book is likely to be read has ever seen a case of smallpox. Surely this is the greatest triumph in the whole of preventive medicine.

The portal of entry of the infection is not known for certain, but it is believed to be the respiratory tract. Headache and persistent pain in the back are characteristic symptoms. After an incubation period of about twelve days the skin lesions appear. At first these are solid papules, but in a few days they become converted into pustules which may cover the face and the entire body. There is swelling and "ballooning" of the epithelial cells, which goes on to liquefaction of the cells followed by suppuration due to streptococcal infection. In chickenpox there is also swelling of the epithelial cells but no infection with streptococci, so that there is no suppuration. The epithelial cells adjoining the lesions contain characteristic cytoplasmic *Guarnieri bodies.* Scabs are formed over the pustules, and as the scabs dry they are cast off and changed into dust, each particle of the dust being covered with the virus. From this it will be seen how important the problem of nursing is, especially in a community that has not been adequately vaccinated. As the pustules heal, scars of varying depth are left in the skin. Thus the dangers of smallpox are twofold: (1) death, and (2) disfigurement.

The patient must be isolated, and contacts are quarantined for 14 days and vaccinated. Discharges from the nose, mouth, and mucous membranes are disinfected or burned. The virus may live in a dried scab for months or years. The skin is covered with petroleum jelly to prevent scaling and dissemination of the infection. The usual general precautions are taken, such as the use of a mask and gown, washing the hands, separate dishes for the patient, and the disinfection of the bed and body linen.

Vaccination, however, is the chief means of prevention (Fig. 46). The vaccine employed is the living virus of cowpox (*vaccinia*), the corresponding disease in the cow but much milder. We owe the method to the English physician, Jenner, at that time a country practitioner, who observed that milkmaids who had had cowpox were immune from smallpox. The live virus is inoculated into the skin, and this is followed by the development of a papule, then a watery vesicle, and finally a pustule, looking to the eyes of Jenner like "a pearl upon the rose leaf." Immunity following vaccination lasts a number of years, but it is not lifelong. To ensure complete immunity the child should be vaccinated before the age of seven, again at the age of fifteen, and once during

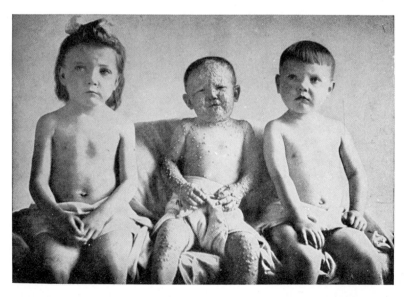

Fig. 46. The value of vaccination. Three of a family exposed to smallpox; the middle one unvaccinated, the other two vaccinated one year before. (Schamberg and Kolmer.)

adult life. When there is no smallpox in the country these extreme measures are hardly necessary. *If the nurse has to attend cases of the disease it is safer to be revaccinated every few years.*

CHICKENPOX (VARICELLA).   This is a mild but extremely infectious virus disease of childhood. Immunity is lifelong. The vesicles frequently do not develop into pustules. In spite of its name, the virus is not related to the pox group, but is identical with the virus of herpes zoster.

HERPES ZOSTER.   As we have just seen, the virus causing this condition is closely related to, or the same as, that of varicella. The disease is marked by severe nerve-root pains usually passing in zonal fashion around the trunk (hence the name), and by the development of vesicles similar to those of varicella along the course of the nerves, the condition known as *shingles.* The primary lesion seems to be in the root ganglia of the sensory nerves involved.

HERPES SIMPLEX.   The virus responsible for this condition is one of the most widely distributed in the general population. The reason for this is that after the initial attack the virus continues to live and multiply in the cells in a latent stage. It often escapes from the buccal mucosa of healthy persons into the saliva, and the infection is transmitted by close contact, as in kissing. The characteristic lesions are on the skin and mucous membrane, particularly lips. This is a jackal virus, as indicated by the use of the common names "cold sore" and "fever blister," indicating the relation between some resistance-lowering infection and activation of the virus.

MEASLES (RUBEOLA).   Measles, because of its extreme contagiousness, is one of the commonest diseases in the world. All races and all ages are susceptible. Practically all city dwellers acquire the disease during childhood, and are subsequently immune. In rural districts it is not so common, but when young adults from such districts are brought together in military or other camps they are very apt to develop the disease. In aboriginal communities where the disease has been unknown it behaves with the fury of smallpox, and the mortality is high.

The virus is contained in the nasal secretions, and it is probably acquired through the respiratory tract. The average incubation period is from 10 to 14 days. *Unfortunately the patient is infective for five days before as well as for five days after the appearance of the rash. It is this which makes the disease so difficult to control.* The *chief symptoms* are fever, the characteristic rash, and signs of an acute catarrhal inflammation of the upper respiratory tract and eyes. The rash covers the face and the whole body, but as there is no tissue destruction it leaves no scars when it clears up. The mouth shows lesions that are of value in diagnosis in difficult cases; these are known as *Koplik's spots,* and are small white areas on the mucous membrane due to thickening of the epithelium. The great danger to be prevented is bronchopneumonia, which is often fatal. Even if the patient recovers from the bronchopneumonia, he is in danger of developing an acute form of pulmonary tuberculosis owing to lowered resistance. An even more to-be-dreaded complication is encephalitis, which may either kill the child or leave him mentally retarded. It is against such a complication that preventive vaccination (see below) is so imperative.

A *rapid laboratory diagnosis of measles* can be made from urinary sediments stained with fluorescent antibody. The measles antigen is detected in urinary epithelial cells giving a positive fluorescent-antibody reaction.

The immunity following an attack of measles is associated with the presence of antibodies in the serum, and these can be used as a means of treatment and prevention. Measles is an outstanding example of a virus disease that can be controlled by immune serum therapy. Now that the virus can be grown in tissue culture, prevention can be even better achieved by the use of *live* attenuated vaccine. As measles kills twice as many children in the United States from a complicating bronchopneumonia as does poliomyelitis, the importance of prevention is self-evident.

GERMAN MEASLES (RUBELLA).   There is only one reason—but it is a very good one—for considering such a mild infection as rubella in this Introduction. There is hardly any fever, a rash resembling measles, and a characteristic enlargement of the lymph nodes. It is less common in children than is measles, with the result that persons in early adult life are more likely to be infected. *If that person is a young woman in the first three months of pregnancy, there is a very real danger that the baby may be born with congenital heart disease, or with other congenital malformation.* How the virus produces these effects on the developing fetus is quite unknown. It may be that the nucleic acid of the virus combines or interferes with that of some genes with these tragic results. In any case it is evident that a woman in the first trimester of pregnancy must be guarded against infection with German measles, a task often easier said than done. This is the very good reason referred to above.

RESPIRATORY TRACT

COMMON COLD.   *Common colds seem to be caused by a number of viruses, or at any rate by a number of strains.* This may serve to explain the remarkably transient immunity, and the fact that reinfection can take place within three weeks of apparent recovery. No laboratory animal is susceptible, but the virus can be grown on tissue culture of human and monkey embryo kidney, in which it produces recognizable degenerative changes in the cells, a technical advance of the first importance. The disease itself is discussed in more detail on page 299.

INFLUENZA. Influenza is the most puzzling of all the virus diseases. Usually the infection is so mild that it is lightly referred to as "a touch of the flu," but several times in a century it will sweep through the world as an epidemic, killing millions of people. The great pandemic of 1970 filled the hospitals of London and Europe to overflowing. Epidemic influenza is caused by two viruses, A and B, of which A is by far the commoner. Although none of the ordinary laboratory animals is susceptible to direct inoculation from man, the infection has been conveyed to ferrets and also to swine. Both viruses can be grown on tissue culture and on the chick embryo (fertile egg), which they kill within three days, *the virus being increased one million times in the course of two days.* Agglutination of red blood cells is produced by dilute suspensions of the virus, and this hemagglutination is inhibited by a known influenza antiserum, a test which is sharply specific in differentiating between closely related strains. The pathological lesions of influenza, including influenzal pneumonia, are described on page 307.

PSITTACOSIS. This is a viral disease of South American parrots and parakeets (*psittakos,* parrot), often known as *parrot fever,* which may be transmitted to man. When a pandemic occurs among the birds, small epidemics are certain to appear in the countries to which the parrots are exported. Unfortunately birds may carry the virus and be infective without showing any evidence of disease. *It is extremely infective for laboratory workers investigating the disease,* even though they have not come in actual contact with diseased birds, the air in the vicinity of the cages being contaminated by nasal discharge and feces of infected birds. The chief lesion is a patchy pneumonia, with a remarkable swelling and proliferation of the epithelium lining the pulmonary alveoli.

NERVOUS SYSTEM

A large and rather indefinite group of *neurotropic viruses* cause inflammation of the brain, meninges, and spinal cord. Two of the best defined of these viral diseases are poliomyelitis and rabies.

POLIOMYELITIS. Although the name suggests inflammation of the gray matter (*polios,* gray) of the spinal cord, infection with the virus is very much commoner than the disease. Most people so infected are symptomless carriers, or merely have a mild fever and symptoms pointing to the upper respiratory or the gastrointestinal tracts.

The virus grows readily in cultures of human and monkey tissue, producing a cytopathogenic effect. This effect is neutralized by specific immune sera. There are three types of virus, which can be differentiated by animal inoculation. Thus Type 1 can be transmitted only to the monkey, while Type 2 can be transmitted to mice as well as to the monkey. Type 1 comprises the majority of epidemic strains; Type 2 is present in the occasional sporadic case; and Type 3 is of minor importance. A vaccine should include all three strains. To make the *Salk vaccine* the virus in grown in tissue culture of monkey kidney and killed with formol; it is given by injection. The *Sabin vaccine* consists of an attenuated *live* virus; it has the great advantage of being given by mouth.

The virus is present both in the nasopharynx and in the feces of the patient and also of contacts. It is evident, therefore, that infection may be acquired either by inhalation or ingestion, but the latter is probably the more important. The virus can survive for several months in sewage. In monkeys a viremia or blood spread of the virus precedes invasion of the nervous system, and it seems probable that in man infection usually spreads to the spinal cord by the blood stream and not by the peripheral nerves as used to be believed. Agglutination of red blood cells in the test tube by the patient's serum is a very valuable simple test. The lesions and clinical picture of poliomyelitis are described on page 500. It must be realized that these lesions and the tragic clinical effects which accompany them are a thing of the past in those communities which employ the Salk prophylactic vaccine. Thus in 1952, just before the first Salk vaccine became generally available in the United States, there were 3,145 deaths and 21,269 cases of paralysis, whereas in 1969 there were only 19 cases of paralytic polio and not a single death.

RABIES.   The popular name of this disease is *hydrophobia,* indicating an aversion or repulsion to water. It is primarily a disease of animals, dogs, cats, and wolves, being rarely transmitted from a rabid animal to man. The virus of rabies is found in the saliva of the rabid animal, and gains entrance to man through wounds from bites or scratches. It is now realized that bats are carriers of the rabies virus, and may transmit the disease through bites or scratches. Their urine, which they spray when flying, contains the virus, and even the air of densely populated bat caves may be dangerous to breathe.

Like poliomyelitis, rabies is a disease of the central nervous system, and the virus passes from the infected wound along the nerves to the spinal cord, in much the same way as the tetanus toxin travels. The time this takes is the incubation period, and fortunately it is long, from 40 to 60 days.

The principal *symptoms,* whether in animal or man, are terrific cerebral excitement and rage, spasm of the muscles of the pharynx, especially at the sight of water, so that the patient is unable to drink, and generalized convulsions. *It is one of the most terrible of all diseases, and when symptoms have developed all cases die.*

The *lesions* are entirely microscopic, for the brain appears normal to the naked eye. Microscopically there is degeneration of the nerve cells and collars of inflammatory cells around the small vessels, but the pathognomonic feature is the presence of *Negri bodies,* which are large inclusion bodies in the cytoplasm of the ganglion cells at the base of the brain (Fig. 44, p. 174). When a dog suspected of rabies has bitten a person, it must be killed and its brain examined for Negri bodies.

It is remarkable that the modern *treatment* of rabies is that introduced by Pasteur, who knew nothing of filterable viruses. He found that the spinal cord of rabbits infected with the disease was rich in the infective agent (the nature of which he knew nothing), as shown by the results of animal inoculation. He also found that he could lower the virulence by drying the cord—the longer the drying, the lower the virulence. He then used the material of low virulence as a vaccine, with which he inoculated repeatedly the person bitten by the rabid animal. By this means he built up resistance to the virus, so that by the time it reached the spinal cord some two months later the patient had become immune. If the Pasteur treatment was commenced immediately after the bite, there was complete prevention in every case. Surely a stroke of pure genius in the earliest days of bacteriology! And Pasteur was a chemist, not a doctor of medicine!

LIVER

Yellow Fever. *Yellow fever is primarily a disease of monkeys and other jungle animals, but it is readily transmitted to man.* The virus can be grown in tissue culture. The varying susceptibility of animals is of interest. The monkey is readily infected, as in the young mouse; adult mice can only be infected by the intracerebral or intranasal route; in both young and adult mice the virus will only multiply in nervous tissue; rats and rabbits are completely resistant. Diagnosis of the disease can be made by intracerebral inoculation of the serum into mice. If the mouse dies of encephalitis, the test is positive. The virus attacks the capillaries, liver and kidneys, so that the stomach and intestine may be full of blood, and there are marked urinary disturbances. The most characteristic **lesions** are in the *liver,* which shows *areas of necrosis, inclusion bodies,* and *rupture of the biliary passages* with *escape of bile into the blood.* The chief **symptoms** are *fever, vomiting, diarrhea,* and *intense jaundice,* so that the skin turns yellow. In epidemics there is a mortality of 80 per cent, so it is little wonder that it was dreaded by Europeans. As with many other viral diseases, if the patient recovers he has a lifelong immunity. Natives living in the tropics develop an acquired immunity.

The real interest, indeed romance, of yellow fever is not so much the virus that causes it, as the means by which the virus is transmitted. Until 1900 it was believed that the disease was due to unsanitary conditions, the infection being probably conveyed from the sick to the healthy by intestinal discharges. In that year the American Yellow Fever Commission under Walter Reed determined to put to the test the theory that a mosquito might carry the infection, as had already been shown to be the case in malaria. At that time no animal was known which was susceptible to the disease, so human volunteers had to be used. These allowed themselves to be bitten by mosquitoes which had already fed on yellow fever patients. One member of the Commission, Dr. Carroll, developed yellow fever and nearly died; a second, Dr. Lazear, became even more desperately ill and finally did die.

The centuries-old problem of yellow fever had at last been solved. The disease was transmitted by a mosquito, the female stegomyia (a different variety from the anopheles which carries malaria). If the stegomyia could be destroyed, the scourge of the tropics could be eradicated. How this was done by General Gorgas cannot be related here, but success was complete. The control of yellow fever has opened up South and Central America, has made Rio de Janeiro habitable, and the Panama Canal possible.

INFECTIOUS HEPATITIS. This very common epidemic disease is now known to be viral in nature. For a long time investigators have been frustrated by an inability to isolate the virus and grow it on tissue culture, but now at last this has been done, and the virus has been photographed (Fig. 47), but the virus has not yet been cultivated or transmitted to any animal. It is present in the blood and feces during the acute phase of the disease, as has been shown by the administration of infective material to human volunteers by feeding and intravenous injection. Neutralizing antibodies to the virus are present in great numbers of the general population, showing that subclinical infection must be widespread.

Serum Hepatitis. This is a viral liver disease similar to that which we have just considered, but transmitted by blood transfusions, the injection of plasma, or even the use of an inadequately sterilized needle in a doctor's or dentist's office. It is believed that in some 1 per cent of apparently healthy individuals the virus responsible for this form of hepatitis circulates in the blood, unable to do harm because of the immunity that has developed. If, however, contaminated whole blood or plasma is injected into a nonimmune person, hepatitis results. *The virus is not the same as the virus of infectious hepatitis,* for there is no cross-immunity between the two diseases, and the incubation period of serum hepatitis is from 60 to 120 days, compared with that of infectious hepatitis, which is 10 to 40 days.

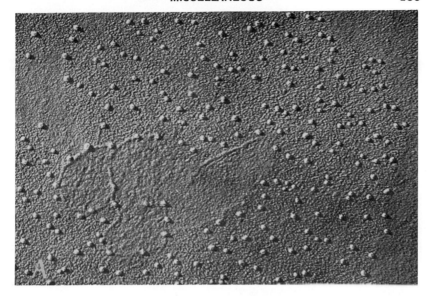

Fig. 47. Partially purified concentrate of hepatitis virus particles obtained from eleventh passage of infectious tissue culture cell fluid by means of ultracentrifugation and fluorocarbon treatment. Chromium shadowed; magnification 53000 ×. (Rightseln *et al.;* courtesy of J.A.M.A.)

Lesions, symptoms, and sequelae of viral hepatitis are discussed in Chapter 20.

MISCELLANEOUS

MUMPS. Mumps is an inflammation of the *parotid gland* on either side, and occasionally of the other salivary glands. The virus can be demonstrated in the saliva. It is essentially a disease of childhood. When the infection occurs in the adult it is more likely to involve other organs such as the *testis* (orchitis), the *pancreas* (acute pancreatitis), and the *meninges* (aseptic meningitis).

CAT SCRATCH DISEASE. This disease, although only recognized in 1951, appears to be of wide distribution. It is probably caused by a virus. There is always a history of an association with cats, but in spite of the name, there may be no evidence of a scratch or bite. There is usually an initial skin lesion with enlargement of the local lymph nodes, but there may be enlargement of the nodes without any obvious skin lesion. In such cases an intradermal skin test with an antigen prepared from infected human tissue is of diagnostic value. The infection nearly always pursues a benign course, with recovery in a few weeks, but in rare cases it may cause fatal encephalitis.

RICKETTSIAL DISEASES

Rickettsiae are minute bacterium-like organisms just visible with the light microscope. They were first observed in 1909 by H. T. Ricketts in the blood of patients with Rocky Mountain spotted fever and in the tick that carries that disease. The next year Ricketts found similar but not the same minute bodies in the intestinal canal of lice that had fed on a typhus patient, and later still others were described. It seems fitting that this group should bear the name of Ricketts, all the more so as he died while investigating one of these infections (typhus).

The rickettsiae seem to be on the borderline between bacterium and virus. They can be seen with the light microscope like bacteria, but like viruses they lack enzymes, so that they do not grow on artificial culture media, demanding the presence of living cells in tissue culture or the developing chick embryo, that is to say they are intracellular parasites. On the other hand they do have a period of intracellular growth in the intestinal tract of their insect vectors, namely such blood-sucking arthropods as lice, rat-fleas, mites, and ticks, which spread the infection to man.

TYPHUS FEVER.   Typhus is an acute infectious fever that used to be one of the great scourges of man. It is caused by *Rickettsia prowazeki,* and it may be noted that Prowazek also died of the disease. *The infection is carried by the louse,* and until this apparently simple discovery was made we were powerless to control this plague, or explain the historic association of typhus epidemics with wars, famines, and wretchedness. But it left unanswered the problem of the smouldering embers of the infection in interepidemic periods, for the human louse soon dies of intestinal hemorrhage on being infected with typhus. *The secret reservoir of infection was found to be the domestic rat, transmission from animal to animal being through the agency of the rat flea.* If the rat dies and the rat flea is hard put to find a new host, he may bite man. The louse now has its chance, and if the victim is lousy and lives in a lousy community, the result is an epidemic. The patient may survive, but the poor louse is doomed. Any reader who may wish to know more about the fascinating story of typhus in war and history should turn to Zinsser's delightful and entertaining *Rats, Lice and History.*

The onset of the disease is acute, with high fever, great weakness and prostration, a hemorrhagic rash, and mental apathy passing into stupor. The characteristic microscopic lesion is a *swelling of the vascular endothelium* throughout the body, including the skin and the central nervous system, the cytoplasm of the cells being crowded with rickettsiae. This is accompanied by *thrombosis and hemorrhage* which account for the symptoms. Curiously enough, in the louse the organisms are confined to the *epithelial cells* lining the gut, so that the excreta are swarming with rickettsiae which, when deposited on the skin, may enter through scratches and abrasions. Bacot, one of the leading workers in this field, died of typhus although he never was bitten.

I feel that I should apologize for devoting so much space to a disease that I sincerely hope the reader will never encounter, but I have been carried away by the fascination of the subject.

OTHER RICKETTSIAL DISEASES.   Five other diseases are known to be caused by rickettsiae. These will merely be mentioned. (1) *Tsutsugamushi fever* is a typhus-like infection, also known as *scrub typhus*. It is endemic in Japan, Malaya and the East Indies and the infection is transmitted by the bite of the infected larva of certain *mites* that live in rotting vegetation and tall grass, hence the name scrub typhus. (2) *Rocky Mountain spotted fever* bears a remarkable resemblance to typhus fever in regard to symptoms, lesions, and bacteriology. It used to be thought that the disease was confined to the Rocky Mountain region of the United States, but it is now known that the infection may be acquired over a considerable part of the United States and in southern Canada. The disease is conveyed by a *wood tick*. As in the case of typhus, laboratory workers may acquire the disease without being bitten by the tick. (3) *Trench fever* is so-called because it was the commonest of all the diseases affecting the troops in France during the trench warfare period of World War I. Infection was carried by the body louse. The mortality was so low that nothing is known of the lesions in man. (4) *Rickettsial pox* is a new rickettsial disease recognized in New York in 1946. The name is due to an eruption not unlike that of chickenpox. Infection is caused by the bite of a tick. The prognosis is uniformly favorable. (5) *Q fever* is a rickettsial disease that derives its name from having been first described in Queensland, Australia. The infection is carried by rodents and is spread by ticks. The remarkable feature of the disease, which is widespread throughout the world, is the absence of any relation between the lesions, which take the form of pneumonic patches in the lungs, and the clinical picture, which is that of a typhoid-like state with a complete absence of respiratory symptoms. The mortality is very low.

FURTHER READING

BURKE, D. C., and SKEKEL, J. J.: Brit. Med. Bull., 1967, *23*, No. 2, p. 109. (Interferons and other cell products influencing viral multiplication.)

BURNET, F. M.: Lancet, 1968, *2*, 610. (Measles as an index of immunological function.)

GAJDUSEK, D. C., GIBBS, C. J., JR., and ALPERS, M. (Eds.): *Slow, Latent and Temperate Virus Infections,* 1965, Washington, D.C.

HORSFALL, F. L., JR.: Can. Med. Ass. J., 1955, *73*, 778. (Virus reproduction and spread.)

HOWATSON, A. F.: Can. Med. Ass. J., 1962, *86*, 1142. (The structure and development of viruses as revealed by the electron microscope.)

LARKE, R. D. B.: Can. Med. Ass. J., 1966, *94,* 23. (Interferon: a changing picture.)

MERIGAN, T. C.: New Eng. J. Med., 1967, *276,* 913. (Interferon of mice and men.)

RHODES, A. J., and VAN ROOYAN, C. E.: *Textbook of Virology,* 5th ed., 1968, Baltimore.

RIVERS, T. M., and HORSFALL, F. L., JR.: *Viral and Rickettsial Infections of Man,* 3rd ed., 1959, Philadelphia.

ZINSSER, H.: Rats, Lice and History, 1935, Boston.

Chapter 10

Fungal Infections

Actinomycosis	Histoplasmosis
Blastomycosis	Moniliasis
Cryptococcosis	Dermatomycoses

Fungi, including yeasts and molds, are plants, although higher in the scale of life than bacteria. As they lack chlorophyll, they cannot manufacture their own food, and are therefore either saprophytes or parasites, living on and at the expense of other plants, animals, and man. Fungi are omnipresent in the air, so that they are apt to contaminate culture media, to grow as molds on food, and to be generally troublesome. Fortunately only a few are pathogenic. For growth they require a high humidity, warmth, and a free supply of oxygen. Any gardener trying to grow roses and prevent "black spot" knows this. *The warmth and humidity of the tropics are particularly favorable for their multiplication, so it is natural that fungal diseases should be much commoner in tropical countries and in the southern United States.* The lower forms reproduce only by budding, but in the higher types repeated budding with failure to separate gives rise to long branching filaments known as *hyphae,* which form masses called *mycelia.* The fungus causing an infection can be grown on culture media or demonstrated in the tissue, preferably with special stains such as P.A.S. (periodic acid–Schiff).

The subject of fungal infections, known as the *mycoses* or mycotic diseases, is rapidly acquiring a new importance by reason of the use and abuse of multiple antibiotics. **These wipe out the harmless bacteria with which the fungi are accustomed to live, and which serve to restrain their growth. With elimination of the bacteria the fungi come to occupy the field, to multiply without restraint, and to assume the role of pathogens.** The damage to the tissues is not caused by toxins, but is the result of allergic necrosis due to sensitization to the proteins of the fungi. Skin tests for hypersensitivity to these foreign antigens are of great value in many instances. Fungi are more resistant than bacteria

189

to drying and the action of antibiotics, which, after all, are derived primarily from fungi. The fungi that cause *superficial infections* spread from animals to man, while those that cause *systemic* infections seem to come from the soil, vegetation, and bird droppings. Only a very few of the pathogenic fungi will be considered in this Introduction.

ACTINOMYCOSIS

The disease is a chronic inflammation, not unlike tuberculosis, but differing from that disease in that there is pus production. The infection, which is much commoner in domestic animals (cattle, horses, pigs) than in man, is caused by *Actinomyces bovis* or *ray fungus,* so-called because of the radiate arrangement of threads at the edge of the colonies. The actinomyces is first cousin of the mycobacteria of tuberculosis and leprosy. The common site is the head and neck. A firm mass develops, usually under the lower jaw; this breaks down to form abscesses, which discharge on the skin (Fig. 48). The pus contains tiny yellow bodies known as *sulfur granules;* under the microscope these are seen to consist of a mass of ray fungus, and therefore form an important means of diagnosis. There is a rarer *abdominal form* of the disease which starts in the bowel in the region of the appendix. The disease is much commoner in farmers and other country dwellers, but there is no evidence that it is conveyed directly from animals to man. The fungus probably becomes an inhabitant of the mouth or intestine in country dwellers,

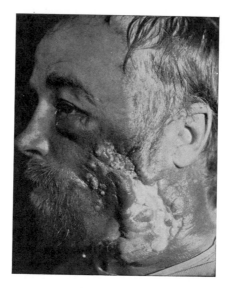

Fig. 48. Actinomycosis of the neck. (Bell, *Textbook of Pathology;* Lea & Febiger.)

and enters the tissues through some break in the mucous or skin surface.

Penicillin and the sulfonamides, together with surgical treatment, when necessary, have effected improvement and cures in many cases, particularly the more localized infections.

BLASTOMYCOSIS

This is a chronic granuloma caused by a yeast-like fungus known as blastomyces. The organisms are spherical, two or three times the diameter of a red blood cell, and show two characteristic features: (1) a clear double contour, and (2) budding-like yeast cells. The disease and the fungus that causes it occur in different forms in different parts of the world. Thus there is North American, South American, and European blastomycosis. The last is better named cryptococcosis, which is described below.

The *North American form* may be cutaneous or systemic in type. In the *cutaneous* (the common) variety skin papules, which later ulcerate, develop more especially on the face, the back of the hand, and the front of the leg. The disease spreads over the surface, so that a large area may be involved. In the *systemic* and naturally much more dangerous variety infection spreads by the blood stream throughout the body, setting up nodules and abscesses usually in the lungs, but any organ may be involved.

South American blastomycosis, a chronic granulomatous disease of the skin, viscera, and lymph nodes which is commonest in Brazil, is caused by a much larger fungus with numerous buds. The most characteristic feature is enlargement of the lymph nodes, particularly those of the neck, which is present in practically every case.

CRYPTOCOCCOSIS (TORULOSIS)

Cryptococcosis or torulosis is a subacute or chronic infection caused by *Cryptococcus neoformans* (Torula histolytica), which *may involve the lungs, skin, and other parts, but has a special predilection for the meninges and brain, so that it is always very dangerous.* In the lungs the smaller lesions are easily mistaken for tubercles, but sometimes they are as large as an orange. Once the yeast has broken through the blood-brain barrier and entered the cerebrospinal fluid, it is quickly seeded over the central nervous system with a fatal result. The causal organism is a blastomyces, so that the disease is also known as European blastomycosis, an unfortunate term, because the disease has been reported from every quarter of the world where laboratory facilities are available. The cryptococcus resembles the other blastomyces, but it is characterized by a heavy gelatinous capsule, which in sections is seen as a clear

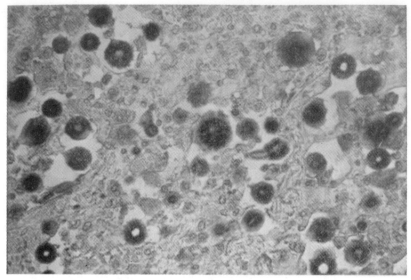

Fig. 49. Cryptococcosis neoformans. The thick capsules of the organisms have been preserved by mounting in glycerin-jelly, omitting dehydration. Alcian blue stain. (Kindness of Dr. R. W. Mowry in Boyd, *Pathology for the Physician.*)

space around the organism. The capsule is best brought out with the aid of the Alcian blue stain (Fig. 49). When meningitis has developed the cryptococcus can be identified in smears or by culture, and a correct diagnosis made.

HISTOPLASMOSIS

Histoplasmosis is a disease with a quite extraordinary history. The organism was first demonstrated in three fatal cases in the Panama Canal Zone in 1906. The causal agent, named at that time *Histoplasma capsulatum,* was believed from its appearance to be a protozoon animal parasite and the disease to be confined to the tropics and uniformly fatal. Some thirty years later the organism was cultured and shown to be a fungus, not a protozoon. This proved to be the breakthrough, for the culture of the fungus was used as the antigen for a histoplasmin skin sensitivity reaction, to be followed shortly by a complement fixation test. These procedures proved to be revolutionary, for they showed that *infection with the fungus was extremely prevalent in the northeastern and central part of the United States, the central Mississippi Valley in particular,* and that in much lesser degree it was worldwide in distribution. From the skin tests it soon became apparent that there were **two different forms of the disease—one mild, localized, and common; the**

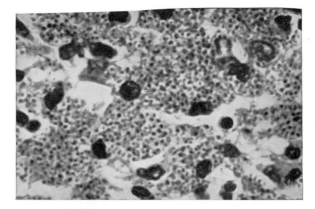

Fig. 50. Reticuloendothelial cells of lymph node packed with *Histoplasma capsulatum.* × 510. (From a section by Dr. W. A. D. Anderson in Boyd, *Textbook of Pathology.*)

other severe, disseminated, rare, and nearly always fatal. In endemic areas histoplasmin tests show that up to 75 per cent of the population may be infected by the fungus without any clinical evidence of disease. The infection does not appear to be transmitted directly from person to person, but to be inhaled in dust from the soil, where the fungus can be demonstrated. Many domestic animals are susceptible to infection, and several epidemics have been associated with contamination of the soil by animal excreta, especially that of pigeons and chickens.

The *mild form* is a benign inhalation infection of the lungs. *At least 95 per cent of cases are asymptomatic.* It is startling to find roentgenographic evidence of extensive infiltration in the lungs with no symptoms or physical signs. The lymph nodes at the hilus of the lung are nearly always enlarged. A few patients have cough, fever, and loss of strength.

The rare *progressive form* is an entirely different story, with a nearly always fatal finish. *Acute disseminated histoplasmosis* is generally the result of a heavy infection with the fungus or poor resistance in young children and debilitated elderly persons. Tubercle-like nodules and necrotic foci are found in the lungs, liver, spleen, and kidneys, together with ulcerating lesions of the mouth, larynx, and intestine in many cases. Microscopically the reticuloendothelial cells are crowded with the organisms, which bear a remarkable resemblance to the protozoa causing Leishmaniasis (Fig. 50).

MONILIASIS

This condition is caused by the fungus *Candida* (*Monilia*) *albicans,* so that an alternative name is *candidiasis*. It is also known as *thrush* when it occurs in the mouth. *Moniliasis is an excellent example of the truth that infection depends not only on the virulence of the invader, but also on diminished resistance of the host,* for it is seen in children and in persons whose resistance has been lowered by wasting diseases. Conditions of moisture favor the growth of the fungus, so that the common sites of infection are the mouth, vagina, urinary tract, and axillary folds.

The *lesions* involve the skin and the mucous membranes. They consist of white patches made up of growing mycelia, which penetrate into the underlying tissue. The fungus consists of branching mycelial filaments with budding yeast-like cells which have thin walls. The infection is a surface one, and does not involve the internal organs.

It will be apparent that pathogenic fungi are the supreme jackals of the microbial world. They patiently await their opportunity, and when they see tissue weakened by reason of infancy before resistance has had time to be established, of old age, of chronic debilitating illness, or of the displacement of the normal friendly bacterial inhabitants by antibiotics, then they move in, and the balance is tilted still more decisively from health to disease. The descriptive term *opportunist fungus infections* has been applied to these cases.

DERMATOMYCOSES

As the name implies, this is the group of fungal diseases of the skin. They are also known as *ringworm,* a name that suggests a single disease marked by the formation of rings due to widening of the area of infection; in reality it is a group of diseases, in many of which there is no ring formation. These infections are all markedly contagious, and are communicated by means of contaminated clothing and structures such as the floors of rooms. Although not dangerous, they are notoriously difficult to treat. The following are some of the more common forms.

RINGWORM OF THE SCALP.   Also known as *tinea* (not to be confused with taenia or tapeworm). For some reason it affects only children. It is highly contagious, and in schools and institutions it may assume epidemic proportions. The fungus, known as *trichophyton* (Greek *thrix,* hair; *phyton,* plant) invades and lives in the hair and the roots of the hair; this explains why it attacks the scalp, why it produces bald patches, and why it is so difficult to eradicate.

RINGWORM OF THE GROIN.   Not nearly so common. The fungus invades the epidermis, and is therefore known as an *epidermophyton.*

INTERDIGITAL RINGWORM.   This form occurs between the fingers and toes, and has recently become very common indeed, because of the increased use of gymnasiums, locker rooms, showers, swimming pools, and the like. The frequency of the disease has in places assumed epidemic proportions. The association of the disease with various sports is the reason for its common name, "athlete's foot." The fungus usually responsible is *epidermophyton.*

FURTHER READING

Carson, R. P.: Am. J. Med., 1955, *19*, 410. (Histoplasmosis.)

Christie, A.: Ann. Int. Med., 1958, *49*, 544. (Disease spectrum of human histoplasmosis.)

Conant, N. F., *et al.: Manual of Clinical Mycology,* 2nd ed., 1954, Philadelphia.

Cope, V. Z.: *Actinomycosis,* 1938, London.

Littman, M. L., and Zimmerman, L. E.: *Cryptococcosis,* 1956, New York.

Chapter II

Animal Parasites

Protozoa	**Cestodes or Tapeworms**
Entamoeba Histolytica	*Taenia Saginata*
Plasmodium Malariae	Beef tapeworm
Trypanosomiasis	*Taenia Solium*
Nematodes or Round Worms	Pork Tapeworm
Ankylostoma Duodenale	*Diphyllobothrium Latum*
Hookworm	Fish tapeworm
Ascaris Lumbricoides	*Taenia Echinococcus*
Roundworm	Hydatid tapeworm
Enterobius Vermicularis	**Trematodes or Flukes**
Pinworm	*Schistosomiasis*
Trichinella Spiralis	Bilharzia
Muscle worm	**External Parasites: Arthropods**
Filaria	*Acarus Scabiei*
Blood worm	*Pediculi*
	Fleas

An animal parasite is a member of the animal kingdom (the bacteria being vegetable) which has acquired the power of living in the body of another animal known as the host. The parasite may or may not produce disease in the host. Here we are only concerned with the human host and with pathogenic (disease-producing) parasites. *Most parasites have developed one very remarkable habit: they spend one part of their life cycle in one host (man) and another part of the cycle in another host (an animal).* The second host may be of any size, from a cow to a mosquito, but each parasite has its own particular animal host; the cow and the mosquito are not interchangeable. Moreover, the second host is a necessity, not a luxury; unless it can be found the race of that particular parasite will die out. It is evident that this invaluable knowledge places a very powerful weapon in the hands of those engaged in the prevention of parasitic diseases. Finally, the second host may be responsible for conveying the disease to man, as in the case of the mosquito and malaria.

One of the most remarkable features of the parasite's life cycle is that the eggs produced in the body of an animal or man do not develop in the same animal. They may develop into larvae in the soil, but usually they must be ingested by another host and develop there. The *definitive host* is the host of the adult parasite (sexual cycle), and the *intermediate host* is the host of the embryo (asexual cycle). Man is the definitive host of the common tapeworms, but the intermediate host of the malaria parasite.

It will be agreed that the animal parasite has evolved a remarkable and perilous method of completing its life cycle, for unless the appropriate intermediate host comes along the family of the parasite is doomed, as the eggs cannot develop in the definitive host. To meet this hazard the parasite has learned to produce eggs in numbers which in some instances are astronomical. Thus the fish tapeworm of man lays several million eggs *daily* and lives for several years, whereas the stomach worm of the sheep lays an egg every 10 to 20 seconds. The problem of reproduction has been simplified in some tapeworms by the male being dispensed with entirely, a somewhat disturbing thought.

Before taking up the various animal parasites, we may look at the question of parasitism from the point of view of the parasite. When an animal decides to adopt this way of life, it must be prepared to make certain sacrifices, including freedom. The host provides the parasite with all the comforts of life, so that organs of locomotion and those of special sense required for hunting prey or avoiding enemies disappear. *The parasite does not necessarily damage the host; the two may live in harmony for many years. Indeed the successful parasite is the one that does not jeopardize the survival of the host, because in so doing it jeopardizes its own survival.* However, it is the pathogenic parasites that must occupy our attention. These are of common occurrence even in temperate climates, and when the tropical parasites are included we meet some of the most widespread diseases of mankind. Only a few of the more important will be considered here. *Disease-producing parasites belong to two great groups, protozoa or unicellular organisms and worms. The worms are divided into round worms, tapeworms, and flukes.*

PROTOZOA

Entamoeba Histolytica.   This is the cause of amebic dysentery, an inflammation of the colon. *It is a single large cell, which is recognized by its motility in a fresh specimen of feces.* It often contains ingested red blood cells. In chronic cases, such as are seen in temperate climates, the ameba becomes globular and is converted into a cyst with a thick outer capsular layer. The cysts are the infective form of the parasite,

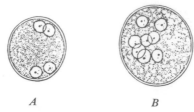

A   *B*

Fig. 51. *A,* Cyst of *E. histolytica* stained with iodine, showing four nuclei; *B,* cyst of *E. coli* with eight nuclei. (Blacklock and Southwell, *Human Parasitology;* H. K. Lewis & Co.)

for the active form is killed by the gastric juice as it passes through the stomach. Multiplication in this simplest of all animals is by direct division; there is no sexual stage.

Differentiation of *Entamoeba histolytica* from the *Entamoeba coli,* which also occurs in the stools, may be difficult, but the latter does not contain red blood cells. The cystic forms are much more easily differentiated than the active forms, for the cysts of *E. histolytica* have four nuclei, whereas those of *E. coli* have eight nuclei (Fig. 51).

Infection may be the result of fecal contamination of water supply or food. *The chief danger is from a carrier rather than from a patient suffering from the active form of the disease.* There are two reasons for this. In the first place the danger from the patient is obvious, and precautions can be taken to prevent the spread of the infection, whereas the carrier is unsuspected. The second reason is that the parasites discharged from the carrier in the form of cysts are much more resistant to the action of the gastric juice than those from the patient with the active disease. For this reason they are able to pass through the stomach and reach the large bowel, where they set up fresh lesions of the disease.

Another means by which infection may be carried is through the agency of flies. The flies have access to infected discharges from the body, their feet become contaminated, and thus they may transfer the infection to food. It is obvious that this method of spread is of much greater importance in rural districts than in large cities.

The lesions and clinical features of amebic dysentery are described in Chapter 19.

The *diagnosis* is made by finding the amebae in the stools, but in order that they may be recognized they must be living and moving. On being passed from the body they soon lose their power of movement, especially when they are chilled. A specimen of stool (only a very small amount is required) must therefore be placed in a warm receptacle, which is then wrapped so as to prevent chilling and immediately dispatched to the laboratory, where it should be delivered directly to the pathologist, and not merely laid down on a table where it may be overlooked for some time. Unless these precautions are taken it will be impossible to detect the amebae.

PLASMODIUM MALARIAE. Malaria is caused by a minute unicellular parasite, known as a plasmodium. *Part of the life cycle is spent in man and part in the anopheles mosquito. Destruction of this type of mosquito will therefore be followed by the disappearance of malaria.* The disease is the most widespread serious malady affecting the human race, although necessarily confined to those parts of the world infested by the anopheles. Greece, a land of heroes, fell in a few centuries to be a land of slaves, largely because the shaking finger of malaria had touched the people. *The disease still constitutes the greatest public health problem in the world.* In certain tropical regions everyone is infected with malaria from the time he is a few days old until he dies. Such persons never know for a single day the feeling of perfect health. Malaria is responsible, either directly or indirectly by weakening resistance, for about two million deaths every year in India alone, and it is estimated that about 100 million suffer annually from the disease in that country.

When an infected mosquito bites man it injects the parasites into the blood stream. Each parasite enters one red blood corpuscle and multiplies inside it until it destroys the corpuscle, which then bursts and liberates the new parasites into the blood. These attack new red corpuscles, multiply inside them and destroy them. It is obvious that in this way billions of parasites may be produced, and billions of red blood corpuscles may be destroyed, so that the patient will develop a profound anemia. The time taken by the parasites to multiply in the blood cells is always the same, so that the billions of blood cells all burst at the same time and liberate the new parasites into the blood stream at the same time. This massive discharge of parasites into the blood produces *sudden high fever* and an attack of shivering known as a *rigor*. The temperature rapidly falls, and may remain normal until the next batch of parasites are liberated. One form of parasite completes this part of its life cycle every 48 hours, and so the fever and chill occur every other day; as this is every third day (counting the day of the attack), this form is known as *tertian* malaria. In another form the life cycle occupies 72 hours, the attack of fever occurs on the fourth day (counting the day of the attack), so that the disease is known as *quartan* malaria.

The human part of the life cycle is asexual, *i.e.,* two sexes are not necessary for reproduction. But this can go on only for a certain time. Unless rejuvenation of the parasite occurs by sexual reproduction, for which the mosquito is necessary, the parasite will die out. *Sexual forms, male and female, are present in human blood, but they are unable to unite. Their chance comes when the mosquito bites a malarial patient and sucks his blood into her stomach* (it is only the female of the species that does the biting). The male and female forms now unite, and the fruit of the union is a fresh brood of rejuvenated parasites, which make their way to the mosquito's proboscis and await their chance to enter the blood of the next man the insect happens to bite. Thus the mosquito not only carries on the life cycle of a parasite but conveys it from person to person.

The *diagnosis of malaria* is suggested by the chills and regular repeated attacks of fever, but it can only be made with certainty by finding the parasites in the red cells in a smear of the patient's blood. The best time to make the blood examination is just before the onset of a chill. The spleen is very large, and in acute cases it is extremely soft and diffluent, but in chronic cases it becomes very hard.

The *control of malaria* in the districts of the world in which it is common has been aided by intensive campaigns against the mosquito by measures such as drainage of marshes and the treatment of stagnant water with oil or D.D.T. to kill the larvae of the mosquito. It is of interest to recall the original meaning of the word malaria. It means bad air (*malo,* bad; *aria,* air), and a reminder of the days when the disease was thought to be transmitted by the miasmic vapors of marshes. It was the mosquitoes, not the miasmas, that lived in the marshes.

There are many drugs that are used in the treatment of a patient with malaria, and these have been improved greatly during recent years. The common drugs in use are quinine, chloroquine, pentaquine, mepacrine, and pamaquine. An important advance has been the introduction of mepacrine and chloroquine as means of suppression of the disease during times of exposure in malarial countries.

TRYPANOSOMES. Trypanosomes are spindle-shaped protozoan parasites characterized by a macronucleus in the center, a micronucleus at one end, and undulating membrane, and a flagellum (Fig. 52). Sexual development occurs in an invertebrate host, the *tsetse fly,* which transmits the infection from one person to another. Asexual reproduction occurs in the blood of the intermediate host, namely man and many wild animals. There are many varieties of trypanosomes and many tsetse flies. *Trypanosomiasis,* the disease caused by trypanosomes, is confined to tropical Africa, for the simple reason that that region is the habitat of the tsetse fly.

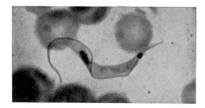

Fig. 52. Trypanosoma gambiense. × 1500.

Human trypanosomiasis or *African sleeping sickness* is caused by *Trypanosoma gambiense* (called after the Gambia river, in which district the fever is prevalent), and is carried by the tsetse fly, *Glossina palpalis.* The trypanosomes live in the blood, causing fever, weakness, emaciation, and enlargement of the cervical and other lymph nodes. It is only later that they invade the central nervous system and cause true sleeping sickness with its characteristic lethargy and coma. The trypanosomes are easily demonstrated in the blood during attacks of fever, and in the cerebrospinal fluid when symptoms of sleeping sickness have developed.

Other diseases produced by parasitic protozoa, which will only be mentioned in passing, are *leishmaniasis* and *toxoplasmosis.*

NEMATODES OR ROUND WORMS

We now leave the protozoa and come to the metazoa. The metazoal parasites which infect the tissues are the *helminths* or worms, some of which are very long, while others are minute. The parasitic worms can be divided into 3 main groups: (1) nematodes or round worms, (2) cestodes or tapeworms, and (3) trematodes or flukes. **Eosinophilia in the peripheral blood is often present. This is always suggestive of a helminth infection, being part of an allergic reaction to the foreign protcin of the worm.** In the case of the nematodes, which form the largest group, with a few exceptions no intermediate host is required for completion of the life cycle.

ANKYLOSTOMA DUODENALE (*Hookworm*). Hookworm disease or ankylostomiasis is one of the most prevalent diseases in the world. It has been estimated that there are some 100,000,000 cases. It is a disease of warm and tropical climates and used to be very prevalent in the southern part of the United States. The worm, which is less than 1 inch in length, occurs in large numbers in the duodenum and jejunum. The mouth is armed with four teeth or hooklets which serve to attach it to the wall of the duodenum and which give it its name (*ankylos,* hooked, *stoma,* mouth). *The method by which it reaches the duodenum is one of the romances of medicine.* The young embryo worm lives in warm moist ground, bores through the skin of the bare feet of natives, enters a vein, and is carried by the blood to the lung where it is arrested. Here it escapes into the bronchi and starts to climb up the trachea. When it reaches the upper end it descends the esophagus, passes through the stomach, and reaches the end of its long journey in the duodenum. Large numbers of hookworms arrive here, and fasten themselves to the wall of the bowel. *In time they produce a marked anemia with profound lassitude and weakness.* This is not remarkable, seeing that hundreds, sometimes thousands, of the little worms have been found hanging on to the wall of the intestine sucking the blood as a baby would suck milk (Fig. 53). No intermediate host is required for

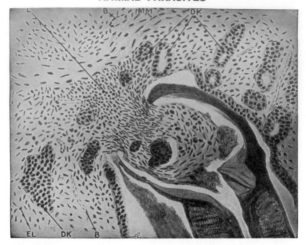

Fig. 53. Section through human intestine, showing method of attachment of hookworm to the wall. (After Oudendal, in *Transactions of Biennial Congress of Far Eastern Association;* John Bale Sons & Danielsson, Ltd., London.)

the development of the hookworm. As many as 10,000,000 eggs may be laid at one time, and if these are deposited in warm moist soil they develop into active embryos, which await a passer-by with bare feet, so that they may penetrate the skin and start on their Odyssey to the duodenum where they complete their life cycle.

Ascaris Lumbricoides (*Roundworm*). The roundworm resembles the earthworm in size and shape, and is a common inhabitant of the intestine, especially in children (Fig. 54). It usually produces no symptoms in the adult, but in children it may cause nervous disturbances. Infection is due to swallowing the eggs of the worm on uncooked vegetables.

This sounds very simple, but the reality is far from simple. The capacity of the uterus has been estimated at about 27,000,000 eggs, and the daily output for each female at 200,000, quite a difference from the human female. Indeed the ascaris seems to be bent on an "exploding population." But when the developing eggs hatch into larvae in the intestine, they are not content to develop there without following the strange example of the hookworm. So they penetrate the wall of the bowel, are carried to the heart and then the lungs, where they are filtered out, and pass up the trachea and down the esophagus into the intestine! With this voyage of discovery behind them they are content to develop peacefully into adult worms. **We can wonder how on earth such a method of development could have been evolved, but we are left without an answer.** If we knew the answer the story would lose its appeal.

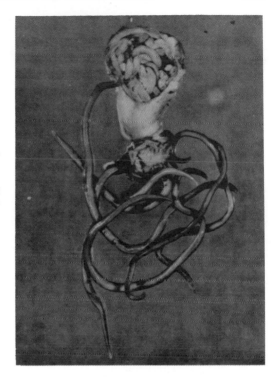

Fig. 54. *Ascaris lumbricoides* in the appendix. (Kindness of Dr. C. H. Lupton, Jr.; Boyd's *Textbook of Pathology*.)

ENTEROBIUS VERMICULARIS (*Oxyuris vermicularis, pinworm, threadworm*). These worms of many names, particularly pinworms and threadworms, are very common parasites in the intestine of children. The worm is only ¼ inch long, and when passed in the stools it resembles a moving piece of white thread. They cause marked irritation and itching of the skin around the anus, and in weak children they may excite nervous disturbances and convulsions. Infection is due to the swallowing of contaminated vegetables and fruits. Masses of pinworms may be found in the vermiform appendix, but they are not responsible for acute appendicitis, as was at one time believed.

TRICHINELLA SPIRALIS (*Muscle Worm*). Every parasitic worm seems to take pride in developing a special way of life, and trichinella, or trichina as it used to be called, is no exception. The disease *trichinosis* is caused by a tiny round worm which passes its complete life cycle in the body of one animal, but unless the host be eaten by another animal the embryos will all die. *Surely a curious arrangement to have been evolved by a worm, but apparently a satisfactory one.*

The parasite infects a variety of animals, in particular the rat, the pig, and man. The pig becomes infected by eating the rat, and man becomes infected by eating the pig, but the life cycle comes to an end with man, because he is not eaten. Epidemics occur, particularly in Germany, from eating imperfectly cooked pork in sausages, etc. The embryos ingested in the infected pork develop in the intestine into tiny adult male and female worms, only 1 to 3 mm. long. The resulting ova develop into embryos, which are discharged into the blood, are carried to all parts of the body, and invade the various organs. **But they can only develop in the voluntary muscles and die out elsewhere (Fig. 55).** Every muscle in the body may be infected, but full development of the embryo into an adult worm is not possible unless the parasite finds itself in the digestive canal of *another* animal. In man the embryos cause *myositis, an acute inflammation of the muscles, which become hard, swollen, and often extremely painful. Fever* is a common symptom, and there is *a marked and very characteristic eosinophilia, which is of great diagnostic value. Final diagnosis is made by muscle biopsy and demonstration of the embryos.*

FILARIA.   *Filariasis is an infection by a nematode worm in which the adult worm lives in the lymphatics while the larvae travel in the blood.* It is a disease of tropical countries, because the culex mosquito is necessary for completion of the life cycle as well as transmitting the infection.

The life history and habits of the filaria are remarkable even for an animal parasite. The adult worm, only 0.5 to 1 cm. in length and extremely thin, lives in the lymphatics, especially those of the groin and pelvis. The male and female live together, and the ova develop in the

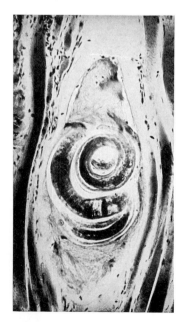

Fig. 55.   Trichinella spiralis in muscle. $\times$ 175. (Boyd's *Textbook of Pathology.*)

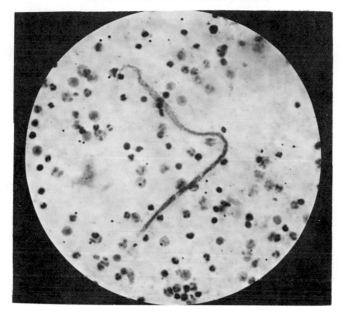

Fig. 56. Microfilaria in blood. × 300.

uterus of the female into active larvae, known as microfilariae, which
are little eel-like bodies so thin that they pass through the smallest capillaries. They are therefore found in the blood (Fig. 56) but **only at
night,** because it is at night that the culex makes its appearance, sucks
the blood of the patient, and thus allows completion of the life cycle
of the parasite. This beautiful piece of timing is made possible by the
fact of a daily cyclical parturition by the females and rapid death of
the microfilariae. Before midday the turgid females are crammed with
microfilariae, but after 2 P.M. the uterus is empty until next day, for
the larvae are in the blood awaiting the mosquito at sundown. They
do the patient no harm, and this nocturnal periodicity may go on for
years. *When the mosquito bites an infected person, the larvae pass with
the blood into its stomach. They penetrate the stomach wall and lodge
in the thoracic muscles. Here they develop into young worms, which
make their way to the base of the proboscis and await injection into
man, where sexual development may be attained and reproduction take
place.*

Although the larvae in the blood do no harm, the adult worms are
apt to produce *lymphatic obstruction,* especially as they are present in
masses. **Elephantiasis** may develop as a result of obstruction to the
lymphatics. This is a condition in which the tissues become enormously
thickened and indurated, the legs resemble those of a young elephant

(hence the name), and the scrotum is huge. The diagnosis of filariasis is made by demonstrating the larvae in the blood at night, but it is elephantiasis caused by the adult worms which constitutes the real disease.

CESTODES OR TAPEWORMS

We now pass to a very different type of worm. Tapeworms are of various kinds, but they all pass part of their life cycle in man and part in another animal. A tapeworm gets its name from its shape, for it is long and narrow like a piece of tape (Fig. 57). The head is very small and the body very long. **There are four tapeworms of importance in human pathology.** Three of these pass the sexual or adult stage in man and the asexual or cystic stage in an animal; hence the name cestode. The fourth passes the adult stage in an animal (dog) and the cystic stage in man. *The easiest way to remember the somewhat difficult names of tapeworms is by the name of the animal that acts as the second host.* All of these worms are known by the generic term, taenia.

The beef tapeworm (Taenia saginata, Taenia mediocanellata) is the common tapeworm of the United States and Canada. It may be 30 feet long, but its head is only 2 mm. in diameter. It lives in the intestine, and the body of the female is crowded with eggs which are discharged in the stools. If these are swallowed by cattle they are carried to the

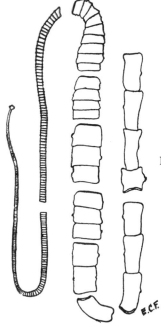

Fig. 57. Tapeworm showing the small head and some of the segments. (Faust, *Human Helminthology;* Lea & Febiger.)

muscles, where they pass through a second phase of the life cycle and develop into cysts. If the beef from an infected cow is eaten imperfectly cooked, human infection will result, and the cystic parasite will grow into the full-length adult in the intestine. The *diagnosis* is made by examining the stools for fragments of the worm (segments) which become broken off and discharged.

The *pork tapeworm* (*Taenia solium*) is a similar but smaller worm only 10 feet long. The second host is the pig, and human infection results from eating infected pork which contains the tiny cysts.

The *fish tapeworm* (*Diphyllobothrium latum*) is very long, and passes the cystic stage in some of the larger freshwater fish, such as pike and perch. There is no danger in eating these fish provided they have been properly cooked, and the same is true of the beef and pork. Infestation used to be found chiefly among the fish-eating peoples in the Scandinavian countries, Russia, and parts of Asia, but more recently it has been imported into the United States and Canada, and is now indigenous in the districts around the Great Lakes and Lake Winnipeg. The eggs are discharged from the ripe segments at the rate of 1,000,000 a day, but the segments are empty and shriveled when shed, in this respect differing from the other two tapeworms. It follows that in stool examinations the presence of ripe segments indicates the beef or the pork tapeworm, the presence of eggs indicates the fish tapeworm.

The *dog tapeworm* (*Taenia echinococcus*) *is entirely different from the other three in the following respects:* (1) *It is extremely small, only ¼ inch long.* (2) *It is the cystic stage which is passed in man; the adult stage occurs in the dog.* (3) *The cysts often cause serious symptoms in man and may prove fatal.* Human infection is usually due to ingestion of unboiled vegetables soiled by the excreta of dogs. The dogs are infected by eating the flesh of infected sheep. The disease in man, which is most prevalent in Australia, South America, and other great sheep-raising countries where infected dogs and men come into very close contact, is called hydatid disease, and the cysts are known as *hydatid cysts*. These cysts are formed principally in the liver, but may occur in any of the organs. They may attain a large size, and sometimes cause the death of the patient. The fluid of the cysts is clear and sterile, but it contains a toxic substance, which must not be allowed to escape during removal of the cysts. Intradermal injection of the fluid is said to give a specific skin reaction in cases of hydatid disease.

TREMATODES OR FLUKES

The flukes are small, flat, leaf-shaped unsegmented worms. There are many varieties of flukes, infesting both animals and man in the Orient, of which the liver fluke in China and the lung fluke in China and Japan may be mentioned. The life cycle of trematodes cannot continue without an intermediate host, which is a water snail.

Schistosomiasis is the most common of the diseases caused by flukes. Again there are several varieties. The only one we shall mention is *Schistosoma hematobium,* commonly referred to as *bilharzia.* This fluke causes widespread disease in Egypt and other parts of northern Africa. The flukes live in the veins of the pelvis and bladder, and the ova, which are armed with a sharp spine, are laid in the wall of the bladder, where they produce an intense reaction, with continual passage of blood in the urine and *a marked tendency to cancer of the bladder wall.*

EXTERNAL PARASITES: ARTHROPODS

The parasitic arthropods, so called because they have jointed legs, are numerous and cause many skin troubles, particularly in the tropics. Some are also carriers of disease. The commonest skin parasites are acarus, the "itch insect" causing scabies, lice, and fleas. The bites of arthropods always itch to some degree, the itching being due to the development of hypersensitivity to the saliva which is deposited at the site of the bite. The hypersensitivity may be so extreme that the itching becomes almost intolerable.

ACARUS SCABIEI. The itch insect, which is the cause of *scabies,* is shaped like a turtle, but is only 0.5 mm. long. The impregnated female bores a tunnel into the skin between the fingers, at the wrists, or in the axillae, laying her eggs at the end of the tunnel where the young are hatched. These in turn bore new tunnels, so that the irritation and itching may be intense. The male remains quietly on the surface and causes no trouble.

PEDICULI. Various pediculi or lice may infest the skin. The *head louse, P. capitis,* lives on the scalp, and causes some irritation. The "nits" we observe are ova, minute bodies attached to the hairs. The *body louse, P. corporis,* lives on the surface of the skin and breeds in the clothing. Not only does the body louse produce much greater irritation than the head louse, but it is responsible for carrying the infection of typhus fever, relapsing fever, and trench fever. It does this by biting first a sick man and then a healthy person.

FLEAS. The common flea is of little significance in relation to disease. The rat flea, on the other hand, is of great importance, because it conveys plague not only from one rat to another, but also from rat to man.

ARTHROPODS AS DISEASE CARRIERS

In the course of our study of infection, whether of bacteria, rickettsiae, viruses, or protozoa, we have seen that an arthropod *vector* or conveyer, usually an insect, is necessary in many instances for the continuation of the infection. A vector may be mechanical or biological. The **mechanical vector** merely picks up the infecting agent from the body or excreta and deposits it on exposed food (house flies in relation to typhoid, or to bacillary and amebic dysentery), or conveys infection through contamination of the biting organ (flies and mosquitoes in relation to anthrax). The **biological vector** plays an essential part in the completion of the life cycle of the pathogen rather than merely offering it a free ride. **In many instances it is only the female that transmits disease,** *an illustration of the old saying that the female of the species is more deadly than the male.*

FURTHER READING

ASH, J. F., and SPITZ, S.: *Pathology of Tropical Diseases, An Atlas,* 1945, Philadelphia.

BLACKLOCK, D. B., and SOUTHWELL, T.: *A Guide to Human Parasitology for Medical Practitioners,* 4th ed., 1940, Baltimore.

CAMERON, T. W. M.: *Parasites and Parasitism,* 1956, London.

FAUST, E. C., RUSSELL, P. E., and JUNG, R. C.: *Clinical Parasitology,* 8th ed., 1970, Philadelphia.

Neoplasia

Of all the disease processes that we have to study in this book, none is more intriguing, more fascinating, and more perplexing than neoplasia. The term means new growth. There are, of course, various forms of new growth such as repair, the formation of granulation tissue, and compensatory hypertrophy of an organ. But the word neoplasm is reserved for the formation of benign and more particularly malignant tumors or cancer. In previous editions this chapter was entitled Tumors, but *tumors are things, and it is the process rather than the thing with which we should be concerned.* Tumor is a clinical term signifying a swelling or lump, but there are many lumps that are not neoplasms.

The normal organs and tissues of the body are composed of cells that are strictly under the control of the laws of growth. An organ like the liver or a bone increases in size, not by the individual cells of which it is composed, becoming larger, but by continual division and multiplication of these cells. In youth this multiplication is rapid, but in adult life it is only sufficient to make good the slow wastage that is continually occurring. Hypertrophy of an organ may occur in response to a demand for more work. Thus if one kidney is removed the other kidney doubles in size in order to do double the amount of work; if one half the thyroid gland is excised the remaining half replaces that which has been removed. This growth of new cells performs a necessary function and is governed by the laws of growth.

A neoplasm is a mass of new cells, which proliferate without control and serve no useful function. This lack of control is particularly marked in malignant tumors (cancer). *Cancer cells are the anarchists of the body, for they know no law, pay no regard for the commonweal, serve no useful function, and cause disharmony and death in their surroundings.* It used to be thought that cancer was a peculiarly human disease, but we now know that it occurs throughout the entire vertebrate animal kingdom. Nor is the popular idea that cancer is rapidly increasing founded on fact. Much of this increase is due to improved methods of diagnosis, and also to the fact that more people now live to the age at which cancer is likely to develop. There are instances, however, such as cancer of the lung, in which there seems to be a real increase.

NATURE OF NEOPLASIA

There is much vague and empty talk about the mystery of cancer, as if it were the only mysterious process in the entire realm of disease. But inflammation is mysterious, and we have not solved the mystery by inventing such words as irritation and chemotaxis; diabetes is a mystery that has not been solved by the discovery of insulin; multiple sclerosis and schizophrenia remain mysteries without even the suggestion of a solution. *A normal cell is concerned more with function than with growth, but the cancer cell is concerned more with growth, in the sense of reproduction of itself, than with function. The capacity for growth has supplanted that for function.* The nerve cells of the human brain represent the highest in specialization of function, but they have lost the power of reproduction. Neoplasms of the brain consist not of nerve cells but of neuroglia or supporting cells.

Cancer is a disorder of cell growth, and the cancer cell is merely a modified normal cell. Unfortunately, we do not know the mechanism of normal growth and its regulation, so it is small wonder that we do not understand cancer. The cancerous modification comprises loss of the more specialized functions, plus the acquisition of increased growth function, an increase that results in invasion of the surrounding tissue and the formation of the secondary growths at a distance which we call *metastases.* We have already seen that normal function is the result of chemical activity governed by enzymes situated for the most part on the mitochondria in the cytoplasm, these enzymes in turn being under the control of the chromosomes in the nucleus with their associated genes. Since cellular growth is a chemical process, it would appear that the abnormal growth we call cancer must reflect some basic alteration in this chemical process. The problem is: What is the basic alteration?

Some forty years ago Warburg introduced the first great generalization concerning tumor growth. The carbohydrate metabolism of a normal cell consists of two processes, *glycolysis* (splitting of the sugar molecule) and *respiration* (utilization of oxygen for further breakdown of the carbohydrate into carbon dioxide and water). Warburg showed in the laboratory that the cancer cell derives its energy mainly from anaerobic glycolysis, whereas the metabolism of the normal cell depends mainly on oxidation. The normal cell breathes, while cancer cells do not breathe but ferment. It was suggested that a difference in chemical behavior might explain differences in morphology and function. Unfortunately Warburg's thesis, while true for some tumors, proved an overgeneralization, for anaerobic glycolysis is absent in some tumors and it is present in many normal tissues, more particularly the retina.

Another concept is concerned with *enzyme systems* normally involved in *regulating synthesis of substances essential to cell division*. Loss or disruption of such systems would make normal regulation of cell division impossible, with resulting unrestricted growth, that is to say, neoplasia. Carcinogens or cancer-producing agents, whether chemicals or radiation, could be responsible for damage to enzyme systems. The end result would be loss of function and gain in ability to multiply.

A difference between the metabolism of cancer cells and normal cells may explain why a cancer, given sufficient time, kills its host unless treated promptly and efficiently. Of course it may do this by blocking a natural passage such as the esophagus, or causing ulceration of a mucous membrane with fatal hemorrhage. *But apart from these complications cancer causes loss of weight, wasting, emaciation, and finally death.* It does this by virtue of what may be termed the *competitive struggle* or *nitrogen trap*. A large neoplasm acquires nitrogenous building blocks from the body stores to satisfy the continual demand for protein synthesis, but the supply of these blocks is not unlimited. Cancer cells appear to exercise priority over the demands of normal tissues for amino acids, thus constituting a nitrogen trap. If amino acids marked with radioactive isotopes are fed to animals with rapidly growing neoplasms, the nitrogen trap can be observed in operation. Small wonder that wasting and cachexia are so characteristic a feature of the later stages of malignancy.

CAUSES OF CANCER

Cancer is in essence a change in cell metabolism, and the regulator of enzymal activity, the governor of the engine, is nucleic acid. The intricate mechanism of chromosomes and genes with their nucleic acid, which controls cellular reproduction as well as metabolism, can be upset in various ways. The interference may lead to permanent changes or "mutation" in the genes, and if the change is such as to permanently speed the rate of mitotic division, the result will be cancer. Just as the regulator of a watch may be moved to fast or slow, so may the mitotic rate be permanently accelerated by carcinogens or retarded by radiation and colchicine. As one cell will produce 60,000 daughter cells after 16 divisions, it is apparent that even a slight increase in the rate and rhythm of cell division will soon produce a tumor.

The exact cause of cancer is not known. *It is very doubtful, indeed, if there is any one universal cause of all cancers, any more than we would expect to find any one universal cause of all inflammations.* Both inflammation and cancer are processes, not diseases, whereas inflammation of the appendix and cancer of the stomach are diseases in the ordinary sense of the term. Again, just as it would be absurd to expect to discover one method of treatment which would cure all infections, so it is probably useless to hope for a single cure of all cancers. The alliteration of "the cause of cancer" and "the cure of cancer" is unfortunate, because it has implanted deep in the mind of the public the fixed idea that there must be *one* cause and *one* cure, so that they tend to reject the information that great advances have been made both in our knowledge of the causation and the treatment of malignant disease. As a matter of fact there are many chronic pathological conditions such as arteriosclerosis, emphysema, and Bright's disease which are far more incurable than cancer. Tumors form a group, just as do the infectious diseases, and each one has to be considered by itself. We do know a good deal about certain factors which play a part in the production of cancer, just as we do know a good deal about treatment of the disease. *The possible factors in carcinogenesis are six in number:* (1) *chemical carcinogens,* (2) *ionizing radiation,* (3) *viruses,* (4) *hormones,* (5) *heredity,* and (6) *environment.* This does not mean that there may not be others, or that only one is responsible in a given case. It will be noticed that some of the factors may be termed external, others internal. *Cancer, like inflammation, is a fire that burns continuously, and there are many methods of starting a fire, some physical and some chemical.*

CHEMICAL CARCINOGENS

The first observation on chemical carcinogenic agents was that of Sir Percival Pott in 1775, who noticed that cancer of the skin was especially common in men who worked with *tar,* and he offered the commonsense suggestion that the tar acted in some manner as a causal agent. In 1915, that is to say 140 years after Pott's paper, Yamagiwa in Japan put this idea to the test by painting tar on a rabbit's ear every day for six months, and he succeeded in producing cancer of the skin. This was an epoch-making discovery, because for the first time it was possible to produce a malignant tumor at will in an experimental animal. It may be noted that if Yamagiwa had used a rat instead of a rabbit he would have failed. Eventually, the mouse proved to be a much more suitable animal than the rabbit.

Tar is a highly complex substance containing a great variety of chemical agents. Again a number of years had to pass before the first carcinogen was isolated from the tar. This was the hydrocarbon benzpyrene. Soon it was discovered that a number of hydrocarbons synthesized in the laboratory were also powerfully carcinogenic, one of the most used being 1:2:5:6 dibenzanthracene. These synthetic carcinogenic hydrocarbons all have a benzene six-membered ring structure. It is perhaps significant that **a very slight change in the chemical structure of a substance may convert it from a noncarcinogen into a carcinogen.** Any of these carcinogens can produce carcinoma (epithelial cancer) or sarcoma (connective tissue cancer) at the site of application. Some can even convert a tissue culture of fibroblasts into a culture of cancer cells.

We have already seen that the giant molecule of DNA is pictured as a double spiral or helix with thousands of turns, and that there are thousands of these molecules in each chromosome (p. 12). It is evident that a structure of such complexity may easily become deranged, not only by polycyclic hydrocarbons, but by ionizing radiation and viruses, many of which are merely aggregates of DNA molecules wrapped in a coat of protein that is left behind when the virus enters a living cell.

IONIZING RADIATION

Of the physical as opposed to the chemical carcinogens the most striking is ionizing radiation. Even a single dose of 600 r is followed by a wide variety of benign and malignant tumors of the skin, connective tissue, and viscera in the experimental animal. The early workers with *x-rays* developed cancer of the skin of the hand many years later, because they were unaware of the danger. The long latent period is of particular interest. Leukemia, a malignant condition of the blood-forming organs, is an occupational hazard of radiologists at the present time, and the survivors of the first Hiroshima and Nagasaki atomic blasts show a ten-fold increase in leukemia in the heavily exposed group. The miners in Schneeberg and Joachimsthal for centuries have suffered from a high incidence of carcinoma of the lung; this is now known to be due to *radioactive uranium. Actinic light radiation* is also carcinogenic, thus explaining the high incidence of cancer of the skin and lip among field workers in the white population of the tropics, Australia, and the southern United States. This form of cancer is very rare in the Negro, who is protected by the high pigment content of his skin. The carcinogenic effect of radium seems to be due to interference with the structure and function of the chromosomes and genes.

VIRUSES

We now come to one of the most exciting of the more modern aspects of carcinogenesis, namely the part played by viruses. It is a huge subject with a vast literature, and it can only be touched on in the most superficial way. As far back as 1911 Rous showed that a *cell-free filtrate* of a sarcoma of fowl could produce a new tumor when injected into another fowl of the same breed. This was the breakthrough, but it aroused no enthusiasm, for the only similar tumors were confined to birds. Then in 1932 a tumor due to a filter-passing viral agent was described in a wild rabbit. A short time later Bittner proved that cancer of the breast in mice can be transmitted to the newborn by an agent in the mother's milk. The agent was known as the *Bittner transmissible milk factor*. At the present time the production of malignant tumors of a variety of types by cell-free filtrates in laboratory animals has become commonplace. It is even possible to induce cancer in cultures of human cells by the addition of the polyoma virus (see p. 216). But such experimental evidence must not be applied without reserve to human cancer; a drug such as benzedrine, which produces cancer with ease in man, is powerless to do the same in the dog. *It seems only natural that a virus, which like an enzyme is a self-perpetuating nucleoprotein, could produce tumors by disrupting the normal regulating mechanism of chromosomes and genes, which themselves are masses of nucleic acid.* It may well be that a molecule of viral nucleic acid, without its protein overcoat, might so closely resemble a gene that it could slip into the cell's chromosomal line-up, displacing a normal gene, and make the cell reproduce abnormally. *Moreover a virus may remain latent, just as may a saprophytic bacterium, and a latent virus may mutate to an active state, this activation being brought about by a variety of agents.* We have already seen that the herpes simplex virus, which is acquired in early life, may pass into a latent state from which it may be awakened at any time by various bacterial infections or even a rise in temperature. Is it possible that at least some carcinogens act by awakening a latent virus?

A major advance in our thinking on the subject of the viral origin of cancer is represented by Gross' concept of *vertical transmission*. A laboratory animal suffering from a bacterial or viral disease will readily spread the infection to its neighbors of the same generation. This may be termed "horizontal transmission." But this is not true of a viral neoplasm, such as leukemia or mammary carcinoma in the mouse. *Leu-*

kemia in mice is an example of a latent virus infection which produces a neoplastic disease that develops in an inbred strain when they reach early adult life. **Gross has shown that the carcinogenic agent is transmitted vertically, that is to say from one generation to another,** through the germinal cells. In the case of the mouse mammary gland carcinoma the virus is transmitted through the mother's milk. The agent may remain latent throughout the life span of the host, which remains healthy, and yet carries and transmits the seeds of disease.

That the seeds are there can be shown by inoculating cell-free filtrates into *newborn* mice of a low-leukemic strain (which would not develop the disease spontaneously) with the production of leukemia when the animals reach adult life. The reason the newborn animal is used is that the fetus is unable to make antibodies against antigens to which it is exposed, an inability that persists for a few hours or days after birth. We have already examined this subject in connection with autoimmunity (p. 120). When the virus of leukemia or the Bittner milk virus is inoculated later in life, it is destroyed by antibodies, so that no neoplasm develops. This suggests the thought that a virus present in the body at birth may live in the cells for years until some external factor combines with it to turn it into a true carcinogen. If the reader wishes to get really confused, he may like to learn that some of the low leukemic strain mice injected with cell-free extracts of leukemic tissue would develop not leukemia, but carcinoma of the parotid gland or fibrosarcoma of connective tissue. Still more startling was the discovery by Sarah Stewart that when the same leukemic agent was grown in tissue culture and a cell-free extract was injected into newborn mice, the animals developed a broad spectrum of more than a dozen apparently unrelated tumors. For this reason the agent was named the *polyoma* (multiple tumor) *virus* (Fig. 58). What this all means I leave the thoughtful reader to guess.

So far we have been speaking of neoplasia in the laboratory animal. Up to the present no virus has been isolated from a human cancer. It must be realized, however, that viruses may be highly specific, so specific indeed that a virus will infect and cause disease in only one kind of cell and one kind of animal. A virus long adapted to human cells could hardly be expected to grow readily in most animal cells, and it is by such growth that the etiological role of viruses in animal neoplasms has been demonstrated. We can induce leukemia by inoculating a newborn mouse, but hardly a newborn baby.

HORMONES

Hormones can act as carcinogens, but they differ from other carcinogens in two respects: (1) they induce tumors only in those organs on

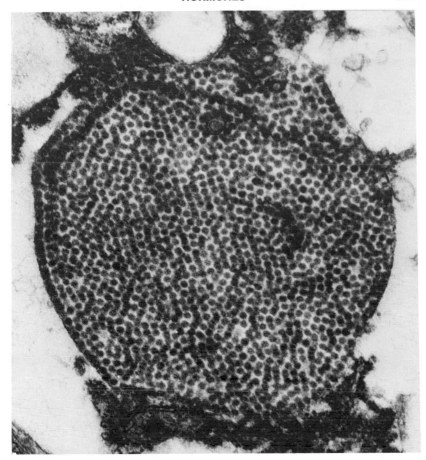

Fig. 58. Polyoma virus. The nuclear material of a cell from the kidney of an infected hamster has been almost completely replaced by virus. × 60,000. (Kindness of Dr. A. F. Howatson.)

which the hormone has a physiological effect, and (2) prolonged exposure of the susceptible tissue is required. Moreover, the cancer is at first *hormone-dependent* on the endocrine imbalance which initiated the process. *Sex hormones* provide the most striking example of a carcinogenic action. Indeed the structural resemblances between the carcinogenic hydrocarbons and the female sex hormones might suggest similar physiological activities. *Thus carcinogenic substances can be estrogenic, and estrogenic substances can be carcinogenic.* Estrogens frequently require the cooperation of one or more additional agencies, the most important of which is heredity. Thus removal of the ovaries at an early age in mice of a high cancer strain will prevent the occurrence of spontaneous *mammary cancer,* but hormonal administration will cause cancer to develop. In the *prostate* there seems to be little doubt that an endocrine dysfunction is an etiological factor in the production of cancer in man; the hormones may be gonadal or adrenal in origin.

The subject of hormonal-dependent tumors has come to assume great clinical importance in relation to the treatment of cancer of the breast in women by removal of the ovaries, and of cancer of the prostate in man by the administration of estrogens, by adrenalectomy, or as a last resort by hypophysectomy, *i.e.,* removal of the hypophysis or pituitary which stimulates the adrenals to activity. *The whole outlook in these cancers has been changed for the better to a remarkable degree by the adoption of one or more of these measures.* It is evident that benefit from hormone therapy or removal of endocrines can only be expected when the tumor is still hormone-dependent.

HEREDITY.   In the experimental animal where pure strains can be bred with ease the genetic constitution may be a factor of supreme importance. Thus we have high cancer strains and low cancer strains of mice for one particular tumor and organ. It is not possible to apply the results of breeding experiments in mice to men for obvious reasons, but a few human tumors show so marked a familial tendency that every member of the family may die of the disease if he lives long enough. Such tumors are neuroblastoma of the retina and malignant papilloma of the large bowel. The historic example of a familial tendency is that of Napoleon, who died at St. Helena of cancer of the stomach. His father, his grandfather, his brother, and his three sisters all died of the same disease.

As a matter of fact cancer, including leukemia, is now one of the leading causes of nonaccidental death in children between the ages of 3 and 14 in the United States and Canada. These cancers differ from those in adults in clinical features, sites of origin, and types of tumor. Tumors of embryonic origin (embryonic tumors) are very common in infants and young children, but correspondingly rare in adults. Four out of five of these tumors in children arise from the nervous system, the urinary system, or the lymphopoietic system, whereas in adults four out of five cancers arise from the alimentary, respiratory, or genital systems.

ENVIRONMENT.   Endless papers and some books have been written on the relation of environment, including occupation, to cancer, but little need be said here on the subject, because so little is known that is universally accepted and beyond dispute. Here we are at the mercy of statistics. It is certainly the case that some forms of occupation bear a striking relation to cancer in particular sites. This is a subject of increasing importance in the industrial age in which we live, and in which workmen's compensation claims a corresponding degree of attention. Mere mention need be made of workers with coal tar and petroleum distillates, aniline dyes, x-rays and radioactive material, and many other raw materials and products. **The truth is that throughout life we seem to swim in a sea of carcinogens, and it is more by good fortune than good management that some of us escape to die from causes other than cancer.** *Chronic irritation* used to be a favorite scapegoat, but it is seldom heard of now, although a few examples come to mind. Cancer of the gallbladder is usually associated with gallstones, cancer of the urinary bladder is common in persons infected with Schistosoma ova, and cancer may develop in the edge of a very chronic ulcer in which prolonged destruction of tissue demands constant replacement of parts with disturbance of the normal growth mechanism.

Geographic Cancer. This is part of the general subject of the geography of disease, a fascinating topic to which one might well devote a lifetime of study. The incidence of different forms of cancer certainly varies greatly in different parts of the world. Sometimes we know the reason for this, but in most instances we do not. *Cancer of the bladder* is very common among Egyptian farm workers, and we have already seen that this is related to the high incidence of Schistosoma hematobium infection in Egypt, although how the presence of the ova of the parasite in the wall of the bladder causes cancer we do not know. We have already seen that *cancer of the skin* is common in white-skinned persons living in the tropics, because of actinic light radiation. Endless other examples could be given, usually with no explanation. *Cancer in Africa* provides one of the most exciting and challenging examples of the geographic pathology of cancer. The pattern of cancer in that continent differs profoundly from that in Europe and North America. There must be good reasons for these differences, but with a few exceptions we are ignorant of them. Two of the most striking examples are cancer of the liver and tumors of the jaw. China also offers many examples of cancer which to most of us are quite bizarre.

Burkitt's lymphoma provides the newest and most dramatic feature of the exciting story of cancer in Africa. A young English observer, armed only with a pencil, a notebook, and the power to draw conclusions from what he saw, pointed out that very great numbers of children in Africa on the line of the equatorial belt running from coast to coast suffered from a neoplasm of the lymphoid tissue, most frequently in the jaws, but also in many of the abdominal and thoracic organs. The most probable cause is a virus, which is also found in the mosquitoes that abound in this zone. In many respects the tumor resembles the multiple neoplasms produced by the appropriately named *polyoma virus* when injected into newborn mice (see p. 216).

CHARACTERISTICS OF MALIGNANCY

Tumors can be divided into two great classes: the one innocent or *benign,* the other *malignant.* Sometimes a benign tumor may develop into a malignant one. A malignant tumor differs from a benign one in the following particulars.

1. A malignant tumor if untreated will kill the patient wherever it occurs, even in the hand or foot. A benign tumor will only cause death if it happens to grow in a vital organ such as the brain.

2. A malignant tumor infiltrates the surrounding tissue. It sends claws into it like a crab (Fig. 59). The word cancer means a crab. A benign tumor grows by expansion, as a toy balloon does when blown up, and is usually separated from the surrounding tissue by a capsule so that it can be shelled out, or at least readily removed.

3. When a malignant tumor is excised it may recur. This is because some of the outlying parts have not been completely removed; they are so minute that they cannot be seen by the surgeon, but they may soon grow to the size of the original tumor. When a benign tumor is removed it does not recur.

4. Speaking generally a malignant tumor grows much more rapidly than a benign one, although some cancers are remarkably slow in growth, especially in old people. The rapid growth is due to the fact that the tumor cells are dividing rapidly. This cell division is called *mitosis,* and it can be recognized under the microscope by the fact that the chromosomal network of the nucleus becomes divided into small particles which are grouped together to form *mitotic figures.* The process has already been described on page 12. Thus the presence of numerous mitotic figures indicates to the pathologist that the tumor is almost certainly a malignant one. The character of the mitotic figures may also be seen to be abnormal.

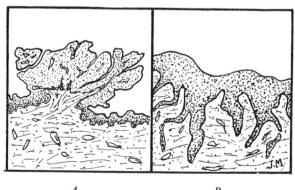

A   *B*

Fig. 59. *A,* Benign tumor (papilloma); *B,* malignant tumor (epidermoid carcinoma).

5. A malignant tumor sets up secondary growths or *metastases* in lymph nodes and in distant organs. This is because the cancer has invaded the lymph vessels or the blood vessels and the tumor cells are carried by the lymph or blood stream to other parts of the body, where they settle down and form new tumors. When this happens no operation on the primary tumor can hope to save the patient.

There are microscopic differences which are of great importance to the pathologist in the task of determining whether the tumor removed by the surgeon is or is not cancer, but they need not be detailed here. Suffice it to say that a benign tumor tends to reproduce the structure of the organ from which it grows, whereas a malignant tumor, being beyond the pale of the law, fails to do so. This is a histological distinction, a failure in arrangement. In addition the individual cells of the malignant tumor may show a lack of normal differentiation, a reversion to a more primitive and undifferentiated type, which is known as *anaplasia*. Both the *histological* and *cytological changes* may be so great that the pathologist can diagnose the case as one of cancer the moment he looks down the microscope. In other cases a decision may be very difficult, and different pathologists may disagree in their interpretation of the microscopic picture.

CARCINOMA-IN-SITU. In the previous editions of this book no mention has been made of the condition about to be described, a serious omission for which I must apologize. An important step in the fight against cancer is the recognition by the pathologist of the very earliest beginnings of the malignant process. When metastases have occurred it is too late. When invasion of the deeper tissues can be recognized it *may* be too late. But when the malignant change is still *cytological* rather than *histological* the disease is curable. This state of affairs is known as *carcinoma-in-situ* or *preinvasive carcinoma*. The cells appear restless, as if looking for a way to get out. The condition may be reversible, but in very many cases the *in situ* state develops into an invasive one. *It is in carcinoma of the cervix uteri that recognition of preinvasive carcinoma is of the greatest practical importance,* and has already saved the lives of countless women.

Some of the principal distinguishing features between benign and malignant tumors are given in Table 2. It must be understood that these are generalizations to which there are frequent exceptions.

SPREAD OF TUMORS

This subject has already been referred to. An innocent tumor increases in size but can hardly be said to spread. A malignant tumor, on the other hand, spreads locally and to distant parts. The local spread is due to the invasive character of the growth, the cancer cells worming

Table 2.   *Characteristics of Benign and Malignant Tumors*

Characteristics	*Benign*	*Malignant*
1. Growth	Slow, expansive, often encapsulated	Rapid, invasive, nonencapsulated
2. Metastases	Absent	Frequent
3. Recurrence after removal	Absent	Frequent
4. Histology	Relatively normal	Abnormal to a varying degree
5. Cytology	Normal	Varying degrees of anaplasia
6. Mitoses	Absent	Often numerous and abnormal
7. Constitutional effects	Rare, apart from endocrine adenomas	The rule

their way into the surrounding tissues, and growing along the lymphatics. This *permeation* of the lymphatics is particularly well seen in cancer of the breast (Fig. 60). This presents a serious problem for the operating surgeon, for if he takes out merely what he can see of the tumor he is certain to leave behind many tumor cells, and soon the patient will return with a *recurrence*.

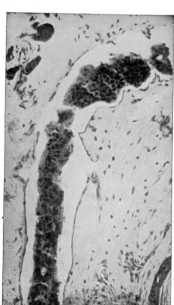

Fig. 60. Lymphatic permeation by carcinoma. × 125. (Boyd, *Textbook of Pathology,* Lea & Febiger.)

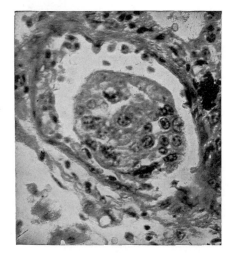

Fig. 61. Tumor embolus in blood vessel.

The other method of spread is by *tumor embolism,* the cancer cells forming emboli and being carried by the blood stream to distant parts in the same way as thrombi may become detached and converted into emboli (Fig. 61). If the *lymphatic vessels* are invaded the tumor cells are carried to the nearest (regional) lymph nodes, where they are arrested and form new tumors similar to the primary one. In the surgical treatment of cancer of the breast the lymph nodes in the axilla, which receive the lymph from the breast, are removed together with the breast. This is done even though they are not enlarged, for they may contain cancer cells which have not yet had time to form a visible tumor.

In embolism by the *blood stream* the tumor cells are carried to some other organ where they are arrested in the capillaries and start secondary growths or *metastases.* In abdominal organs such as the stomach the secondary growths are usually in the liver, because the blood from the digestive tract is carried first to the liver. In the case of other organs the metastases commonly occur in the lungs, but any organ in the body may be involved.

Having reviewed some of the general aspects of tumor pathology, we may now briefly consider a few of the more important varieties of tumors. Many of these will be described more in detail in connection with the organs in which they occur. It is difficult to give an interesting or even intelligible account of tumors without reference to the microscopic structure and the use of a large number of technical terms, but this will be avoided as far as possible, for microscopic descriptions are nothing but a mass of words unless one has the opportunity to study the microscopic sections themselves.

BENIGN TUMORS

The general characteristics of a benign tumor have already been outlined, so they need not be repeated here. In describing benign tumors, and the same is true of malignant tumors, it is best to name them after the tissue from which they arise, adding the suffix -*oma,* which indicates tumors, just as -*itis* indicates inflammation. Some of the principal tissues are as follows: (1) *Epithelium,* which makes up the skin, the mucous membranes which line the mouth, stomach, intestine, uterus, etc., and the glandular organs, such as the breast, liver, and uterus; (2) *fibrous* or *connective tissue* which forms a general framework of the body and therefore occurs in all organs; (3) *fat;* (4) *bone* and *cartilage;* (5) *muscle;* (6) *blood vessels;* (7) *nervous tissue;* (8) *lymph nodes.*

PAPILLOMA. This is a benign epithelial tumor which grows as a projecting mass from an epithelial surface (Fig. 59*A*). Its common site is the skin, but it also occurs in the mouth, large intestine, and bladder. Sometimes a papilloma, especially when irritated, may develop into cancer.

ADENOMA. This is also a benign epithelial tumor, but it is glandular in structure, that is to say, the cells are arranged around gland spaces. It naturally occurs in organs that are themselves glandular, such as the breast and thyroid gland.

FIBROMA. This is a tumor of fibrous tissue, and therefore dense and hard. As fibrous tissue is universally present, a fibroma may occur in practically every part of the body, and yet strangely enough fibromas are distinctly uncommon tumors. Perhaps the commonest site is under the skin.

LIPOMA. This is a soft fatty tumor growing from fat (adipose tissue). It may occur wherever fat is present, but is most common in the neck, shoulders, back, and buttocks, in all of which places fat is abundant.

OSTEOMA AND CHONDROMA. An osteoma arises from osseous tissue or bone, and consists of bone; a chondroma arises from cartilage and consists of that tissue. In the embryo the bones consist of cartilage which is gradually converted into bone. As long as bone is growing in length some cartilage remains at each end. It is natural, therefore, that both osteomas and chondromas should grow from the ends of bones.

MYOMA. This is a tumor composed of muscle. There are two kinds of muscles in the body: (1) Voluntary or striated muscles, which are under the control of the will and form the ordinary muscles of the limbs and trunk; (2) involuntary or unstriated (plain) muscles, which are not under the control of the will and are found in the walls of the stomach and intestine, the blood vessels, and the uterus. Curiously enough myomas are of great rarity in voluntary muscles, but they are extremely common in the uterus where they are known as *fibroids,* because of the large amount of fibrous tissue that is mingled with the muscle.

ANGIOMA. An angioma is a tumor composed of vessels, usually blood vessels but sometimes lymph vessels. It is therefore usually of a bright or dark red color, although a lymphangioma is colorless. Its common site is the skin, especially of the face or neck, where it forms a red patch known as a *port-wine stain* or *birthmark*. The latter term is used because the tumor is usually present at birth. An angioma may form an unsightly swelling of the lip in children.

NEVUS. A nevus is a tumor of the skin composed of epidermal cells filled with melanin pigment, being usually dark in color and sometimes jet black. It is therefore a melanoma. There are two varieties of melanoma, benign and malignant. The nevus is a *benign melanoma,* its common name being a *mole,* which simply means a mass. Moles are so common that nearly everyone has at least one tiny one, and many people have a large number. A nevus is a congenital condition, but it may not be apparent at birth. The common sites are the face, neck, and back. They are probably under hormonal influence, for they tend to increase in size at puberty. They may grow slowly for a time, remain quiescent for a long period, and then gradually atrophy. The beginning of a malignant change in later life is indicated by an increase in size and pigmentation, the presence of a pink halo due to congestion, and itching. The tumor has now become a *malignant melanoma. It is customary to refer to the benign form as a nevus and to the malignant form simply as a melanoma, the malignancy being taken for granted.* The dangerous sites are the palm, the sole of the foot, the fingers and toes, the genitals, and places exposed to continued trauma. The transformation is often slow and insidious, for melanoma enters by stealth like a thief in the night, but any sudden increase in the rate of growth should arouse a suspicion of malignancy, and the tumor should at once be removed. A mole that shows no change need not be touched except for cosmetic reasons, but chronic irritation and trauma must be avoided at all costs. The malignant melanoma is discussed again on page 228.

MALIGNANT TUMORS

From every tissue of the body that can give rise to a benign tumor a malignant tumor also may arise. In practice, however, nearly all malignant tumors can be divided into two great groups, carcinoma and sarcoma, both of which are included under the common term *cancer.* This simplification of nomenclature is due to the fact that the epithelial tumors are called carcinoma, whereas the name sarcoma is applied not only to connective tissue tumors but also to tumors of bone, cartilage, fat, and muscle, which are derived from or closely related to connective tissue. The carcinomas form a more compact group, the sarcomas a more miscellaneous one.

CARCINOMA. This is the commonest of all malignant tumors, very much commoner than sarcoma. *It spreads principally by the lymph stream,* so that secondary involvement of the regional lymph nodes is extremely common and has to be considered by the surgeon in every case. *Spread by the blood stream is also common,* and it sometimes happens that the first indication of cancer in an organ such as the lung is the development of a secondary tumor in the brain, the secondary tumor naturally being mistaken for the primary one until the original is discovered. **It is evident that when tumors are present in two organs it may be difficult to say which is primary and which secondary.**

Carcinoma may arise either from the skin or from glandular organs (breast, liver, etc.), including the secreting glands in the mucous membranes of the stomach, intestine, and uterus. The *microscopic structure* differs in the two cases. In skin cancer there is some attempt at repro-

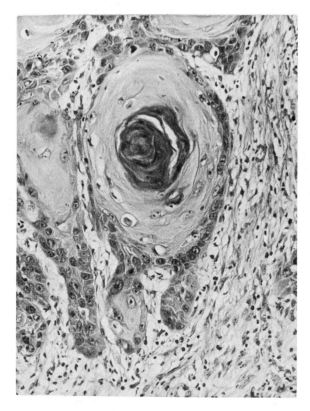

Fig. 62.   Epidermoid carcinoma of skin, showing downward invasion. $\times$ 200.

ducing the normal arrangement of the epithelial cells in layers, so that this tumor is known as *epidermoid carcinoma* (resembling the skin or epidermis), an older name being *epithelioma* (Fig. 62). In glandular cancers there is an attempt at arrangement of the cells around gland spaces, so that the tumor is known as *adenocarcinoma* (Greek *aden,* gland) (Fig. 63). In both forms masses of tumor cells invade the deeper structures.

The degree to which carcinoma can resemble the normal skin or glandular structure varies greatly. There may be absolutely no approximation to the normal arrangement of cells; such a tumor is said to be *undifferentiated* or *anaplastic*. These anaplastic tumors are naturally highly malignant, and as they are rapidly growing they are the most sensitive to radiation. Or the tumor may reproduce the normal structure with a fair degree of success, and is then said to be *differentiated*. It is evident from what has been said previously that if a tumor is highly differentiated the pathologist may have difficulty in distinguishing it from a benign epithelial tumor (adenoma, papilloma). The more highly differentiated the tumor, the less will be its malignancy and the less will it respond to radiation. **Speaking generally, highly anaplastic tumors are better treated by radiation, highly differentiated**

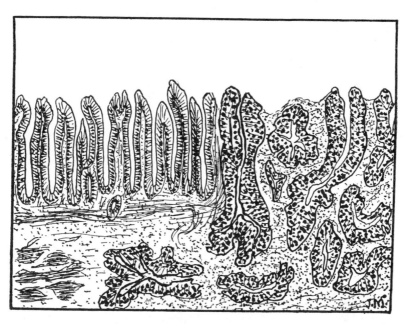

Fig. 63. Adenocarcinoma of bowel, showing sudden change from normal regular glands to malignant irregular glands. The cancer is invading and destroying the deeper part of the wall of the bowel.

tumors by surgical removal. The degree of differentiation is expressed as four grades, Grade 1 being the most differentiated, Grade 4 the most anaplastic.

The *common sites* of carcinoma are the skin, mouth, lung, stomach, breast, and uterus. *Skin cancers* as a rule are not highly malignant, and early removal is followed by a high percentage of cures. A special type of skin cancer is known as *rodent ulcer* (Fig. 64); this is confined almost entirely to the face, is of slow growth, long duration, and low malignancy, and is therefore very amenable to treatment. The microscopic picture is called *basal cell carcinoma,* because the tumor is composed of cells resembling the basal cell layer of the epidermis, and differing from epidermoid carcinoma in which the cells tend to become cornified or keratinized like those of the superficial layers of the normal skin. *Mouth cancer* occurs chiefly on the lower lip and tongue, usually on the basis of some previous site of irritation. *Cancer of the lip* is usually of low-grade malignancy and has a good prognosis, whereas *cancer of the tongue* tends to be a higher grade with a correspondingly bad prognosis. Cancer of the other organs will be described when the diseases of those organs are considered.

SARCOMA.   A sarcoma is a malignant tumor of connective (fibrous) tissue, and of those structures such as bone and cartilage which are derived from connective tissue. While we say that a sarcoma is a tumor of connective tissue, we must keep in mind that it is a tumor of connective tissue *cells,* not connective tissue fibers. The term is also applied loosely and incorrectly to certain other malignant tumors. Sarcomas may occur in any part of the body, as connective tissue is present everywhere, but the principal sites are bone, subcutaneous tissue, and muscle. These tumors are quite uncommon compared with carcinoma. A sarcoma infiltrates the surrounding tissue, just as does a carcinoma, but it seldom spreads by the lymph stream to the local lymph nodes. Distant spread is by the blood stream, and the metastases are usually in the lungs.

LYMPHOSARCOMA.   This is a malignant tumor of the lymph nodes. *Its two chief characteristics are its wide distribution and its extreme sensitiveness to radiation.* The disease spreads from one group of nodes to another, so that it may involve in turn the nodes in the neck (Fig. 65), axilla, and groin, as well as the nodes in the chest and abdomen. The response to radiation is remarkable, large masses of tumor melting away in a few days or weeks like snow before the sun. Some cases can be cured and many held in check for a long time by means of radiation in the form of roentgen rays.

MALIGNANT MELANOMA.   We have already encountered this neoplasm as a malignant development of a nevus, which is a benign mel-

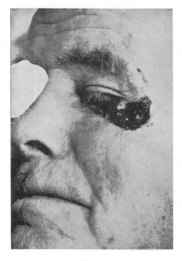 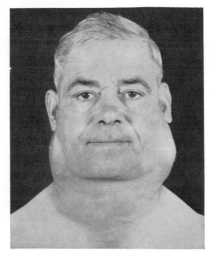

Fig. 64 Fig. 65

Fig. 64. Rodent ulcer; at the outer angle of the eye.
Fig. 65. Lymphosarcoma. Bilateral enlargement of cervical lymph nodes.

anoma, but it is customary to reserve the term melanoma for the malignant variety. The change from nevus to melanoma never takes place before puberty, suggesting that hormonal stimulation plays an important part in the development of the malignancy. As the name implies, the tumor cells are loaded with black melanin pigment, more particularly in the cytoplasm (Fig. 66). *The great danger of malignant melanoma is not local destruction, as is seen in carcinoma and sarcoma, but early invasion of the lymphatics and blood vessels, causing widespread dissemination and the formation of metastases throughout the body.* Perhaps the most dangerous site of origin is the foot. A pigmented lesion is less likely to attract attention there than on the hand or face. *The melanoma, unfortunately, is completely radioresistant.* In the occasional case the tumor arises from the pigment cells not of the skin, but of the eye.

GLIOMA. This is a malignant tumor of the glia or neuroglia of the brain which separates the nerve cells from one another, and therefore acts as a kind of connective tissue. Brain tumors are quite common, but such tumors practically never arise from nerve cells, always from neuroglia. The gliomas vary much in malignancy, but even the least malignant ones show no attempt at encapsulation and merge with the surrounding brain tissue. This makes the task of the brain surgeon a peculiarly difficult one, because even when he has exposed the tumor he finds it hard to know how much of the surrounding brain to remove.

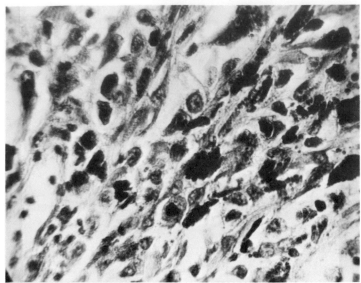

Fig. 66. Malignant melanoma showing abundance of black pigment in the tumor cells. (Kindness of Dr. N. K. Patoria, Nagpur, India.)

LABORATORY DIAGNOSIS. **The final diagnosis of cancer, that is to say, whether a lump is a neoplasm, and whether that neoplasm is innocent or malignant, must be made in the laboratory.** *The clinician can be suspicious, but he cannot be certain.* The laboratory, or rather the man who works in the laboratory, can employ a number of techniques.

Biopsy. When a tumor is removed by a surgeon in the operating room it must be sent to the pathology laboratory, where it is fixed, imbedded in paraffin, sectioned, and stained. *It is on the microscope examination of these sections that the final diagnosis is made by the pathologist as to whether or not the lesion is a malignant one.* Under some circumstances, particularly in the case of lumps of the breast, it may be highly desirable for the surgeon to have a report on the nature of the lesion *during the course of the operation,* so that he may determine the extent of his subsequent procedure. For this purpose the *frozen section* on unfixed tissue stained with polychrome methylene blue enables a "rush diagnosis" to be made on a "rapid section" in the course of a few minutes. **The responsibility laid on the pathologist is heavy.** If he says that the lesion is benign, nothing more need be done. If he says that it is malignant, the entire breast and regional lymph nodes must be removed. If the lesion is in a limb, the pathologist's opinion may decide whether or not the patient shall lose an arm or a leg.

Exfoliative Cytology. Cancer cells lose the adhesiveness characteristic of normal cells, so that they tend to be cast off or exfoliated from a surface very early in the disease, even in the preinvasive stage. These cells are found in exudates, secretions, washings, and scrapings. This diagnostic method, often referred to loosely and inaccurately as cytology, has opened up new vistas in the early diagnosis of cancer. Its greatest value at present is in cancer of the cervix and bronchus, where it is easy to obtain fresh cells which have not yet degenerated. By this means it is possible to detect very early cancers. Curiously enough, in advanced cancer the test may be negative, because the cells have become necrotic and therefore unrecognizable. *The test is always associated with the name of Papanicolaou,* although he first introduced his smear method for the study of cells in animal vaginal secretions, and not for cancer.

In the laborious task of "screening" large numbers of presumably normal persons for carcinoma, more particularly for cancer of the cervix uteri, *fluorescence microscopy* has proved a time-saving measure. This procedure has the additional advantage that it can be done by physicians or technicians without special training in exfoliative cytology. The method employs *cytochemistry,* with special relation to the cytoplasm, whereas the conventional method depends on *cytomorphology,* with particular attention to the nucleus. Using the fluorescence dye *acridineorange* the deoxyribonucleic acid (DNA) of the nucleus appears green under the fluorescence microscope, while the ribonucleic acid (RNA) of the cytoplasm appears brown, orange, or flaming red. **Malignant cells usually contain large amounts of cytoplasmic RNA, associated with the extremely active protein synthesis, so that they display brilliant orange or red cytoplasmic fluorescence, and are readily distinguished from the normal cells displaying green or brown fluorescence.** Study of the cells by the standard method is essential in the cases showing a suggestive fluorescence reaction.

Cancer Cells in the Blood. By the use of special techniques it is now possible to demonstrate cancer cells in blood removed from a vein in many cases of cancer, particularly when the vein drains the organ in which the cancer is situated. These observations are of particular interest in relation to the question of metastases. The method is not used for the simple diagnosis of cancer.

Chemical Tests. An enormous amount of time and money has been spent on the search for a chemical test of the blood or secretions which would indicate that neoplasia was in progress. We need a method such as the Wassermann test for syphilis or the test for hyperglycemia (high blood sugar level) in diabetes. The results have been uniformly disappointing. It is true that in individual instances the tests may be of clinical value, as in the high serum acid phosphatase level in carcinoma of the prostate with massive metastases in the bones, due to the marked ability of the normal epithelium of the prostate to elaborate this enzyme. *But the fact remains that we still have no chemical test for neoplasia as such.*

SYMPTOMS OF CANCER. *The most important single fact about the clinical picture of cancer is that in the early stages the disease is painless.* If it were as painful as toothache, far fewer people would die from the disease. The symptoms will vary with the location of the tumor, but in most cases there are likely to be such general constitutional symptoms as weakness, loss of weight, anemia, and pain later in the disease. In a superficial part such as the lip or breast a lump may be felt. When the affected organ communicates with the surface there may be a discharge as in cancer of the uterus. In cancer of the stomach the first evidence may be loss of appetite, in the case of the kidney there may be blood in the urine. There may be no symptoms of any kind for a considerable period, as is shown by the fact that a malignant tumor of some size may be discovered incidentally at autopsy, although the patient presented no evidence suggestive of any malignant disease.

Finally it must be remembered that the symptoms may not be due to the primary tumor, which may remain latent, but to metastases. One of the best examples of this very confusing occurrence is that of a silent carcinoma of the lung which metastasizes to the brain, so that the patient comes to the doctor with symptoms of a brain tumor, but no cough, shortness of breath, pain in the chest, or spitting of blood.

So far we have spoken of the clinical effects of cancer as those due to the local lesion and to metastases. But the most puzzling, indeed mysterious effects are those known as *systemic manifestations.* These are too multiform to be enumerated, but they may be *dermatological,* including various inflammations of the skin; *vascular,* more particularly thrombophlebitis migrans; *hormonal disturbances* involving estrogens; and *neuromuscular* symptoms suggesting lesions of the nerves and muscles. For these, unfortunately, we have no explanation.

TUMOR IMMUNITY

Before the discovery of the chemical carcinogens all the experimental work consisted of transplanting malignant tumors that occurred spontaneously in animals into other animals. The second animal had to be another member of the same species (homotransplantation). The tumor would not grow in an animal of another species (heterotransplantation), because the tumor tissue acted as a foreign antigen, which stimulated the formation of specific antibodies that destroyed the antigenic tumor tissue. For this reason it was impossible to successfully transplant human cancer to laboratory animals. Resistance to heterotransplantation has now been overcome in two ways: (1) *preliminary radiation of the animal,* (2) *administration of cortisone.* Both of these methods appear to depress antibody production to heterologous antigens in the transplanted tumor, probably due to a great reduction in the number of lymphocytes which are known to produce antibodies. The result of these procedures has been exciting, for it is now possible to transplant human cancer to such animals as the rat, guinea pig, and rabbit, and maintain it over successive generations.

SPONTANEOUS REGRESSION. Of all the ugly words we know in medicine, none is more repellent than cancer, the crab. When we think of cancer in general terms, we are apt to conjure up a process characterized by a steady, remorseless, and inexorable progress in which the disease is all-conquering, and none of the immunological and defensive forces that help us to survive the onslaught of bacterial and viral infections can serve to arrest the faltering footsteps to the grave. The idea that antibodies may be produced against neoplastic tissue has aroused fresh interest in the subject of the *spontaneous regression of cancer.* We are apt to think of a cancer as growing continuously and at a uniform rate. This is true of a tissue culture of cancer cells, but it is not true of neoplasia either in the experimental animal or in man. *A cancer often grows by fits and starts, and it may apparently stop growing for a period. This arrest is almost certainly due to something in the environment rather than to a change in the cancer cells.* We have already seen the control that hormones exert on neoplasia. The accelerated growth of breast cancer during pregnancy has long been recognized. Cancer in man may be made to regress either by the administration of hormones or by removal of endocrine glands. In rare instances this regression may be *spontaneous,* the tumor not only ceasing to grow, but actually disappearing. I have collected and reported a series of such cases, in all of which the diagnosis of cancer had been confirmed previously by microscopic examination. In many of them there has been a history of *partial* surgical removal, palliative radiation therapy, or the occurrence of some acute bacterial infection. *In all of these instances there seems to have been some change in the immunological relationship between the tumor and the host,* which may be regarded as the converse of the depression of immunological resistance induced by the use of cortisone.

The object of this brief discussion of tumor immunity is to suggest that the cancer problem is not quite so hopeless as it is customary to believe, and that the body can develop some degree of resistance, either local or general, to the neoplasia that threatens its life. In my own case, to which reference is made below, the cancer cells must have been held in abeyance for 17 years before they again manifested themselves. The immunity (resistance) of skeletal muscles to metastases is remarkable, for they must receive countless tumor emboli, yet rarely show metastatic growth. Future work may enable us to so influence the environment in which the cancer cells grow that the balance in favor of the body is restored and recovery becomes possible.

CANCER THERAPY

At the present time cancer can be treated effectively by surgical removal or by radiotherapy or both, and in some cases palliatively by hormonal therapy or chemotherapy. Unfortunately it is impossible to avoid the destruction of normal tissue both by the surgeon's knife and by the even more lethal weapon of radiation. The ideal therapeutic agent would be one with a selective action on malignant cells while leaving normal cells untouched, just as antibiotics lead to the destruction of bacteria in the tissues.

Innocent tumors are treated with complete success by local removal, that is to say, only the tumor itself needs to be removed and none of the surrounding tissue. *With malignant tumors the reverse is the case.* Not only the tumor but as much of the surrounding tissue as is feasible must be excised, for it may harbor cancer cells that cannot be detected by the eye or hand, but only by the microscope. A cancer of the breast may be no larger than a pea in size, yet the whole breast has to be removed. The regional lymph nodes also may have to be removed, but cancer of each organ must be considered as a separate entity, and what is true of one is not necessarily true of another. Thus the regional lymph nodes, although apparently normal, are always removed in cancer of the breast, but not necessarily in cancer of the lip. The presence of distant metastases (blood spread) is an indication that surgical treatment can offer no hope of cure.

It should be emphasized that every cancer is curable in the early stage before it has begun to spread. This is particularly true of cancer of the skin, lip, and other places where it can be readily seen. Other tumors may eventually recur after, say, five years, but to give a man or woman of sixty years another five years of life is surely something worth while. I had carcinoma of the parotid salivary gland in 1948 which was removed by operation immediately after being observed, followed by the implantation of 18 radium needles. I remained in perfect health for 17 years till the tumor recurred in 1965, and again twice later, but with efficient treatment I have been well until the present time (1971). Naturally the affected area is checked every few months.

A stitch in time saves nine. The great difficulty at present is to diagnose cancers of the internal organs before they have extended too far to be operable or have set up metastases.

Radiation is a well tried and very valuable method of treating certain forms of cancer. It may be used either in the form of roentgen rays or radium. This treatment is made possible by the fact that radiations have a greater destructive action on rapidly growing cells than on normal cells. They therefore have a *selective action* on cancer cells compared with that on the surrounding tissue. It is possible, however, to kill *all* the tissue by radiation and this danger has constantly to be borne in mind by the radiotherapist. His aim is to use the maximum amount of radiation on the cancer but to stop just short of damaging the normal tissue. *This requires quite as much skill and special training as it does to cut the tumor out with a knife.*

Radium gives off radiations (gamma rays) that are similar in nature to x-rays and have a similar action on tumor tissue. Both may be used for attacking some tumors, but in most cases one or the other is preferable. X-rays may be of low voltage (50,000 to 100,000 volts) or high voltage (usually around 220,000 volts, though in some machines very much higher). The low voltage rays are known as *soft;* they have only slight penetrating power and are therefore suitable only for surface tumors. High voltage rays are known as *hard;* they have great penetrating power, which makes them ideal for treating deep-seated tumors. It may be necessary to press the treatment until a marked and sometimes painful inflammatory reaction is produced.

Radium may be used in three ways: radon seeds, radium element, and radium bomb. *Radon* is the name given to an emanation or gas given off by radium and compressed into capillary tubes of gold or platinum. Radium continues to give off this emanation indefinitely, which can be collected in tubes every day. It soon loses its radioactive power. *Radium element* is a salt of radium, minute quantities of which are put into platinum tubes or needles. Both the radon and radium element needles are introduced directly into the tumor. The *radium bomb* is a large amount of radium (4 grams or more) used at some distance from the body. It produces some of the penetrating effects of hard x-rays. It is evident that some form of radium will be useful for tumors in certain positions, whereas other forms will be preferable for tumors in other positions.

Tumors vary tremendously in their response to radiation. Some, such as lymphosarcoma, are highly radiosensitive; others such as malignant melanoma are as highly radioresistant. *An intimate knowledge of tumor pathology is therefore necessary before treatment of cancer by radiation can be attempted.* The tumors that are most sensitive to radiation are those in which the cells are dividing most rapidly, which are furthest removed from normal structure, and which are therefore the most malignant. The rays have no discriminating action on innocent tumors, as these resemble normal tissues in structure. Speaking generally, roentgen rays are used for the treatment of widely diffused tumors such as the malignant growth of lymph nodes known as lymphosarcoma, and also for deep-seated tumors such as cancer of the lung. Radium, on the other hand, is planted directly into the tumor and kills all the cancer cells within reach. *Cancer of the cervix of the uterus, one of the commonest and most dreaded forms of cancer in women, has proved particularly susceptible to treatment by radium.* Frequently the various forms of treatment, surgery and radiation, are combined.

Some tumors may be treated successfully by various types of radiation. The source of the radiation may be an x-ray tube, a naturally occurring isotope such as radium, or a man-made isotope such as cobalt-60. There is no difference between the gamma rays which come from a radioactive source and the x-rays which come from an x-ray machine.

In the past, x-rays generated from 50,000 to 400,000 volts were used to treat tumors, the low voltage for skin tumors, the higher voltages, because of increased penetration, for deep-seated tumors. Even with 400,000 volts, it was often not possible to treat the tumor to a high enough dose without damaging the skin excessively. To overcome this, high energy machines ranging from 2,000,000 to 25,000,000 volts were developed. With these machines, skin reactions are avoided and adequate doses to the tumor are possible. With the development of nuclear reactors, a whole host of new radioactive isotopes have been produced. Some of these, such as cobalt-60 and cesium-137, can replace the x-ray tube as the source of gamma rays and isotope units may be used in place of an x-ray machine. For example, the rays from a cobalt-60 unit treating at a distance of 80 cm. are equivalent to the rays from a 3,000,000 volt x-ray machine. Most deep-seated tumors today are treated with some type of cobalt-60 unit.

A word about so-called *cancer cures* and quack remedies. Most of these remedies are in the form of cancer pastes which are applied to external growths. They contain powerful irritants such as arsenic, which may kill the superficial part of the cancer and which irritate the deeper part to increased activity, so that by the time the surgeon is consulted the case has become hopeless. Sometimes one hears of cancers that have been cured by such remedies. In every case it will be found that no microscopic examination of the tumor has been made. Unless a biopsy is done, and a microscopic examination of the piece removed is made, it is impossible to be certain if the supposed cancer really is a tumor or merely an inflammatory mass.

FURTHER READING

ANDREWES, SIR CHRISTOPHER: Brit. Med. J., 1966, *1,* 653. (Tumour-viruses and virus-tumours.)

BASERGA, R., and SAFFOTTI, W.: Arch. Path., 1955, *59,* 26. (Blood spread of metastases.)

BEAN, R. H. D., and TRAILL, M.: Lancet, 1967, *1,* 364. (Microscopy of the cancer cell as a guide to chemotherapy.)

BITTNER, J. J.: Science, 1936, *84,* 162. (Milk factor in mammary mouse cancer.)

BOYD, W.: *The Spontaneous Regression of Cancer,* 1966, Springfield, Ill.

BURKITT, D., and HUTT, M. S. R.: International Pathology, 1966, *7,* 1. (Geographic pathology in developing countries.)

BURKITT, D., and O'CONOR, G. T.: Cancer, 1961, *14,* 258. (Malignant lymphoma in African children.)

COLE, W. H., McDONALD, G. O., ROBERTS, S. S., and SOUTHWICK, H. W.: *Dissemination of Cancer. Prevention and Therapy,* 1961, New York.

EVERSON, T. C., and COLE, W. H.: *Spontaneous Regression of Cancer.* 1966, Philadelphia.

GROSS, L.: Cancer Res., 1958, *18,* 371. Brit. Med. J., 1958, *2,* 1. (Vertical transmission of cancer.)

HORSFALL, F. L., JR.: Bull. New York Acad. Med., 1966, *42,* 167. (Cancer and viruses.)

RHOADS, C. P.: Ann. Roy. Coll. Surg. of England, 1957, *20,* 139. (The soluble puzzle of cancer control.)

SIMINOVITCH, L.: Can. Med. Ass. J., 1962, *86,* 1137. (The chemical basis of heredity in viruses and cells.)

STEWART, S. E., *et al.:* Virology, 1957, *3,* 380. (Viral production of cancer.)

STOKER, M.: Endeavour, 1966, *25,* 119. (Viral carcinogenesis.)

SULLIVAN, J. D., and RONA, G.: Can. Med. Ass. J., 1964, *91,* 647. (Systemic effects of non-endocrine tumors.)

WARBURG, O.: *The Metabolism of Tumors,* English translation, London, 1930. Science, 1956, *123,* 369.

WILLIS, R. A.: *Pathology of Tumours,* 4th ed., 1967, London.

Ionizing Radiation

The fundamental feature of ionizing radiation is the detachment of an electron from an atom. It is the most powerful of all physical irritants, for it injures not only organs and cells, but the very molecules and atoms of which the cells are composed. We have long been familiar with the effects produced by x-rays and radium, but in the atomic age with its varied uses of nuclear energy we have unfortunately to face other sources of radiation.

THE ATOM

The atom consists of (1) a central *nucleus* made up of *positively charged protons* and *neutrons without charge,* and (2) a *cloud* of *negatively charged electrons* which fly in orbit around the nucleus. The number of negative electrons equals the number of positive protons, so that the electric charges balance, with resulting neutrality. The proton is 1800 times more massive than the electron, and the neutron is still larger. The atom is like a miniature solar system with the nucleus taking the place of the sun and the electrons following orbits around it, as do the planets. The orbit of the electrons around the nucleus is 10,000 times as large as the nucleus itself. As the electrons are widely separated, it follows that the atom, and matter which is composed of atoms, is largely empty space.

If the nucleus contains an excess of either protons or neutrons it is radioactive, because there is a redistribution of the particles with emission of energy in the form of radiation. An *ion* is an electrically charged particle given off from the atom. As particles with the same charge tend to repel one another, like humans associating too closely in a closed community, they must be held together by extremely powerful forces. It is these so-called "nuclear forces" which when released constitute the new power factor in peace and war. We say "new," but actually atomic energy is the source of 99 per cent of all energy known to man, both stored in fuels as previous energy from the sun or streaming all the time as solar radiations.

The *neutron* must not be underestimated, merely because it does not have a positive charge like a proton or a negative charge like an electron. As a matter of fact it is the neutron's electrically neutral character as well as its large size which make it the ideal instrument for producing disintegration or fission of the nucleus, as it does not have to overcome electrical repulsion like the protons. It is the use of accelerators such as the cyclotron and betatron that have made it possible to bombard nuclei with protons as well as neutrons. Isotopes are made in an atomic pile reactor through bombardment with neutrons.

RADIOACTIVITY

High energy radiation represents a stream of very small particles which have escaped from the atomic nucleus and are traveling at very high speeds. Radioactive materials emit three types of radiation, known respectively as alpha, beta, and gamma rays. *Alpha rays* consist of positively charged particles (protons) and neutrons, which are several thousand times as heavy as electrons. On account of their large mass they collide very early with atoms which they encounter, and only penetrate for a fraction of a millimeter. This is fortunate, because they produce devastating injury. *Beta rays* are streams of electrons released from many radioactive elements, as well as from cathode-ray tubes. Being very much smaller than alpha particles they penetrate the tissues for two or more millimeters, but they have less ionizing power. *Gamma rays* are similar to high-energy x-rays, the only difference being one of length, the gamma rays being shorter and therefore having more energy, deeper penetration, and greater power to cause ionization by detaching an electron from the atom on which they impinge.

IONIZATION. Ionizing radiations produce electrically charged particles—ions—on their passage through any matter, living or nonliving. When an electron is ejected from an atom, it leaves the electrically unbalanced residue of the atom as a positively charged ion. This is the essence of ionizing radiation. The detached electron may become attached to some other atom, which also loses its electric neutrality, and thus becomes charged or ionized. Either the loss or the gain of an electron may alter the chemical behavior of the molecule affected.

RADIOACTIVE ISOTOPES. *Isotopes are elements having the same atomic number* (the sum of the protons) *but different atomic weights* (the sum of the protons and neutrons). Radioisotopes are normally stable elements made radioactive in atom smashers. The *half-life* of a radioactive element is the time required to lose 50 per cent of its radioactive atoms which have broken down. The difference in the half-life of various materials is simply fantastic. Thus in the case of uranium the time is 4 billion years, while with iodine-138 it is only six seconds. It is evident that for clinical use the half-life must be short, otherwise permanent radiation damage would result.

Radioactive isotopes are used in medicine in two very different ways, as "tracers" or in therapy. (1) **Isotopes as tracers** depend on the fact that a radioactive isotope of an element is *chemically* identical with the nonradioactive form, and can therefore be substituted for it in a chemical compound. This is known as "tagging," the radioactive atoms being demonstrated by means of a Geiger counter. The tagged molecules can now be followed through complex chemical and metabolic processes. This has proved invaluable in the investigation of both normal and diseased function. (2) **Isotopes in therapy** are used in much larger doses. The method depends on the selective concentration of an element in a particular organ or tissue. The best example is the use of radioactive iodine in hyperplasia and cancer of the thyroid gland, since any iodine administered is concentrated to an overwhelming degree in the thyroid. Radioactive isotopes obviously provide us with a method of applying radiation locally to internal organs for cancer and other hyperplastic conditions.

They are even more important in the early diagnosis of cancer, for their concentration in certain organs and tissues makes possible the detection of a neoplasm sometimes many months before it is evident in conventional roentgenograms. This is particularly true of tumors of the lung and brain. The new radioisotopes are fortunately short-lived, only hours or at most a few days. Their presence is shown by a gamma-ray detector, a technique known as *scanning*.

BIOLOGICAL REACTIONS

Chemical molecules are held together by interactions between the outer orbital electrons of the atoms. The loss or the acquisition of an electron by an atom in the process of ionization results in a transfer of energy from the radioactive agent to the cells, causing damage that may prove fatal. The electron bullets may hit one of the 46 chromosomes in the *nucleus* with their thousands of genes, or an enzyme molecule attached to a mitochondrion in the *cytoplasm*. In the latter case the biological result will be small, as there are many more similar molecules to carry on the function, but if the target is large, as in the case of a gene, the result may be serious, resulting in a mutation. The effects of ionizing radiation are most evident during mitosis, because at this time the chromosomes present discrete targets. *It is for this reason that rapidly dividing cancer and other cells are more radiosensitive than those that seldom divide.* A large dose of radiation arrests mitosis permanently and results in death of the cells. On the other hand long-continued exposure to sublethal doses of irradiation may result in neoplasia.

COMPARATIVE RADIOSENSITIVITY. *Different tissues differ widely in their sensitivity to radiation.* Different kinds of animals also vary in a similar and, at present, quite inexplicable manner. In general terms it may be said that those cells are especially radiosensitive which normally continue to multiply throughout life, owing to their own short life span. Such are the cells of the lymphatic and hematopoietic or blood-forming systems, and the germinal cells of the gonads. We would expect a lymphocyte, with its life span of a few hours, to be more sensitive to radiation than a nerve cell that never divides.

Cancer Cells. The cells of a neoplasm, like the normal cells from which they originate, differ widely in their response to irradiation. (Irradiation is the deliberate use of radiation.) Rapidly dividing cells may be expected to respond well. But the radiotherapist must beware of generalizations and know the peculiarities of individual tumors. Thus such tumors as malignant melanoma and osteogenic sarcoma may be teeming with mitoses and yet be quite radioresistant. Lymphosarcoma, composed of short-lived lymphocytes, is particularly radiosensitive, and may melt away as quickly as the proverbial snowball in hell. *Unfortunately there is a profound difference between radiosensitivity and radiocurability,* for even the most radiosensitive of tumors have often a small proportion of cells that survive and transmit the property of resistance to their progeny, so that eventually the entire mass may be radioresistant. We have already seen the same thing happening in the case of antibiotics and bacteria.

RADIATION HAZARDS

There never has been a time when the question of radiation hazards was of graver concern or closer to the hearts of men than the present. These hazards are of three kinds, which in their order of importance may be termed diagnostic, therapeutic, and fallout hazards. *Diagnostic radiation,* when used with judgment, presents so small a hazard to health that it is completely outweighed by the potential for good. If overdone and repeated too frequently it may be a source of danger. The growing ends of bone in children are easily injured by radiation, and we have come to realize the insidious danger of fluoroscope installations in shoe stores, which give such a fascinating view of the bones of a child's foot in the shoe being fitted. *Therapeutic radiation* obviously involves greater hazard, because the radiotherapist's object is to disable or kill cancer or other undesirable cells, and in the process the normal tissue may easily be injured. In some cases the injury may be much more serious and devastating than that inflicted by the surgeon's knife. The effect of radiation depends on (1) size of dose and (2) sensitivity of tissue, to which must be added the area involved in the radiation. The dosage is expressed as roentgens or r, in honor of Roentgen, who first observed the rays or radiations from the vacuum cathode tube. *Fallout radiation,* which gives rise to total body radiation, may be the result of atomic or hydrogen bomb bursts in war, of atomic weapon tests, or of accidental leakage from atomic energy installations. A dose of 400 r over the total body surface is believed to be enough to kill half of a given human population.

SKIN. The skin is most frequently involved, because all therapeutic external radiations must pass through the skin. *Acute radiodermatitis* is really a burn of the skin, but one that takes many days or a week or two to develop. It is equally slow in healing, and scarring may go on for many months, causing marked deformity. *Chronic radiodermatitis* is likely to be the result of frequent small doses. It was a common lesion on the hands of radiologists before the danger was realized and efficient screening was practiced. The epidermis is thinned and devitalized, so that minor injury may result in localized areas of necrosis which often take months to heal. The surrounding capillaries are dilated, so that the skin is red. Finally, carcinoma may develop, often after an interval of many years since the last exposure to radiation.

LYMPHOID AND HEMATOPOIETIC TISSUES. *These are the most sensitive to radiation.* Damage to these tissues is most likely to be seen in total body radiation. As the life span of the lymphocyte is only a few hours, extensive injury to lymphoid tissue is immediately followed by a marked drop in the number of lymphocytes in the circulating blood. The hematopoietic cells of the bone marrow are even more sensitive than the lymphocytes. There is a striking drop in the number of circulating granular leukocytes and blood platelets, the maximum effect being seen about the end of the first week of total body radiation. By that time the bone marrow is almost acellular (Fig. 67). If the patient survives he is sure to suffer from recurring infections due to the lack of leukocytes as well as failure in antibody formation owing to the loss of lymphocytes, and from frequent hemorrhages due to the lack of platelets. Long-continued exposure to small doses of ionizing radiation may cause neoplasia rather than destruction of the marrow cells resulting in leukemia, an occupational hazard of radiologists before this danger was recognized. Leukemia is also liable to develop in patients receiving

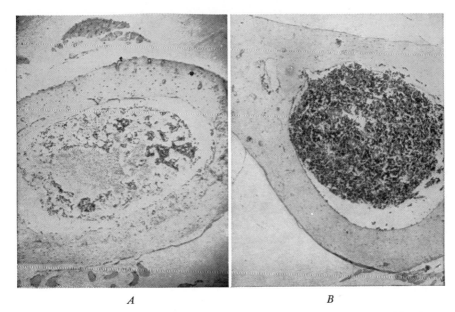

A   *B*

Fig. 67. *A,* Shaft of femur of a mouse ten days after irradiation with 600 r x-rays. *B,* Shaft of femur of control mouse. (Mole, courtesy of Société de Chemie Physique.)

long-continued heavy radiation for the disabling disease of the spine known as ankylosing spondylitis.

GASTROINTESTINAL TRACT. The epithelium of the stomach and intestine is continually being renewed, so that it belongs to the highly radiosensitive class, but the deep location of these structures serves to protect them against external radiation of moderate intensity. When radium is implanted for the treatment of carcinoma of the cervix, the mucosa of the rectum and colon may be seriously injured, with changes comparable with the lesions of radiodermatitis. In about 2 per cent of presumably oversensitive persons, inflammatory lesions with ulceration may develop in the anterior wall of the rectum from six months to several years after completion of the treatment. These ulcers are painful and the partitions between the rectum, bladder, and vagina may break down with distressing results. Even if the lesions heal there may be extensive scarring with stricture (narrowing) of the rectum.

GERM CELLS. The germinal cells of the ovary and testis are highly radiosensitive, so that these organs have to be shielded with particular care in persons liable to be exposed to radiation, more especially workers with radioactive material. The testicles are naturally more exposed than the deeply situated ovaries. If the cells are killed, sterility is the result. If, on the other hand, one of the chromosomes or even one of its genes is damaged, the result may be a mutation which becomes hereditary, being transmitted to future generations. This is the basis of the *genetic hazard* of fallout radiation resulting from atomic bomb explosions or tests.

ACUTE RADIATION SYNDROME. This syndrome, caused by whole body radiation due to atomic fallout from the air, must be distinguished from *radiation sickness,* the result of intensive local radiotherapy, which is characterized by loss of appetite and nausea, but rarely by vomiting. The essential lesion of total body radiation is cell depletion. This applies particularly to the intestine, the bone marrow, and the testes, but with a marked difference in the time element. After a single small total body exposure, the maximum damage to the small bowel occurs within a few days, to the granulocytes of the marrow in three to five weeks, while the sperm cells reach their minimum number in about one year. In the *low-dose range* (100 r) death is due to depression of the bone marrow; in the *middle-dose range* (500 r) it is due to damage to the gastrointestinal tract; in the *high-dose range* (2000 r) it is the result of failure of the central nervous system. There is a wide variation in individual susceptibility both in the experimental animal and in man. There were many thousands of survivors of the Hiroshima and Nagasaki blasts who resumed their previous occupation with full vigor. Of these we hear little.

The *clinical picture* is as follows. Within two hours of exposure there is a sudden onset of anorexia (loss of appetite), nausea, fatigue, malaise, and drowsiness. By the third day the patient feels well. Some three weeks later he begins to suffer from chills, fever, malaise, and shortness of breath. These are followed in a day or two by (1) *diarrhea* and other evidence of ulceration of the bowel, (2) *hemorrhages into the skin and from the mucous membranes* due to destruction of the megakaryocytes in the bone marrow which make the blood platelets, (3) severe infections in the mouth and elsewhere due to the disappearance of the polymorphonuclear leukocytes and of the lymphocytes which make antibodies, and finally (4) severe anemia due to destruction of the blood-forming cells of the marrow.

A moving account of the development of the acute radiation syndrome in an entire community representing the last survivors of a world war fought with atomic weapons will be found in Nevil Shute's novel, *On the Beach.*

In the above account of the radiation effects of atomic blast no reference has been made to late sequelae such as cataract, leukemia, and a variety of neoplasms, nor to the danger of the incorporation of the radioactive isotope strontium-90 into vegetation and thus eventually into milk.

FURTHER READING

ARONOW, S.: New Eng. J. Med., 1962, *266,* 1145. (A glossary of radiation terminology.)

CROW, J. F.: Bull. of the Atomic Scientists, 1958, *14,* 19. (Genetic effects of radiation.)

GERSTNER, H. B.: United States Armed Forces Med. J., 1958, *9,* 313. (Acute radiation syndrome.)

HOYT, R. C.: Bull. of the Atomic Scientists, 1958, *14,* 9. (What is radiation?)

TABERSHAW, J. R.: J. Chr. Diseases, 1959, *9,* 134. (Industrial hazards of ionizing radiation.)

TAYLOR, R. M.: Can. Med. Ass. J., 1962, *86,* 521. (The somatic effects of radiation.)

WEBSTER, E. W.: Radiology, 1959, *72,* 493. (Hazards of diagnostic radiology.)

Chapter 14

Heredity in Disease

MEDICAL GENETICS

In the causation of disease two great factors always demand consideration; these are environment and heredity. In Chapter 3 on The Causes of Disease we have only been concerned with what may be called the environmental diseases caused by bacteria, poisons, trauma, hunger, ionizing radiation, etc. These are the aspects of disease that have engaged the attention of medical investigators during the past one hundred years. Now heredity has suddenly marched into the forefront, largely on account of recent technical advances.

Actually the date of the birth of the *science* of genetics is 1866, when the Austrian monk, Gregor Mendel, crossed a red pea with a white pea in a tiny plot in a monastery garden in a small country town. In the second generation four plants bore red flowers, but in the third generation three were red while one was white. Mendel enunciated the concept of a *dominant* (red) and a *recessive* (white) *character,* the latter being present but hidden in the second generation. The application of Mendelian principles to the practice of horticulture and husbandry has proved invaluable, for it has made possible the elimination of undesirable characters in animal stock and crops, and the selection and cultivation of desirable traits. There are obvious difficulties in the application of these principles to human society. This epoch-making discovery attracted absolutely no attention until the beginning of this century, when it was realized that the very large chromosomes of the salivary gland of the fruit fly provided ideal material for studies in heredity. The present era dawned with the discovery of technical methods which rendered possible a precise study of *human* chromosomes, and the changes they may show in hereditary disease.

Heredity is the transmission of a quality, character, or defect from one generation to another. As in the case of Mendel's peas, this character may be dominant or recessive. A recessive character may be transmitted indefinitely for many generations in the germ plasm without coming to light until it meets a similar recessive trait from another strain; in such a case it may be impossible to recognize the hereditary character of the transmission in human material, owing to the necessarily long lapse of time. Disease factors in man are generally dominant, but they may be recessive or sex-linked (see below).

We must not confuse congenital with hereditary. A *congenital defect* is one which is present at birth, although it may only develop later to a sufficient degree to be detected clinically, as in the case of congenital cystic kidneys. *The defect may be hereditary, but frequently it is acquired in utero,* in which case it is in no sense genetic. Thus congenital syphilis is acquired from the mother before the baby is born. It is now recognized that *viral infections* of the mother during pregnancy may result in congenital defects, which may be evident at birth or may only become apparent later. The worst offender is *rubella* (German measles), which is apt to result in congenital heart disease if the infection strikes during the second and third months of pregnancy, as well as other congenital defects, such as blindness, deafness, or mental retardation. Mumps appears to be next in line as a crippler *in utero*. It seems probable that many other environmental factors during the early stages of pregnancy, such as radiation fallout, exposure of the mother to x-rays during pregnancy, poor maternal diet, and accidents *in utero* or at birth, may be responsible for many congenital defects which in the past have been regarded as truly hereditary or genetic in origin.

The study of the mechanism of heredity constitutes the science of genetics, which in turn is dependent on the behavior of the *genes,* countless particles of nucleic acid (DNA) arranged along the chromosomes. As the masterword of heredity is the DNA of the chromosomes, we must consider in more detail these structures which were merely mentioned in Chapter 1.

CHROMOSOMES. The chromosomes of man are 46 in number, not 48 as used to be thought before the introduction of modern chromosomal technique, although each species of animal and plant has its own characteristic number. Of these 44 are somatic (*soma,* body), and are known as *autosomes,* the remaining 2 being *sex chromosomes.* **Both the autosomes and the sex chromosomes are arranged in pairs, one member of each pair being maternal and the other paternal in origin.**

There are therefore 22 pairs of autosomes and one pair of sex chromosomes. *It is only during mitosis that the chromosomes become visible as separate units under the microscope.* They appear short and thick, but they are believed really to be long filaments along which the genes are arranged. When seen in a microscopic section of cells undergoing mitotic division the characteristics of individual chromosomes cannot be distinguished clearly, because they are bunched together on the spindle.

Recent technical methods have now surmounted this obstacle. Tissue cultures of dividing cells are used, first bone marrow cells obtained by sternal puncture, but now the white cells of the blood. Colchicine is added to the culture; this stops mitosis in full course, so that the chromosomes accumulate and are easier to find. Colchicine also breaks up the spindle and allows the chromosomes to spread out. The cells are then made to swell by means of hypotonic salt solution, and finally squashed firmly on the slide. The so-called *squash preparation* of chromosomes is shown in Figure 68. For a lucid description of the modern work on chromosomes the reader is referred to a delightful paper by Bernard Lennox entitled Chromosomes for Beginners.

It will be seen that even at this early phase of mitosis each chromosome has split into two longitudinal halves called *chromatids,* which remain adherent at only one point, the *centromere.* At the crucial moment of division the centromere splits, the chromatids travel into the daughter cells, and become their chromosomes. In looking at Figure 68 it will be seen that the chromosomes vary much in size and that the position of the centromere also differs, so that the "arm" may be short and the "leg" long, or vice versa. Using these facts as a basis, it is now possible to arrange the individual chromosomes (one of each pair) as an *idiogram* or order of length, and give them numbers by which, like convicts, they are known (Fig. 69).

Sex Chromosomes. Each of the 44 chromosomes (autosomes) contributed by a male gamete is homologous with a corresponding chromosome contributed by a female gamete. *In addition there are two chromosomes which determine the sex of the individual;* these are known as the X and Y sex chromosomes. In the female somatic cells there are two *homologous* X-chromosomes, whereas in the male the arrangement is *heterologous,* with one X- and one Y-chromosome. With a stretch of the imagination it might be said that the essential difference between Romeo and Juliet was that Romeo had a Y-chromosome in place of a double X. The Y-chromosome is as small as the smallest of the autosomes and carries very few genes (Fig. 69). The distinction between the two is easy to recognize in the giant chromosomes of the salivary gland of the fruit fly.

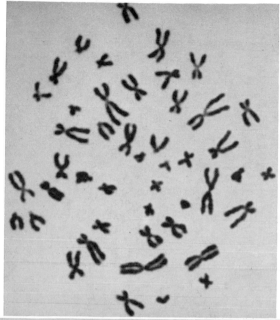

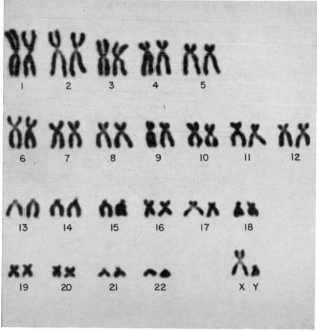

Fig. 68. The chromosome complement of a normal male (44 autosomes and an XY sex chromosome complex). (Barr and Carr; Canad. Med. Assn. Jour.)

HEREDITY IN DISEASE

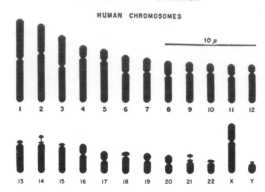

Fig. 69. Idiogram of human chromosomes. (D. Yi-Yung Hsea; New Eng. J. Med.)

In the *reduction division* (*meiosis*), which precedes the formation of a gamete or sex cell, there are naturally two kinds of spermatozoa, one set with one X-chromosome, which on fertilization will result in a female offspring, the other with one Y-chromosome will result in a male. The father passes on the Y-chromosomes received from his father to all his sons, and the X-chromosomes received from his mother to all his daughters. Both of the sex chromosomes carry additional non-sexual genes which are known as *sex-linked genes.* As the female has 2 X-chromosomes, she will be heterozygous and therefore a mere carrier for a mutant gene in a single X-chromosome, whereas the male with a single X-chromosome will be homozygous for the mutant gene, so that the trait will become apparent. The gene in question may be passed from father to daughter and from mother to son, but if it is recessive it is only in the male, in which it is unmasked, that it will become apparent. *The abnormality is thus confined to the male, but is transmitted by the female.* In the female the recessive abnormal gene (X) will be masked by the dominant normal gene on the other X-chromosome. This explains what is at first sight the peculiar sex distribution of hemophilia, "the bleeding disease," which is the finest and most famous example of a sex-linked inherited disease. Only the male is affected and only the female transmits the disease, another illustration of the old saying that the female of the species is more deadly than the male.

The question of *sex chromatin* has already been discussed on page 33. This simple method of determining the true sex by the examination of cells is of particular value in doubtful cases of intersex, and also in the determination of the chances of fertility.

Sex anomalies due to errors of development are fortunately uncommon, although of supreme importance to the unhappy victim. Even in the most normal person neither sex represents a state of absolute uni-sexuality. Usually one sex predominates to such an extent that no doubt exists, but although the genitalia are an important criterion of sex, they are often unreliable indicators of chromosomal sex. Most of the anom-alies are examples of *sex reversal,* a condition in which *chromosomal sex differs from anatomical sex.* True *hermaphroditism* (*Hermes,* mes-senger of the gods, and *Aphrodite,* goddess of love), in which testes and ovaries are both present, is very rare. In *pseudohermaphroditism* only testes *or* ovaries are present, but there is an intersexual anatomy of the rest of the reproductive system. This is the condition known as sex reversal, and is not uncommon. Two examples are described below in connection with chromosomal abnormalities.

Chromosomal Abnormalities. Loss of an entire chromosome, known as *monosomy* because only one of a pair remains, is nearly al-ways fatal. To this there is one exception, namely sex chromosome monosomy, in which there is a single X or, as it is expressed, XO. *Tri-somy,* the presence of three chromosomes of a kind instead of the nor-mal pair, is also damaging but not nearly as bad. Again nearly all the cases with more than one extra chromosome have involved the sex chromosomes. There are four well-established and fairly common syn-dromes, three involving sex chromosomes and one an autosome, three being trisomies with 47 chromosomes, one a monosomy with 45.

Mongolism or Trisomy-21 is that pathetic condition in which auto-some No. 21 is in triplicate, and the newborn child has mongoloid (slanted) eyes, hyperextensibility of the finger joints, imbecile facies, and, as becomes apparent only too soon, an imbecile mind. The trisomy is believed to be due to the failure of a pair of homologous chromo-somes to segregate or undergo *disjunction* at a meiotic division during the formation of gametes, a condition known as *nondisjunction.* Other examples of trisomic syndrome are coming to light, some of them incom-patible with life.

The *Klinefelter syndrome* is the commonest of the sex anomalies. *The basic feature is the addition of a sex chromosome, so that the sex chromosome complex is XXY.* The testes are small, with resulting infer-tility, the breasts may be enlarged, there are eunuchoid features, and the presence of sex chromatin (female) in smears of the buccal mucosa serves to clinch the diagnosis. The gonads of the early embryo have developed into testes rather than ovaries as they would do normally. *Mental deficiency* is a common feature of the Klinefelter syndrome as it is in other sex reversals.

Turner's syndrome is a fortunately rare condition in which there is *a single X-chromosome, often written as XO.* It forms an interesting contrast to the sex anomaly just described, for *just as Klinefelter's syn-*

drome may be regarded as a masculinization of the female, so Turner's syndrome is a feminization of the male. The nuclei therefore lack sex chromatin. The nuclear sexing test shows that the majority of these "girls" are really males with absence of testicular tissue, so that secondary sex characters fail to develop at puberty, as does menstruation.

GENES. *The genes, as we have already seen, appear to be chemical particles of DNA located along the chromosomes.* The gene acts as a *biochemical carrier of biological information from one generation to the next.* As in the case of the chromosomes, the genes are in pairs known as *allelomorphs* or *alleles* (*allelon,* one another), one member of the pair being maternal, the other paternal in origin. Allelic genes from father and mother are situated at the same spot or *locus* on the two members of the same pair of homologous chromosomes. **Fundamentally genes control enzymes, and enzymes control the chemistry of life.** If any mutation or change takes place in the structure of a gene, there will be a functional disturbance somewhere in the body. This is the basis for the rather rare group of conditions first described in 1908 as "inborn errors of metabolism" by Garrod, who, with remarkable insight at a time when biochemistry and genetics were in their infancy, regarded these disorders as genetically transmitted biochemical defects in which there was deficiency of enzymes necessary to normal metabolism.

Genes are of differing grades of potency, the more powerful being known as *dominant* and the weaker as *recessive. Both genes of a pair* producing a similar trait and occupying the same locus on the homologous chromosomes may be dominant or both recessive, a *homozygous* condition, or *one may be dominant and the other recessive,* the resultant being *heterozygous.* (These names are necessary in our subsequent discussion). If the gene is dominant, the individual will show the corresponding characteristic, whether the arrangement is homozygous (double dose) or heterozygous (single dose), because the strong gene does not need to be reinforced. If, however, it is weaker (recessive), the gene has to be duplicated (homozygous) before it can make itself apparent. When the gene is recessive and single, the corresponding character is not evident, and the individual plays the part of a passive *carrier.* The single recessive gene holds its place on the chromosome, biding its time in obscurity. It may have to wait for many generations (a short time in the case of the fruit fly, but in the case of humans, hundreds of years) before it gets its chance by being freed of suppression by a dominant gene. It is small wonder that some hereditary diseases of man are not recognized as such.

Dominance may not be as pure as suggested by what has just been said. It is not necessarily a matter of all or nothing. The degree of dominance, the grade of potency, is expressed by the term *penetrance.* When a dominant gene fails to manifest itself in the individual carrying the gene, there is said to be *partial penetrance*. A dominant gene with 80 per cent penetrance will express itself in only 80 per cent of cases; the remaining 20 per cent carrying it will skip a generation.

Mutation. Each gene is made up of millions of atoms, so it is natural that occasionally a rearrangement of the atoms may occur, giving the gene fresh properties. Such a change is called a mutation which is believed to represent a haphazard change in the DNA structure of the gene. Mutant genes must produce their effects by some alteration in biochemical function, and the loss or alteration of a single enzyme may have widespread and diverse effects. The best examples of the effect of mutant genes in single or double dose are conditions associated with abnormal hemoglobins. In the case of *sickle cell anemia* (see p. 467), if the gene is heterozygous (single dose) the person only manifests what is known as the *sickle cell trait,* that is to say, the red blood cells become sickle-shaped when the blood is deoxygenated in the laboratory. Sickle cell hemoglobin is exactly like normal hemoglobin except for a single alteration, a single amino acid out of nearly 300, and this results in the fatal red blood cell condition.

The majority of new mutants are harmful or even lethal, because in a delicately balanced system like the gene complex, as in the engine of a motorcar or a television set, almost any change is likely to be for the worse. **On the other hand mutation can be regarded as the masterword in evolution,** for helpful mutants are inherited just as are normal genes, and without them life would never have advanced. Animals with protective coloration owe their protection to a helpful mutation, although the black sheep of a white flock may blame its color on mutation, and the same might be said of the black sheep of a human family. In addition to the spontaneous variety, mutation may be *induced* by external influences, of which the best example is radiation.

INHERITANCE OF DISEASE

The transmission of hereditary defects from parents to offspring, defects which may manifest themselves as disease, may be chromosomal or genetic in origin. We have already considered some of the main results of chromosomal anomalies, involving both the autosomes and the sex chromosomes, the latter with their associated genes giving sex-linked inheritance of disease traits. We now turn to the very much larger field of diseases due to defects in the genes themselves. It has become apparent that a large number of disease conditions are due to gene mutations. To give a list of these conditions would be obviously absurd at this stage of our studies; indeed many of the rarer ones will not even be mentioned

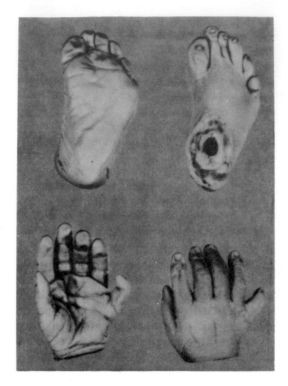

Fig. 70. Polydactyly of hands and feet in the newborn infant of a 19-year-old girl. (Kindness of Dr. C. H. Lupton, Jr.; Boyd's *Textbook of Pathology.*)

in the chapters that follow dealing with diseases of individual organs. Suffice it to say that all the inborn errors of metabolism, the problem of blood groups and the Rh factor, diseases of the blood such as sickle cell anemia, sex-linked blood disorders such as hemophilia, many chronic progressive diseases of the nervous and neuromuscular systems, and a host of anomalies and malformations of the skeleton have a firm genetic foundation. The inheritance may be autosomal dominant or autosomal recessive. The question of *sex-linked inheritance* has already been discussed.

DOMINANT INHERITANCE. This is naturally the easiest type to recognize, for each affected person has an affected parent and grandparent. The character can be transmitted by a parent of either sex to a child of either sex. If one parent has the dominant gene, two out of four children will inherit this gene and, although the condition is heterozygous, they will show the trait. The other two children did not receive the dominant gene and are homozygous for the recessive gene, so that they will appear normal. Examples are *brachydactyly* (short fingers and toes), which has been traced through very many generations, *polydactyly,* in which there are too many digits on the hands and feet

(Fig. 70), *multiple polyps of the colon, sickle cell anemia, diabetes insipidus,* and countless other conditions.

RECESSIVE INHERITANCE.   This type of inheritance is naturally much more difficult to recognize. The defect is only obvious in a homozygous individual, one in whom a double dose of corresponding genes determines the same defect. It must therefore have been inherited from heterozygous parents, neither of whom exhibited it, merely acting as carriers. A lethal recessive gene may be paired with a normal dominant gene, but its possessor goes through life happily unconscious of the fact that genetically he is half dead. The condition may thus remain unsuspected for many generations, until a homozygous mating brings two recessive genes together. This is most likely to happen with a marriage of first cousins. If two people, each carrying the same abnormal recessive gene, happen to marry, the offspring have one chance in four to be abnormal, one to be normal, and two to appear normal but carry the trait. The most striking example of recessive inheritance is the disease with the tragically descriptive name, *amaurotic* (blind) *family idiocy.* A moving account of this condition will be found in H. G. Wells' short story, "The Valley of the Blind," written very many years ago. The parents are always normal, although both must carry the recessive gene. No affected person ever grows up to be a parent, as the disease is fatal in early life. Another example of recessive inheritance is *albinism,* a startling defect in pigmentation which leaves the skin, eyes and hair a varying degree of white. An albino will usually marry someone who does not carry that particular and unusual gene; all the children will be heterozygous carriers. If he marries a girl who is a heterozygote, half the children will be albinos and half unaffected heterozygotes. If two albinos marry, all the children will be albinos.

The five possible results of mating dominant with recessive autosomal genes are shown in the following table, where D represents a dominant gene and r a recessive one.

1. $DD \times DD = DD$
2. $rr \ \times rr \ \ = rr$
3. $DD \times rr \ \ = Dr$
4. $DD \times Dr \ = \frac{1}{2} DD + \frac{1}{2} Dr$
5. $Dr \ \times Dr \ = \frac{1}{4} DD + \frac{1}{2} Dr + \frac{1}{4} rr$

Although only the surface of the subject has been scratched, I trust it will be apparent that great advances have been made in our knowledge of the heredity of disease since Mendel worked at his peas in the monastery garden, although the practical applications of this knowledge still lie for the most part in the future.

FURTHER READING

ALLEN, E. V.: Ann. Int. Med., 1934, *7*, 1000. (Sex and disease.)

BARR, M. L.: Can. Med. Ass. J., 1966, *95,* 1137. (Sex chromatin and sex chromosomes.)

CLARK, C. A.: *Genetics for the Clinician,* 2nd ed., 1964, Oxford.

CREW, F. A. E.: *Genetics in Relation to Clinical Medicine,* Edinburgh, 1947.

FORD, E. B.: *Genetics for Medical Students,* 5th ed., 1961, London.

HSIA, D. Y.-Y.: *Inborn Errors of Metabolism,* 2nd ed., 1966, Chicago.

LENNOX, B.: Lancet, 1961, *1,* 1046. (Chromosomes for beginners.)

PENROSE, L. S.: Lancet, 1967, *1,* 298. (Finger-print patterns and the sex chromosomes.)

THOMSON, J. S., and THOMSON, M. W.: *Genetics in Medicine,* 1966, Philadelphia.

Part Two

THE ORGANS AND
THEIR DISEASES

Chapter **15**

Heart

GENERAL CONSIDERATIONS

From the earliest of times our ancestors have realized the importance of the heart to life itself. Our language testifies to this fact, particularly the language of the poets. We say that a man is brokenhearted, or wounded to the heart, or that he wears his heart on his sleeve, or that it is in his throat or in his boots. Our knowledge of the anatomy and physiology of the heart has advanced in recent years to an incredible degree. We can pass catheters into its cavities, record the electrical changes in its muscle, and estimate its enzymes during life. But we still do not understand how it is that one man may have extensive myocardial fibrosis without suffering unduly, while in another who dies apparently of sudden heart failure no adequate explanation can be found at autopsy. It is probably a question of enzyme function.

STRUCTURE. The general structure of the heart has already been considered in Chapter 1. The average *weight* is 300 grams in the male, 250 grams in the female, but these figures will be considerably greater in a big, muscular laborer, or reduced in a tiny fragile woman. It is composed of muscle and valves (Fig. 71). The valves consist of an extraordinarily thin and delicate membrane, the **endocardium,** which also lines the cavity. Although so thin, they prevent a single drop of blood leaking through when closed. On the right side of the heart the *tricuspid*

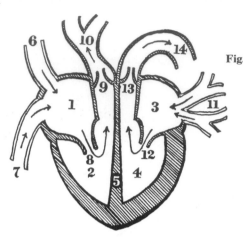

Fig. 71. Interior of heart. 1, Right atrium; 2, right ventricle; 3, left atrium; 4, left ventricle; 5, septum; 6, superior vena cava; 7, inferior vena cava; 8, tricuspid valve; 9, pulmonary valve; 10, pulmonary artery; 11, pulmonary veins; 12, mitral valve; 13, aortic valve; 14, aorta. (After Rabin, *Pathology for Nurses;* W. B. Saunders Co.)

valve divides the chamber into an *atrium* or *auricle,* which receives the venous blood from the body, and a *ventricle,* which sends the impure blood to the lungs by the pulmonary artery, whose mouth is guarded by the *pulmonary valve.* The left side is divided by the *mitral valve* into an atrium, which receives the purified blood from the lungs, and a ventricle, which sends this blood out into the great artery, the aorta, whose mouth is guarded by the *aortic valve.* Valvular disease of the heart nearly always affects the mitral and aortic valves. The function of the valves is to prevent backflow of blood between the beats. These functions are gravely interfered with in valvular disease.

Just as the interior of the heart is lined by the endocardium, so its outer surface is covered by a similar delicate membrane, the **pericardium.** The part of the chest in which the heart is situated is lined by a second layer of pericardium, so that between the two layers there exists a space, the *pericardial cavity,* in which the heart can contract and expand.

The heart muscle or **myocardium** must have an abundant blood supply. This is much more important than in the case of other muscles, because, unlike them, it can never for a moment rest. This blood supply is provided by two arteries, the right and left *coronary arteries,* which arise from the aorta immediately above the aortic valve and carry blood to every part of the heart muscle. Contrary to what might be expected, very little of the blood that is continually flowing through the chambers of the heart takes any part in supplying the muscle with blood. As we have just seen, if the myocardial pump ceases to work, life ends. Coronary sinus catheterization now enables us to look into the physiology of the myocardium and cardiac metabolism in a way never before possible. Physiologists have even begun to explore the electric activity of single heart muscle cells by inserting a microelectrode into the interior of a cell.

FUNCTION.   The heart is a hollow muscular pump whose function it is to cause the blood to circulate throughout the body. It sends impure venous blood to the lungs, where fresh oxygen is taken up and carbon dioxide given off, and then pumps the oxygenated blood to the tissues where the oxygen is used. The essential meaning of respiration is this delivery of life-giving oxygen to the tissues. *It is evident, therefore, that the heart is concerned with respiration just as much as are the lungs,* so that the principal symptom of heart disease is shortness of breath or *dyspnea.*

We do not actually know what makes the heart beat, although we know a lot about what regulates its rate. What we call the beat is a contraction, like that of other muscles, but unlike other muscles, the beat can go on after the nerves that supply the heart are cut, and even after the animal (or person) is dead. I was once much startled to feel the heart begin to beat in my hand on the autopsy table, the patient having been dead a number of hours. The contraction of the myocardium which drives the blood out of the atria and ventricles into the arteries is known as *systole.* The succeeding relaxation during which the cavities become refilled with blood from the veins is called *diastole* (Fig. 72). In health the various valves prevent a back flow of blood from the arteries into the right and left ventricles, and from the ventricles into the atria. The *sinoatrial* (auricular) *node,* a small area of specialized tissue in the upper part of the right atrium close to the entry of the superior vena cava, is called the **pacemaker.** Each time the heart beats, a current of electricity passes through the myocardium from the sinoatrial node. Impulses pass out in all directions, reaching the ventricle where they are carried by a specialized branch of muscular and nervous tissue called the *atrioventricular bundle of His.* If this bundle is interfered with by disease, the result is known as *heart block,* which is characterized by a very much slower rate of contraction.

There are two ways in which medical treatment can influence the pacemaker, one old, namely digitalis, originally an infusion or brew made from the leaves of the purple foxglove, Digitalis purpurea or ladies' fingers (hence the name), the other very new, the electric pacemaker. When the heart is diseased, a quivering of the atria in place of a regular beat often sets in, this is known as *atrial* or *auricular fibrillation.* Impulses now pass into the bundle of His so rapidly that the ventricles respond very irregularly and ineffectively. **Digitalis** make a chemical union with the bundle of His, blocks passage through the bundle, and thus protects the ventricles from the incessant bombardment of the auricular impulses. Digitalis has been regarded in the past as a cardiac

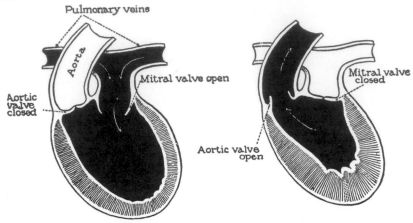

Fig. 72. Diastole and systole in the left heart. Note the positions of the two valves in both cases. Diastole to the left, systole to the right. (From Clendening, *The Human Body;* Alfred A. Knopf.)

stimulant, but now that its true action is understood it will be apparent that it is a regulator rather than a stimulator.

The **electric pacemaker** has been used in those serious cases of heart block known as *Adams-Stokes disease* (also called Stokes-Adams disease) with a very slow pulse rate, which may be associated with severe congestive heart failure. The condition may be a late after-effect of myocardial infarction involving the bundle of His. A tiny transistorized pacemaker driven by a long-life battery is placed under the skin of the abdominal wall and connected with electrodes implanted in the heart muscle. The heart block is now overcome and a new rate established. The cardiac output may be best at induced rates different from that of the natural sinoatrial pacemaker. *From what has been said it will be seen that the use of digitalis may be regarded as a method of imposing a form of heart block on a fibrillating heart, whereas the electric pacemaker overcomes heart block.*

An electric current is normally generated in the contracting myocardium, and this is measured by the electrocardiographic machine and recorded in the **electrocardiogram,** which shows a series of waves known by the letters of the alphabet. The *P wave* is caused by contraction of the atria, and the *Q, R, S waves* by contraction of the ventricles. In heart disease the waves may show a change in shape and position, which may help the physician to arrive at a correct diagnosis.

When the normal heart is listened to with the assistance of a stethoscope applied to the chest wall, two *heart sounds* are heard. The first sound is longer, softer, and of deeper pitch than the second sound. The irst sound, which is caused partly by contraction of the heart muscle, partly by closure of the valves (mitral and tricuspid) between the atria and ventricles, is likened to Lubb; the second sound, short, hard and of a higher pitch, is represented by Dup. A change in the quality of these sounds is an indication of disease of the valves.

The **rate** of the heart beat, *i.e.*, the *pulse*, varies. *The normal rhythm of the heart is dependent on the balance of two sets of nervous impulses, one tending to slow, the other to accelerate the heart's action.* Both nerves belong to the involuntary or autonomic nervous system. The *vagus nerve* is responsible for the **retarding impulses,** and we now know that a chemical substance, *acetylcholine,* is liberated at the nerve endings of the vagus and that this acts on the heart muscle. The **accelerating impulses** pass along the *sympathetic nerve fibers,* and another chemical substance is probably liberated at their nerve endings. The quickening of the heart beat that results from emotion, the feeling that your heart is in your mouth or in your boots, is due to an upset of the exquisite balance which normally exists between these two sets of influences.

The rate of the heart also depends on the demand of the tissues for oxygen. The runner's heart beats faster and he breathes more quickly in response to an increase in this demand. Muscular work is an expenditure of energy, and energy is obtained from the burning of food. As food cannot be burnt without oxygen, the heart beat is quickened and breathing becomes deeper and faster to supply this need.

The condition of the blood vessels must also be taken into account in any consideration of the heart's action. When the heart pumps blood into the arteries it does so against a certain amount of resistance. This is called the *peripheral resistance.* As the result of disease this resistance may become too high or too low. Both have an injurious effect on the heart's action. The resistance is increased by prolonged contraction of the muscular walls of the small arteries, the arterioles, resulting in the condition known as *high blood pressure* or *arterial hypertension.* No organ works at its maximum capacity; it has a large amount of *reserve force* in order to cope with emergencies. When hypertension develops the heart becomes larger and more powerful so that it can cope with the increased amount of work, a process known as *compensation.* In the course of time or because of disease of the heart muscle this power may fail, and *decompensation* sets in.

The clinical symptoms of heart disease may be caused by lesions of the valves or the myocardium, and the nature and site of these changes may be indicated if due attention is paid to the electrocardiogram, the sounds heard through the stethoscope, and the character of the pulse.

Transaminase. The myocardium is rich in enzymes, of which the most important from the clinical standpoint is transaminase. Its full name is glutamic oxaloacetic transaminase, which indicates its various biochemical activities, but this is shortened to GOT for convenience. This enzyme is widely distributed in the body, but the greatest concentration is in the heart. The normal serum level is low, from 4 to 40 units, but in myocardial infarction due to coronary artery occlusion a large amount is released into the blood, so that the serum level is a sensitive and very valuable index of recent necrosis of the myocardium Transaminase levels are determined either by paper chromatography or by the faster and more accurate spectrophotometric method.

HEART DISEASE. Of all the ailments that may blow out life's little candle, heart disease is the chief. There are three main ways in which the action of the heart may be interfered with, three ways in which heart disease may be produced: (1) The valves of the pump may be damaged by inflammation, a condition known as endocarditis. (2) The muscle of the pump may not receive sufficient nourishment owing to narrowing of the coronary arteries, sometimes associated with thrombosis. (3) The pump may have too much work to do and finally give way through exhaustion. This is apt to occur in long-continued arterial hypertension.

Heart disease heads the causes of death. Its mortality is twice that of cancer, its nearest rival. The statistics of the Metropolitan Life Insurance Company show that 600,000 people die of heart disease in the United States every year. The incidence has been steadily rising, partly, at least, because of the increased life span. As we grow older our coronary arteries get narrower, just as our hair grows gray or even white.

There are five main forms of heart disease. These are: (1) *rheumatic heart disease,* (2) *bacterial endocarditis,* (3) *coronary artery occlusion,* (4) *hypertensive heart disease,* and (5) *congenital heart disease.* Of these much the commonest are hypertensive heart disease and coronary artery occlusion; then comes rheumatic heart disease; very much less common are bacterial endocarditis and congenital heart disease. Syphilis used to be ranked with the important causes of heart disease, but modern therapy has completely changed the picture.

RHEUMATIC HEART DISEASE

Rheumatic fever is caused by infection with Group A hemolytic streptococci, but it is not a simple streptococcal disease like scarlet fever, for no bacteria can be demonstrated in the blood or the lesions. It is an autoimmune antigen-antibody reaction which results in a focal allergic necrosis with accompanying response characteristic of the collagen diseases (p. 122). All parts of the heart are involved, endocardium, myocardium, and pericardium. This universal involvement is called a pancarditis, but the valves are the chief sufferers.

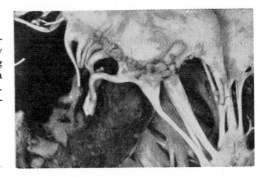

Fig. 73. Rheumatic endo-
carditis. A bead-like row
of vegetation runs along
the line of contact of a
cusp of the mitral valve.
(Boyd's *Textbook of Pa-
thology.*)

As a result of the infection the *valves* (commonly the mitral) become
inflamed, and from the blood flowing over it blood platelets and fibrin
are deposited on the inflamed valve. These form little nodules called
vegetations, each about the size of a pin's head, which form a row along
the margin of the cusps (Fig. 73). The inflamed cusps, normally almost
as thin as gossamer, become markedly thickened, and tend to adhere
to one another, just as do inflamed loops of bowel when brought in
contact. As the inflammation subsides, fibrous tissue takes the place of
the inflammatory exudate, and this slowly contracts, causing retraction
of the cusps.

The result of all this on the function and use of the valve may be
of two kinds, although often both are combined. Owing to the adhesions
between the thickened cusps they are unable to open properly when
the blood flows through the valvular opening, so that this opening becomes permanently narrowed, a condition known as **stenosis** (Fig.
74C). This narrowing may become so extreme that finally the opening
is no larger than a buttonhole, whereas normally it should admit two
fingers. *The mitral valve is the common site of rheumatic endocarditis,*
and **mitral stenosis** is one of the most serious forms of heart disease,
for not enough blood can flow from the left atrium into the left ventricle, and so is dammed back first in the lungs, then in the right side
of the heart, and finally in the veins of the body. It is three times commoner than all other rheumatic heart lesions. The second possibility is
incompetence of the valve (Fig. 74B). Here the retraction of the cusps
is much more marked than their sticking together. The result is that
the cusps are unable to meet when the valve tries to close, and the blood
escapes back from the ventricle into the atrium in the case of the mitral
valve, from the aorta into the ventricle in the case of the aortic. From
the point of view of the patient incompetence of the aortic valve is more
important than incompetence of the mitral. What used to be a commoner and even more serious form of **aortic incompetence** is that pro-

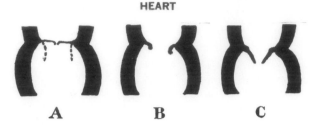

Fig. 74.   Heart valve lesions. *A*, Normal valve in closed and open (dotted lines) position; *B*, incompetence; *C*, stenosis.

duced by *syphilis*. In this condition syphilitic inflammation followed by scarring not only causes retraction of the cusps but also injures the wall of the aorta to which the cusps are attached, so that it gradually dilates to such a degree that the cusps are unable to come together and close the opening. Modern therapy has made this late sequel of syphilis a rarity.

It is important to realize that a person with chronic valvular disease of the heart is not necessarily an invalid, nor should he be encouraged to consider himself as such. The evidence of a valvular lesion is a murmur heard by the stethoscope over the heart, but *a person with a cardiac murmur may lead a full and vigorous life.* If the heart muscle is healthy it is able to compensate for the valvular lesion, unless the latter is marked and progressive.

In addition to causing inflammation of the valves, rheumatic fever also damages the *heart muscle* and pericardium. Small areas of inflammation and destruction known as *Aschoff bodies* or nodules are scattered through the muscle, and later these become converted into scar tissue. Such a scarred myocardium cannot fail to be weakened. On account of the damage to the wall of the atrium the peculiar condition known as *atrial fibrillation* is apt to develop, especially in mitral stenosis. Normally the *atria* beat at the same rate as the ventricles; this is natural, because normally the wave of muscular contraction starts in the atria and passes on to the ventricles; it is the beat of the ventricles that produces the pulse. In atrial fibrillation the atria no longer contract in a regular manner; they seem to be trembling instead of contracting. The result is that the ventricles contract in a rapid and irregular manner, this irregularity being reflected in marked irregularity of the pulse. The ventricles tend to become exhausted, with resulting heart failure, the symptoms of which are palpitation and dyspnea. The administration of digitalis prevents the irregular impulses from the atria from reaching the ventricles, which then commence to beat in a much slower and more regular manner, with immediate relief to the patient.

The *pericardium* also becomes inflamed, a condition of *pericarditis,* and the two inflamed layers of pericardium may stick together and form adhesions which may seriously cripple the heart's action. The truth of the remark made in the general discussion of rheumatic fever will now be evident, that it is a disease which licks the joints but bites the heart, for the patient is left with permanent lesions which may cripple his heart to the day of his death, although that day may be far removed. "The moving finger writes, and having writ moves on."

BACTERIAL ENDOCARDITIS

In the continually changing picture of disease it would be difficult to name a condition that has altered its appearance more completely in recent years than bacterial endocarditis. It used to be a malady in which the heart was beating muffled marches to the grave, in quick time in the acute form, with a slower but just as deadly rhythm in the subacute variety. **Now, thanks to antibiotics, it has become a curable disease when treated early. This, indeed, is one of the great triumphs of antibiotic and chemotherapy.** A sharp distinction has been drawn in the past between the acute and subacute forms of bacterial endocarditis. The importance of this distinction has rather faded, and more emphasis is laid on the infecting agent. It is, however, still convenient to speak of acute and subacute varieties, of which the latter is much the more common.

SUBACUTE BACTERIAL ENDOCARDITIS. This form of endocarditis is much less common than the rheumatic form but it used to be very much more fatal. Until the introduction of antibiotic therapy the mortality was practically 100 per cent.

The disease used to run its course in a number of months, sometimes a year. It is caused by a variety of nonhemolytic streptococcus (*Streptococcus viridans*) which reaches the heart from the throat. One peculiarity is that the disease is usually superimposed on an old rheumatic endocarditis, previously healthy valves being seldom affected. The inflammation is very much more severe than in the rheumatic form, the *vegetations* are large and extremely friable (Fig. 75), and the cusps of the valve are sometimes destroyed. The vegetations are teeming with streptococci, and these are discharged into the blood stream where they can be detected by blood culture, so that this procedure is of great value in the diagnosis of difficult cases.

The most striking feature of the disease is the formation of large numbers of *emboli* due to the breaking off of fragments of the friable vegetations. These sail off in the blood stream and stick in various organs where they give rise to some of the characteristic symptoms of the disease. Some of the emboli are large, and if these lodge in the brain they may cause paralysis, etc., while in the kidney they may cause blood

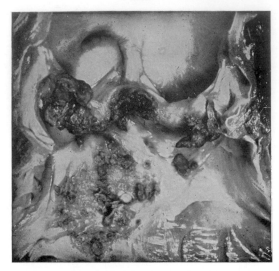

Fig. 75. Subacute bacterial endocarditis. The friable vegetations, the mural spread, and the old thickening of the aortic cusps are all very characteristic. (Boyd, *Textbook of Pathology;* Lea & Febiger.)

to appear in the urine. Sometimes they are minute, but if these tiny emboli should lodge in the smallest vessels of the skin they will cause these vessels to rupture, with the formation of multiple pinpoint hemorrhages known as *petechiae*. The petechiae in the skin, the blood in the urine, and the streptococci in the blood culture, together with enlargement of the spleen and long-continued fever are some of the principal clinical features.

Acute Bacterial Endocarditis. This is a much rarer form of endocarditis caused by enormous numbers of pyogenic bacteria such as *Staphylococcus aureus* and *Streptococcus haemolyticus*. The cusps of the valves are rapidly destroyed (hence the terms acute and ulcerative), and the patient *used* to die in less than six weeks without antibiotic therapy.

CORONARY ARTERY OCCLUSION

In a previous chapter we studied the effect of cutting off the arterial blood supply to an organ not provided with a good collateral circulation, and we found that the effect depended on whether the closure of the artery was slow or sudden. Gradual closure due to narrowing of the lumen of the artery by atherosclerosis led to slow atrophy and death of the specialized cells of the part (*e.g.,* heart muscle) and their replacement by scar tissue. Sudden closure by embolism or thrombosis caused the formation of an infarct, an area in which all the tissue was killed by the sudden ischemia.

The coronary arteries supplying the heart muscle with blood are unfortunately among the vessels most subject to *atherosclerosis* with consequent narrowing of the lumen. This is very common after middle age, but may occasionally occur before the age of thirty. The scarring of the heart muscle caused by the cutting off of the blood supply leads to great weakening of the heart's action. Penetration of the atheromatous lesion in the intima of the artery by new capillaries can be demonstrated in a large proportion of the cases. Hemorrhage can occur into the arterial lesion from these new capillaries. Such hemorrhage may result in: (1) complete occlusion of the lumen of the artery by expansion of the atheromatous lesions, or (2) rupture of the atheroma with subsequent thrombus formation in the lumen of the artery.

Frequently **thrombosis** is added to the atherosclerosis, the thrombosis suddenly closing the already narrowed vessel. Two things may happen: (1) The patient may die suddenly, sometimes in his bed; this is likely to happen if the main branch of the left coronary is occluded. (2) If a smaller branch is blocked the patient may survive, but an infarct of the heart is produced which severely cripples the organ. The infarct, consisting of dead tissue, is a weak spot in the heart wall which may in time bulge outward and finally rupture, causing sudden death. Or the patient may have several attacks of thrombosis in different branches of the coronary arteries, any of which may prove fatal.

Although the public speaks of a "coronary attack," from the standpoint of the patient the essential feature is the presence or absence of a **myocardial infarct.** An infarct may occur without thrombosis, the lumen of the coronary artery being greatly narrowed by atherosclerotic thickening of the inner coat (intima), and the final obstruction produced by rupture of the soft atheromatous material into the lumen. Or thrombosis may occur without the production of an infarct, because the area of cardiac muscle is supplied with blood from one of the other coronary arteries, such a supply being designated as a collateral circulation. *It is the infarct of the heart muscle, not the thrombosis of the coronary artery, that produces the symptoms and distress from which the patient suffers.* The infarct is a soft, yellow area of dead muscle in the wall of the left ventricle, varying greatly in size (Fig. 76). The softness of the dead tissue makes it a weak spot in the wall of the ventricle which may rupture during the first week of the attack, or at a later date may bulge outward and rupture, in both instances resulting in sudden death (Fig. 77).

CLINICAL PICTURE. When the blood supply to a muscle is suddenly cut off, very *severe pain* will be experienced if the muscle continues to be used. In the case of the heart complete rest is impossible, and the result is the agonizing pain known as *angina pectoris,* and a sense

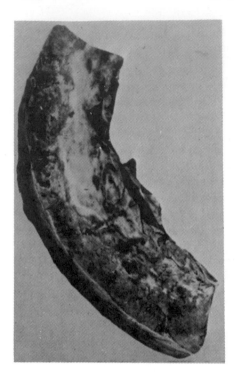

Fig. 76. Infarct of heart. The white necrotic areas stand out against the normal dark muscle. (Boyd's *Pathology for the Physician.*)

of suffocation as if the chest was held in a vise. *The sudden pain is felt in the region of the heart and frequently passes down the left arm.* It may, however, be felt in the epigastrium, the upper part of the abdomen, and when not too severe is often mistaken for acute indigestion. **When a person suffers a supposed attack of acute indigestion and dies shortly afterwards, he is almost certain to have had coronary occlusion.** The victim of an anginal attack experiences a feeling of impending dissolution, one of the most terrible accompaniments of the disease. His face is an ashy gray, and is bathed in a cold sweat. Occasionally pain is absent, but the patient still has a sense of suffocation and marked *dyspnea* or shortness of breath, which, indeed, is the most constant of all the symptoms. Sometimes the attack of pain is sudden and short; in other cases it may last for many hours. The explanation of these differences is difficult, and cannot be entered into here.

The importance of **transaminase,** an enzyme whose name signifies that it transfers amino groups from one amino acid to another, has already been referred to. In myocardial infarction the enzyme is liberated from the muscle fibers and passes into the blood. Serum transaminase activity may rise from 2 to 20 times the normal within 24 hours of

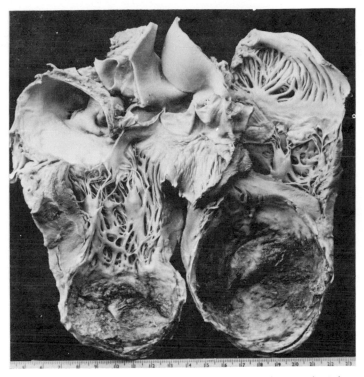

Fig. 77. Huge aneurysm of the heart, rupture of which resulted in sudden death. (Kindness of Dr. N. K. Patoria, Nagpur, India.)

an infarction, not returning to normal levels for three to six days. In a doubtful case an estimation of serum transaminase activity is obviously of very great value.

The **prognosis in coronary artery occlusion** varies greatly, depending on the size of the artery that is blocked, the extent of the damage to the heart muscle, and the question of collateral circulation. The patient may die instantaneously; this, indeed, is the commonest cause of sudden death. But if the heart survives the shock, as is frequently the case, the neighboring arteries pour blood into the ischemic area and a collateral circulation is in time established. When this occurs the patient may make a reasonably satisfactory recovery, but the heart will be permanently crippled, and his future life must be adjusted with this fundamental fact in mind. The immediate mortality of coronary thrombosis is believed to be around 10 per cent. *If the patient survives the attack the infarcted area needs at least six weeks to become strengthened by scar tissue. The patient must therefore be kept at complete* *rest in bed for this period and in some cases for a good deal longer.* Once the infarct has healed the patient may live for 15 or 20 years in good health provided he observes the rules of the game.

In *angina pectoris* the patient should be advised to live within his exercise tolerance, *i.e.,* he should do no more activity than he can perform without production of anginal pain. The use of nitroglycerin may give relief to the anginal pain at the time of its occurrence, but does nothing toward relieving the underlying cause.

HYPERTENSIVE HEART DISEASE

If the heart pump has to work for years against a greatly increased resistance in the shape of high blood pressure it will gradually become exhausted and fail. The strain naturally falls principally on the left ventricle, and for a time the wall of this ventricle becomes thicker (hypertrophied) so as to be able to overcome the increased resistance. When the heart is grasped at autopsy it feels like a closed fist. Finally, however, this power is lost, the heart fails, the ventricle becomes dilated, and the end picture is very much like that of other forms of heart failure. The condition is known as hypertensive heart disease. The symptoms are similar to those of heart failure from other causes such as valvular disease and coronary artery disease. *It must be pointed out, however, that very many persons with hypertension live vigorous lives for many years without developing signs of heart failure. Such people would be happier if they were ignorant of the fact that they had high blood pressure.*

The principal causes and varieties of hypertension are discussed in the next chapter. In the common form, known as *essential hypertension,* the small arteries throughout the body are contracted with narrowing of their lumen, and this leads to increase of the peripheral resistance to the blood flow so that the pressure of the blood in the large arteries rises. The patient with hypertension may not die of heart failure, but as the result of the bursting of a blood vessel in the brain (cerebral hemorrhage, apoplexy). The narrowing of the small arteries to the kidneys may lead to atrophy of these organs, and the patient may die of renal failure. *Death in hypertension may thus be due to disease of the heart, the brain, or the kidneys.*

CONGENITAL HEART DISEASE

Heart disease may be congenital rather than acquired. The child is born with cardiac defects due to failure in the process of development. **An important predisposing cause is German measles in the mother during the first three months of pregnancy.** The condition has for the first time assumed practical importance, because surgical operations have been developed for the treatment of several of these defects. A great variety of congenital abnormalities of the heart may occur, some very rare, others incompatible with life. Only those amenable to surgical treatment will be described.

The key to most of the defects lies in variations in the formation of the septum, which divides the heart into a right and a left side. The all-important feature of congenital heart disease is the possibility of an intermingling of the blood in the systemic and pulmonary circulations as the result of an arteriovenous shunt. The *three common causes of left-to-right shunts* are (1) *atrial septal defect,* (2) *ventricular septal defect,* and (3) *patent ductus arteriosus.* In all of these the lungs become overloaded with blood. An equally important clinical distinction is between *cases with cyanosis and without cyanosis.* Cyanosis will be caused by a right-to-left venous-arterial shunt, because poorly oxygenated venous blood then enters the systemic circulation.

Congenital defects are points of weakness against bacterial infection. Not infrequently the patient with congenital heart disease dies of subacute bacterial endocarditis.

At least 90 per cent of the patients with congenital disease of the heart and great vessels fall into one of four groups. These are, in their order of frequency although not in their order of discussion: (1) *septal defects,* (2) *coarctation of the aorta,* (3) *patent ductus arteriosus,* (4) *the tetralogy of Fallot. All of these are amenable to surgical treatment.*

SEPTAL DEFECTS. *Atrial septal defects* may be trivial or very serious. *Patency of the foramen ovale,* the opening in the septum between the two atria which is normally present at birth, is the commonest and the least important of congenital cardiac anomalies. As the opening is very small and oblique, little blood can pass from one side to the other. A *true septal defect* due to failure of development is quite another matter. The opening may be very large, and blood passes readily from the left to the right side where the pressure is lower, so that both the right atrium and the right ventricle become greatly dilated and hypertrophied. There is *no cyanosis* until cardiac failure sets in, and the patient may live from 30 to 50 years.

Ventricular septal defects may be uncomplicated by other cardiac anomalies. The opening is usually small, situated in the membranous part of the septum, and causes little disturbance. Here again *cyanosis will be absent* except as a terminal phenomenon. *Bacterial endocarditis,* however, occurs at the margin of the opening in many cases, so that surgical closure of the defect is indicated. When the defect is small the characteristic physical sign is a loud systolic murmur.

TETRALOGY OF FALLOT. *This is the most important congenital lesion of the heart,* and the most common of the lesions causing *cyanosis* for reasons which will soon become obvious. The essence of this condition is *pulmonary stenosis.* The pulmonary valve is markedly narrowed, so that the blood is unable to pass in sufficient quantity from the right ventricle to the lungs. Fallot described three other changes in addition to the pulmonary stenosis. (1) The septum, which separates the left side of the heart from the right, is shifted to the right, thus farther narrowing the pulmonary opening; (2) a gap is present in the septum (patent interventricular septum) through which the blood can pass; (3) the wall of the right ventricle is hypertrophied by reason of the increased work it has to do in forcing the blood through the narrow pulmonary opening. The combination of these four is the reason for the rather pedantic word tetralogy (*tetra,* four) (Fig. 78). The tetralogy of Fallot

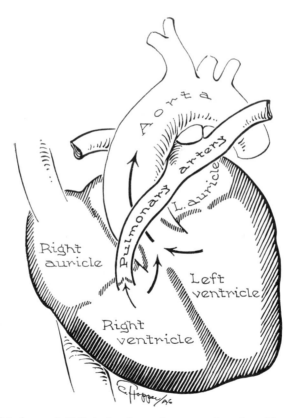

Fig. 78. Tetralogy of Fallot showing pulmonary stenosis, wide aorta, hypertrophied right ventricle, and defect in interventricular septum. (Boyd, *Pathology for the Surgeon;* W. B. Saunders Co.)

is the most common cause of the condition known as the "blue baby," a name given because of the extreme degree of cyanosis, the blue color being most marked on the lips, ears, cheeks, and hands. The principle of the operation is to bypass the obstruction at the opening of the pulmonary artery. This is done by anastomosing the left subclavian artery, a branch of the aorta, to the pulmonary artery beyond the obstruction, so that the blood now reaches the lungs, although from the left instead of the right ventricle. Reference to Figure 79 may make the matter more clear, although the branches of the aorta are not shown in the diagram. The improvement in the child's condition is immediate and dramatic, the cyanosis and shortness of breath being often improved by the time the patient is returned to bed from the operating room.

PATENT DUCTUS ARTERIOSUS. The ductus arteriosus is a short vessel which passes from the bifurcation of the main pulmonary artery into its two main branches to the arch of the aorta. During intrauterine life the blood from the right side of the heart passes along this channel into the aorta without passing through the lungs, as these organs are not used for respiration while the child is still within the womb. The ductus should become closed a few weeks after birth. It may, however, remain open or patent. In this condition the blood flows from the aorta into the pulmonary artery owing to the pressure being higher in the former than the latter. The blood therefore receives sufficient oxygen from the lungs, and there is *no cyanosis* except in cases complicated by other congenital defects. Although the condition is compatible with a long and active life, in the great majority of cases life expectancy is considerably shortened. The great danger is the development of streptococcal endarteritis at either end of the ductus. The treatment is surgical division of the ductus, a relatively simple operation.

COARCTATION OF THE AORTA. This is a narrowing of the aorta (*coarctare,* to press together) in the region where it is joined by the ductus. This is beyond the origin of the large arteries to the head and arms, so that there is an abundant flow of blood to these parts and the blood pressure in the arm is high. Very little blood passes through the narrowed aorta to the abdomen and legs, where the blood pressure is low and the pulse can hardly be felt, although some blood manages to bypass the obstruction through abundant collateral vessels which open up (Fig. 79). Recognition of this collateral circulation by means of radiography greatly assists the doctor in making a correct diagnosis. The surgical treatment consists in clamping the aorta above and below the obstruction, excising the narrowed segment, and sewing the divided ends of the aorta together. This dramatic operation is usually attended with complete success.

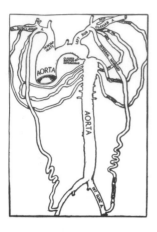

Fig. 79. Coarctation of aorta with collateral circulation. (Maude Abbott and Dawson, *International Clinics;* J. B. Lippincott Co.)

The *clinical features* of congenital heart disease are considered in outline on page 280.

CHRONIC VALVULAR DISEASE

In our discussion of diseases of the heart various references have been made to lesions of the valves. The general subject of valvular disease may conveniently be considered here. We have already seen that there are four valves in the heart, two on the left side and two on the right. We shall confine our attention to the valves on the left side, namely the mitral and the aortic. Either of these may be too narrow (stenosed) or too wide (insufficient or incompetent). There are thus four possibilities.

MITRAL STENOSIS. Most, if not all, cases of mitral stenosis are *rheumatic* in origin. The condition is much commoner in women than in men. The valve opening may be a mere buttonhole, which will hardly admit the tip of the little finger (Fig. 80), whereas the normal opening should admit two fingers with ease. The valve looks like a deep funnel, the walls of which are formed by the fused cusps. The blood rushing through this rigid funnel on its way from the left atrium to the ventricle causes a vibration of its walls, which is responsible for the characteristic diastolic murmur heard and thrill felt. If the reader will pause to think of the anatomy of the heart and the direction of the blood flow (Fig. 71, p. 260) he will not need to be told that owing to the obstruction the left atrium and the right side of the heart are greatly dilated. A thrombus may form in the dilated left atrium, and this may become detached and give rise to cerebral embolism. The *general effects* of mitral stenosis are those of chronic venous congestion.

The stenosis can now be treated surgically by valvotomy and reconstruction of the valve. In assessing the value or desirability of the opera-

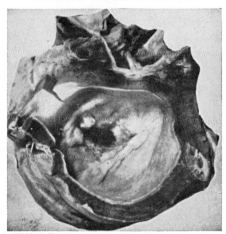

Fig. 80. Mitral stenosis. The thickened cusps have fused so as to cause extreme narrowing of the opening. (Boyd, *Textbook of Pathology;* Lea & Febiger.)

tion it must be remembered that the condition is not necessarily progressive, and that well over 50 per cent of the patients survive without operation for 20 years or more, many showing little change in their clinical condition.

MITRAL INSUFFICIENCY.   This is the least well defined of the four principal valvular lesions. The incompetence is caused by sclerosis and contraction of the cusps or by dilatation of the valve ring. The common cause is *rheumatic endocarditis,* but *subacute bacterial endocarditis* will also cause some degree of incompetence. The condition of the heart is similar to that of mitral stenosis except that the left ventricle is also much dilated.

AORTIC STENOSIS.   Pure *aortic stenosis* usually occurs in *men* over fifty years of age, whereas *mitral stenosis* is commoner in *women* at an earlier age. Can this difference have a sex hormone basis? The stenosis is of the calcified nodular type, best called *calcific aortic stenosis.* The cusps adhere together to form a kind of diaphragm as in mitral stenosis, but the most striking feature is the presence of warty calcified masses which may cover the cusps (Fig. 81). The entire valve is incredibly hard and rigid. It is generally believed that the condition is the *result of rheumatic infection,* although this is hard to prove. Calcific aortic stenosis is certainly being encountered more frequently than formerly. It is seldom associated with mitral stenosis, which is rather puzzling. The heart shows a perfect example of pure or concentric hypertrophy of the left ventricle. The most characteristic physical sign is a *rough rasping systolic murmur and thrill at the aortic area.* Cardiac

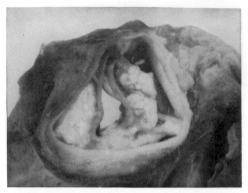

Fig. 81. Calcific aortic stenosis. (Boyd, *Textbook of Pathology;* Lea & Febiger.)

surgery promises relief with a reasonable degree of safety. The roentgen-ographic demonstration of calcification in the area of the aortic valve may serve to confirm the diagnosis. It must be noted that calcific aortic stenosis is often tolerated quite well into old age even after evidence of severe obstruction to the aortic outflow has been noted.

Aortic Insufficiency.   Insufficiency or incompetence of the aortic valve may be due to endocarditis of the valve cusps or to dilatation of the aorta and the aortic ring. The former is likely to be caused by *rheumatic endocarditis* or *subacute bacterial endocarditis,* the latter used to be a common result of *syphilitic aortitis* before the days of the modern treatment of syphilitic infection. It was the syphilitic form which used to give the classic picture of the disease, but this is now becoming a rarity.

The condition of the heart is the opposite of that in mitral stenosis. Here the heart is all left ventricle which is greatly hypertrophied as well as dilated, on account of the regurgitant flow of blood from the aorta into the ventricle through the incompetent valve during diastole. On this account the arteries contain too much blood during systole (from the dilated ventricle), and too little blood during diastole (owing to the backward flow). This accounts for the *"water-hammer pulse"* of leaping character felt at the wrist. The *loud diastolic murmur* which is the most characteristic physical sign is due to the rush of blood back into the ventricle during diastole.

The five important diseases of the heart have been outlined, together with the four principal valvular lesions. Practically nothing has been said about diseases of the myocardium, apart from its involvement in coronary artery occlusion, nor about the pericardium, which may be involved in various forms of inflammation in addition to rheumatic pericarditis. Such discussions would be out of place in this Introduction.

It may be mentioned, however, that tumors of the heart, both benign and malignant, fortunately are curiously rare.

BASIS OF SYMPTOMS OF HEART DISEASE

Of all the ailments that may blow out life's little candle, heart disease is the chief. But it will be realized from the foregoing account that the symptoms may be widely varied. These symptoms may be those that point to the heart itself, or they may be the result of failure of the circulation, which again may be chiefly arterial or chiefly venous. In valvular disease such as mitral stenosis or aortic incompetence the heart becomes enlarged from both dilatation and hypertrophy. The *dilatation* of the chambers is to accommodate the increased volume of blood which either is dammed back into the left atrium in mitral stenosis or escapes back into the left ventricle through an incompetent aortic valve. The *hypertrophy* of the heart muscle is a *compensatory* mechanism by virtue of which more work is done in order to overcome the valvular defect. For a while this compensation is successful and no symptoms of heart disease develop, although physical examination of the heart may reveal to the physician the true state of affairs. The compensation may be wonderfully successful and the patient may enjoy good health for many years, *especially if he regulates his life with discretion*. Sooner or later, however, especially with the approach of age, compensation is likely to fail and a stage of *decompensation* is entered upon, with the development of the symptoms known as congestive heart failure.

The introduction of cardiac catheterization and angiocardiography have greatly increased the accuracy of diagnosis. *Cardiac catheterization* reveals the pressure and oxygen content in the various chambers and great vessels, whereas *angiocardiography,* as the name suggests, provides visualization of the chambers of the heart, the aorta, and the pulmonary artery. But these new devices do not replace the time-honored methods of clinical examination.

Of the **cardiac symptoms** of heart disease the chief are pain, palpitation, and disorders of rhythm. *Pain* has already been discussed in connection with coronary occlusion. *Palpitation,* a condition in which the patient becomes aware of the forcible beating of his heart, may be a symptom either of valvular or myocardial disease. Frequently, however, it does not indicate any organic heart disease, being caused by purely nervous disorders. *Disorders of rhythm* may take the form of increased rate (tachycardia) or irregularity of rhythm, occasional beats being missed. *Murmurs,* which may be heard with the stethoscope, are caused by the blood leaking back through an incompetent valve or forcing its way through a stenosed one. *Heart block* is a condition in which the pulse rate drops to about one-half the normal, and is caused by scars due to coronary artery disease interfering with the "conduction bundle," which carries the electric impulse necessary for muscular contraction from one part of the heart to the other.

Of the **symptoms due to interference with the circulation,** the commonest is *dyspnea*. The shortness of breath is due to the fact that the failing heart is unable to purify the blood properly by sending it through the lungs; when the impure blood reaches the brain it stimulates the respiratory center, causing the patient to breathe rapidly and feel short of breath. *Fainting attacks* may occur in aortic incompetence because part of the blood, instead of going to the brain, escapes back into the left ventricle. This causes cerebral anemia (ischemia) which is the essential cause of all fainting attacks. *Congestive heart failure* is a picture presented by patients the right side of whose heart is becoming exhausted, and is particularly well seen in mitral stenosis. There is damming back of the blood in the veins that empty into the right atrium, so that the veins in the neck stand out prominently; the liver is enlarged and tender because the blood accumulates in its substance. The lips, ears, and fingers are *cyanosed* or blue because of insufficient oxygenation of the blood flowing through them, for it is the presence of oxygen that imparts to the blood in the arteries its bright red color.

Edema or dropsy is evidence of congestive heart failure, although it may also be caused by other conditions such as Bright's disease. In heart disease it occurs when the blood serum that accumulates in the congested veins gradually passes out and collects in the tissues; it is most marked in the feet and legs, where it causes a swelling in which a hole can be made by steady pressure of the finger (pitting on pressure). The reason for this transudation of fluid from the blood vessels is partly the increased pressure in the capillaries and small veins caused by the back pressure from the heart, and partly damage to the vessel walls with an increase of their permeability owing to an insufficient supply of the oxygen that is necessary for their health.

Congenital heart disease has its own special symptoms. *Cyanosis* is the most characteristic of these symptoms, sometimes being present from the moment the blue baby makes its appearance in the world, but usually developing later. *Dyspnea* on exertion is equally common, but may range from the slightest to the most severe. *Polycythemia* (increased number of red blood cells), which is compensatory in nature, serves for a time to offset the deficiency in oxygen. The size of the red cells is also increased for the same reason. *Clubbing of the fingers* (Fig. 82), one of the most striking of the physical signs, is due to a disturbance of nutrition of the tissues which affects both the terminal phalanges and the nails, the latter being thickened and curved. *Cerebral symptoms,*

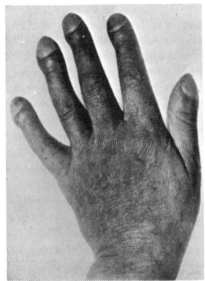

Fig. 82. Clubbing of the fingers. (Boyd's *Pathology for the Physician.*)

such as faintness, dizziness, and even syncope, are frequent owing to the anoxia.

Perhaps the most important fact to remember is that the majority of people with structural heart disease are able to lead useful lives. Many patients with heart disease are kept in bed quite unnecessarily. The discovery that a cardiac murmur is present does not mean that the patient's whole mode of life has to be changed. A man with valvular disease of the heart may live comfortably for many years on account of the compensating power of the heart muscle. It must be remembered that the essential part of the heart is the muscle, not the valves.

One can do little about the underlying heart disease, but the occurrence of the edema can be prevented in many cases by adequate treatment. The most important part of the treatment is the use of *a diet which is low in salt.* In heart failure salt tends to accumulate in the body fluids. This concentration results in the retention of water and production of swelling in various regions. The restriction of salt intake to very low levels tends to prevent the accumulation of this swelling. *Digitalis* is an important drug in the treatment of heart failure, particularly in cases where atrial fibrillation has occurred. Salt and water can be eliminated from the body by the use of *diuretics,* the most important of which are the mercurial diuretics, which are given by injection. After an attack of heart failure the patient may be again able to resume activity, but he must be instructed to limit his exertion to reasonable limits within his exercise tolerance. Education of the patient with heart disease as to the mode of life best suited to him is a most important item in the treatment. Too great solicitude on the part of the patient can be almost as unfortunate as too great recklessness.

Finally it must be remembered that no organ is influenced to so marked a degree by *nervous stimuli* and what are commonly referred to as the *emotions*. The simple everyday words of our language testify to the truth of this statement. We say that the person is heavy-hearted, hard-hearted, heartless, good-hearted, that his heart aches with loneliness, flutters with alarm or stops with fear. It is evident that cardiac symptoms may have an emotional rather than an organic basis, and to confuse one with the other is a serious matter both for the physician and the patient.

HEART TRANSPLANTATION

The general subject of tissue transplantation has already been discussed in Chapter 7. Transplantation of the heart has naturally aroused keener interest and greater excitement than in the case of any other organ. The supreme problem is rejection of the transplanted heart, a problem that has not yet been solved, in spite of the use of a wide variety of immunosuppressive drugs. Indeed the heart seems more vulnerable to rejection than the kidney. The rejection may be *early,* in one to four weeks, or *late,* in weeks or months with occlusion of the coronary arteries. It is evident that immunosuppressive therapy must become more efficient without destroying the patient's resistance to infections if the future is to be as bright as we hope.

The rejection problem is not likely to be solved in the near future. In the meantime it seems probable that a plastic artificial heart equipped with a lightweight external source of power will be available, so that a human transplant will no longer be needed.

FURTHER READING

ADOLPH, E. F.: Scient. Amer., 1967, March, *216,* 32. (The heart's pacemaker.)

DURLACHER, S. H., FISH, A. J., and FISHER, R.: Am. J. Path., 1953, *29,* 558. (Coronary artery lesions in sudden death.)

GOULD, S. E.: *Pathology of the Heart,* Springfield, Ill., 2nd ed., 1960.

HUDSON, R. E. B.: *Cardiovascular Pathology,* London, 1965.

NORA, J. J., *et al.:* New Eng. J. Med., 1969, *280,* 1080. (Rejection of the transplanted human heart.)

SURAWICZ, B., and PELLEGRINO, E. D.: *Sudden Cardiac Death,* New York, 1964.

TAUSSIG, H. B.: *Congenital Malformations of the Heart,* Cambridge, Mass., 1960.

Chapter 16

Blood Vessels

Arteries	*Disseminated Lupus*
Arteriosclerosis	*Erythematosus*
Atherosclerosis	*Thromboangiitis Obliterans*
Medial Calcification	*Syphilis*
Arteriolosclerosis	Aortitis
Arterial Hypertension	Arteritis
Essential Hypertension	**Aneurysms**
Secondary Hypertension	**Veins**
Arteritis	*Varicose Veins*
Polyarteritis Nodosa	*Hemorrhoids*

ARTERIES

A sound heart is greatly to be desired, for it has to pump from nine to ten tons of blood every day, but without sound arteries it is severely handicapped. An artery, whether small or large, consists of three coats: (1) a very thin inner coat or *intima,* including the delicate lining endothelium; (2) a middle coat or *media,* composed mainly of muscle, although in the aorta and larger arteries it also contains much elastic tissue; (3) the outer fibrous coat or *adventitia,* in which inflammatory changes may be particularly evident.

We must not forget, however, that the 60,000-mile network of the blood vessels of the body is composed largely of capillaries, which form connecting links between the arteries and veins, and which do the detailed work of the vascular system. These links are about three-thousandths of an inch in diameter and their walls are only one ten-thousandth of an inch thick, an ideal structure for the passage of nutriment and oxygen between the circulating blood and the tissues.

Diseases of the arteries are among the most common causes of invalidism and death in those of middle age and later life. These diseases belong to two great groups: (1) degenerative (arteriosclerosis) and (2) inflammatory (arteritis). As the former group is by far the more common and important, it will be considered first.

Arteriosclerosis

Before commencing the study of this common and obscure condition, it may be well to mention that the arteries can be divided into three main groups: (1) the *large* or *elastic arteries,* such as the aorta and its main branches; (2) the *medium-sized* distributing or *muscular arteries,* which carry the blood from the main trunks to the various organs and tissues; (3) the small *arteries* and *arterioles,* which extend from the ends of the distributing arteries to the capillary beds. Arteriosclerosis, a general and rather vague term which really signifies hardening of the arteries, can also be divided into three main forms, which differ sharply in microscopic appearance and to some degree in distribution. These are: (1) *atherosclerosis,* a patchy, fatty degeneration of the intima; (2) *medial calcification,* commonly called Mönckeberg's degeneration, which involves the media of the middle sized vessels; and (3) *arteriolosclerosis* which is a diffuse intimal thickening of the smaller visceral arteries. It is possible that these represent different diseases or degenerations.

ATHEROSCLEROSIS. Atherosclerosis is a degenerative process which used to be called atheroma, but it is better to reserve that term for the local lesion in the wall of the artery. It is a nodular type of arteriosclerosis which affects the large arteries, especially the aorta and its main branches, and also the small arteries, particularly the coronaries and cerebrals. It is the fact that these arteries supply the myocardium and the brain respectively, and that this is the only form of arteriosclerosis which commonly predisposes to thrombosis, that lends to atherosclerosis a sinister significance.

It is in essence a patchy or nodular thickening of the intima of the artery with a great accumulation of lipid largely in the forms of cholesterol crystals and resulting narrowing of the lumen at one or more spots (Fig. 83). The blood supply may be cut down to the danger point, and a thrombus is apt to form on the diseased wall and obstruct the narrowed lumen. This is the mechanism of production of coronary thrombosis, cerebral thrombosis, and thrombosis in the arteries of the leg. Atherosclerosis is an extremely common condition and is the chief cause of ischemia of the heart muscle, the brain, and the leg.

Etiology. It is a remarkable fact that in spite of the frequency of the condition and the enormous amount of time and money expended in the investigation, we know as little about the cause of atherosclerosis as about the cause of cancer. This lack of knowledge has proved an insurmountable obstacle to devising some method of preventing this crippling and often fatal condition, which is the curse of the declining years of life. It is perhaps better to speak of the pathogenesis of atherosclerosis, its mode of production, rather than the etiology, which sug-

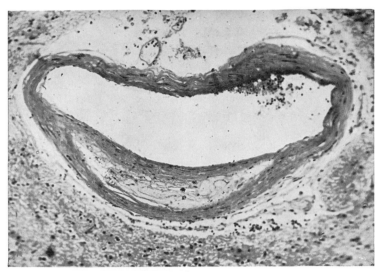

Fig. 83. Atherosclerosis of a cerebral vessel. The thickened intima shows accumulation of lipid in its deeper layers, and there is some atrophy of the media underlying the thickened plaque. × 125. (Boyd, *Textbook of Pathology;* Lea & Febiger.)

gests one causal agent. The very large amount of experimental work has brought forth three main lines of thought, but unfortunately the natural condition is almost exclusively a human disease, and does not occur spontaneously in the laboratory animal.

(1) The **blood lipids** have been incriminated. We have already seen that the most striking feature of the lesion is the great accumulations of lipids, cholesterol in particular, in the intima of the vessel. It seems reasonable to suppose that these lipids have come from the circulating blood, and that the blood lipids are derived from the food. Modern so-called civilized man with increasing wealth consumes more food rich in animal fats and indulges in less physical activity, which he now prefers to watch. In some experimental animals such as the rabbit it is easy to raise the blood lipids by means of a diet rich in cholesterol, and this is followed by the formation of lesions in the aorta similar to those of human atherosclerosis. *But this does not prove that a faulty diet is responsible for the disease in man, because the cholesterol metabolism in man and the rabbit is quite different. The amount of atherosclerosis varies greatly in different countries,* being very much more common in affluent communities where there is a high consumption of animal fats and of dairy products, both of which are rich in cholesterol, than among less fortunate (?) peoples who are relatively free from atheroma. The fallacy of such reasoning is that we are dealing with

different races, in whom genetic factors may be more important than dietary differences.

(2) The **vessel wall** must play some part, or rather local factors such as enzymes in the vessel wall. One of the most striking peculiarities of atherosclerosis is its patchy distribution. One artery is heavily involved and another is spared. Almost more remarkable is the patchy distribution of the lesions in a single vessel, such as one of the coronary or cerebral arteries. This should be contrasted with the diffuse distribution of the lesions in arteriolosclerosis. Unfortunately a single lesion, no matter how small, is able to inflict irreparable damage on the heart or brain; when a tap in a water pipe is shut down it does not have to be large in order to stop all flow of fluid.

(3) **Mural thrombosis** was suggested in 1852 by Rokitansky as a key to thrombosclerosis. For very many years the idea was forgotten, but now it has been rejuvenated. This idea envisaged the deposition of thrombus-forming material on the intima, vascularization of the new thrombus, hemorrhage from the new vessels, and liberation of cholesterol from the released blood platelets. Normally these deposits of thrombotic material are removed by fibrinolysin, but if the person has an unbalanced fibrinolytic system, where lysis is delayed, the consequences may be serious.

Accessory factors must also be taken into consideration. One of the most important of these is *age*. Atherosclerosis is a degenerative condition of advancing years, just as is graying of the hair. The blood vessels begin to feel the effect of the sharp tooth of time. Occasionally, however, it may begin before the age of thirty, and a person of advanced years may be singularly free from the disease, so that the saying that "a man is as old as his arteries" is profoundly true. *Heredity* without doubt may play a part. In some families deaths are commonly due to coronary occlusion, while in others they are due to strokes caused by cerebral hemorrhage. Other people seem to inherit arteries with an enzymatic architecture so sturdy that the various atherogenetic factors make no impression on it. *Stress* or *strain* may injure vessels, with resulting deposition of lipids. This is seen in the localization of the lesions at the origin of branches or the bifurcation of arteries. The coronary arteries are more frequently involved with atheroma and at an earlier age than any other artery. This may be related to their origin directly from the aorta, there being no opportunity to step down the high pressure they receive directly from the main arterial trunk.

The discussion on the pathogenesis of atherosclerosis in the medical literature is endless. Its length is a testimony to our confusion of thought on the subject. When the answer is known it may perhaps be expressed in a sentence.

MEDIAL CALCIFICATION. This condition, often called *Möncke-berg's sclerosis*, is the type of arteriosclerosis that is observed by the clinician when he feels the arteries, for it is the vessels of the limbs, arteries of the muscular type, which are affected. The pipe-stem radials, the tortuous and prominent temporals, belong to this class. The visceral arteries (*e.g.,* mesenteric) are seldom involved. The calcification of the media seems to bear little relation to the other forms of arteriosclerosis, nor does it cause serious narrowing of the lumen of the vessels.

ARTERIOLOSCLEROSIS. The arterioles are the smaller arteries within the viscera, such as the kidneys, what have been called the intimate vasculature. *There is a diffuse thickening of the wall of the arterioles* (in contrast to the nodular thickening of atherosclerosis) *with accompanying narrowing of the lumen.* There is none of the cholesterol accumulation which is so characteristic a feature of atherosclerosis. Arteriolosclerosis is a common accompaniment of *hypertension,* but it may also occur in old age, even though the blood pressure remains normal. In younger persons hypertension and arteriolosclerosis often go hand in hand. It is particularly in disease of the kidneys (nephritis) that thickening and narrowing of the renal arterioles assumes a position of great importance, as we shall see in due time.

Arterial Hypertension

The blood pressure in a state of health is the resultant of a number of forces, among the chief of which are the contractions of the heart and the peripheral resistance provided by the arterioles. In spite of the fact that these factors are constantly changing under ordinary conditions, any sudden change in pressure is rapidly restored to normal.

Hypertension or high blood pressure is defined by the life insurance companies as any elevation of the systolic pressure above 140 mm. of mercury and of the diastolic pressure above 90 mm. of mercury. This may be true statistically, but it does not follow that these figures can be applied to every individual and thus label him as a hypertensive. **A rise in the diastolic pressure is very much more important than a similar rise in the systolic pressure.** The condition is at present divided into two forms, *primary* or *essential,* where the cause is unknown, constituting about 90 per cent of all cases of hypertension, and *secondary,* where there is some associated lesion such as chronic nephritis or tumor of the adrenal cortex, which is presumed to be responsible for the raised blood pressure.

ESSENTIAL HYPERTENSION. This is the commonly used term for the primary variety. It is divided in turn into so-called benign and malignant forms. The *benign form* is characterized by a gradual onset and a long-continued course, often of many years. The *malignant form,* fortunately very much less common, is frequently of abrupt onset, and runs a course measured in months rather than years, so that it justifies its name. It often ends with renal failure (uremia), but not necessarily so.

Etiology. The very names primary and essential indicate our ignorance of the etiology of the condition, but that does not forbid us from speculating as to possibilities. There is evidence, both experimental and human, to suggest that the kidney and the adrenal cortex exert some regulating effect on the blood pressure. It was over one hundred years ago that Richard Bright pointed out the association between *chronic nephritis* (Bright's disease) and work hypertrophy of the left ventricle indicating raised blood pressure. When the arteries to both kidneys in the dog or one kidney in the rat are gradually constricted by a clamp, the resulting *renal ischemia* is associated with hypertension. The same thing happens in man when the main renal artery to one kidney is constricted by disease. The *adrenal cortex* apparently exerts its influence on blood pressure by regulating the salt content and therefore the water content in the walls of the smaller arteries, thus affecting their lumen. One of the most striking features of Addison's disease, which is caused by destruction of both adrenals, is the very low blood pressure. *It seems probable that both the kidney and the adrenal are associated in the control of blood pressure in health,* and that an upset in this balance may be responsible for so-called essential hypertension. The difference between the essential and the secondary forms is that in the former no constant lesions can be demonstrated at autopsy either in the kidneys or the adrenals. *Heredity* plays a part in determining whether or not a patient will develop essential hypertension. The hereditary tendency is generally transmitted as a Mendelian dominant, so that it is easy to recognize.

SECONDARY HYPERTENSION. Raised blood pressure may be associated with renal disease, endocrine tumors, and constriction of the arteries. *Renal lesions* have already been referred to. They may take the form of (1) *glomerulonephritis* which causes diffuse glomerular ischemia, (2) *chronic pyelonephritis,* and (3) *stenosis of the main renal artery* on one or both sides by atheroma in the elderly. *Endocrine tumors* may be (1) *pheochromocytoma of the adrenal medulla* producing a vasoconstricting hormone, (2) *adenoma of the adrenal cortex* producing a salt-retaining hormone with resulting *aldosteronism,* and *pituitary basophil adenoma. Constriction of the arteries* may take the form of *coarctation of the aorta* (p. 275), in which the hypertension is naturally restricted to the upper part of the body and the upper limbs, a principal cause of hypertension in childhood, and one readily cured by operation. *Polyarteritis nodosa* causing widespread narrowing of the small arteries is described below. The *arteriolar narrowing of age* is associated with hypertension, but which is cause and which effect it is very hard to say.

ARTERITIS

So far we have been considering the degenerative conditions to which the arteries are liable. We may now turn to the very much less common inflammatory lesions. A number of these appear to be manifestations of allergy or hypersensitivity, although little or nothing is known about the substances to which the person is allergic.

POLYARTERITIS NODOSA.   This is one of the *diffuse collagen diseases* (p. 122), and is also known as *periarteritis nodosa* by reason of the periarterial inflammatory exudate that is often a prominent microscopic feature. It is an acute inflammation that involves the small arteries to the viscera rather than those to the limbs. The cause is unknown, but *there is strong evidence to suggest that this disease represents a type of hypersensitivity.* The disease often runs an acute course with fever and prostration, ending fatally in the course of a few weeks or months. The symptoms are extremely varied, depending on which arteries are involved. The principal vessels affected are those of the gastrointestinal tract, the kidney, and the heart. There may be acute abdominal symptoms due to involvement of the mesenteric arteries, acute cardiac symptoms from coronary artery involvement, or neuritic pains due to lesions of the arteries supplying the peripheral nerves.

DISSEMINATED LUPUS ERYTHEMATOSUS.   In this confusing name the word "lupus" originally signified wolf, but is now taken to denote the distribution of the facial rash mentioned below. This is another of the collagen diseases, similar in many ways to polyarteritis nodosa, for it involves the small vessels to the viscera. The heart, kidneys, skin, and serous membranes are also involved. *A butterfly-like red rash over the bridge of the nose and both cheeks is a common and striking feature.* A peculiar occurrence is the finding of what are known as LE (lupus erythematosus) cells. These are polymorphonuclear leukocytes containing a large homogeneous inclusion mass (Fig. 84). They indicate an underlying autoimmune mechanism. The LE cells were first found in the bone marrow of patients suffering from the disease, but it is now known that the phenomenon depends on the presence of some factor in the patient's blood serum which acts upon the cells. When a test is made for the LE phenomenon, the patient's blood serum is mixed with his white blood cells, and a smear is made and searched for the development of LE cells. It must be realized that the phenomenon is an *in vitro,* not an *in vivo* one, being probably activated by the breakdown of platelets during coagulation when the blood is drawn.

THROMBOANGIITIS OBLITERANS.   This is in essence a thrombotic occlusion (obliteration) of the vessels of the legs in relatively young men

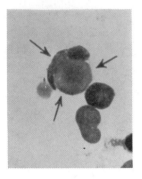

Fig. 84.   LE cell. (Kindness of Dr. A. J. Blanchard.)

with resulting gangrene of the toes and then the feet. It was Buerger who in 1908 brought the condition to the attention of the medical profession, so that it is commonly referred to as *Buerger's disease*. **The sex incidence is striking, for the disease is practically confined to men.** It is a disease of young adult life, is particularly common in Jews, and usually affects the arteries of the legs, although those of the arms may also be involved. The cause is unknown, but it is believed that there is a condition of allergic hypersensitivity in the arterial wall, as a result of which an acute inflammatory reaction develops. *Patients seem to be specially hypersensitive to tobacco, and the sufferer is often found to be a very heavy cigarette smoker.* In the treatment of the disease one of the most important points is to give up tobacco. The disease has an acute and a chronic stage. It is the chronic form which is more likely to give rise to serious symptoms, because the vessels are more widely and seriously involved by that time. The walls of both the arteries and the veins are inflamed, and the lumen of both these vessels is blocked by thrombi. The result is ischemia of the more distant parts of the leg and foot. Buerger called the lesion an angiitis, meaning an inflammation of vessels, both arteries and veins, but at the present time *thrombosis* is coming to be regarded as the dominant feature of the disease rather than inflammation, so that perhaps Buerger's disease (a noncommittal name) should not be considered here.

The first symptoms are usually indefinite pains in one foot or cramp-like pains in the calf after walking a short distance, a condition known as *intermittent claudication* (*claudicare,* to limp). No pulse can be felt at the ankle. When the foot hangs down it becomes bright red and throbs painfully. When the foot is raised it becomes more blanched than normal. Later in the disease ulcers and gangrene of the feet may develop, so that amputation may have to be performed. The tragedy of the condition is that the process tends to extend upward along the leg so that amputation may have to be done at an ever higher level.

SYPHILIS. Syphilis attacks two important sets of vessels: (1) the thoracic aorta, more especially the ascending portion, and (2) the cerebral arteries.

Syphilitic Aortitis. This used to be one of the commonest and most important of the lesions of syphilis, but modern antibiotic therapy has made the condition a rarity. The destruction caused by the *Treponema pallidum* in the wall of the aorta may produce aortic insufficiency or aneurysm. *Aortic insufficiency* or *incompetence* is caused by infection of the aortic ring to which the cusps of the aortic valve are attached. This results in destruction of the elastic tissue that forms one of the chief constituents of the wall, so that gradual stretching and dilatation occur, the valve becoming incompetent. The three cusps of the valve are shrunken, and show a characteristic cord-like thickening, becoming separated from one another, and thus further adding to the incompetence. The smooth intimal surface of the aorta becomes pitted, scarred, and wrinkled like the bark of a tree. *Aneurysm* is a localized or diffuse dilatation of the wall of the thoracic aorta caused by damage to the elastic tissue of the wall. Syphilitic aneurysm is considered below, together with other varieties of aneurysm.

Syphilitic Arteritis. This is best seen in the small arteries at the base of the brain. In addition to an inflammatory reaction in the adventitia, the all-important lesion is uniform thickening of the intima with marked narrowing of the lumen, which may lead to thrombosis and cerebral softening. Syphilis used to have to be considered in every case of these tragic occurrences, but such is no longer true.

Aneurysms

An aneurysm is a localized dilatation of an artery. This dilatation may be **saccular,** an outpouching of the vessel at one point (Fig. 85), or **fusiform,** a uniform dilatation of an entire segment of the artery. Every aneurysm is caused by weakening of the arterial wall. As a rule, it is the media that is damaged. *Syphilis* used to be the most important cause of aneurysm of the aorta and its main branches. With the modern control of syphilis and with the increasing age of the population *atherosclerosis* has come to replace it. *Polyarteritis nodosa* may weaken the artery and lead to the formation of multiple small aneurysms. Finally, *congenital weakness* of the media in the arteries at the base of the brain has been suggested as a cause of so-called congenital aneurysms in this region, although when we come to the chapter on diseases of the nervous system we shall see that this concept has been challenged. We shall confine our attention here to aneurysms of the aorta.

AORTIC ANEURYSM. Aneurysm due to *atherosclerosis* occurs at a later age than the syphilitic form, it generally affects the abdominal

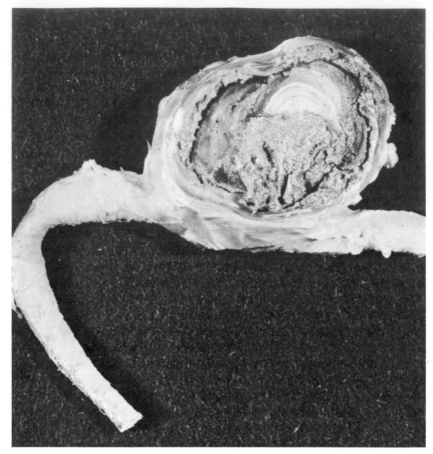

Fig. 85. Saccular aneurysm of the femoral artery. The laminated character of the clot, due to its being formed at intervals, is unusually distinct. (Boyd's *Textbook of Pathology.*)

aorta, and it usually causes diffuse dilatation of the vessel. The site of election is the lower part of the aorta below the origin of the vital renal arteries. This is singularly fortunate, because it makes possible the replacement of the aneurysm by an aortic homograft or a plastic tube, which may be a lifesaving procedure. A friend of mine, a surgeon, has had this replacement done on two separate occasions with excellent results. Unfortunately the aneurysm may press on the lower dorsal and lumbar vertebrae, with disastrous results (Fig. 86). A *syphilitic aneurysm* occurs at an earlier age, involves the ascending aorta or the arch, is usually saccular, and presses on the surrounding structures, causing pain in the back, dyspnea, and difficulty in swallowing. It may rup-

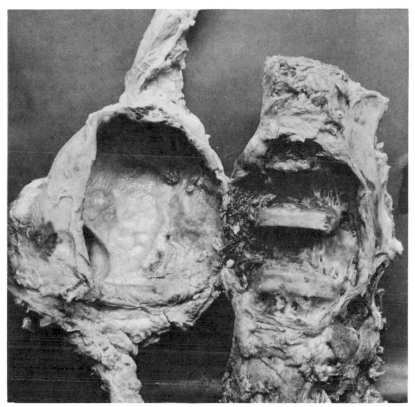

Fig. 86. Aneurysm of aorta involving levels from the eleventh dorsal to second lumbar vertebrae. Note the erosion of the vertebral bodies. Death was due to rupture of the aneurysm. (Kindness of Dr. N. K. Patoria, Nagpur, India.)

ture on the surface or internally, killing the patient at once. *Dissecting aneurysm* is not a true aneurysm, as the vessel is not dilated. A hemorrhage occurs in the media of the aorta at a point of weakness, and spreads along the vessel dissecting the media into two layers. The *symptoms of dissecting aneurysm* are characteristic. The patient is seized with a sudden sharp or excruciating pain in the chest or the abdomen, accompanied by prostration. He often experiences what he describes as a tearing sensation. The pain passes off, but in a typical case death occurs some days later from the bursting of the aneurysm into the chest or the abdominal cavity.

VEINS

The pathology of the veins is entirely different from that of the arteries. Veins differ from arteries as regards structure in two respects, both of which have a bearing on the development of disease. (1) They

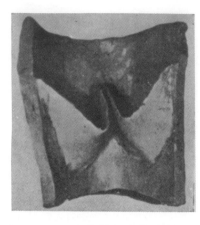

Fig. 87. Valve in saphenous vein (Edwards and Edwards, courtesy Am. Heart J.)

have *valves* (Fig. 87). Failure of the valves is one of the important features of varicose veins. (2) They have *lymphatics,* which accounts for the fact that malignant growths invade veins with the greatest ease, but seldom invade the walls of arteries, which are lacking in lymphatics. Bacteria from without can also readily penetrate the vein wall by way of the lymphatics.

Phlebitis or inflammation of the veins used to be of extreme importance, but antisepsis and chemotherapy have changed the picture completely. The great danger of phlebitis used to be an associated *thrombosis,* septic in character. This has disappeared, but **venous thrombosis** unassociated with phlebitis still remains a great threat and an unsolved problem. This question has already been discussed in Chapter 4. Two conditions especially affecting the veins in which thrombosis is common and often serious, namely varicose veins and hemorrhoids, will be considered here. The two really belong to the same group, for hemorrhoids or piles are merely varicose veins at the lower end of the intestinal canal.

VARICOSE VEINS. A varicose vein is one that is dilated and tortuous (Fig. 88). The dilatation may be extreme in degree, so that the valves which normally guard veins and prevent a backflow because of gravity become incompetent and cease to function. As a result of this the stagnation and accumulation of blood in the vein becomes increasingly great. The common site of varicose veins is in the superficial veins of the leg just under the skin. Bluish knuckles of veins can be seen pushing the skin in front of them. These are liable to injury, with resulting **hemorrhage** into the surrounding tissue. **Thrombosis** is liable to occur due partly to the slow flow in the dilated vessels, partly to the frequency of injury to the vessel wall. The circulation in varicose veins is gravely interfered with, the legs become swollen, and **varicose ulcers** are formed

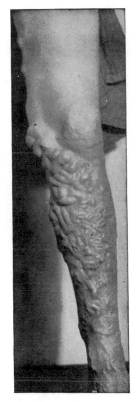

Fig. 88. Varicose veins. (Boyd, *Pathology for the Surgeon;* W. B. Saunders Co.)

in the lower part of the leg. These ulcers used to be extremely chronic and difficult to treat, but the outlook has been completely changed by modern methods of treating the varicose veins.

The **causes** of varicose veins are obscure. *Heredity* undoubtedly plays a part and the condition may run in a family for generations. The active factor is *increase of pressure* in the vein. This may be due to prolonged standing, muscular straining (in the case of piles), or the pressure of a tumor in the pelvis, a pregnant uterus, or even a continually loaded rectum.

The **treatment** of varicose veins is directed to the relief of the congestion, the accumulation of stagnant blood, in the dilated vessels. This may be accomplished by the application of a uniform support to the leg in the form of an elastic bandage or stocking; this should extend to the groin rather than to the knee which is the common practice. If this fails to relieve the condition the veins may be obliterated by the injection of irritating solutions (*e.g.,* sodium morrhuate) which injure the vessel walls, leading to thrombosis and finally fibrosis. The varicosity only affects the superficial veins, and as these communicate with the deep veins of the leg by small collateral channels, the circulation is re-established through the leg veins. For the same reason there is no danger of emboli passing from the superficial veins into the general circulation.

HEMORRHOIDS. Hemorrhoids or **piles** is a condition in which the veins at the lower end of the rectum become varicose and enlarged. *Internal hemorrhoids* are those covered by the mucous membrane of the lower end of the rectum; they may "come down" through the anal opening and appear on the surface, although they can be replaced by pressure. *External* hemorrhoids are covered by the skin in the neighborhood of the anus.

The **causes** are those of varicose veins, *i.e.,* heredity and increased pressure in the vein. The commonest cause of increased pressure is chronic constipation accompanied by undue muscular straining while the bowel is being emptied. A condition that must always be borne in mind, especially in a man past middle age, is cancer of the rectum, which may produce piles by causing pressure on the veins coming from the lower end of the bowel. In this case the piles are merely a symptom of a much more serious condition.

The possible **effects** which may render the condition serious are hemorrhage, phlebitis, and thrombosis. *Hemorrhage* when the bowels are moved is usually small in amount, but may be continued over a long period, so that a grave degree of *anemia* may be produced without the patient's suspecting its cause. *Phlebitis* or inflammation of the dilated veins together with inflammation of the surrounding tissue is commonly referred to as an "attack of the piles." Its danger is that it may lead to the formation of an infected thrombus, which readily becomes converted into an embolus.

The **treatment** of hemorrhoids is partly indirect, partly direct. By indirect treatment we mean keeping the bowels loose by means of bland laxatives and suitable food. Direct treatment is directed against the dilated veins. These may be closed by the injection of sclerosing solutions, and no more may need to be done. In more severe cases operative removal of the hemorrhoids may be necessary.

FURTHER READING

ALDERSBERG, D., and SCHAEFER, L. E.: Am. J. Med., 1959, *26,* 1. (Interplay of heredity and environment in atherosclerosis.)

DUGUID, J. B.: Brit. Med. Bull., 1955, *11,* 36. (Mural thrombosis in pathogenesis of atherosclerosis.)

GOLDBLATT, H.: *Renal Origin of Hypertension,* American Lecture Series, Springfield, Ill., 1948.

PAGE, I. H.: Circulation, 1954, *10,* 1. (Pathogenesis of atherosclerosis.)

ROBERTSON, P. W., *et al.:* Lancet, 1962, *2,* 567. (Essential hypertension.)

WOOD, J. E.: Scient. Amer., 1968, *218,* 86. Jan. (The venous system.)

Chapter 17

Lungs

STRUCTURE AND FUNCTION

It is obvious that the lungs form part of the respiratory system, so that this chapter might be given the name of that system. I wish, however, to concentrate attention on the lungs, although some of the other structures and their diseases will be mentioned.

The essential business of the lungs is purification of the blood, a business in which the heart and lungs are partners. The impure blood laden with the waste products of the body in the form of carbon dioxide is brought to the lungs where the carbon dioxide gas is given off into the air and fresh oxygen is taken up into the blood. This is done by means of respiration. Respiration is the first essential of life; when it ceases, so does life itself. The purified blood returns directly to the heart, and is then sent through the arteries to supply the needs of the body. The lungs constitute the great mixing place of air and blood, and they have a corresponding structure. Each lung is a honeycomb, with air in place of honey in the cells of the comb, and an infinite number of blood capillaries in their walls. *These walls are so thin that gases (carbon dioxide and oxygen) can readily pass through in either direction* (Fig. 89). The

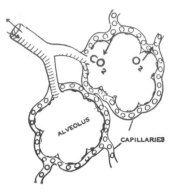

Fig. 89. Bronchiole going to two alveoli. The small circles in the capillaries are red blood cells. (Best and Taylor, *The Human Body;* Holt & Co.)

air is carried to the air spaces or *alveoli* by the bronchi and their terminations, the bronchioles, which subdivide and ramify throughout the entire lung.

The quantity of *oxygen* that could be carried in the fluid part of the blood, the plasma, would not maintain life for a second. It is the red blood cells, of which there are 25,000,000,000,000 in the blood of a man of average size, which carry the oxygen by reason of a chemical combination with the hemoglobin of which the red cells consist. The *carbon dioxide* (CO_2), on the other hand, is carried mainly in the plasma combined with sodium as sodium bicarbonate ($NaHCO_3$). The CO_2 is dissolved and combined with water to form carbonic acid (H_2CO_3). This process is greatly speeded by an enzyme in the red blood cells known as *carbonic anhydrase.* The same enzyme acts in a reverse direction when the blood reaches the pulmonary capillaries, with breakdown of the H_2CO_3 into CO_2 and H_2O, the gas being eliminated in the expired air. The most remarkable feature of this beautiful mechanism is that **it is the CO_2 in the blood flowing through the respiratory center in the medulla at the base of the brain which provides the stimulus for the muscles of respiration. Even a slight increase in the amount of CO_2 in the blood will increase the rate and depth of breathing,** as becomes evident whenever you run faster than you should. Thus a waste gas which must be removed from the body stimulates the mechanism required for its removal, surely a *tour de force* of precise automation.

It is now realized that the alveoli are lined by a film of lipoprotein called *surfactant,* so named because it is surface-acting. This lowers the surface tension and thus prevents collapse of the alveoli. The ability of the lungs to retain air therefore depends on the special properties of this film.

It must not be supposed that respiration, which in the last analysis is oxygenation of the tissues, is the only function of the lungs any more than excretion is the only function of the kidneys. Both are concerned with maintenance of the acid-base balance. When that balance is temporarily upset it can be restored to normal much more quickly by blowing off CO_2 than by the excretion of acid by the kidneys.

It will be evident that none of the wonderful mechanism serving respiratory function is of any value if anything interferes with the exchange of oxygen and carbon dioxide across the membrane which constitutes the alveolar walls. When the alveolar membranes become thickened owing to disease the result is *alveolar-capillary block*. Such interference may be marked in emphysema, the dust diseases, pulmonary edema, and other pathological conditions which we are about to study.

Owing to the rhythmic movements of the chest during respiration air is being continually sucked into and expelled from the lungs. One great disadvantage of this arrangement is that the interior of the lungs is in communication with the outside air, so that infecting germs are liable to enter and cause inflammation, although most of them are held back in the nose and throat. This is not the case with any of the other organs of the body, and for this reason inflammation and tuberculosis are far commoner in the lungs than in organs like the heart and kidney.

The lung, like the heart, is covered by a thin membrane, the *pleura*, and a similar membrane lines the chest wall. Although a potential space, the *pleural cavity*, exists between the layers, in health these layers are in contact with one another. It is evident that inflammation of the lung may easily extend to the pleura and set up inflammation in that membrane, a condition known as pleurisy.

COMMON COLD

The limits of this book make it impossible to consider diseases of the nose, throat, larynx, and trachea, which form the upper part of the respiratory tract, but brief mention must be made of so universal an ailment as the common cold.

Although this is the commonest of all infectious diseases, it is only during the last few years that any certain knowledge has been gained as to its causation. The causal agent is a *filterable virus*, which can be grown on tissue of human and monkey embryo kidney, in which it produces recognizable degenerative changes. No animal has been found that is susceptible, so that "the cold" is a peculiarly human disease. The virus is spread with extreme readiness from one person to another, so that epidemics of colds are frequent. Unlike most other filterable viruses, it fails to confer any immunity upon the infected person, so that he may suffer from several attacks in the course of a winter. It is now recognized that several groups of viruses may be involved in different epidemics. It is little wonder, then, that one attack does not immunize a person against a second attack. *Contributory factors,* as is well known, play an important part. Of these the most important is chilling of the body as the result of sitting in a draught, wet feet, and the like.

The infection produced by the virus is an acute one, and like other acute infections it may clear up in the course of a few days. Only too often, however, *secondary invaders* follow upon the primary infection, and these convert the acute into a chronic disease which may drag on for many weary weeks. The commonest of the secondary invaders are pneumococci, staphylococci, and streptococci.

The virus of the common cold and also the secondary invaders attack first the nose and throat, and later they may spread down to the larynx, trachea, and bronchi, and up into the sinuses which open into the nose. For the first day or so the mucous membrane lining the nose and throat is swollen, red and dry, giving the well-known "stuffed-up" feeling, but soon a watery fluid is poured out which runs from the nose continually. If the secondary invaders gain a hold, the inflammation becomes suppurative in type, and the watery secretion is replaced by a purulent one, which may continue to be discharged for many weeks.

BRONCHITIS

Bronchitis may be of an acute or a chronic form. The acute form usually involves the trachea as well as the larger bronchi.

Acute tracheobronchitis. The irritant responsible for the acute inflammation may be bacterial, mechanical (various dusts), or toxic (poisonous gases). The mucous membrane is red and swollen, and the lumen is filled with pus. When the irritant is removed, the inflammation is likely to subside.

Chronic bronchitis. This is a much more confused condition. It is seldom a primary entity, but rather a complication of some pre-existing pathological state, such as chronic heart disease, infection in the nasal sinuses, and prolonged cigarette smoking. In Britain it outranks all other respiratory diseases as a crippler and a killer, being four times as common in men as in women, perhaps connected with heavy cigarette smoking. The mortality is five times greater among unskilled laborers than in the professional classes. This suggests the important part played by inhaled noxious agents which cause paralysis of the cilia and bronchospasm. The chief clinical feature is excessive secretion of mucus from the bronchial tree. This is associated with hypertrophy of the bronchial mucous glands. Such a combination naturally leads to obstruction to the outflow in the bronchial tree, with the pulmonary alveoli as the real sufferers, resulting in chronic obstructive emphysema and bronchiectasis (see below). The advanced cases are described in the United States as bronchiectasis and emphysema rather than chronic bronchitis.

BRONCHIECTASIS

Bronchiectasis is a condition of dilatation of one or more of the smaller bronchi (Fig. 90). It is similar to aneurysm of an artery, and like an aneurysm *it is caused by weakening of the wall of the bronchus by infection.* The two important *causal factors* are *infection* and *bronchial obstruction.* **A single agent is seldom sufficient to produce the condition.** It is commonest in children following such viral infections as whooping cough or measles, in both of which the bronchial walls are inflamed, but it often occurs in young adults, and may persist into middle life. The *most significant lesion* is the destruction of the musculature and elastic tissue, for it is these that weaken the wall of the bronchus and allow the dilatation to occur. The bronchus dilates and forms a cavity in which septic matter collects. In time a regular cesspool is formed, the wall of the bronchus is destroyed, and an abscess results.

The *chief symptom* of bronchiectasis is the coughing up at intervals of great quantities of purulent material which may be very foul-smelling. In abscess, also, large quantities of pus are brought up and the breath may be foul. The latter is particularly likely to happen when gangrene, *i.e.,* putrefaction, of the lung develops. The disease may be confined to one or more segments, a point of great importance when it comes to a question of surgical removal of the lesion. (A segment is a section of lung parenchyma more or less completely separated from neighboring segments and supplied by a separate bronchus.)

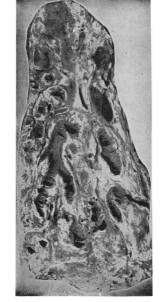

Fig. 90. Bronchiectasis. The bronchi are markedly dilated.

The diagnosis is made by the combined use of a radiopaque contrast material and x-ray examination. When such a material is introduced into the bronchial tree it soon spreads, and an x-ray film will now show a beautiful picture of all the bronchi, and any tell-tale dilatation can at once be detected.

Bronchiectasis is one of the tragic diseases of childhood, for it can be arrested in the early stages, whereas in the later stages it is much more hopeless than tuberculosis, and the frequent expectoration of large quantities of pus accompanied by a disgusting smell make the condition a peculiarly distressing one. If the disease had a simple but alarming name such as "lung rot" parents might be more careful of their children when they manifest continued cough and expectoration after measles and whooping cough.

BRONCHIAL ASTHMA

This difficult and distressing disease is well named, for it is derived from the Greek word meaning panting. Bronchial asthma, as opposed to cardiac and other forms of asthma, is *allergic* in origin, so that it has been discussed in Chapter 7 on Immunity and Hypersensitivity. A second etiological factor is *heredity,* there often being a family history of asthma or some other form of allergy. Finally a *psychosomatic factor* may be evident, the asthmatic attack being precipitated by some form of emotional stress. The smaller and medium-sized bronchi are occluded with thick, tough, and tenacious mucus, so that it is little wonder that the patient suffers from severe respiratory distress during the attack. Some of the allergens that may be responsible are indicated on page 119.

EMPHYSEMA

Emphysema is one of the most important of pulmonary diseases. The word actually means overinflation. It is not only by far the commonest chronic disease of the lungs, but the most crippling over a long period and therefore the most to be feared, for the patient does not die quickly, but drags out a miserable existence for years, a trial and a tribulation to himself, his family, and his doctor. He suffers with every breath he takes, and he must breathe some 20,000 times in 24 hours. It has been said that perhaps the most compelling of human appetites is the need for air, and probably no distress is so agonizing as that which results from the inability to breathe adequately. Emphysema is frequently associated with chronic bronchitis, so that the term *emphysema-bronchitis complex* is often used. It has become the single most important cause of disability in the working population of the United States, and the most rapidly rising cause of death. It is even more prevalent in Britain, where chronic bronchitis is a factor of supreme importance.

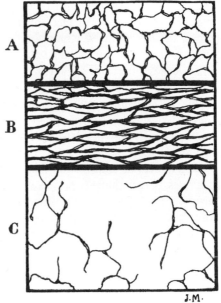

Fig. 91. *A,* Normal lung; *B,* atelectasis; *C,* emphysema.

J.M.

The lungs are voluminous and pale, and often present large blebs or bullae which project on the surface. Rupture of one of these bullae is the commonest cause of spontaneous pneumothorax. The walls between the air spaces are atrophied and many disappear, so that one large space is formed from many smaller ones (Fig. 91*C*). The condition is the reverse of atelectasis or pulmonary collapse, which is considered on page 317. Emphysema may be diffuse or focal, the former being much the more common.

The pathogenesis of emphysema, sad to relate, is still an unsolved problem. None of the many theories explain *all* the facts. There appears to be no single cause, but two factors demand special attention: (1) *increased intraluminal pressure,* and (2) *degeneration of the walls of the alveoli.* Increased pressure is due to obstruction of the check-valve type, which allows air to be drawn in during inspiration, but prevents it passing out during expiration. A very minor degree of stenosis of these narrow passages over the months and years may have disastrous effects on the alveolar passages that lie beyond. The cough that accompanies chronic bronchitis intensifies the tension within the alveoli. The chronic bronchitic may cough several hundred times a day for many years. There is therefore a close relationship between chronic bronchitis, bronchial asthma, and emphysema. The great increase in the incidence of the emphysema-bronchitis complex in recent years, particularly in

Britain, seems to be associated with the marked increase in heavy cigarette smoking, together with pollution of air by dust and fumes. In the sudden London smog of December, 1962, some 4000 deaths from respiratory failure occurred within a few days. Some cases in younger people show a marked familial tendency, suggesting a genetic predisposition. These cases often have a *severe deficiency of alpha-1-antitrypsin in the blood;* this, as its name indicates, is a serum protein which inhibits the action of trypsin, a powerful digestive enzyme. It has been suggested that the lack of antitrypsin may allow the trypsin, believed to come from bacteria and inflammatory cells, to digest the lung parenchyma. Of this at present there is no proof.

The effects of emphysema may be serious and far-reaching. The chest becomes barrel-shaped, respiratory movements are diminished, and expiration is difficult and prolonged. Owing to the widespread atrophy and destruction of the alveolar walls, the small blood vessels that run in them are obliterated, with resulting obstruction to the flow of blood from the right side of the heart in the pulmonary artery. The back pressure on the heart may become so extreme that great cardiac and respiratory distress develops, with marked cyanosis and finally fatal heart failure.

BACTERIAL PNEUMONIAS

Pneumonia signifies **an inflammatory consolidation of the lung,** a pneumonitis, the consolidation being either diffuse or patchy. The lung is the one organ in the body that is in direct contact with the outside air. It is but natural, therefore, that bacterial infection is frequent. The most important causes of acute bacterial pneumonias are *Diplococcus pneumoniae, Streptococcus hemolyticus, Staphylococcus aureus,* and *Friedländer's bacillus.* The diffuse or lobar form of pneumonia is nearly always caused by the pneumococcus, while the patchy or bronchopneumonic form is likely to be due to one of the other organisms just enumerated.

LOBAR (PNEUMOCOCCAL) PNEUMONIA.   The normal habitat of the pneumococcus is the mucous membrane of the upper respiratory tract (nose and throat), from which it may pass down into the lungs. About 40 per cent of healthy people carry pneumococci in their throat and nose. Infection is acquired from another person, usually one who harbors pathogenic pneumococci in the throat (a carrier) rather than one suffering from the acute disease. As in the case of other infections, **predisposing causes** are of great importance. Anything that lowers the resistance may act as a predisposing cause, but some of the most important weakening agents are *chill, a severe injury* (*e.g.,* fracture of the femur), and *a surgical operation under a general anesthetic.*

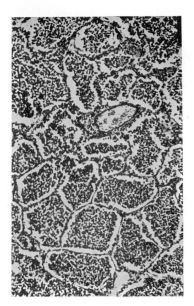

Fig. 92. Lobar pneumonia, showing air spaces (alveoli) filled with inflammatory exudate.

When a person with pathogenic pneumococci in the throat is exposed to one of the predisposing causes, the pneumococci pass down the trachea and bronchi and invade the air spaces or alveoli in the walls of which they cause acute inflammation. As the thin-walled blood vessels in the walls are in such intimate relation with the alveoli, an abundant acute inflammatory exudate pours from the vessels into the air spaces. This exudate consists of the various elements which have already been described in the chapter on Inflammation, but the predominating elements are polymorphonuclear leukocytes and serum, with formation of abundant fibrin threads from the latter. It is indeed in essence a *fibrinous exudate.* Many of the capillaries give way, so that red blood corpuscles are added to the exudate. **The result of all this is complete replacement of the air in the alveoli by the exudate,** so that the affected part of the lung is no longer air-containing but solid (Fig. 92). This part is now said to be *consolidated.* The inflammation spreads throughout a lobe, and may involve the entire lung. Often, however, the consolidation is confined to one or two lobes; hence the term lobar pneumonia. Such a consolidated lung is about as different from the normal spongy structure as it is possible to imagine. The infection reaches the pleura, and the beautifully smooth membrane is now covered with a shaggy exudate, a condition of *pleurisy.*

Lobar pneumonia usually runs its course in about a week. By the end of that time, provided the patient survives (which he usually does), the pneumococci are all killed; the exudate disintegrates, becomes softened, and is finally removed by being coughed up in the sputum. This removal, which is called *resolution,* is extraordinarily complete, and in a few weeks the lung is restored to its normal spongy condition, the alveoli being filled with air instead of with exudate.

The above description applies to the classic case of lobar pneumonia before the days of sulfonamides and antibiotics. Naturally, if the infection is nipped in the bud, the characteristic lesions will not have time to develop, nor will the case come to autopsy.

BRONCHOPNEUMONIA. This may be caused by staphylococci, streptococci, or pneumococci. *It is primarily a bronchitis,* an inflammation of the bronchi, and is widespread throughout one or both lungs. Here and there the infection penetrates into the alveoli and produces a small patch of inflammatory consolidation. These patches may be felt throughout the lung, but they are separated by an abundance of air-containing lung tissue. Such a lung is not said to be consolidated.

Bronchopneumonia is very much commoner than lobar pneumonia. It occurs at the extremes of age, being most frequent in young children and in the aged. It is a frequent accompaniment of the infectious fevers of childhood, and is so commonly found at postmortem examination as a terminal condition that it hardly attracts the attention of the pathologist unless it is very marked. Nevertheless it must often serve like some ministering angel to snuff out the flickering flame when life is ebbing away.

In these days of prevalent staphylococcal hospital infections, bronchopneumonia has assumed a new twofold significance. (1) Persons suffering from some pre-existing lung disease when admitted to hospital readily become infected with the antibiotic-resistant staphylococci in the ward, and the resulting bronchopneumonia may prove fatal. (2) Such staphylococcal lesions, especially if associated with lung abscess, may act as an important reservoir and source of hospital infection which is widely disseminated by the coughing of the patient.

VIRAL PNEUMONIAS

It is now recognized that viral pneumonias outnumber all other pneumonias, especially during epidemics. In addition to the pneumonitis complicating such viral infections as influenza and measles, there are many cases of primary lung infection caused by a variety of different viruses for which no very appropriate names have so far been suggested, so that these cases are given the rather ambiguous name of *primary atypical pneumonia.*

INFLUENZAL PNEUMONIA. Influenza is an acute inflammatory disease of the upper respiratory tract (throat, trachea, and bronchi), associated with marked general debility and sometimes accompanied by pulmonary complications. The special peculiarity of influenza is that usually it is the mildest of infections, lightly referred to as "a touch of the flu." At long intervals it assumes a virulent form, and like "a blast from the stars," as an old writer said, great epidemics sweep across the world killing millions of people. At such times, as in the 1918–1919 pandemic, it seems, as John Bright remarked in another connection, that "the Angel of Death is abroad in the land; you can almost hear the beating of his wings." In the 1918–1919 pandemic there were some 500,000,000 cases throughout the world, of whom 15,000,000 died. By comparison the more recent pandemic of Asian influenza was comparatively mild. It is in these virulent outbreaks that pulmonary complications in the form of influenzal pneumonia acquire a fearful significance. These epidemics may spread with extraordinary rapidity. In one of the United States Army camps in 1918 there were three cases one day and 3000 on the next!

The *cause* of influenza *is a filterable virus of various strains or groups* (p. 181). This virus is inhaled, and sets up an acute inflammation in the nose and throat, which may spread upward into the sinuses and downward into the trachea and bronchi, causing the feeling of rawness behind the breast bone which is so familiar to everyone. The virus causes not only a characteristic feeling of profound weakness and lassitude, but in some cases lowers the resistance of the lungs, so that other bacteria, secondary invaders like the seven devils of Holy Writ, pass down into the lungs and produce influenzal pneumonia. This is much more likely to happen during the great epidemics, thus explaining the high mortality on these occasions. It differs from lobar pneumonia in that both lungs are always involved, and in place of being consolidated and dry as a result of containing a more or less coagulated exudate, they are wet and water-logged. *When the lung is examined at autopsy it is found to be intensely congested with blood, so that it is a bluish-purple color and when it is incised frothy blood-stained fluid pours from the cut surface and from the bronchi.* Under the *microscope* the alveoli are seen to be filled with inflammatory serum which has not coagulated to form fibrin, leukocytes of varying kinds, and red blood corpuscles due to rupture of the capillaries in the walls of the alveoli. The exudate is essentially watery and hemorrhagic. *Abscesses* are apt to form throughout the lung, and if one of these is situated just under the pleura it may rupture into the pleural cavity causing *empyema,* a condition in which there is a large collection of pus in the pleural cavity. These complications naturally add greatly to the gravity of the disease.

Among the *symptoms* the dry, hacking *cough,* which is so common, is caused by acute irritation of the trachea and large bronchi. The profound *prostration* is due to a general toxemia. In *influenzal pneumonia* there is marked *cyanosis* (blueness of lips and face) and *dyspnea*. This is due to the large amount of inflammatory fluid that is poured into the alveoli and prevents the interchange of gases, which should normally occur and keep the blood purified. This watery exudate mingled with hemorrhage is the reason for the profuse, watery, *frothy, hemorrhagic sputum* which almost flows out of the patient in striking contrast to the viscid, stringy expectoration of lobar pneumonia. *Fever* is present as in all acute infections, but on account of the prostration it may not be high.

PRIMARY ATYPICAL PNEUMONIA. This relatively new arrival among the pneumonias appears to be a group rather than an entity, being caused by a variety of related viruses, which can be isolated from the sputum, and to which antibodies can be demonstrated in the blood between the second and third week of the illness. The disease may appear in small epidemics, usually in schools and army camps where young people are congregated. There is an acute inflammation of the upper respiratory tract, only involving the lungs to a minor degree, so that although the morbidity is high, the mortality is low. Even when pneumonia does develop the physical signs are largely negative, a characteristic feature, but there is roentgenographic evidence of a patchy ill-defined consolidation seldom involving more than a part of a lobe. The course is usually mild, recovery occurring in two or three weeks.

Basis of Symptoms of Pneumonia. Lobar pneumonia will be taken as the type. Most of the symptoms can be explained by the pathological lesions. The face is flushed, the breathing rapid, shallow, and painful, there is cough with blood-streaked sputum, fever and leukocytosis are present, and examination of the chest reveals changes in the lung. The **dyspnea** and rapid breathing are caused by interference with the free interchange of gases between the blood and the air owing to the exudate in the alveoli. The **cough** is due to irritation of the bronchi. The **sputum** is sticky so that it can be pulled out in strings and is a characteristically red or rusty color. The stickiness is caused by the inflammatory serum, and the color by the red blood corpuscles in the exudate. The sputum consists largely of polymorphonuclear leukocytes (pus cells) and contains large numbers of pneumococci. The **pain on breathing** is an indication of pleurisy, the rough and inflamed surfaces of the pleura being rubbed together each time the patient takes a breath. **Fever** is caused by the toxins produced by the pneumococci. **Leukocytosis** is the natural result of the demand for enormous numbers of leukocytes to be poured into the alveoli of the lung. When the healthy chest is percussed a drum-like note is heard, but when the lung is consolidated there is **dullness on percussion,** owing to replacement of the air by exudate.

ABSCESS

In lobar pneumonia there is no true suppuration, for suppuration implies destruction of tissue, and in pneumonia the walls of the alveoli are not destroyed. It is this that makes the complete structural recovery of the lung possible. Sometimes, however, especially when accessory factors are present which weaken resistance, suppuration develops, the lung tissue is destroyed, and abscesses are formed. This is more likely to happen in bronchopneumonia, and, as we have already seen, hospital staphylococcal infection is often responsible.

Abscess of the lung can be divided into three groups, depending on the method of causation. These are the inhalation, the embolic, and the pneumonic groups.

The **inhalation group** is the largest and most important. Lung abscess is a constant threat in operations on the mouth, nose, and throat, especially tonsillectomy and extraction of teeth. Infected material passes down the trachea and bronchi. Abscess is commoner in the right lung, which has a more vertical bronchus, and in the lower lobe. Stomach contents may be vomited during general anesthesia and inhaled into the lungs. Foreign bodies, especially peanuts and coins, may pass from the mouths of children down the trachea and cause lung abscess.

The **embolic group** is due to a septic thrombus being carried by the venous blood to the right side of the heart, and then via the pulmonary artery to the lung. Two sources of an infected blood clot which may be mentioned are the veins of the female pelvis (in puerperal sepsis) and the lateral venous sinus of the skull which becomes infected in inflammation of the middle ear and mastoid.

The **pneumonic group** represents a complication of pneumonia, usually streptococcal or influenzal in type; abscess formation is rare in lobar pneumonia.

The *chief symptoms* are fever, cough, and copious expectoration of pus, foul breath, and foul sputum. *An important complication of lung abscess is the formation of an abscess of the brain,* due to infected material being carried by the blood from the lung to the left side of the heart and thence to the brain. This is also liable to happen in bronchiectasis.

PULMONARY TUBERCULOSIS

The general principles that govern tuberculous infection have already been discussed in Chapter 7, together with the question of the reduction in the incidence of the disease. As the infection is acquired in the vast majority of cases by inhalation, it is natural that the lung should be by far the commonest site of the disease. We have seen that tuberculosis is a struggle between attack and defense, usually on fairly even terms but with the odds considerably in favor of the defense. When infection is established there are three possible courses: (1) *healing with scarring;* (2) *fibrocaseous tuberculosis;* (3) *acute tuberculous pneumonia.* The result depends on the size and frequency of the dose of tubercle bacilli on the one hand and the natural powers of defense on the other. It is important to distinguish between *primary infection* and *reinfection,* often called secondary infection.

PRIMARY INFECTION. The first infection usually occurs in childhood, but now as the result of public health measures it may be delayed until adult life. The primary or **Ghon lesion** is a small caseous focus, seldom more than 1 cm. in diameter, *situated in any part of the lung.* In this it contrasts sharply with the secondary lesion, which nearly always makes its first appearance at the apex. Infection spreads along the lymphatics, so that the regional lymph nodes become enlarged and caseous, again in contrast to what is found in secondary infection. *The patient with primary infection either recovers or dies;* the disease does not become chronic, nor is there any cavity formation. Recovery is marked by disappearance of the pulmonary and lymph node lesions, or their conversion into fibrous tissue with calcification. *But the patient is rendered hypersensitive or allergic to a subsequent infection as shown by the tuberculin test.* If healing fails to occur there may be generalized blood infection with fatal miliary tuberculosis or invasion of a bronchus with rapidly fatal bronchopneumonia.

REINFECTION. There is a curious immunity between the ages of five and fifteen, and death from pulmonary tuberculosis during these years is extremely rare. The reaction of the now allergic tissues to reinfection is quite different from that of the primary infection. The right lung is attacked much more often than the left, and the lesion is nearly always just below the apex. There are now four possibilities: (1) healing with fibrosis, (2) chronic fibrocaseous tuberculosis, (3) acute tuberculous caseous pneumonia, and (4) acute miliary tuberculosis. The result will depend on the size and frequency of the dose of tubercle bacilli on the one hand and the natural powers of defense on the other.

Healing with Scarring. This fortunately is by far the commonest course for the infection to run, as shown by the frequent presence of old tuberculous scars at the apex of one or both lungs in persons who come to autopsy. For some reason which is not clear the infection nearly always starts at the apex. There is a limited amount of destruction of tissue, but if the dose is not large and the person is in good health the healing process asserts itself, the bacilli are overcome, fibrous tissue surrounds and invades the area, and finally only a scar is left in which lime salts are often deposited. Even during the active stage the patient shows no symptoms, and is quite unaware that he has acquired tubercu-

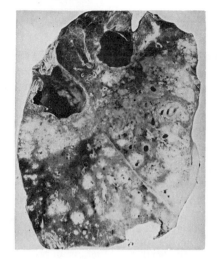

Fig. 93. Tuberculosis of lung, showing two large cavities in the upper part, consolidation (white) and small tubercles in the lower part.

losis, but the positive tuberculin test of the skin will show that this is the case.

Fibrocaseous Tuberculosis. This is the usual form in the person who shows active signs of tuberculosis. The name shows that both of the main processes are at work. There is fibrosis indicating healing and caseation indicating destruction. The basic lesion as usual is the tubercle. The tubercles coalesce to form caseous or cheese-like masses. The caseous material becomes softened, liquefied, discharged into a bronchus, and finally expectorated as tuberculous sputum filled with tubercle bacilli. A *cavity* is formed in the place formerly occupied by the caseous material (Fig. 93). This cavity may be small, or it may be so large as to involve the greater part of a lobe. Sometimes an artery is left traversing a cavity. Should this vessel finally rupture, very profuse *hemorrhage* may occur. In time numerous cavities are formed. The intervening parts of the lung show *tuberculous consolidation,* the alveoli being filled with inflammatory cells and caseous material. If the progress of the disease is slow, fibrosis may be quite marked as shown by white strands, especially around the cavities, but true healing does not occur. The disease spreads from the apex downward, so that the oldest and most advanced lesions are at the top. In a case with extensive lesions there may be cavities in the upper part of the lung, consolidation in the middle, and separate tubercles at the base. Pleurisy is always present, and adhesions are formed between the two layers of the pleura.

Acute Tuberculous Pneumonia. Here the infection overwhelms the resistance, and runs through the lung like a forest fire, giving rise to the clinical picture of galloping consumption or acute phthisis (wasting). There are no discrete tubercles, but in their place a diffuse pneumonic process. There is no fibrosis, no attempt at limitation of the infection. Acute cavities are formed. The disease may prove fatal in a few months or even weeks.

Acute Miliary Tuberculosis.   This is a fourth possibility, which may be regarded as a complication of any of the previous three. The tuberculous process may penetrate the wall of a blood vessel and discharge large numbers of bacilli into the blood stream. These are carried throughout the body, where they cause the formation of an infinite number of miliary tubercles in all the organs. The lungs are no exception, so that in addition to a small lesion at the apex of one lung, both lungs may be peppered with fine miliary tubercles.

BASIS OF SYMPTOMS.   The *general symptoms,* such as fever, loss of weight, and weakness, are due to the absorption of toxins. They become more marked when secondary infection with pyogenic bacteria is added to the pure tuberculous infection (again an example of the seven devils). *Cough* is a bronchial symptom due to irritation of the larger bronchi. *Pain in the side* is due to tuberculous pleurisy. The character of the *sputum* depends on the nature of the lesions. In acute miliary tuberculosis there may be no sputum. Until cavities have formed it is scanty and may contain no bacilli. After cavity formation it is copious, purulent owing to secondary infection, and contains large numbers of bacilli. The more rapid the disease the more bacilli will there be, the more stationary the disease the fewer are their numbers.

Hemoptysis, the coughing up of blood, is due to erosion of a blood vessel. It has been said that hemoptysis marks the end of the beginning or the beginning of the end of the disease. At the beginning there may be erosion of a small vessel in the early process of softening, and the sputum becomes blood-streaked. In the advanced stage a large artery crossing a chronic cavity may give way causing a severe and possibly fatal hemorrhage.

It must not be forgotten that the patient with pulmonary tuberculosis is a potential source of danger to those with whom he comes in contact. This danger may remain potential and not become actual if he is educated in the principles of hygiene. The two sources of danger are sputum and coughing at close quarters. If sputum is safely disposed of and the danger of coughing infected droplets in the direction of another person recognized, the tuberculous patient need not be a source of infection to those with whom he lives. But the danger is always present, and precautions must not for a moment be relaxed. The price of safety is eternal vigilance.

DUST DISEASES

The long-continued irritation of certain dusts may cause a chronic interstitial pneumonia known as *pneumoconiosis* (*konis,* dust). These dusts are encountered as the result of certain industrial processes. The dangerous element in the dust is silica.

SILICOSIS. Silicosis is the most widespread, the most serious, and the oldest of all occupational diseases. It provides a serious hazard in the *gold-mining* industry in certain districts such as the South African Rand and northern Ontario. If, in *coal mining,* hard rock has to be drilled through, coal miners may also suffer. Other occupations in which there is danger are *tin mining, stone working, metal grinding,* and *sand blasting.* In all of these cases, dust containing fine particles of silica may be inhaled over long periods of time.

The silica dust is carried by phagocytes from the bronchioles into the septa of the alveoli. There the dust acts as an irritant which stimulates the formation of large amounts of connective tissue. This fibrosis goes hand in hand with destruction of the lung structure. At first there are discrete nodules of fibrous tissue, but in the course of time these coalesce to form large fibrous areas, which are completely useless from the point of view of respiratory function. These fibrous areas give a characteristic x-ray picture, by means of which an accurate diagnosis can be made.

We have spoken as if the silica particles explained everything. Another concept, the antigen theory, has come into fashion. Silica, instead of having a simple toxic effect on the tissue, is now believed to combine with body protein to form an antigen, so that there may be some of the element of an antigen-antibody reaction in the producing of fibrosis.

The condition is a progressive one, and the patient continues to get worse even after he has been removed from the source of dust for a number of years. Most silicotics die of tuberculosis because the presence of silica in the tissues favors the growth of tubercle bacilli to an astonishing degree. There is gradually increasing shortness of breath, with developing heart failure owing to the difficulty which the right ventricle has in pumping blood to the densely fibrosed lungs. This is one of the few conditions for which there is absolutely no treatment, and it is evident that in this case prevention is all-important. This can be done by paying attention to adequate ventilation of factories and providing miners with masks that will filter out the dust. Silicosis, however, remains one of the great industrial hazards.

OTHER DUST PNEUMONIAS. *Anthracosis* is a condition in which the lung becomes filled with coal dust. If the coal is hard coal, damage will result, because the rock from which the coal was mined contains a certain amount of silica. *Asbestosis* is an important disease caused by the inhalation of asbestos dust. The disease may be acquired either during the crushing of asbestos rock or in the process of the manufacture of asbestos. As the great bulk of asbestos comes from the province of Quebec, it is natural that most of the cases should be found in this locality. The lung shows the same airless and fibrous condition that is so characteristic of silicosis. Both in asbestosis and in silicosis there is a marked tendency to the development of pulmonary tuberculosis.

BRONCHOGENIC CARCINOMA

Cancer of the lung does not arise from the pulmonary tissue, which does not contain epithelium, but from the bronchus, as the name implies. At the present time bronchogenic carcinoma is perhaps the most interesting and challenging of all malignant tumors. It is interesting because of the problems it presents with respect to: (1) *increased incidence,* (2) *possible relation to external carcinogens.* It is challenging because of the fact that of all the malignant tumors of internal organs it is the most readily seen by means of the bronchoscope, and yet the prognosis is among the worst.

When I was a student in Edinburgh the tumor used to be regarded as a rarity. In fact I do not remember seeing a case either in the ward or in the autopsy room, but I do remember seeing many cases that were called mediastinal lymphosarcoma invading the lung. During the past quarter of a century bronchogenic carcinoma has become one of the commonest, if not the commonest, of the killing cancers, especially in the male. There can be little doubt that there has been a real increase, but it is equally true that what we know we see. It was not until the beginning of the present century that coronary thrombosis and myocardial infarction were recognized. No one suggests that the disease started then, yet the lesions, which any medical student can now tell at a glance, were not appreciated by such masters as Virchow and Rokitansky, who probably gave them different names. The modern radiologist is responsible for very many of the correct diagnoses made at the present time.

If there were differences of opinion as to the question of an increased incidence of cancer of the lung, these differences are multiplied many times when we come to the matter of *causation.* The trouble is that there are so many possible carcinogens. The *exhaust gases and soot from automobiles,* especially when idling at stop lights in the city, are rich in carcinogenic agents. The same is true of *radiation fallout,* although that is an ultramodern hazard which can hardly be blamed for the development of cancer 25 or more years ago.

Cigarette smoking is the etiological agent that has aroused the greatest interest and the most heated debate. The statistical evidence certainly supports the idea that excessive smoking is a factor of importance. Although there is still no *proof* in the usual sense of the word that cigarette smoking is a cause of lung cancer, statistics show that cigarette smokers have a greater risk of dying of lung cancer than have nonsmokers, and

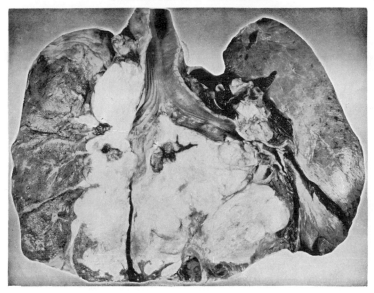

Fig. 94. Primary carcinoma of the lung. Part of the new growth is the lung tumor, but part is the greatly enlarged bronchial lymph nodes. (Boyd's *Textbook of Pathology.*)

the risk increases with the number of cigarettes smoked. It is awkward that women, who have become such inveterate cigarette smokers for many years, still show no increase in the incidence of lung cancer.

LESIONS.   The tumor grows into and surrounds one of the main bronchi, gradually narrowing the lumen until it becomes completely blocked (Fig. 94). Two results follow from this blockage. (1) In the first place the part of the lung supplied by the bronchus is cut off from a fresh supply of air, the air in this part of the lung is gradually absorbed into the blood, and finally the affected area of the lung undergoes *collapse*. This collapse can readily be recognized in the roentgenogram even though the tumor itself may be invisible, and by this means a correct diagnosis can be made. (2)   The second result is *bronchiectasis* and abscess formation. This is due to the fact that the secretions in the blocked part of the bronchus cannot escape and therefore stagnate and undergo putrefaction, so that the wall of the bronchus is weakened and dilates, a condition of bronchiectasis. Cancer cells from the surface of the tumor that projects into the lumen of the bronchus are shed off and coughed up in the sputum. *Examination of the sputum for these cells, either by making smears or by coagulating the sputum into a block of tissue and cutting microscopic sections, is an extremely valuable means of making an early diagnosis, especially in cases where the tumor cannot be seen by the bronchoscope.*

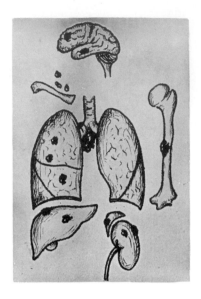

Fig. 95. Diagram to illustrate sites of metastases in bronchogenic carcinoma. (Boyd's *Textbook of Pathology*.)

One of the chief features of the disease is the formation of **metastases.** Even when the tumor in the bronchus is comparatively small, the cancer cells may spread by lymph vessels to the lymph glands in the chest, where they form a large tumor mass, and by the blood stream to distant organs such as the liver, brain, and bones (Fig. 95). The first indication that the patient has a cancer of the lung may be swelling of the abdomen due to a large tumor in the liver, severe headache due to a brain tumor, or a fracture caused by weakening of a bone from the presence of a secondary tumor. The adrenal and kidney are often involved. In addition to distant metastases the tumor may spread widely throughout the lung and involve the pleura.

BASIS OF SYMPTOMS. The symptoms are due to pressure and obstruction. The *persistent cough* is due to irritation of the bronchus by a growth. When a patient in the cancer age, particularly a man, has suffered from a cough and expectoration without obvious cause for more than a few weeks, it is always wise to suspect carcinoma and to examine the sputum for cancer cells or to pass a bronchoscope and inspect the lining of the bronchi. *Bloody sputum* is caused by the tumor in the bronchus opening into a blood vessel. *Dyspnea,* one of the commonest symptoms, is due to the cutting off of air from the lung, pressure by the enlarged glands, and interference with the heart's action. *Pain* in the chest and back is caused by pressure on the nerves. *Pleural effusion* is common, and is due to irritation of the pleura by spread of the tumor. Other symptoms may be due to metastases in the brain and elsewhere.

There are other tumors of the lung, both benign and malignant, in addition to bronchogenic carcinoma, but by comparison they are uncommon and unimportant—unless you happen to develop one of these tumors in your own lung.

ATELECTASIS

Atelectasis means collapse of the lung. The lung is a sponge filled with air. When this sponge is compressed it collapses. Before birth there is, of course, no air in the lungs, and they are therefore completely collapsed, a condition of *congenital atelectasis*. As soon as the child breathes after birth the lungs become expanded with air. In medicolegal work the absence of atelectasis is a proof that the child has lived after birth.

Apart from the congenital form, collapse of the lung may be produced in two entirely different ways: by compression of the lung or by obstruction of a bronchus. **Compression of the lung** may be caused by pleural effusion, empyema, or the presence of air under pressure in the pleural cavity (pneumothorax). **Obstruction of a bronchus** may be caused in a variety of ways. A foreign body such as a peanut, coin, or tooth, may pass down the trachea and become lodged in a bronchus. No air can now enter the part of the lung supplied by the blocked bronchus; the air already there is absorbed into the blood, and the lung collapses. In debilitated children suffering from bronchitis mucus may collect in the bronchi in such large amount that obstruction and atelectasis results; owing to the debility the mucus is not expelled by vigorous coughing. For the same reason areas of collapse may develop after an abdominal operation, because mucus collects in the bronchi owing to the irritation of the anesthetic, and coughing is interfered with by the abdominal wound. In bronchogenic carcinoma the tumor often obstructs a bronchus so that the distal part of the lung undergoes collapse, a condition that can be recognized in the roentgenogram, and is of great help in making a diagnosis.

In all forms of atelectasis the lung presents the same appearance. A part or the whole of the lung is collapsed like a compressed sponge; it is firm, airless, and dark owing to the air being squeezed out of it. Microscopically the walls of the alveoli are pressed together, so that the lumen is almost obliterated (Fig. 91*B*).

PLEURISY

The pleura, that delicate membrane which embraces the lung so intimately, is naturally involved in the infections that attack the lung. Inflammation of the pleura, or pleurisy, is therefore a common accompaniment both of pneumonia and of tuberculosis. Inflammation of serous membranes, of which the pleura is an example, is characterized by *the*

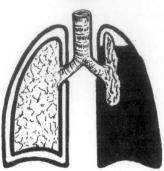

Fig. 96. Pleural effusion. The left pleural cavity is almost completely filled with fluid causing marked collapse of lung.

formation of a shaggy inflammatory exudate consisting of fibrin. This exudate forms a rough layer on the smooth surface of the pleura covering the lung and may also involve the pleura lining the chest wall. These two rough surfaces rub together each time the lung moves during respiration, producing *sharp stabbing pain in the side.* In time the two inflamed surfaces may stick together with the formation of temporary or permanent adhesions. Fluid poured out in the exudate may accumulate in the pleural cavity between the two layers, a condition known as **pleurisy with effusion. In dry pleurisy,** a more common condition, there is little or no fluid in the pleural cavity. If the fluid is large in amount it will press the air out of the lung and cause partial or complete *collapse* of that organ (Fig. 96). The fluid exudate of pleurisy with effusion is serous in character, that is to say it consists mostly of blood serum with only a slight admixture of inflammatory cells.

EMPYEMA. Empyema is a purulent pleurisy, in which the pleural cavity is filled not with watery serous fluid but with pus. It is therefore synonymous with pus in the pleural cavity. Before the days of the sulfonamides and antibiotics empyema used to be a common and dangerous complication of intrathoracic disease. Now it has become uncommon and even rare. A frequent cause used to be the formation of an abscess of the lung immediately under the pleura; if this abscess should rupture into the pleural cavity with an outpouring not only of pus but of enormous numbers of bacteria, empyema will result. Empyema may complicate lobar pneumonia, especially in children, but is more likely to follow streptococcal bronchopneumonia such as may occur in the course of influenza.

PLEURAL FLUID. The pleural cavities are normally empty, but as a result of disease they may contain a large amount of fluid. This fluid may be either an exudate or a transudate. In both cases the fluid comes from the blood vessels. An *exudate* is formed as the result of inflammation (pleurisy, empyema), which renders the walls of the vessels more permeable so that an inflammatory exudate pours out. We shall therefore expect an exudate to resemble the blood in containing much albumin and leukocytes (pus cells) and in having a high specific gravity. A *transudate* is formed as the result of back pressure in the veins and capillaries, which causes the watery part of the blood to escape through the vessel walls. This occurs in congestive heart failure. A transudate is more watery than an exudate, contains little albumin and few cells, and has a low specific gravity. In an exudate the albumin is over 3 per cent, the specific gravity is above 1.018, and the fluid may be turbid on account of the presence of large numbers of pus cells. In a transudate the albumin is under 3 per cent, the specific gravity is under 1.015, and the fluid is clear.

Pleural fluid may be a clear transudate, or a fairly clear exudate (pleurisy with effusion), or thick purulent fluid (empyema). Pleurisy with effusion is usually due to pulmonary tuberculosis. As an exudate is caused by bacterial infection, the fluid is cultured in the laboratory, so that it must be collected in a sterile container. It is preferable to add a little sodium citrate to the container to prevent the fluid from clotting.

PNEUMOTHORAX

Pneumothorax is air in the pleural cavity. The air may come from the lung, usually as the result of rupture of an emphysematous bulla, very occasionally a tuberculous cavity on the surface. More rarely it may come from the outside, as in a perforating wound of the chest or fracture of a rib. Whatever the cause of the pneumothorax, the air accumulates in the pleural cavity and compresses the lung, causing collapse in just the same way as an accumulation of fluid may lead to collapse. The presence of air can easily be detected by the physician by the physical signs it produces and by the appearance in the roentgenogram.

FURTHER READING

Doll, R., and Hill, A. B.: Brit. Med. J., 1956. *2*, 1071. (Relation of smoking to bronchogenic carcinoma.)

Flick, A. L., and Paton, R. R.: Arch. Int. Med., 1959, *104,* 518. (Smoking and chronic bronchitis.)

Gray, Jr., F. D.: *Pulmonary Embolism.* Philadelphia, 1966.

Hinshaw, H. C., and Garland, L. H.: *Diseases of the Chest,* Philadelphia, 1956.

Reid, L.: *The Pathology of Emphysema,* London, 1967.

Rosenblatt, M. B., and Lisa, J. R.: *Cancer of the Lung,* New York, 1956.

Spencer, H.: *Pathology of the Lung,* London, 2nd ed., 1968.

Chapter **18**

Upper Digestive Tract

The digestive or alimentary canal extends from the mouth, through which food enters the body, to the anus through which the residue escapes. Its function is two-fold: (1) To convert the food into a digestible form in which it can be assimilated; (2) to absorb the food thus digested. More briefly, the functions are digestion and absorption. Digestion is begun in the mouth and continued in the stomach. Absorption is accomplished by the intestine, although digestion also takes place in the upper portion of that tube. The digestive tract has been compared with a modern factory, for it is completely automated, and the owner's job merely consists of ordering bulk supplies and disposing of the output.

We may, therefore, divide the alimentary canal into an upper part, the mouth, esophagus or gullet, and stomach, and a lower part, the small and large intestine. The distinction is convenient on account of the difference in the diseases that affect the two portions. The common diseases of the upper part are inflammation and tumors.

MOUTH

The principal structures in the mouth are the lips, tongue, tonsils, and teeth.

CANCER OF THE LIP. As the lips are covered by skin and gum, both of which are epithelial structures, the common tumor is carcinoma. Cancer of the lip is uncommon in women and extremely rare in the upper lip. It occurs principally in men past middle age, and begins as a thickening at the junction of the skin and mucous membrane (the red part of the lip) which may or may not be raised above the surface (Fig. 97). It is usually preceded by some chronic inflammatory lesion such as an ulcer or crack which may have been present for months or even years. The irritation produced by excessive smoking may be a factor. *The most important single fact about cancer of the lip is that it is remarkably amenable to treatment.* Surgical removal or treatment by radium usually brings about a complete and lasting cure. The worst thing to do is to apply some form of caustic or irritant with the idea of burning off the nodule, for such treatment only serves to stimulate the growth of the tumor. If the condition is untreated it will gradually destroy the lip, and the tumor cells will be carried to the local lymph nodes under the jaw and in the neck, enlargement of which will form a large hard lump. When this occurs the prospects of successful treatment are greatly lessened.

CANCER OF THE TONGUE. As might be expected, the appearance of the lesion and the etiological factors concerned are similar to those of cancer of the lip. Chronic irritation in the form of a jagged tooth or a badly fitting plate is an important factor. The tumor usually begins on the edge of the tongue, and is felt as a lump which finally breaks down to form an ulcer. The tumor spreads much more rapidly than in the case of cancer of the lip, so that the presence of a lump in the tongue, however small, demands immediate attention. *The prognosis is much worse than in cancer of the lip,* particularly in cancer of the pos-

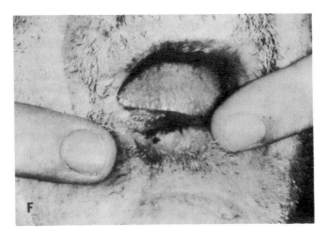

Fig. 97. Cancer of lower lip. (Zegarelli et al., Diagnosis of Diseases of the Mouth and Jaws.)

terior part of the tongue, but radium treatment has served greatly to lighten the gloom of the picture.

CANCER OF THE MOUTH. Carcinoma may arise from the gum of the jaws and cheeks, from the palate, and from the throat. In the front of the mouth the tumor is of the same character as cancer of the lip and tongue, and is again associated with chronic irritation. At the back of the mouth and in the throat the tumor may present two special characteristics: (1) The local lesion may remain small and indeed undiscoverable for a long time, but the lymph nodes in the neck become greatly enlarged. (2) The tumor (mass in neck) is highly radiosensitive, although it is seldom that a cure can be effected by this means.

TONSILLITIS. The tonsils are masses of lymphatic tissue, one on each side of the throat. They are full of little recesses or *crypts,* and as the mouth is teeming with bacteria it is natural that infection should be frequent. The infecting agent is commonly the streptococcus. As a result of the acute inflammation the tonsils become markedly swollen, narrowing the opening of the throat, and causing great pain and difficulty in swallowing. The surface may be covered with pus. *Quinsy* is a very severe suppuration of the entire tonsil, frequently with spread of the infection to the surrounding tissues of the throat and abscess formation. One attack of tonsillitis tends to predispose to another, and a state of chronic infection may be established within the crypts. Acute or chronic sore throat, like tonsillitis, is due principally to streptococcal infection.

TEETH

STRUCTURES. A tooth is composed of four structures: (1) enamel, (2) dentine, (3) pulp, and (4) cementum (Fig. 98). The *enamel* is the outer covering or crown of the tooth. It is calcified and extremely hard, so that it can stand the wear and tear of a long life and can enable a dog to crunch bones without itself becoming worn away. It forms a perfect covering for the dentine, but unfortunately it is brittle and easily cracked. Moreover, fissures may form in the course of development, and through these fissures infection may reach the underlying dentine. The *dentine* forms the main bulk of the tooth. Like the enamel it is calcified. It is traversed by large numbers of minute channels, the dentinal tubules, which pass from the pulp and travel to the enamel. It is along these channels that infection may find its way once it has reached the dentine. The *pulp* consists of soft connective tissue filled with blood vessels and nerves.

CARIES. Caries or dental caries is one of the most widespread of diseases. It is found in the teeth of Egyptian mummies, so that it is no new affliction of mankind, and it is world-wide in its distribution,

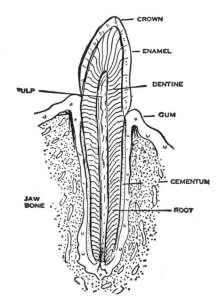

Fig. 98. Section through a tooth to show its structure. (Best and Taylor, *The Human Body and Its Functions;* Henry Holt & Co.)

although certain races such as Eskimos and African natives are remarkably exempt. It is principally a disease of childhood and adolescence; when that period is past the threat of caries becomes very much less. Both the deciduous teeth and the permanent teeth are liable to the disease, but it is most likely to attack the permanent teeth after continued exposure to refined carbohydrates coupled with inadequate oral hygiene. The molars are most frequently affected.

There is no single cause of dental caries, but its essence is decalcification of the inorganic salts of which the tooth is composed. Anything which endangers the integrity of the enamel covering is liable to lead to caries. The factors may be exciting or predisposing. The *exciting cause is bacterial infection with acid-producing organisms,* which by enzyme action cause fermentation of refined carbohydrates retained as food debris in stagnant areas around the teeth with the elaboration of organic acids that attack the enamel. Of *predisposing causes faulty diet* is all-important. Caries is essentially a disease of civilization, and it is the diet of civilization, particularly finely ground white flour, sugar and starchy foods, which is the culprit.

The *lesions* of caries can only be appreciated when the structure of the tooth is understood. Like the caries of bone tuberculosis, it is a gradual eating away of the tooth. All the elements of the tooth may be affected. The acids produced by the bacteria enter the enamel through cracks and defects, and gradually dissolve away the calcium of this hard substance. In time they reach the dentine, which is now exposed by the erosion of the enamel not only to the acids but to the bacteria themselves. Destruction of the dentine occurs much more rapidly and widely, so that a large cavity may be formed in the dentine although there is only a small defect in the overlying enamel. The bacteria readily pass along the dentinal tubules and thus reach the pulp where they set up a true and often a violent inflammation. It is this inflammatory reaction in the pulp that is responsible for the pain of caries. The infection may pass down through the opening in the root of the tooth through which the dental nerve enters the pulp, and may give rise to a *root abscess* (Fig. 99).

Other common conditions are periodontitis and gingivitis, but they will only be mentioned. *Periodontitis,* as the name indicates, is a disease of the surroundings of a tooth, not of the tooth itself. It is the greatest single cause of loss of teeth in the adult, for a gap is formed between the root of the tooth and the bone. *Gingivitis* is inflammation of the gingiva, the mucous membrane surrounding the neck of each tooth. The gums are swollen and inflamed, and may bleed when the toothbrush is used too vigorously.

ESOPHAGUS

The esophagus, considering its length and the variety of highly irritating fluids and solids that pass along it, is remarkably free from disease. The only function of the esophagus is swallowing, and we shall consider only two pathological conditions, varices and carcinoma.

ESOPHAGEAL VARICES. Esophageal varices are dilated tortuous veins in the wall of the esophagus, usually just below the surface and most marked in the lower third. Their importance lies in the fact that *rupture of the veins may result in massive hemorrhage, which may well prove fatal.* Apart from the bleeding they cause no symptoms, so that their presence may go unsuspected. They are the result of hypertension in the portal system of veins, the portal hypertension in turn being caused by cirrhosis of the liver. Modern surgery has made such advances in the treatment of portal hypertension that it is now important to diagnose esophageal varices before they become a threat to life. In cases of cirrhosis the two most valuable methods are *barium x-ray studies* which show multiple filling defects produced by the varicosities, and *esophagoscopy,* which reveals longitudinal tortuous masses of veins (Fig. 100).

CANCER OF THE ESOPHAGUS. The only important tumor of the esophagus is carcinoma. This usually occurs in men past middle age, although it is also met with in women. The tumor surrounds the muscular tube, producing narrowing of its lumen, so that difficulty in swallowing is the chief symptom. The common site is the middle, where

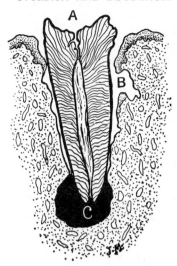

Fig. 99. Dental disease. *A,* Caries affecting crown of tooth and penetrating down to the pulp. *B,* Periodontitis; shrinking of bone and gum away from tooth. *C,* Root abscess.

the esophagus is crossed by the left bronchus, followed rather closely by the lower end. The only treatment is surgical removal of the tumor, and this is possible in very few cases and can only be undertaken by the most skillful of surgeons.

STOMACH AND DUODENUM

STRUCTURE AND FUNCTION.   The stomach and the first part of the duodenum above the site of entry of the bile duct and the pancreatic duct have very much in common. Both have a similar developmental origin and blood supply. The first part of the duodenum, being above the entrance of the alkaline bile and pancreatic juice, is exposed like the stomach to the acid gastric juice. These factors have a bearing on the incidence of peptic ulcer. In other respects the stomach and duodenum are very different, particularly with regard to the frequency of carcinoma, which is very common in the stomach and very rare in the first part of the duodenum, only an inch or two away, a difference that remains an enigma.

The stomach is an elongated muscular bag situated in the upper part of the abdomen (epigastrium) under the ribs. Its capacity is about 1½ quarts. The end that opens into the duodenum is called the *pylorus.* At the pylorus there is a circular band of muscle, the *pyloric sphincter,* which is usually contracted, but relaxes to allow food that has been properly liquefied by the gastric juice to pass into the duodenum. If it

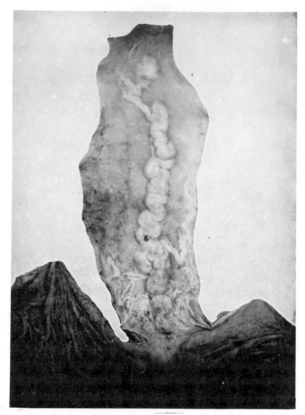

Fig. 100. Esophageal varicosities which caused severe hematemesis. (Boyd, *Textbook of Pathology;* Lea & Febiger.)

refuses to relax, the stomach becomes dilated. The most frequent cause of *dilatation of the stomach* is an ulcer or cancer at the pylorus. When an ulcer becomes chronic or heals, much scar tissue is formed, which contracts and narrows the opening (*pyloric stenosis*). The mere irritation of the ulcer may cause the muscle of the sphincter to go into spasm, thus keeping the opening closed. Sometimes abnormal nervous stimuli will produce the same result even though no lesion can be found in the stomach. This "functional obstruction" is known as *pylorospasm*. The normal stomach should empty itself in one to seven hours, depending on the nature of the meal. If the stomach is not empty at the end of seven hours as shown by the x-ray examination, *retention* is said to be present. In marked organic obstruction the stomach may become enormously dilated, and may fill the greater part of the abdomen, causing great distress and continuous vomiting.

The only function of the esophagus is swallowing. The function of the stomach, on the other hand, is to initiate the process of digestion, to prepare the food mechanically and chemically so that it can be received into the small intestine for more complete digestion, and to eject the prepared material slowly and in small quantities into the duodenum.

The gastric juice contains (1) a digestive ferment, *pepsin,* which acts only on the proteins of the food, and (2) *hydrochloric acid,* which is necessary for the proper functioning of the pepsin. Both are produced by the gastric mucous membrane in response to certain nervous and chemical stimuli. The **nervous stimulus** is brought about by the attractive appearance, taste, and odor of the food. If these are unattractive, or if the eater gives no consideration to the things eaten, this nervous stimulus is lost and digestion suffers. *It is not the mouth only that waters at the sight or even the thought of delicious food; the stomach also "waters."* Food must be enjoyed to be digested properly, and a good cook is one of the stomach's most valuable assistants. The **chemical stimulus** is a hormone produced at the pyloric end by the action of meat extracts on the mucous membrane. For this reason soups and meat juices form the proper beginning of a dinner. The hydrochloric acid ceases to be produced in cancer of the stomach and in certain grave anemias, particularly pernicious anemia. This absence of hydrochloric acid, as shown by analysis of the stomach contents (gastric analysis), is of great diagnostic value.

Reference has just been made to the effect of nervous stimuli on gastric secretion. Food does not need to actually enter the stomach for the gastric glands to be stimulated. The mere presence of food in the mouth is sufficient for the stomach to respond in anticipation. This was proved by the great Russian physiologist Pavlov, who divided the esophagus in the neck of a dog, brought the end above the division out through the wound, and gave the dog as much to eat as he wished. The empty stomach poured out a plentiful supply of gastric juice, even though it received no food. The profound influence which psychic stimuli and stress have on the human stomach has been demonstrated by observations on patients in whom the interior of the stomach has been exposed to inspection over a long period as the result of an accidental gunshot wound.

It must be appreciated that food in the stomach and bowel has not really entered the body and come into contact with the tissues for which it is intended. It is merely in the alimentary canal, which runs through the body from the mouth to the anus. The large molecules of proteins, carbohydrates, and fats have to be broken down by the process of digestion before the food can be absorbed. The stomach and bowel represent the kitchen in which the food is prepared for use by the tissues. Neither water nor food are actually absorbed by the stomach itself. Both are taken up by the small intestine, and water by the large intestine.

In addition to secreting the gastric juice so necessary for digestion, the gastric mucosa elaborates what is called the *intrinsic hematopoietic* (blood forming) *factor,* which prevents pernicious anemia. It does so by facilitating the absorption of vitamin B_{12} from the intestine with consequent maturation of the red blood cells. We shall return to this subject in the study of pernicious anemia.

Vomiting is the sudden ejection of the gastric contents caused by contraction of the muscular wall of the stomach. This may be brought on by the action of an acute irritant such as concentrated alcohol (cocktails) on an empty stomach. Gastric retention is frequently accompanied by vomiting. Even nervous influences such as a nauseating sight, violent emotion, or the giddiness of seasickness or airsickness may cause the stomach to contract and thus produce vomiting.

Organic disease of the stomach is commonly accompanied by "indigestion" or **dyspepsia,** a feeling of bloating, fullness, or actual pain. In many cases, however, these symptoms are caused by lesions in some other organ such as the gallbladder, duodenum, or appendix. These organs are supplied by branches of the same nerves that go to the stomach, and *the stomach is so sensitive an organ that it may cry aloud in sympathy with its suffering neighbors.* Sometimes these cries are so loud that they drown those of the organ really involved, and this sometimes makes the correct diagnosis of abdominal diseases a matter of extreme difficulty. The patient should sympathize with his doctor as well as the doctor with his patient.

The three common organic diseases of the stomach are gastritis, ulcer and cancer.

GASTRITIS. When we consider the extraordinary assortment of substances, both fluid and solid, hot and cold, sweet and sour, alcoholic and aerated, to which the gastric mucosa is exposed, it is a wonder that we do not all have inflamed stomachs. Gastritis may be acute or chronic. In chronic gastritis the signs of inflammation have faded into the past, leaving an atrophic mucosa. We shall confine our attention to the acute variety.

Acute gastritis may be caused by powerful surface irritants. The commonest of such irritants, of course, is *alcohol.* Acute gastritis must be present to some extent after every severe alcoholic bout, and this is largely responsible for the too familiar "morning after" feeling. Chemical poisons swallowed accidentally by children or with suicidal intent by adults, dietary irritants, and bacterial and viral general infections may be accompanied by acute gastritis with dyspepsia. Food poisoning involves the intestine rather than the stomach. The mucous membrane is red, swollen, and infiltrated with inflammatory cells. If the acute attacks are repeated, as in the habitual alcoholic, the lesions become those of chronic gastritis and eventually gastric atrophy.

PEPTIC ULCER.   An ulcer of the stomach is called a *peptic ulcer,* because the peptic or digestive juice plays an all-important part in its production. But a similar ulcer occurs in the part of the duodenum next to the stomach, so that *duodenal ulcer* will be considered together with gastric ulcer under the common heading of peptic ulcer.

The **cause** of peptic ulcer can be stated in part, but only in part. When for any reason a small area of gastric or duodenal mucous membrane is injured and becomes necrosed, the acid gastric juice digests the dead tissue just as it would digest any piece of dead meat. In this way a depression or hole is made which extends for a varying depth into the wall of the stomach or duodenum. The chemical conditions are the same in the first part of the duodenum as in the stomach, for the acid gastric juice is poured into that part of the bowel when the pyloric sphincter relaxes. At about three inches along the duodenum the pancreatic duct and bile duct open on the mucous membrane, and as the juices from these ducts are strongly alkaline the acidity of the gastric juice is neutralized. For this reason peptic ulcer is confined to the first part of the duodenum. The role of the gastric juice in the production of peptic ulcer is easy to understand. But we are still in the dark as to the *cause of the initial necrosis* of the mucous membrane. A bewildering variety of theories have been suggested such as blood-borne bacterial infection, hyperacidity of the gastric juice, abnormal nervous impulses passing along the vagus nerve from the hypothalamic region of the brain to the stomach (vagotomy, *i.e.,* bilateral division of the vagus nerves, may give spectacular therapeutic results), hormonal stimulation, and so on. In spite of all the theories peptic ulcer remains a mystery. The patient with peptic ulcer is usually nervous and high-strung, restless and irritable, prone to worry, and upset by strain. These characteristics are not the result of the ulcer; they are much more probably its cause and have to be considered by the physician who undertakes the treatment of a case.

The **site** of the ulcer is usually at the pyloric end of the stomach or along the upper border (lesser curvature). In treating an ordinary ulcer of the skin, treatment consists in putting the part at rest and preventing irritation of the ulcer. But in the stomach the organ is made to work every time a meal is taken, and the hydrochloric acid acts as an acute irritant so that the area of necrosis tends to become deeper. This necrotic tissue is in turn digested and in time the hole may penetrate the whole thickness of the wall so that *perforation* into the abdominal cavity occurs, a condition that will prove fatal if not treated by immediate operation.

Fortunately, however, protective forces are at work that tend to prevent this catastrophe and limit the spread of the ulcer. The continued irritation stimulates the formation of fibrous tissue in the floor of the ulcer and this offers marked resistance to its spread. *A chronic peptic ulcer is therefore a circumscribed hole, usually not more than one inch in diameter, funnel-shaped, of varying depth, with a hard fibrous base.* When the ulcer is still small healing may take place, but when it is deep this is unlikely to occur. The abundant scar tissue at the base of the ulcer may contract to such a degree that obstruction of the pylorus is produced, or if the ulcer is in the middle of the stomach the contraction may divide that organ into two compartments, a condition known as *hourglass stomach.*

Basis of Symptoms. The great symptom of peptic ulcer, whether gastric or duodenal, is **pain,** relieved by the taking of foods and alkalis. The pain may be a mild feeling of discomfort known as *dyspepsia,* or it may be extremely severe. It bears a characteristic relation to food, being relieved by the taking of food for about an hour and then coming on again. The triple rhythm of pain-food-relief shows a remarkable regularity. An alkali such as sodium bicarbonate may relieve the pain to an even greater degree. The usual explanation given for the pain and its relief by food and alkalis is that it is caused by the irritating action of the hydrochloric acid on the raw surface of the ulcer, the acid being neutralized by food and alkali. *Muscular contraction of the stomach wall may be even more important in producing pain than the action of the acid.* Inflammatory foci in the neighborhood of the ulcer cause contraction of the surrounding muscle and spasm of the pyloric sphincter. This all tends to increase the tension within the stomach and thus excite pain. Food and alkalis cause the stomach to relax for a time and thus relieve the pain. A large gastric ulcer sometimes produces no symptoms until it finally perforates, a state of affairs for which no satisfactory explanation can be offered.

Hemorrhage is a frequent symptom, varying from a slight oozing of blood to a copious flooding which may prove fatal. Severe hemorrhage is due to rupture of a large artery in the base of the ulcer. In gastric ulcer there may be vomiting of blood, the vomitus being not red but "coffee-grounds" in appearance, owing to the action of the gastric juice on the blood. Vomiting of blood is known as *hematemesis.* The patient may not vomit but may pass the blood in the stools, imparting to them a blackish color (tarry stools), a condition known as *melena.*

Perforation is a complication rather than a symptom. A hole is made right through the wall of the stomach or duodenum, through which the gastric contents pour into the abdominal cavity. The patient experiences sudden very severe pain, and soon develops a general peritonitis or inflammation of the lining of the abdominal cavity. The condition will prove fatal unless the opening in the stomach can be closed by immediate operation.

CANCER OF THE STOMACH. Cancer is much commoner in men than in women. Indeed, in men cancer of the stomach, together with bronchogenic carcinoma, is the commonest form of carcinoma, although it must be added that there has been a remarkable (and unexplained) decline in the death rate of gastric cancer in the last thirty years. The usual age period is about sixty years, but it may occur much earlier. The tumor is generally situated at the pyloric end of the stomach, but it may occur in any part of the organ. It may form a large mass projecting into the cavity of the stomach (Fig. 101), or it may merely constitute a thickening of the wall in the pyloric region (Fig. 102). Gradually, however, this thickening leads to narrowing of the opening until finally complete obstruction may be produced, causing marked dilatation of the rest of the stomach. The tumor in the stomach is best detected by means of x-ray examination.

Spread may occur by lymphatics or by the blood stream. Cancer cells are carried to the nearest abdominal lymph nodes by the lymphatics, but sometimes the lymph nodes on the left side of the neck may be

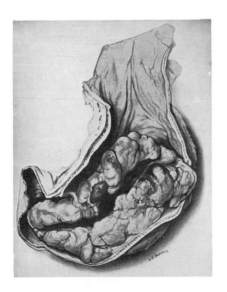

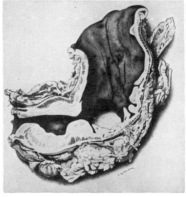

Fig. 101   Fig. 102

Fig. 101.   Cancer of the stomach, papillary form.
Fig. 102.   Cancer of stomach, infiltrating form.

enlarged by tumor growth. The cancer cells may be carried by the blood to the liver, brain, and other organs. *When distant spread has occurred and metastases are formed, no treatment is of any avail.* It is the early spread of carcinoma, often at a time when there are no warning symptoms, which makes the operative removal of the tumor often so very disappointing. In this respect the disease resembles bronchogenic carcinoma.

Basis of Symptoms. Unfortunately *pain* is not an early symptom of cancer either in the stomach or in other parts of the body, although it may be marked in the later stages, especially when pyloric obstruction has set in. *Loss of appetite* and a feeling of repletion before the meal is finished is much more characteristic, and should be regarded as a danger signal in a man in the cancer age period who has previously had a healthy appetite, one who frequently states that up to that time he has been able "to digest nails." *Absence of hydrochloric acid* in the gastric contents obtained by the stomach tube is a sign of great importance. So also is the presence of *blood*. This blood is most easily tested for by examination of the stools. It cannot be seen with the naked eye as it is too small in amount, but it is readily detected by a simple chemical test. Blood that can only be detected by such a test is known as *occult blood,* because it is hidden from the eye. *Anemia* or bloodlessness is a common symptom. This is due only in part to the loss of blood. The ulceration and infection of the tumor which occur in the later stages interfere with blood formation and thus lead to anemia. When pyloric obstruction has developed, *vomiting* from the dilated stomach may be a distressing symptom. The vomitus may be a *coffee-grounds* character owing to the presence of altered blood, as in the case of gastric ulcer. It will be noticed that nothing has been said about the presence of a lump or tumor that can be felt by the doctor. Such a lump can only be felt in the later stages, when it is too late to hope for cure of the patient.

Exfoliative cytology is the newest arrival in the diagnostic field. Gastric secretion rapidly digests any exfoliated cancer cells, and they soon become unrecognizable, so that a preliminary light diet and overnight fasting are essential. The minimum delay in examination of the aspirated material (special technician and laboratory facilities) is also of great importance. The use of an abrasive balloon, which is inflated in the stomach and deflated before removal and rubs off many tumor cells, has greatly increased the number of positive results.

GASTRIC ANALYSIS. The examination of the gastric contents gives three valuable pieces of information: (1) *The emptying time of the stomach, i.e.,* whether or not there is obstruction at the pylorus which prevents the food passing into the duodenum; (2) *the presence or ab-*

sence of hydrochloric acid (HCl), which is secreted by the normal stomach when food is taken; (3) *the presence of blood and tumor cells.* Various methods may be employed by the clinician, but the simplest is to give a standard test meal and remove the stomach contents an hour later by means of the stomach tube. Sometimes a thin tube is left in the stomach for two and a half hours, samples being withdrawn by aspiration every half-hour. If the "fasting contents" are to be examined, the stomach tube is passed first thing in the morning before the patient has taken any food.

Interpretation. In the normal stomach there should be practically no fasting contents. Any considerable *accumulation of fluid* and food particles indicates pyloric obstruction, which may be caused by cancer at the pylorus or by the fibrotic contraction that accompanies a chronic gastric ulcer. *Blood* may be seen with the naked eye diffused throughout the contents. It may be red or brown in color. The brown color is due to conversion of the hemoglobin to acid hematin by the acid in the stomach and indicates that the blood has been in the stomach for some little time. Blood in the stomach in any considerable amount is due to bleeding from a gastric ulcer or cancer. A few streaks of fresh blood are of no significance, being caused by the passage of the stomach tube. For the same reason delicate chemical tests for blood are of no value, as a trace of blood is very likely to be present.

The *free hydrochloric acid,* which should normally be present after a test meal, is absent (achlorhydria) in pernicious anemia, primary hypochromic anemia, and cancer of the stomach. In pernicious anemia the absence is complete, but in cancer of the stomach a small amount may be present. In certain normal persons the nervous excitement of the passage of the stomach tube is sufficient to suppress the secretion of hydrochloric acid. For this reason an addition to the test may be employed, usually the injection of histamine. If after this procedure no free HCl is found, a true achlorhydria is present. In ulcer there is usually an increase in the amount of HCl. This is not due to an increased secretion of acid, but to spasm of the pylorus produced by the irritation of the ulcer, thus preventing the normal regurgitation of alkaline fluid from the duodenum into the stomach which occurs normally and serves to lower the gastric acidity.

Lactic acid may be present in the stomach contents. The indicates that fermentation is going on in the stomach on account of the food being unable to escape into the duodenum. It is usually a sign of cancer obstructing the pyloric end of the stomach.

To Sum Up. Examination of the gastric contents is of value in three diseases: gastric ulcer, gastric cancer, and severe anemia of both pernicious and primary hypochromic type. *In gastric ulcer* there may be blood, an excess of hydrochloric acid, and perhaps gastric retention. *In cancer* there will be little or no hydrochloric acid; blood and cancer cells will probably be present, together with gastric retention and lactic acid if the tumor is near the pylorus. *In pernicious and primary hypochromic anemia* there will be a complete absence of hydrochloric acid even after the use of histamine, but with no blood, gastric retention, or lactic acid.

FURTHER READING

BILLINGTON, B. P.: Lancet, 1956, *2,* 859. (Gastric cancer and blood groups.)

BROWN, C. H., FISHER, F. R., and HAZARD, J. B. Gastroenterology, 1952, *22,* 103, (Malignant change in gastric ulcer.)

COOPER, W. A., and PAPANICOLAOU, G. N.: J.A.M.A., 1953, *151,* 10. (Exfoliative cytology in cancer of stomach.)

COX, A. J. JR.: Am. J. Path., 1943, *19,* 401. (The stomach in pernicious anemia.)

DORAN, F. S. A.: Lancet, 1951, *1,* 190. (Etiology of chronic gastric ulcer.)

DRAGSTEDT, L. R.: J.A.M.A., 1959, *169,* 83. (Cause of peptic ulcer.)

FOOTE, F. W., and FRAZELL, E. L.: Cancer, 1953, *6,* 1065. (Salivary gland tumors.)

ILLINGWORTH, C. F. W.: *Peptic Ulcer,* Edinburgh, 1953.

WOLF, S.: *The Stomach,* New York, 1965.

Lower Digestive Tract

STRUCTURE AND FUNCTION

The lower digestive tract consists of two divisions different in structure and function, named the small and the large intestine. The names apply to their diameter, not to their length, for the small intestine is about 20 feet long and the large intestine about 5 feet long. The *small intestine* consists of an upper short section 12 inches in length, the *duodenum,* into which open the bile duct from the gallbladder and the pancreatic duct, and a long lower section, the upper two-fifths of which are called the *jejunum* and the lower three-fifths the *ileum.* The lower end of the ileum is connected with the large intestine by the ileocecal valve, situated in the lower right part of the abdomen. Just beyond the valve the *vermiform appendix* opens into the large bowel. The *large intestine* begins as a wide pouch, the *cecum,* and continues as the *colon,* which passes up in the right flank, across the abdomen beneath the liver and stomach, and down in the left flank, to become the *sigmoid,* an S-shaped portion, finishing as the *rectum,* which is about 5 inches long and opens on the surface at the *anus.*

The **small intestine** is concerned with the digestion and absorption of the food, and its structure is designed to perform these two very different functions. The mucous membrane lining this part of the bowel contains innumerable glands in the form of simple tubes which secrete ferments that act on the food as it passes along. The *pancreas,* a flat organ that runs transversely across the abdomen behind the stomach, pours a powerful digestive juice into the duodenum at the same point at which the bile enters the bowel. By the action of these juices, not forgetting the enzymes from the stomach, the food is completely lique-fied and converted into a form that can be readily absorbed; in other words it is *digested. Absorption* is accomplished by millions of delicate finger-like projections known as *villi* (Fig. 103). Each villus contains a minute blood vessel, and the liquid food passes through the mucous membrane into these vessels, by which it is carried to the portal vein and in that vessel to the liver. The food is made to pass along the bowel by contractions of the involuntary muscle that makes up the greater part of its wall. The small intestine should be emptied in less than twelve hours.

The **large intestine** conducts the indigestible part of the food, chiefly cellulose, to the exterior, but at the same time it absorbs a large amount of water, so that the contents of the colon are converted into solid masses. The mucous membrane has no villi, but is lined by tubular glands. These do not secrete digestive juices, as digestion is completed in the small bowel, but they do produce a slimy material known as *mucus.* When the large bowel is inflamed this mucus is poured out in great quantities, just as the mucous membrane of the nose pours out mucus in the early stages of a cold, so that the presence of mucus in the stools indicates the presence of inflammation of the large bowel. The rectum is the cesspool of the body, swarming with bacteria. Their toxins are carried to the liver, where they are detoxicated. The discom-fort and headache of constipation are not due to the absorption of poi-sons from the intestinal tract, as was at one time thought, but to the mechanical effect of the overloaded bowel on the nerves of the intestine.

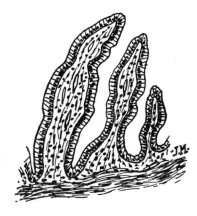

Fig. 103.   Intestinal villi.

TYPHOID FEVER

Although the striking lesions of typhoid fever are intestinal, the infection is really one of the lymphoid tissue in general, so that it has already been described in connection with bacterial infections in general (p. 158). The lesions in the bowel are most marked at the lower end of the small intestine, that is to say in the ileum. The lymphoid masses, the Peyer's patches, in the deeper part of the mucous membrane become acutely swollen, and by the end of the first week the overlying mucosa is desquamated. During the second week the lymphoid tissue undergoes necrosis and is shed off, leaving a deep ulcer (Fig. 39, p. 160). By the end of the third week the ulcers have fortunately healed over, but one of these may extend more deeply and eventually perforate, just as may happen in peptic ulcer.

DYSENTERY

Dysentery is an acute inflammation of the colon, a colitis, accompanied by very frequent diarrhea and the passage of mucus, pus, and blood in the liquid stools. There are two kinds of dysentery due to entirely different causes, although with rather similar lesions and symptoms. These are amebic dysentery, caused by *Entamoeba histolytica,* and bacillary dysentery, caused by the dysentery bacillus.

AMEBIC DYSENTERY. Amebic dysentery is caused by a unicellular organism, that is to say, a protozoon, called *Entamoeba* or *Amoeba histolytica.* The parasite is swallowed in infected (uncooked) food or water, and when it reaches the lower part of the intestine (colon) it invades the wall of the bowel, causing the acute inflammation (colitis) known as dysentery. Amebic dysentery is a disease of the tropics, but it also occurs in temperate regions.

The **chief symptom** is *profuse and painful diarrhea,* the liquid stools containing slimy *mucus, pus,* and *blood.* Large numbers of amebae leave the body in the fecal discharge.

The characteristics of the ameba, together with the mode of infection, have already been discussed in connection with the protozoon parasites (p. 166).

The **lesions** of both forms of dysentery are very similar. *Large and small ulcers* are scattered along the length of the colon, and these are responsible for the pain, the diarrhea, and the mucus, pus, and blood in the stools. In the case of amebic dysentery, the amebae may be found burrowing deeply into the wall of the bowel, and they may invade the branches of the portal vein and be carried to the *liver* where they set up amebic abscesses of that organ. In spite of modern *treatment* with chemotherapy and antibiotics it may not be possible to eradicate the infection in all cases, and some amebae may remain for a long time, even for years, protected by the bowel wall, and the patient may be subject to repeated attacks of dysentery.

BACILLARY DYSENTERY. The *Shigella group* of bacilli, which are responsible for bacillary dysentery, are intestinal parasites peculiar to man. The characteristics of these bacteria and the mode of infection have already been described (p. 163). The character of the lesions is similar to that of the lesions of amebic dysentery outlined above.

CHRONIC ULCERATIVE COLITIS

This chronic, distressing, and intractable condition, characterized by alternating periods of exacerbations and remissions, remains an unsolved problem in spite of a vast amount of investigation. It is equally common in both sexes, and usually begins between 20 and 40 years of age. The lesions, namely, extensive ulceration of the colon and rectum, and the symptoms, namely, diarrhea with mucus, pus, and blood in the stools, are those of the other forms of dysentery. But no causative agent has so far been discovered. The patient appears to be hypersensitive to certain types of food, and is usually of a high-strung, somewhat neurotic temperament. The disease may last for many years, but is marked by remissions and exacerbations. The latter often occur when the patient is subjected to strain, overwork, or worry.

In many cases there seems to be a strong psychogenic factor. The sufferer frequently presents an illusion of serenity and calm, but in reality may be hostile and anxious. It has been said that the sorrow that has no vent in tears may make other organs weep. Treatment has to be directed to the mind as well as to the colon.

The ulcers are usually confined to the colon and rectum. In fatal cases the entire large bowel may be covered with ulcers that vary in size from tiny erosions to ulcers several inches in diameter. Although the ulcers are superficial, occasionally one of them may perforate. The mucosa between the ulcers becomes heaped up into masses, and sometimes, after many years, one of these masses may become malignant.

BASIS OF SYMPTOMS. All the symptoms are caused by the ulcers. The dominant and distressing complaint is **diarrhea,** with **blood, pus, and mucus in the stools,** which vary in frequency from 4 or 5 to 30 a day. It is easy to picture what a threat to occupation and social life the higher figures must mean. *Secondary anemia* and *loss of weight* are very common. X-ray examination shows the so-called *pipestem colon,* a term indicating *loss of the normal haustra* or sacculations produced by normal bands in the normal colon. When viewed with the sigmoidoscope during an exacerbation the ulcers are seen to be scattered over a fiery red mucosa which bleeds at the slightest touch, so it is little wonder that blood in the stools is common. The really remarkable thing is that we are so ignorant as to the cause of this quite remarkable state of affairs.

REGIONAL ENTERITIS

This is a disease of the bowel as mysterious as chronic ulcerative colitis and resembling it in many ways. The distribution of the lesions, however, is quite different, as we shall see. It was first described by Crohn of New York in 1932, so that it is commonly known as *Crohn's disease*. Here again a psychogenic element is apparent. The patient is often frustrated for one reason or another, and emotional storms may precede the onset of the disease and the occurrence of relapses.

The lesions are limited to the small intestine in the great majority of cases, often to the terminal ileum, hence the name enteritis as opposed to colitis. The affected area is thick and rigid like a hose-pipe owing to a progressive fibrosis and scarring. The great thickening of the wall results in marked narrowing of the lumen and chronic obstruction, giving a characteristic *"string appearance"* of the terminal ileum in the roentgenogram. Although ulcers may be present, ulceration does not dominate the picture as it does in chronic ulcerative colitis. The bowel may become adherent to the abdominal wall, followed by slow perforation and the formation of a fistula. One of the most remarkable features is the patchiness of the lesions, areas of normal bowel referred to as "skip areas" alternating with areas of dense fibrosis, so that the term *regional* is well deserved.

BASIS OF SYMPTOMS. *The outstanding clinical features are a mass in the right iliac region, diarrhea, and fever.* The disease may begin with an attack like appendicitis, but there is often *blood in the stools* due to bleeding from the mucous membrane which is intensely congested in the early stage of the disease. The subacute and chronic forms are marked by recurring attacks of diarrhea with mucus in the stools, episodes of abdominal pain, and sometimes vomiting. A peculiarly puzzling feature of Crohn's disease is the recurring nature of the attacks, with intervals of freedom. The condition is certainly an enigma.

TUBERCULOSIS

Tuberculosis of the bowel is usually a complication of tuberculosis of the lungs due to tuberculous sputum being swallowed, but in children it may be due to the drinking of tuberculous milk.

The *lesions,* which take the form of ulcers similar to those of typhoid, first appear at the lower end of the small bowel and the beginning of the large bowel, but from there the infection spreads up and down. The affected part tends to become adherent to neighboring loops of bowel, and these adhesions may cause serious intestinal obstruction.

The *symptoms,* in addition to those of pulmonary tuberculosis, are *abdominal pain, diarrhea, and the presence of pus and blood in the stools.* The onset of intestinal tubercuosis adds considerably to the gravity of a case of pulmonary tuberculosis, but if the lung condition can be treated successfully the intestinal lesions tend to clear up.

APPENDICITIS

The *vermiform appendix* is a small tube about four inches long and as thick as the tip of the little finger, which opens out of the cecum close to the spot where the small and large intestine join. If it has a function it does not appear to be of any importance. It is liable to the same diseases as the rest of the bowel, but the one condition that is of supreme importance from the point of view of both frequency and gravity is acute inflammation.

The **causal factors** are *infection* and *obstruction,* and it is becoming more and more apparent that the latter is the dominant factor. There is a sphincter-like mechanism at the base of the appendix which makes it a potential closed loop. Obstruction may be due to the presence of a concretion at the proximal end, but probably much more frequently to contraction of the sphincter or previous fibrosis at the proximal end. The acute attack has been likened to a knock at the door saying. "Let me out." As a result of the obstruction the lumen becomes distended and the venous return interfered with, so that the wall is poorly oxygenated and invaded by bacteria. The infecting organisms appear to invade the mucosa from the lumen, the chief being streptococci and *E. coli.* In exceptional cases the infection may be by the blood stream from an acute tonsillitis or septic sore throat. It is undoubtedly a fact that appendicitis is seen more in highly developed countries and cities than in backward countries and rural districts. Acute appendicitis in children is becoming particularly frequent. Natives who live on a diet abundant in cellulose are immune to the disease, but when they adopt the diet of civilization they lose that immunity. These and many other similar facts suggest that habits of life, and in particular modes of diet such as meat-eating, are of importance in predisposing toward appendicitis.

LESIONS.   There are all grades of acute appendicitis from the most mild to the most severe, but for purposes of description we shall take the severely inflamed organ that is removed just in time to prevent it from rupturing. Such an appendix is swollen and elongated, sometimes to an extraordinary degree, bright red in color, and covered by an acute inflammatory exudate (peritonitis). The inflammation is usually most marked toward the tip of the appendix. If *gangrene* (death of the tissue) has set in, usually at the tip, the gangrenous part will be green or black. As the process goes on, the wall of the appendix becomes thinned at

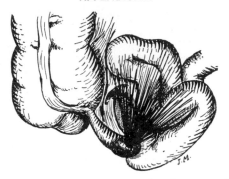

Fig. 104. Acutely inflamed ruptured appendix. Contents of the appendix are sprayed into the peritoneal cavity.

one or more points and may *rupture* (perforation), so that the intestinal contents are poured out into the abdominal cavity causing *general peritonitis* (Fig. 104). A gangrenous appendix is certain to rupture unless it is removed in time. It is hardly necessary to add that antibiotic therapy has changed, to a marked degree, the picture just painted.

The picture so far has been painted in the blackest colors—severe inflammation, gangrene, rupture, general peritonitis, death. Fortunately such a sequence is the exception, not the rule. Most attacks of appendicitis are of a mild character and the patient recovers without operation. Unfortunately no one can tell if a given case is going to result in spontaneous recovery or in gangrene. Rupture does not necessarily mean a fatal general peritonitis, for adhesions to surrounding structures tend to form before the rupture occurs, and these adhesions limit the inflammatory process so that the peritonitis remains local and an abscess is formed around the appendix. When this abscess is subsequently drained it may be found that the appendix has been completely destroyed. This localization of the inflammation and infection is an excellent example of the beneficent effect of adhesions.

BASIS OF SYMPTOMS. The principal symptoms of a severe attack of appendicitis are pain and tenderness in the region of the appendix, nausea and vomiting, fever, and leukocytosis. The *pain* is at first of a general character, a "stomach-ache," but presently it settles in the right lower segment of the abdomen. *Tenderness on pressure* over the appendix is the most important single symptom. The pain and tenderness are caused by the great inflammatory swelling of the appendix with accompanying tension and pressure on the nerve endings. The pain goes on increasing in intensity until rupture occurs, when it is suddenly, completely, and most unfortunately relieved by the sudden cessation of tension when the pus escapes. The relief is unfortunate because it may persuade the patient and the relatives and even the nurse that all is well, whereas the reverse is the case. The *nausea* and *vomiting* are reflex symptoms due to the fact that the same nerve (vagus nerve) supplies the appendix and the stomach, so that pain stimuli pass from the appendix to the brain and back again to the stomach, where they cause nausea and vomiting. The *fever* and *leukocytosis* are general symptoms due to absorption of bacterial toxins from the inflamed appendix. The leukocytosis is a very valuable means of distinguishing between the appendicitis and simple colicky pains in that part of the abdomen unaccompanied by inflammation.

PERITONITIS

The peritoneum is the exquisitely thin layer of serous membrane that lines the abdominal cavity. It consists of two layers, one covering the inner surface of the abdominal wall, the other covering the stomach, intestines, and the other viscera. Between these two layers lies the *peritoneal cavity*. Infection causing inflammation of the peritoneum generally comes from one of the hollow viscera covered by the membrane, but occasionally it is carried by the blood stream. The commonest source of the infection is an acutely inflamed appendix, but rupture of a peptic ulcer in the stomach or duodenum or of a typhoid ulcer will flood the peritoneal cavity with infected material. The common microorganisms are streptococci and *E. coli*.

Peritonitis may be local or general. *Local peritonitis* is inflammation limited to one region, *e.g.,* the appendix and pelvic organs. The inflamed membrane with its covering of fibrin readily sticks to a neighboring part similarly inflamed. These *adhesions* are at first readily broken down and the parts separated, but they are invaluable in limiting the spread of the infection. This is particularly well seen in the case of the appendix where, if adhesions are formed before rupture occurs, a localized abscess in a walled-off space is the result instead of a spreading fatal peritonitis. *General peritonitis* is the result of an infection that is not limited but spreads throughout the peritoneal cavity. The membrane covering the intestine is red and inflamed, and becomes covered with a sticky inflammatory exudate, which glues the coils of bowel together. A large amount of fluid may collect in the cavity and between the loops of bowel. This may be thick pus or thin watery fluid, depending on the organisms responsible for the infection.

The great danger of general peritonitis is *acute intestinal obstruction*. When the wall of the bowel (and the peritoneum forms the outer part of this wall) becomes inflamed, muscular movements are no longer able to pass along it, and the extremely serious condition of acute obstruction develops. It is this that will kill the patient rather than the widespread infection, for reasons to be discussed in a subsequent section. The modern treatment of general peritonitis is largely directed toward the acute obstruction that accompanies it.

INTESTINAL DIVERTICULA

Diverticula of the intestine may occur in any part of the bowel, but *the common sites are the duodenum and more particularly the sigmoid,* which intervenes between the descending colon and the rectum. It is here that they may cause trouble. The diverticulum is a protrusion or herniation of the mucosa and submucosa through the muscular coat at some point of weakness. Diverticula may be present in great numbers, a condition of *diverticulosis* (Fig. 105). The usual size is that of a large pea. In the sigmoid the contents are naturally fecal and sometimes in the form of concretions.

DIVERTICULITIS. The condition of *diverticulosis* is unattended by symptoms, and is often discovered accidentally in the course of a barium series examination by the radiologist. But if inflammation occurs in the diverticula, symptoms will be produced, just as they are in the appendix, which itself is a large diverticulum of the cecum. The inflammation may be acute or chronic. *Acute diverticulitis,* often associated with a hard

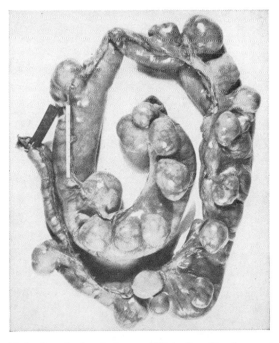

Fig. 105.   Multiple diverticula of the small intestine. Death was due to infection of one large diverticulum. (Bell, *Textbook of Pathology;* Lea & Febiger.)

concretion in the diverticulum, is similar to acute appendicitis, except that the symptoms are on the left side of the abdomen. *Chronic diverticulitis* is much commoner, the characteristic feature being the formation of a large mass of chronic inflammatory tissue on the outside of the bowel which may easily be mistaken for carcinoma in that region.

MALABSORPTION SYNDROMES

Food must be both digested and absorbed. Deficiency in absorption is known as the malabsorption syndrome, so-called because a number of disease entities may be involved. The chief of these are sprue, celiac disease in children, and Whipple's disease, conditions that it would be inappropriate to discuss in detail in this Introduction. They constitute the *primary malabsorption syndrome*. The defect seems to be in the mucosal cells of the small intestine. Biopsy of the mucosa of the jejunum shows blunting and atrophy of the intestinal villi to be a constant feature (Figs. 106 and 107).

The *chief defect is in the absorption of fat,* so that the outstanding symptom is the frequent passage of fatty stools which are unformed, bulky, pale, and greasy so that they float, and give off an unforgettable stench. The character of the stool is summed up vividly by the patient who said that his bowels only moved once a day, "but when they move it fills a bucket and drives everyone out of the house."

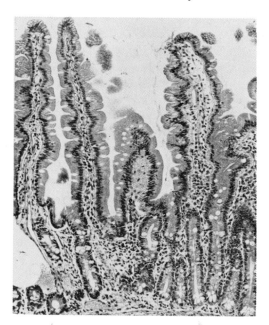

Fig. 106. Jejunal biopsy from a control subject. (Hematoxylin and eosin stain. × 125.) (Yardley, Bayless, Norton, and Hendrix, courtesy of New Eng. J. Med.)

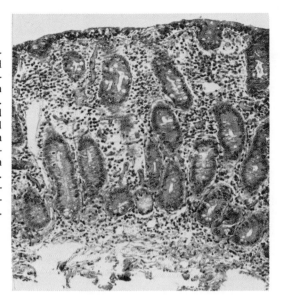

Fig. 107. Jejunum in a patient with untreated malabsorption syndrome. Hematoxylin and eosin stain. × 125. Villi are absent and there are increased chronic inflammation and a deranged surface epithelium, with sparing of the crypts. (Yardley, Bayles, Norton, and Hendrix, courtesy of New Eng. J. Med.)

In addition there may be a *secondary malabsorption syndrome,* in which the chief defect is again in the absorption of fat. This is due to absence of the necessary lipotropic enzymes caused by disease of the stomach, the hepatobiliary system, the pancreas, or the small intestine.

CARCINOMA

The only common tumor of the bowel that gives rise to symptoms is carcinoma, and this is the most important cause of chronic obstruction. It seldom occurs in the small intestine, the usual sites being the rectum and sigmoid and less commonly the rest of the large intestine, especially at the ileocecal junction. The tumor slowly surrounds the bowel and causes gradual narrowing of the lumen and *chronic intestinal obstruction* (Fig. 108). *Cancer of the rectum* remains for a long time confined to the bowel without spreading to neighboring structures or to distant organs, so that *if a reasonably early diagnosis can be made the prognosis is quite hopeful.*

SYMPTOMS. The early symptoms are unfortunately vague, *e.g.,* persistent constipation with occasional attacks of colicky pain. Gradually increasing constipation in a man past middle age who previously has been regular in his intestinal habits is a danger signal and suggests a medical examination by which the diagnosis can easily be confirmed or refuted. *Blood in the stool* is an important sign. Piles may be present owing to pressure on the veins. Alternating attacks of constipation and diarrhea may finally be replaced by complete obstruction. The only

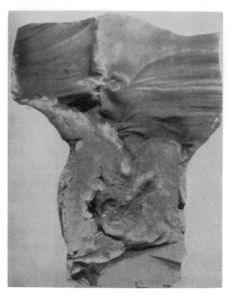

Fig. 108. Carcinoma of the large bowel. There is almost complete obstruction, and above the obstruction the bowel is greatly dilated. (Boyd's *Textbook of Pathology.*)

treatment is surgical removal, which in early cases may give excellent results.

HERNIA

A hernia or rupture is a protrusion of a loop of bowel through an opening or weak point in the abdominal wall. The common site for such a protrusion is in the groin (*inguinal* and *femoral hernia*), occasionally at the navel or umbilicus (*umbilical hernia*). Such a protrusion tends to become larger as time goes on. At first the loop can be pushed back or *reduced,* although it tends to come down again when the pressure inside the abdomen is increased by coughing, straining, or lifting a heavy weight. Eventually adhesions may form and the hernia becomes *irreducible.*

The great danger of every hernia is the possibility of **strangulation** (Fig. 109). The muscular contraction of the bowel may force so much bowel through the narrow opening that acute pressure is exerted by the sharp edges of the opening on the vessels entering the wall of the loop and supplying it with blood. The blood supply is thereby cut off and gangrene will soon develop. At the same time the increasing pressure closes the lumen of the bowel. The patient has therefore developed acute intestinal obstruction, and is in imminent danger of general peritonitis. *Strangulated hernia is therefore one of the acute abdominal catastrophes that demand immediate surgical attention.*

The sharp edges of the opening have to be divided, the injured loop

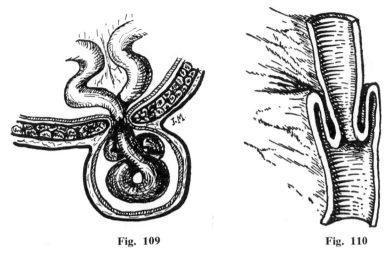

Fig. 109   Fig. 110

Fig. 109. Strangulated hernia. The constricted loop is dark and congested.
Fig. 110. Intussusception.

returned to the abdominal cavity, and the opening closed so that the hernia will not recur. If the loop of bowel is not seriously damaged no more may need to be done. If, however, gangrene has set in, the affected part has to be excised and the cut ends of the bowel sewn together. The success of the operation depends on how early the diagnosis is made and how early the treatment is carried out.

INTUSSUSCEPTION

An important cause of acute intestinal obstruction in children is intussusception. By this we mean that a segment of bowel is pushed into and ensheathed by the succeeding portion, in the same way as the finger of a glove can be pushed down into its hand (Fig. 110). The entering part of bowel is seized by the part it enters and forced along it by peristaltic movements, just as a mass of feces might be pushed along. The usual starting point is the junction of the small and large intestine at the ileocecal valve. The condition generally occurs in boys under one year of age.

The danger of the condition is *strangulation*. The sheath of bowel grips the entering part so tightly that blood cannot escape by the veins and great swelling of the part occurs. This serves to increase the tension so that the arteries are compressed, the blood supply stops, and *gangrene* sets in. Once more the patient is confronted with the double danger of acute intestinal obstruction and general peritonitis.

Immediate diagnosis and treatment are just as necessary as in the case of strangulated hernia.

SYMPTOMS. The symptoms are sudden abdominal *pain* in a child and the passage of *blood* and *mucus* in the stools. The reason for the blood is that the greatly dilated veins in the mucous membrane of the bowel give way and hemorrhage occurs into the lumen. Outpouring of mucus is the usual result of any acute irritation of the mucous membrane of the colon. Although blood and mucus appear, no fecal material is passed on account of the intestinal obstruction.

VOLVULUS

Volvulus is torsion or twisting of an organ. It is commonest in an ovarian cyst with pedicle and in the pelvic colon. It is particularly common in Russia and in the Scandinavian countries, where it constitutes 40 per cent of the cases of acute intestinal obstruction. The cause of volvulus is obscure. The actual twisting may be due to irregular spasmodic contraction of the bowel. The vessels of the mesentery are occluded by the twisting, so that there is intense congestion of the organ followed by gangrene, with acute intestinal obstruction.

· INTESTINAL OBSTRUCTION

Intestinal obstruction is a condition in which the contents of the bowel are unable to pass along its length. The obstruction may be organic or paralytic. **Organic obstruction** is due to some material obstacle, such as tumor, twist, or kink, blocking the bowel. The lumen does not need to be blocked for obstruction to be produced. Passage along the bowel is brought about by a series of waves of muscular contraction known as *peristalsis* which, as it were, milk the contents onward. A tumor or other lesion may interrupt the muscle that forms the greater part of the thickness of the bowel wall and thus stop the peristaltic wave and the onward passage of the contents just as effectively as if a plug had been inserted in the lumen. The most important causes of organic obstruction are tumors, adhesions, hernia, intussusception, and volvulus.

Paralytic obstruction, usually called *paralytic ileus* because the common site is the ileum or lower part of the small intestine, is due to inflammation of a segment of bowel as a result of which *peristaltic movements cannot pass from the segment above to the segment below,* the bowels are unable to move, and the practical result is obstruction as complete as if a string had been tied around the bowel. A common cause is the peritonitis that often complicates acute appendicitis with rupture; a loop of ileum hangs down into a pool of pus and becomes completely paralyzed.

Intestinal obstruction may be acute or chronic. The difference is fundamental, for in the acute form there is immediate danger to life and urgent need of operation, whereas in chronic obstruction there is no urgency.

ACUTE INTESTINAL OBSTRUCTION. This may be organic or paralytic in type. *Organic obstruction* may be caused by a variety of conditions, of which strangulated hernia in the adult and intussusception in the child are the most important; pressure by peritoneal adhesions and volvulus or twisting of the bowel are also important. The common cause of *paralytic obstruction* is general peritonitis, but paralysis of the bowel may result from an abdominal operation. The higher the site of the obstruction, the more dangerous is the condition.

One of the chief *dangers* in acute organic obstruction of the small bowel is that the blood supply to a segment of bowel is cut off; this segment dies and undergoes *gangrene,* and through the dead wall bacteria pour out causing general peritonitis. Or the gangrenous part may rupture, flooding the peritoneum with fecal material. From these considerations it is obvious that the patient suffering from acute intestinal obstruction is in a very serious condition and in need of immediate surgical attention. When the abdomen is opened the bowel above the obstruction is seen to be greatly distended with fluid and gas while the part below is collapsed. If the blood supply is cut off and the affected part has become gangrenous it will be greenish or black in color.

Symptoms. The symptoms of acute intestinal obstruction are very important to recognize. There is *complete constipation.* Once the lower part of the bowel has emptied itself no further fecal matter can be brought away even with the assistance of an enema. No gas (flatus) is passed. Peristaltic movements are vigorous in organic obstruction, but as the intestinal contents cannot be forced past the obstruction the peristaltic wave is reversed, moving in the opposite direction, so that *vomiting* takes the place of emptying of the bowel. First the contents of the stomach are vomited, then the bile-stained contents of the upper part of the small intestine, and finally the foul-smelling contents of the lower part of the intestine (fecal vomiting), depending on the site of the obstruction. The abdomen will become tense and distended on account of the greatly dilated condition of the intestine. *Pain* is at first sharp and spasmodic (colicky); later it becomes continuous. In organic obstruction there are early symptoms of *shock,* as the nerves to the bowel as well as the blood vessels are pinched.

CHRONIC OBSTRUCTION. Here the process is slow and there is no interference with the blood supply. *The usual causes are cancer of the bowel and pressure by peritoneal adhesions.* Although the obstruction is not complete, the bowel above the obstruction is dilated while the part below it is collapsed. *The obstruction is usually in the large intestine,* so that hard masses of feces tend to accumulate above the obstruction. These may irritate the bowel, causing mild attacks of diarrhea. For this reason alternating periods of constipation and diarrhea are very suggestive of chronic intestinal obstruction, and should always arouse a suspicion of cancer of the bowel.

Of particular concern is the question of the restoration of the fluid that the patient has lost by vomiting and by suction. This fluid contains water, protein, hydrochloric acid, sodium chloride, potassium chloride, and other substances that are of great value to the body in maintaining a balance between the fluid in cells and the circulating blood in the capillaries.

Because the patient is usually unable to retain oral fluids, his needs are supplied by the intravenous administration of blood, plasma, or water solutions containing glucose for nourishment, and sodium chloride and potassium chloride in carefully calculated amounts designed to replace what he has lost and to allow a little extra for his daily needs, but with due regard for the dangers of overloading his system with fluids.

DIARRHEA

In our survey of some of the principal diseases of the intestine diarrhea has been noted as a frequent symptom. It may therefore be worthwhile briefly to review this important symptom. Diarrhea, the passage of too frequent and too soft stools, results when the fluid contents of the small intestine are hurried so rapidly through the large intestine that there is not sufficient time for the fluid to be absorbed. It is therefore to be expected that diarrhea will be most marked in an *inflammatory disease of the large bowel* such as *dysentery*. In this condition there is also a copious outpouring of mucus from the glands lining the colon, which makes the stools still more liquid. *Inflammation of the small intestine,* especially when associated with ulcers, may also cause diarrhea.

Irritating foods tend to cause diarrhea. This may be because the food is particularly indigestible and coarse. Or the diarrhea may be caused by *food infections,* bacteria-contaminated foods that have been allowed to decompose or "go bad."

Nervous diarrhea is well known, and is due to excessive nervous stimuli causing an undue amount of peristalsis. Some persons always have a looseness of the bowels when going up for examinations and at other similar but equally inopportune moments.

FECES

In the course of digestion the food passes from the stomach into the intestines, where it meets in the duodenum two powerful digestive agents, the bile and the pancreatic juice, both of which are necessary for the proper digestion of fat. In the small intestine the food becomes completely fluid, owing to the solid masses of food being dissolved and to the presence of the digestive fluids of the bowel. It now passes slowly along the large intestine, where the greater part of the water is absorbed, so that the stools or feces that leave the body are soft, well-formed, brown, cylindrical masses. If the bowel movements are accelerated to any marked degree, there is insufficient time for the water to be absorbed, so that the stools remain fluid, a condition of diarrhea. After the protein, carbohydrate, and fat have been absorbed, there remains indigestible material, chiefly cellular from vegetable food, which acts as "roughage" and stimulates the motility of the bowel. The feces, however, are not just residues of food that have not been absorbed, but are composed in large part of material that has been excreted from the blood. For that reason the bulk of the feces is not much diminished during starvation. It is rather surprising to learn that bacteria make up nearly 10 per cent of the bulk of the feces.

Constipation is usually due to bad habits. The passage of feces into the rectum causes a desire to defecate, which should result in the complete emptying of the rectum. If this call is neglected or suppressed, the desire passes, and water is absorbed from the fecal mass which becomes hard and dry. If this state of affairs is continued for long the rectum, which is only five inches long and should normally be empty, contains feces all the time and comes to lose its sensitivity.

An examination of the feces will reveal many facts of importance with regard to the gastrointestinal canal, the process of digestion, and the many disorders that may affect it.

FORM. The normal form and consistency of the stools depends upon the extraction of water during their passage through the large intestine. If the time of this passage is shortened owing to the increased irritability of the bowel which occurs in such a condition as dysentery, water is not absorbed, and the stools are therefore fluid in character. On the other hand, the feces may remain in the large bowel for an undue length of time owing to chronic constipation. In this case the stools take the form of small, hard, round masses, known as *scybala*. When the stools are narrow and ribbon-like it is probable that there is some marked narrowing at the lower end of the large bowel, usually due to cancer of the rectum.

Mucus and pus are found in large amounts in acute dysentery and ulcerative colitis, often associated with blood. The mucus is produced by the cells lining the mucous membrane of the inflamed large bowel, just as mucus is discharged from an inflamed nose. The presence of pus is natural in an acute inflammation like dysentery. The mucus can be seen with the naked eye as slimy streaks or shreds. Pus is best detected by means of the microscope.

The intestinal parasitic worms causing disease and the entamoeba of dysentery have already been described in Chapter 11.

COLOR. The normal color varies from yellow to brown. When the stool is *large* and *pale* it contains *undigested fat,* the commonest cause of which is obstruction to the flow of bile into the duodenum either by a gallstone impacted in the bile duct or by a tumor. A chemical test for bile will give a negative result. In disease of the pancreas the stool tends to be even more voluminous and greasy, owing to complete suppression of fat digestion on account of the absence of pancreatic juice.

The stools may be colored by *blood*. This blood may be bright red, dark, or black. Red blood comes from the lower part of the intestine. Streaks of bright blood, especially at the end of defecation, are probably due to *bleeding piles*. Bright blood may come from *carcinoma of the rectum* or of another part of the large intestine. During the third and fourth weeks of *typhoid fever* the nurse must watch the stools carefully for bright blood, because a few specks or streaks may be the forerunner of a severe hemorrhage. *Acute inflammation of the colon* (colitis, dysentery) is often marked by the presence of blood in the fluid stools, associated usually with mucus and pus. Dark or black blood has been altered by digestion so that it comes from high up in the alimentary canal, usually the *stomach* or *duodenum,* the lesion being *ulcer* or *cancer*. If the bleeding from the ulcer or tumor is only slight, it will not be possible to detect the blood with the naked eye; it is hidden or occult. When these lesions are suspected, a specimen is sent to the laboratory to be tested chemically for *occult blood*. It is important that the patient be properly prepared before this examination by the omission of all red meat, meat soups, and meat extracts from his diet for at least three days. The inclusion of green vegetables in the diet does not interfere with most of the tests for occult blood. *It must be remembered that the stools may be dark and tarry in appearance for reasons other than the presence of blood, especially the medicinal use of iron or bismuth.*

FURTHER READING

BACON, H. E.: *Ulcerative Colitis*, Philadelphia, 1958.

CROHN, B. B., and YARNIS, H.: *Regional Ileitis,* 2nd ed., New York, 1958.

JACKMAN, R. J.: *Lesions of the Lower Bowel,* Springfield, Ill., 1958.

MACDOUGALL, I. P. M.: Lancet, 1964, *1,* 655. (Cancer risk of ulcerative colitis.)

SLEISENGER, M. H.: New Eng. J. Med., 1969, *281,* 1111. (Malabsorption syndrome.)

Chapter 20

Liver and Gallbladder

LIVER

STRUCTURE AND FUNCTION.   To the ancient Babylonians the liver, not the heart, was the seat of the soul, while in ancient Greece it was considered the central organ of the body. The liver, tucked under the ribs below the diaphragm on the right side of the abdomen, is the largest organ in the body. Its *weight* is 1400 to 1600 grams in the male, 1200 to 1400 grams in the female. It is singularly simple in structure, being composed of columns of cells all apparently absolutely identical, and yet it is remarkably complex in function. It will be recalled that all the blood from the stomach and intestine flows through the liver before passing into the general circulation, being brought there by the portal vein, and that the blood from the spleen also flows into the portal vein. The apparent simplicity of structure is dispelled by the use of the electron microscope, which reveals a multitude of different organelles, while histochemical technique demonstrates a wide variety of enzymes. After all, *it is not what a cell looks like but what it does that matters*. The liver has at least half-a-dozen functions. These may be divided into three main groups:

1. *Metabolism of Food.*   The foodstuffs brought to the liver from the intestine by the portal vein are altered so as to be more suitable for use by the tissue or are stored as in a bank so as to be paid out on demand. It is the proteins chiefly that undergo further preparation, and the waste product urea, which is one of the main constituents of

the urine, is formed in the liver, so that in advanced liver disease the urea in the urine is greatly diminished. The sugar brought from the bowel in the form of glucose is stored in the liver as *glycogen,* and is restored to the blood as glucose when the demand arises.

2. *Production of Bile.* The red blood corpuscles have a relatively short life, on an average about 120 days, at the end of which time they are destroyed and the red pigment or hemoglobin they contain is discharged from the body. It is first converted into a pigment, known as bilirubin, and this is excreted by the liver in the bile. Throughout the entire liver there is a vast network of fine *bile canals,* and the columns of liver cells intervene between blood capillaries on one side and bile capillaries on the other, so that the bile pigment has to traverse these cells in order to pass from the blood into the bile. The liver cells add two other substances to the bile, namely, bile salts and cholesterol, the importance of which will be mentioned presently. The bile is conducted from the liver by the *hepatic duct*, which is joined by the *cystic duct* from the *gallbladder*; the tube formed by the union to the hepatic and cystic ducts is called the *common bile duct,* which opens into the duodenum about three inches from the pylorus at the point where the duct from the pancreas also opens. The bile from the liver does not go straight into the duodenum, but passes back along the cystic duct into the gallbladder, where it is concentrated by absorption of water, stored, and sent down into the common duct and duodenum when a meal, particularly a meal rich in fat, is taken. For the bile, or rather the bile salts that it contains, is necessary for the proper digestion of fat. The bile does not act on the fat directly, but activates the ferment from the pancreas whose function it is to digest the fat. The reason for the bile and the pancreatic juice both entering the bowel at the same spot is thus apparent. It is also evident that if the bile is prevented from entering the duodenum by the presence of a gallstone in the common duct (Fig. 111), the fats of the food will not be digested, an omission that can easily be recognized by the pale fatty color of the stools.

3. *Detoxifying and Antibacterial Function.* Large numbers of bacteria pass with the foodstuffs from the intestine into the portal vein and thus reach the liver, where they are destroyed. Toxic substances that may pass from the bowel to the liver are likewise neutralized. *The male and female sex hormones are excreted into the bile and then reabsorbed.* It is evident that a breakdown of this mechanism may result in a sex hormone imbalance, a matter to which we shall have to return in the discussion of cirrhosis. When the complexity of all the functions of the liver is considered it appears rather unrealistic to expect any "liver pills" to restore to health these functions when disordered.

It is probable that the liver has a number of other functions, but as these have no direct bearing on its behavior in disease they will not

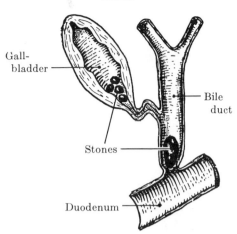

Gall-
bladder

Bile
duct

Stones

Duodenum

Fig. 111. Large stone obstructing the common bile duct; small stones in the gallbladder.

be discussed here. In actual disease of the liver it is wonderful how little the normal functions may be interfered with unless the involvement is extremely widespread. One reason for this is that the liver has great reserve power, so that only a small part of it is sufficient to do the work of the whole organ. Moreover the liver has a great capacity for regeneration; large areas may be destroyed, but new liver cells are formed that take the place of those that are lost. These facts make the diagnosis of liver disease sometimes a matter of great difficulty.

LIVER FUNCTION TESTS. When we remember the multiplicity and complexity of liver functions, it is obvious that no one test can tell us a great deal about disturbance of function. Perhaps for this reason the tests are continually changing in number and variety. In broad terms it may be said that tests for liver function fall into two main groups. (1) The *differential diagnosis of the various types of jaundice.* This matter will be referred to when we come to the subject of jaundice. (2) *The estimation of liver damage in the absence of jaundice.* For this purpose the most sensitive are the excretory tests such as serum bilirubin and the tests for bile pigments in the urine, together with *bromsulfthalein,* which is the best test for estimating the total functioning mass of hepatic tissue in the nonjaundiced patient. It has also been found, more by accident than design, that *flocculation* or *turbidity tests,* particularly *zinc sulfate* and *thymol turbidity,* which are involved with the gamma globulin of the serum, may throw valuable light on liver function.

In addition to the conventional liver tests, observations on the behavior of **liver enzymes that enter the blood** have provided information of marked value. The two most important of these enzymes in indicating some functional change in the hepatic cells are *glutamic oxaloacetic transaminase* and *alkaline phosphatase.*

HEPATITIS

In the liver the ordinary pathological processes such as inflammation, tuberculosis, syphilis, and primary carcinoma are of little significance. The term hepatitis signifies inflammation of the liver, but it is not inflammation in the usual sense of the word with the connotation of inflammatory cells pouring out of the blood vessels to form an exudate in the interstitial tissue. The reaction to irritation in the case of the liver is shown by **necrosis of the hepatic cells.** When the injury is slight and transient the dead cells are quickly removed and replaced by new liver cells, but when it is severe and prolonged there is likely to be a proliferation of fibroblasts resulting in fibrosis, which in the liver is known as *cirrhosis.* We can distinguish three main groups of hepatitis or hepatic necrosis, namely viral, toxic, and deficiency; any of these may terminate in cirrhosis.

VIRAL HEPATITIS.   This is an acute diffuse hepatic necrosis which occurs both in sporadic and epidemic form. The sporadic form is usually very mild and shows itself as a transient attack of jaundice. The epidemic form, which is much more severe, was extremely common among the troops of all armies in World War II. The virus is excreted in the stools, and this is how the infection is spread under the unsanitary conditions of wartime. There are two types of viral hepatitis caused by different although related viruses with a practically identical clinical picture. The first is known as **infectious hepatitis** (I H), the infection being of fecal origin. The second is called **serum** or **syringe hepatitis** (S H), because the virus is transmitted by the intravenous injection of human serum or by a syringe or needle that has become infected by such serum, *the common source of infection being pooled plasma or blood used for transfusion.* It will be evident that in the S H form the stools are not infective, a point of importance in the nursing care.

The **lesions** vary greatly in severity. In the exceptional fulminating case the necrotic liver is extremely soft, bright yellow in color, and may lose half of its weight in the course of a week. These are the cases, known as *acute yellow atrophy,* which end fatally. Complete recovery is the rule, but in the occasional case varying degrees of cirrhosis may develop.

The **symptoms** vary as much as the lesions. In the most severe cases (acute yellow atrophy) the onset is sudden and the course very acute, with vomiting, profound jaundice, bile in the urine, delirium, coma, and death. A low nutrition level greatly aggravates the condition, thus explaining the fact that fulminating cases are commoner in women in the late months of pregnancy when there may be a dietary deficiency due to diversion of protein to the fetus. In the more ordinary well-developed case loss of appetite or *anorexia* is the earliest symptom, and the sight and even the thought of food may be revolting. *Fever* is present in about half the cases. Then comes *jaundice* with the appearance of bile in the urine. The patient is out of the woods in two to six weeks depending on the severity of the attack, but lassitude and fatigue may persist for several months.

TOXIC HEPATITIS. Necrosis of the liver (hepatitis) may be caused by *drugs,* including tranquilizing drugs, *poisons* used for suicidal or homicidal purposes, and *chemicals* used in technical processes, particularly carbon tetrachloride. The lesions and symptoms are similar to those of viral hepatitis.

DEFICIENCY HEPATITIS. Knowledge of this form of liver disease is due to feeding experiments on laboratory animals, and relatively little is known about the condition in man, which is unfortunate. When a rat is kept for a prolonged period on a diet deficient in protein and various special food factors, the liver cells first become greatly distended with fat and then undergo necrosis, with severe cirrhosis completing the picture. In *chronic alcoholism* the diet is nearly always deficient in these protective food substances. The appetite of the chronic alcoholic is impaired by gastritis, and alcohol supplies calories that take the place of food. The liver of alcoholic cirrhosis used to be called the "gin-drinker's liver," but it depended not so much on gin *before* dinner as on gin *instead of* dinner. Dietary deficiency is responsible for the widespread prevalence of cirrhosis in the African Bantu, in whom the cirrhosis is frequently associated with carcinoma. **Kwashiorkor,** an African term meaning red boy, is a widespread nutritional disease in East and Central Africa and in the West Indies. It is prevalent in children as well as adults, and liver carcinoma is often seen in young adults. The striking lesion in the liver is an extreme degree of fatty infiltration with ensuing cirrhosis. For some reason which I do not know the hair and skin show a red pigmentation, especially in children; this is the basis of the name.

CIRRHOSIS

Cirrhosis of the liver is a progressive chronic destruction, diffuse in extent, accompanied by fibrosis. The damage may be due to viral, toxic, or deficiency hepatitis. *Nutritional deficiency, often combined with alcoholism, is the most common etiological factor,* but in many or most cases it is not possible to point with certainty to any one cause.

The *liver* comes to assume a highly characteristic appearance. Although it may be enlarged in the early stages, as the disease develops it becomes smaller and smaller. At the same time the surface becomes nodular due to extensive scarring by fibrous tissue. In this way the surface of the liver becomes covered with little knobs of tissue, so that it is sometimes called the "hob-nailed" liver (Fig. 112). The consistence of the liver becomes very firm and when it is cut with a knife it may feel almost leathery. This is due to the great increase of fibrous tissue.

SYMPTOMS. *The most important effect of cirrhosis of the liver is obstruction to the portal vein.* The pathways by which the blood passes through the liver are distorted and obliterated by the scarring and tissue destruction, so that blood is dammed back and collects in the portal vein and its branches. The portal vein collects blood from the stomach and intestines, from the peritoneum, and from the spleen. All of these organs therefore suffer in cirrhosis. The mucous membrane of the stomach is continually congested with blood so that the patient suffers from *dyspepsia*. The veins in the stomach and to an even greater extent those at the lower end of the esophagus become dilated and tortuous (*varicose veins*) to such an extent that rupture may occur. *Hemorrhage from the stomach and esophagus* is thus a common symptom, and the hemorrhage may be so profuse as to prove fatal. Back pressure in the veins of the peritoneum causes the blood plasma to pass out into the peritoneal cavity where it may accumulate in great amount, a condition known as *ascites*. This fluid causes so much distention and discomfort that it may have to be drawn off, but after each removal it tends to

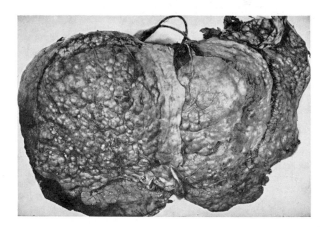

Fig. 112. Nutritional cirrhosis of the liver. The external surface has a coarsely granular hob-nail appearance.

recur. *Enlargement of the spleen* is common on account of the blood that is continually dammed back in that organ. *Jaundice* may develop in the late stages owing to interference with the excretion of bile, which accumulates in the blood and tinges the skin, the whites of the eyes, and the tissues in general a yellowish or green color. Reference has already been made to the occurrence of sex hormone disturbance in diffuse liver disease. In cirrhosis this may show itself in the male by (1) *atrophy* of the *testes,* and (2) *gynecomastia* or marked enlargement of the breasts.

JAUNDICE

Jaundice or *icterus* is a coloration of the skin and sclerotics (whites of the eye) by bile pigment in the blood. The color varies from pale yellow to deep orange, or even green. The pigment of the bile (bilirubin) is formed from broken down red blood cells by the reticuloendothelial system (*e.g.,* lymph nodes, spleen), and is excreted by the liver, passing first by the bile ducts to the gallbladder and then along the common bile duct to the duodenum.

It is evident that there are three very different ways in which bilirubin may accumulate in excess in the blood and so give rise to jaundice.

1. OBSTRUCTIVE JAUNDICE. The liver may excrete the bile normally, but it may be unable to escape into the duodenum owing to some obstruction. The two common causes of obstruction are a gallstone lodged in the common bile duct, and carcinoma of the head of the pancreas, which blocks the opening of the duct into the duodenum. Under these circumstances the bile is dammed back in the liver and is reabsorbed into the blood. Such a condition is called obstructive jaundice. The jaundice may become intense, and the urine is colored with bile. As no bile reaches the intestine the stools are extremely pale and are described as clay-colored. There is a marked tendency to hemorrhage, because absence of bile in the bowel prevents absorption of vitamin K, a substance that is necessary for the formation of prothrombin and normal clotting of the blood. This can be overcome by administering vitamin K and bile by mouth (through a duodenal tube), and when the prothrombin in the blood has returned to normal an operation for the removal of an impacted stone can be performed with safety.

2. HEPATIC JAUNDICE. If the liver is extensively diseased, as in hepatitis, it is unable to excrete the bilirubin brought to it, which therefore accumulates in the blood. The result used to be and still is called *catarrhal jaundice,* which is the commonest of the three varieties. Usually it clears up in a few days or weeks, but if the hepatitis is very severe the jaundice becomes extreme and the case may end fatally.

3. HEMOLYTIC JAUNDICE. If an excessive amount of blood is broken down, more bilirubin will be formed than can be excreted by

the liver, so that it will remain in the blood. This is seen in extensive internal hemorrhage, when the wrong type of blood has been used for transfusion (the injected red cells becoming hemolyzed), and in the disease called congenital hemolytic jaundice in which the red corpuscles are abnormally fragile and easily hemolyzed. The type of jaundice caused by abnormal breaking down of red blood corpuscles (from whatever cause) is called hemolytic jaundice. *In this group bile does not appear in the urine.*

The investigation of a case of jaundice and deciding to which group it belongs is not only of academic interest. It helps to answer the all-important question as to whether medical or surgical treatment is indicated. Laboratory tests and clinical acumen are of equal value, but it is easier for a doctor to order the laboratory tests. These may indicate whether or not the hepatic cells are sick. But to the clinician the age may give a clue; patients past 40 years of age are more likely to have obstructive jaundice due to gallstones in women or to carcinoma in men, whereas the younger they are the more chance there is of viral hepatitis. As regards occupation, bartenders are more likely to have alcoholic cirrhosis than are clergymen. And so on. The appearance of dark urine is the best criterion of the onset of jaundice, especially in colored patients. In infectious hepatitis the stools are likely to be clay-colored for about a week and then to acquire a normal color again.

TUMORS

Primary tumors of the liver, both benign and malignant, are remarkably uncommon. Secondary turmors, on the other hand, are very common, because all the blood from the gastrointestinal canal and pancreas passes through the liver via the portal vein. Primary carcinoma is as rare as secondary carcinoma is common, but to this statement there are some striking exceptions. (1) Carcinoma is not uncommon in advanced cases of cirrhosis. (2) Primary carcinoma of the liver is one of the commonest forms of cancer in certain parts of the world, more particularly among the African Bantu and in certain parts of China. For this there must be a good reason, but so far it has eluded the investigator.

GALLBLADDER

The gallbladder is a small muscular bag with a normal capacity of about three ounces, situated on the undersurface of the liver with its tip projecting beyond the free margin of that organ so that when the gallbladder is much distended it can be palpated by the physician. Bile continually flows into the gallbladder from the liver along the cystic duct, but the bile is only expelled by the gallbladder at intervals when a meal containing fat enters the duodenum. The liver produces 20 times the amount of bile that the gallbladder contains, so that a large amount of water must be absorbed from bile during its stay in the gallbladder. This is easy to understand when we examine the structure of the mucous membrane, for it is thrown into a series of exquisitely delicate folds filled with capillaries, an arrangement that greatly increases the absorbing surface. As a result of the absorption of water there is marked concentration of the bile. One of the early signs of gallbladder disease is loss of this concentrating power. The *visualization test* of gallbladder function is really a test of this power; an organic iodine compound is given which is excreted by the liver in the bile and is opaque to roentgen rays when concentrated sufficiently. This substance fills the gallbladder and is seen on x-ray examination when the gallbladder is concentrating normally. If this power is lost as the result of disease, the test substance is not concentrated sufficiently to be seen radiographically, so that the outline of the gallbladder remains invisible. The gallbladder has the same nerve supply as the stomach, so that the symptoms of gallbladder disease are usually referred to the stomach, which seems to cry aloud in sympathy.

CHOLECYSTITIS. Cholecystitis means inflammation of the gallbladder (*chole,* bile). The chief *cause* of cholecystitis appears to be obstruction to the cystic duct, which connects the gallbladder with the common bile duct. The obstruction may be due to a gallstone or to inflammation of the wall of the duct, which closes off its already narrow lumen. The process appears to be chemical rather than bacterial in origin, and is caused by the action of the bile salts on the wall of the gallbladder. The inflammation may be acute or chronic. *Acute cholecystitis* is comparatively uncommon, but *chronic cholecystitis,* often associated with gallstones, is very frequent and is commonly referred to as gallbladder disease.

GALLSTONES. Gallstones or biliary calculi (Fig. 113) are usually formed in the gallbladder itself, but may originate in the bile passages in the liver. They consist of bile pigment, cholesterol, and calcium, all of which substances are derived from the bile. The most important *cause* is infection of the gallbladder, which allows substances normally in solution in the bile to be precipitated in solid form. Pregnancy, the female sex, and obesity are accessory factors, so that those who are "fair, fat, and forty" are candidates for gallstones. In pregnancy the blood cholesterol is raised, an increased amount passes through into the bile, and the tendency to precipitation is thus increased. The number varies from one to several hundreds, and they may be large or small. It is little dogs that make the most noise, and the same is true of gallstones, for it is the little stones which are apt to pass along the cystic and common bile ducts causing the extreme pain of biliary colic. The stone may be-

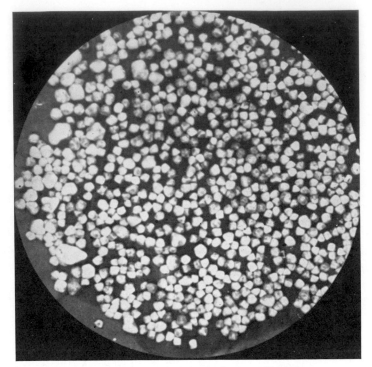

Fig. 113.   Gallstones. There were 1264 stones in the gallbladder.

come lodged or impacted at the lower end of the common bile duct, causing the bile to accumulate on the proximal side of the obstruction and producing marked distention of the common bile duct and hepatic ducts (Fig. 109). The gallbladder may also become distended, but it is probable that the chronic cholecystitis that usually accompanies the presence of gallstones has resulted in such thickening and contraction of the gallbladder that it is incapable of distention.

BASIS OF SYMPTOMS. Cholecystitis and calculi are frequently associated, so that the symptoms will be considered together. The *symptoms of chronic cholecystitis* are for the most part referable to the stomach, *i.e.,* indigestion, nausea, belching of gas, and a feeling of fullness and bloating. These symptoms are aggravated by fatty foods, (*e.g.,* fried foods). Food containing much fat causes the gallbladder to contract and empty itself, and if the wall is inflamed this may cause much discomfort. *Dyspepsia* suggesting disease of the stomach is more often due to cholecystitis than to ulcer of the stomach or duodenum. The stomach suffers because it has the same nerve supply as the gallbladder, and irritation of one branch of the nerve is reflected in the other branch, causing spasm of the pylorus with accompanying retention of food, a *feeling of bloating,* and *belching of gas.*

The *symptoms of gallstones* are in part those of the chronic cholecystitis that accompanies the condition, in part those of biliary colic, and in part those of obstruction. A gallbladder may contain numerous stones without any symptoms on the part of the patient. *Biliary colic* or gallstone colic is the result of the passage of a stone along the cystic duct. The patient is suddenly seized with pain of the most excruciating character, which starts under the ribs on the right side and passes up to the right shoulder. The pain is due to distention of the duct which is abundantly supplied with nerves. The agony endures during the slow passage of the stone along the narrow cystic duct, which to the patient seems endless, becomes eased when it enters the wider common duct, and ceases entirely when it passes into the duodenum. The patient may be mildly jaundiced after the attack. *Obstructive jaundice* occurs in those cases in which the stone becomes *impacted* at the lower end of the common bile duct and fails to pass through the narrow opening into the duodenum. It may remain in this situation for many months. The bile is prevented from passing freely into the duodenum, and accumulates in the liver and finally in the blood.

FURTHER READING

CAMERON, R., and HOU, P. C.: *Biliary Cirrhosis,* Edinburgh, 1962.

CONNOR, C. L.: Am. J. Path., 1938, *14,* 347. (Alcoholic cirrhosis.)

GALL, E. A.: Am. J. Path., 1960, *36,* 241. (Post-hepatic, post-necrotic, and nutritional cirrhosis.)

MacDONALD, R. A.: New Eng. J. Med., 1956, *255,* 1179. (Increased incidence of liver carcinoma.)

SHERLOCK, S.: *Diseases of the Liver and Biliary System,* 4th ed., London, 1968.

WAKIN, E. C.: Am. J. Med., 1954, *16,* 256. (Physiology of the liver.)

Chapter 21

Pancreas

Structure and Function
   Exocrine Function
   Endocrine Function
      Insulin
      Glucagon
   Pancreatic Function Tests

Acute Hemorrhagic Pancreatitis
Diabetes Mellitus
Tumors
   Carcinoma
   Islet Cell Tumors
Cystic Fibrosis

STRUCTURE AND FUNCTION

The pancreas, known in animals as the "sweetbread," is an elongated flat organ that crosses the left side of the abdomen behind the stomach. It is the most powerful digestive gland in the body, and has been called the salivary gland of the abdomen, because, not only does it resemble the salivary glands in structure, being composed of tubular acini, but it pours its secretion into the digestive canal by a duct. The pancreatic duct opens into the duodenum at the same point as the common bile duct enters the bowel; indeed the two ducts usually have a common opening, the importance of which fact will soon become evident. *The pancreas is a remarkable example of a double organ, for it is partly exocrine, producing three digestive enzymes, and partly endocrine, releasing two hormones into the blood.* One of the enzymes prepares carbohydrates for absorption, while the hormones regulate the metabolism of carbohydrates once absorbed. The pathology of the pancreas also assumes a double aspect.

EXOCRINE FUNCTION. The pancreatic juice produced by the acini contains the three most powerful *digestive enzymes* or ferments, one for the digestion of proteins, one for carbohydrates, and one for fats. (1) *Trypsin,* like the pepsin of gastric juice, acts on the proteins, but it carries the process a step further. (2) *Amylase* or amylopsin resembles in its action ptyalin, the enzyme for carbohydrates in the saliva, but it is much more powerful, breaking large molecules of starch into smaller molecules of maltose, which are converted into still smaller

364

molecules of glucose by a ferment in the intestinal juice. The glucose is absorbed and carried by the portal vein to the liver, where it is stored as glycogen, to be reconverted into glucose as needed. (3) *Lipase* (or steapsin) splits ingested fats into fatty acids and glycerol with the aid of bile.

ENDOCRINE FUNCTION. The endocrine part of the pancreas is not visible to the naked eye, being represented by tiny groups of cells called the *islets of Langerhans,* after the man who first described them in 1869, although never guessing their function. The islets are scattered among the acinar tissue throughout the length of the pancreas. Their cells are of two types containing granules that stain differently, so that they are known as A or alpha and B or beta cells. The alpha cells stain red and the beta cells blue. Sixty to 90 per cent of the cells are beta cells, which manufacture insulin. The alpha cells produce glucagon, the other internal secretion.

(1) *Insulin,* secreted by the beta cells, is absorbed directly into the blood that passes through the pancreas. Were it to enter the pancreatic duct it would immediately be destroyed by the pancreatic ferments. It had been known since 1889 that removal of the entire pancreas in animals was followed by a fatal diabetes, but we had to wait till 1922 for the demonstration in Toronto by Banting and his coworkers that an extract of islets would control the diabetes produced by pancreatectomy. They named the substance insulin because it came from the islets (*insula,* an island). The function of insulin is to regulate carbohydrate metabolism; when insufficient insulin is produced, diabetes develops. Insulin acts: (1) by making the storage of sugar possible, especially in the liver and muscles; (2) by enabling the tissues to burn sugar. When the blood sugar in the portal vein carrying blood from the pancreas to the liver is above normal (hyperglycemia), insulin is released into the vein.

(2) *Glucagon* is the alpha cell hormone. It may be regarded as the opposite twin of insulin, for it is released into the portal vein when the blood sugar is below normal. It brings about the breakdown of liver glycogen into glucose, so that there is a prompt rise in the sugar content of the blood leaving the liver.

PANCREATIC FUNCTION TESTS. These depend on an estimation of one or more of the three main digestive enzymes in the blood. The lipase and amylase levels in the serum give invaluable information. *Lipase estimation* occupies about 24 hours, but *serum amylase* can be measured within an hour, so that it is the method of choice in acute pancreatitis, which may constitute an acute abdominal emergency that has to be differentiated from acute appendicitis, perforated peptic ulcer, and biliary colic. These tests are of little help in chronic pancreatitis, but it is here that a high *serum trypsin* level may point to a correct diagnosis, as well as in carcinoma of the head of the pancreas, which obstructs the duct and prevents the escape of the enzyme. Tests for endocrine dysfunction will be considered in connection with diabetes.

The three most important diseases of the pancreas are acute hemorrhagic pancreatitis, diabetes mellitus, and cancer, although others will be mentioned briefly.

ACUTE HEMORRHAGIC PANCREATITIS

The pancreas produces a powerful proteolytic ferment, *trypsin,* but as long as this remains in the duct it does no harm to the pancreas itself. Should the duct become blocked, however, the dammed-up secretion may rupture the finer branches of the duct and leak into the surrounding pancreatic tissue which it will proceed to digest. If bile, particularly infected bile, should enter the pancreatic duct, it may render the trypsin sufficiently active to enable it to digest the wall of the duct and thus act on the pancreatic tissue. The fact that the pancreatic and bile ducts frequently unite before entering the duodenum facilitates the passage of bile into the duodenum, especially when the common opening is blocked by a gallstone. The pancreatic tissue is then broken down by the activated trypsin, *i.e.,* it becomes necrosed, blood vessels are destroyed, and extensive hemorrhage rapidly occurs into the pancreas. The pancreatic ferments are now free to escape into the abdominal cavity, where the fat-splitting ferment acts on the abundant yellow fat in the peritoneum and on the surface of the pancreas, producing little white patches of **fat necrosis.** When the surgeon opens the abdomen and sees these tell-tale white patches he is at once able to make a correct diagnosis even before the deepseated pancreas has been exposed.

From the above account it might be thought that the causation of acute pancreatitis presented no problem. The reverse is the case. In many instances no gallstones are present, and in such cases other factors must be involved. This *Introduction* is no place for a discussion of this contentious matter, but it may be noted that many cases are associated with acute alcoholism.

BASIS OF SYMPTOMS. *The disease is one of the acute abdominal accidents.* The terrific *pain* that is the outstanding symptom usually comes on after a heavy meal when abundant bile is pouring out of the gallbladder. The suddenness of the onset, the illimitable agony that accompanies it, and the high mortality dependent on it render it the most formidable of catastrophes. The pain, more terrible than that of perforated peptic ulcer, causes the sufferer to remain motionless, whereas in gallstone colic he changes his position every minute, seeking the relief that does not come. There is a marked condition of *shock,* and the face assumes a peculiar slate-blue color which is very characteristic.

Serum enzyme estimations are of great value, for the differential diagnosis may be very difficult and the life of the patient may depend on a correct answer. The most valuable single laboratory test is the demonstration of a *raised serum amylase,* the enzyme passing into the veins after injury to the pancreas. It is important to realize that the rise is usually transient, returning to normal in the course of two or three days.

DIABETES MELLITUS

Diabetes means a "running through"; mellitus means "sweet" (literally honeyed). Diabetes mellitus is thus a condition in which there is an excessive outpouring of urine containing sugar. The word diabetes is also used for another disease, *diabetes insipidus,* in which the amount of urine is greatly increased but contains no sugar and is therefore insipid or tasteless. The nomenclature obviously dates from the time, happily now past, when tasting the urine was a recognized part of urinalysis.

As diabetes insipidus is rare, diabetes mellitus is usually known simply as diabetes. The fact that the urine is increased and contains sugar might suggest that this was a disease of the kidneys. This is not so, for the kidneys may be perfectly normal. It is a disorder of carbohydrate metabolism as a result of which the sugar of the food is not burnt by the tissues and converted into energy. The cause of the disorder is a deficient supply of insulin, and the lesion responsible is to be sought in the islets of Langerhans in the pancreas.

It might be thought that everything is known about diabetes that can be known. As a matter of fact the reverse is the case. We do not know the essential *cause* of diabetes, *i.e.,* the factor that damages the islets of Langerhans. The lesions in the islets are the reverse of striking, and may indeed be difficult and sometimes impossible to detect. The cells of the islets are of two kinds known as alpha and beta. In diabetes there is first loss of the granules of the beta cells, and later these cells disappear. Eventually it may be difficult to find any islets.

Heredity is undoubtedly an important factor in the causation of diabetes. Certain persons are born with a diabetic tendency, a genetic defect. Such persons may develop the disease in childhood, or in later life, or not at all, depending on the severity of the effect. The last-named group serve as diabetic "carriers." The inheritance follows a recessive Mendelian pattern. It would appear, therefore, that diabetes mellitus may be regarded as fundamentally **a defect in one or more of the genes that regulate carbohydrate metabolism.** Without treatment the downhill progress is much more rapid the younger the patient is, and the untreated child will not survive for more than a year or possibly two.

We do know, however, that insulin in some way serves as a spark that enables the glucose carried to the tissue cells, particularly the muscles, to unite with the oxygen there and be burnt with the production of energy. Sugar in the form of glucose is to the body as gasoline is to the internal combustion engine. Every time the heart beats or we move a muscle we use up glucose, and just as a spark is necessary to fire the gasoline in the engine, so insulin is necessary to burn up the glucose. Insulin also enables the glucose carried from the intestine to the liver to be converted into glycogen. When insulin is lacking it is evident that glucose will neither be changed into glycogen in the liver nor be burnt up by the muscles, so that it will accumulate in the blood in large amounts. When the blood reaches the kidneys the glucose will flow out into the urine. A diagnosis of diabetes can be made by testing either the urine or the blood for sugar, remembering that some is always present in the blood. The normal blood sugar is 60 to 80 mg. per 100 ml., but in diabetes it may reach 300 mg. or higher.

There is an even greater danger than the failure to burn carbohydrates, namely, a failure to burn fats. For the proper combustion of fat a certain proportion of carbohydrates must be burnt at the same time. In the carburetor of an automobile the correct mixture must be present, else the engine will "smoke" and will miss fire. So also in the tissues if the correct fat-glucose mixture is not present it will "smoke" during combustion, the smoke representing toxic acid substances which are the result of incomplete combustion of the fat. These are known as *ketone bodies,* and the clinical condition is *acidosis* or *ketosis.* We may say, then, that *diabetes is initially a derangement of carbohydrate metabolism, but that this leads to a perverted fat metabolism which if unchecked will result in death.*

BASIS OF SYMPTOMS. The chief signs and symptoms of untreated diabetes are *polyuria* (excessive urination), *glycosuria* (sugar in the urine), *high blood sugar, excessive thirst* and *hunger,* and *marked weakness* and *loss of weight.* Another group of symptoms due to the incomplete combustion of fats are manifestations of *acidosis, e.g., air hunger, coma,* and *ketone bodies in the urine.* Still other accompaniments of the disease are *itching, boils, gallstones, arteriosclerosis,* and *gangrene of the limbs.* Nowadays as the result of insulin treatment most patients do not die of diabetes but of complications and infections.

The *glycosuria* is due to the excess sugar in the blood flowing out in the urine. As much as one pound of sugar a day may be excreted in the urine if a patient with marked diabetes eats all the sugar and starch he wants. The large amount of sugar dissolved in the urine *raises the specific gravity* or density so that it becomes 1.030 or 1.040 in place of the normal of around 1.020. The *high blood sugar* is the natural result of the sugar not being burnt up and not being converted into glycogen. Sugar acts on the kidney as a diuretic or stimulant to secretion, hence the *polyuria.* On account of the large amount of water the urine is characteristically pale in color. The tissues are dehydrated by the excessive loss of water in the urine and this causes great *thirst.* As the tissues are not able to use the sugar there is *hunger, weakness,* and *loss of weight.* The chief cause of the loss of weight, however, is the fact that the tissue protein is converted into sugar; the diabetic is unable to use the sugar in his blood, and so has to draw on his protein reserves for nourishment and fuel. *Itching* is probably due to sugar in the tissues, and the sugar is also responsible for *boils* and *carbuncles,* as it forms an excellent culture medium for bacteria. A carbuncle may be so severe as to prove fatal. **The chief danger to life is from acidosis caused by incomplete burning of the fats.** Ketone bodies appear in the blood and urine, and the presence in the urine of *diacetic acid* and *acetone* is always a danger signal. The onset of acidosis is indicated by the deep sighing respiration known as *air hunger,* and sometimes followed by drowsiness and later unconsciousness, a condition of *diabetic coma,* due to the action of the ketone bodies on the brain. For some reason that is at present unknown *the blood cholesterol is raised;* the cholesterol in the bile is accordingly increased, and this explains the frequency of *gallstones.* High blood cholesterol appears to favor the development of *atherosclerosis,* and the consequent narrowing of the vessels of the limbs together with the devitalization of the tissues by the sugar stored in them tends to result in *diabetic gangrene.*

Insulin has not only increased the span of life, especially in young children in whom there is great danger of coma, but it has added enormously to the happiness, comfort, and usefulness of the great army of diabetics, of whom there are some 3,000,000 in the United States at the present time. Indeed it might be said that if one must have a chronic disease, please let it be diabetes.

Insulin is not a cure for diabetes, but it gives the overworked islets of Langerhans a much needed rest, and as a result of that rest they may regain to some extent the power of attending to the carbohydrate needs of the body. But the essential basis of the disease has not been altered, nor is it possible to restore a perfect carbohydrate balance during every hour of the twenty-four. *The result of treatment with insulin has been a fundamental change in the clinical picture.* No longer is there a risk of death from diabetic coma, as used to be the eventual expected outcome, but the greatly prolonged span of life provides time for the development of *secondary lesions* in the *arteries,* the *kidneys,* and the *retina,* with their accompanying clinical manifestation. Thus diabetics are much more likely to develop *coronary thrombosis* than are non-diabetics. These lesions are secondary to the disturbances of carbohydrate and fat metabolism, and are particularly liable to happen when the diabetes has developed during childhood. Among the most striking of such lesions are microaneurysms of the capillaries of the retina, seen as red spots with the ophthalmoscope, giving rise to *diabetic retinopathy,* with its accompanying threat to vision. In juvenile diabetics who have had the disease for 20 years or more this condition is said to be present in over 90 per cent of cases.

TUMORS OF THE PANCREAS

CARCINOMA. Carcinoma of the pancreas, arising from the acini, usually occurs at the end that is in contact with the duodenum, the part known as the head of the pancreas. This position of the tumor is responsible for the characteristic symptoms of the disease, for it presses on and blocks both the pancreatic and common bile ducts. Owing to pressure on the pancreatic duct the pancreatic juice is prevented from entering the duodenum, so that digestion is interfered with. Like other cancers of the digestive tract, it is much commoner in men than in women. The patient therefore becomes extremely wasted, and much of the food in the stools passes out unchanged. The *stools* are *clay-colored,* owing to the presence of undigested fat. Pressure on the bile duct leads to a gradually deepening *jaundice,* for the bile is unable to escape. This jaundice is usually painless, in contrast with the pain that accompanies jaundice caused by obstruction of the duct by gallstones. This is one of the most serious forms of cancer, and the results of surgical removal are far from encouraging. Occasionally, when cancer involves the head of the pancreas and produces a complete obstruction of the bile ducts, the jaundice becomes so troublesome from itching that surgical treatment will produce relief by joining the gallbladder to the small intestine, thus by-passing the obstruction.

ISLET CELL TUMORS. These tumors form an uncommon but remarkably interesting group for, although they are benign adenomas, often not more than 1 cm. in diameter, they may result in the death of the patient unless a correct diagnosis is made. When that is done the condition can usually be cured promptly. As there are two types of islet cells, alpha and beta, so there are two varieties of adenoma.

Beta Cell Tumor. The tumor is usually a small adenoma 1 or 2 cm. in diameter, and more readily felt than seen by the surgeon at operation, being really a gigantic islet which is easily enucleated. Occasionally there is a general enlargement of the islets, and still more rarely carcinoma with metastases.

The **symptoms are those of hyperinsulinism or insulin shock,** with correspondingly low blood sugar owing to overactivity of the islet tissue in the adenoma. There may be attacks of weakness and unconsciousness when the interval after a meal is too long. In severe attacks the patient may pass into a stupor which may be followed by convulsions. The attack is at at once aborted by the administration of sugar. It will be seen that the condition is the reverse of diabetes. The occupational hazard for airplane pilots, engine and taxi drivers, window cleaners, and the like is all too obvious, and the beneficial effect of enucleation of the adenoma is almost unbelievable to the despairing patient.

Alpha Cell Tumor. In 1955 Zollinger and Ellison of Ohio State University reported two cases of a curious association of (1) *recurring peptic ulcers,* (2) *marked gastric hypersecretion and hyperacidity,* and (3) *an islet cell tumor* that did not produce insulin. This combination is now known as the *Zollinger-Ellison syndrome,* and the tumor is recognized to be an alpha cell adenoma. Severe *watery diarrhea* of long duration may also be a feature. The relation between the clinical condition and the alpha cell tumor is not at present understood. Excess of glucagon production naturally comes to mind, but without explaining anything.

CYSTIC FIBROSIS

This condition, originally called *fibrocystic disease of the pancreas,* was not known 25 years ago, yet it is now recognized to be a common cause of death in children. It is a *familial disease of young children,* the genetic defect being transmitted as an autosomal recessive gene, resembling diabetes in this respect. In a family where both parents carry the recessive gene there is a 25 per cent chance in every pregnancy that the baby will develop the disease. The condition is rare in the Negro. The result of the defect is an increased viscosity of mucous secretions involving perhaps all the mucous glands of the body, but more especially the pancreas, lungs, and liver. It is therefore more correctly also known as **mucoviscidosis.** In six or seven years after the onset of the first symptoms, 99 per cent of the children used to be dead, but modern understanding of the disease has materially improved the outlook.

In the *pancreas* the small and large ducts and also the acini are dilated and converted into small cysts filled with inspissated mucus, which prevents the digestive ferments from entering the duodenum (Fig. 114). The child therefore fails to gain in weight, although developing a remarkably healthy appetite. The normal fecal matter of the newborn consists of a mixture of mucus and bile known as *meconium.* In mucoviscidosis the intestinal mucus may be so inspissated that it forms a plug that blocks the lumen of the bowel, leading to obstruction and even rupture of the ileum, a condition known as *meconium ileus.* This is one of the causes of death. If the child survives, the distended pancreatic acini become replaced by fibrous tissue so that the term cystic fibrosis is well deserved.

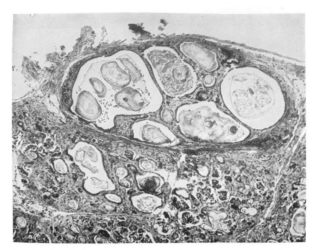

Fig. 114. Cystic fibrosis of the pancreas. (Boyd, *Textbook of Pathology;* Lea & Febiger.)

In the *lung* the mucous glands of the trachea and bronchi are filled with inspissated mucus, which blocks the air passages causing atelectasis and emphysema. A few years elapse before the development of marked pulmonary symptoms such as cough, wheezing, shortness of breath, and recurring staphylococcal infections that may readily produce a fatal bronchopneumonia.

In the *liver* evidence of obstruction of the bile ducts is still later to develop. If the patient lives long enough the final result may be cirrhosis with portal hypertension, but this is quite exceptional.

It is evident that despite its name cystic fibrosis is not fundamentally a disease of the pancreas, but one in which this organ is frequently, although not necessarily, involved. *It is pulmonary involvement that dominates the clinical picture and determines the outcome.* The deficient pancreatic enzymes can be supplied daily, although at a cost that may well be imagined. With the aid of antibiotics the threat of staphylococcal pneumonia may be held off, so that the child may have time to grow up.

A simple and very reliable clinical test depends on the fact that the *sweat glands* are involved in nearly every case. There is excessive perspiration with a corresponding loss of sodium, potassium, and chloride, so that the patients are unduly susceptible to heat exhaustion in hot weather. The test indicates the presence of excessive chloride on the skin. The *"sweat test"* has shown that adults as well as children may show the hereditary defect and may manifest mild forms of the disease.

FURTHER READING

BAGGENSTOSS, A. H.: Minn. Med., 1958, *41*, 599. (Pathogenesis of acute pancreatitis.)

BODIAN, M.: *Fibrocystic Disease of the Pancreas,* London, 1953.

HAMILTON, J. D.: Diabetes, 1953, *2*, 180. (Pathology of diabetes.)

MARBLE, A., WHITE, P., BRADLEY, R. F., and KRALL, L. P.: *Joslin's Diabetes Mellitus,* 11th ed., Philadelphia, 1971.

LEVINE, R.: Arch. Path., 1964, *78*, 405. (History of the etiology of diabetes.)

VOLK, B. W., and LAZARUS, S. S.: Am. J. Path., 1958, *34*, 121. (Diabetogenic hormones.)

WARREN, S., and LeCOMPTE, P. M.: *The Pathology of Diabetes Mellitus,* 4th ed., Philadelphia, 1967.

Genitourinary System

The genitourinary system includes the urinary system, itself composed of upper and lower tracts, and the male genital system. In this place we shall consider the urinary and genital systems separately. From the point of view of disease, by far the most important member of the urinary system is the kidney.

URINARY SYSTEM

Structure and Function

The urinary system is designed to remove waste products from the blood, particularly those containing nitrogen, *e.g.,* urea. Excretion is accomplished by means of a filtering mechanism in the *kidneys* that removes water and solid material from the blood in the form of urine, which passes from each kidney in the corresponding *ureter* to the *bladder* (Fig. 115), and thence through the *urethra* to the exterior. The urinary bladder differs from the gallbladder in that it is merely a reservoir and does not absorb or concentrate the fluid that it contains. Such absorption and concentration does, however, go on in the kidney

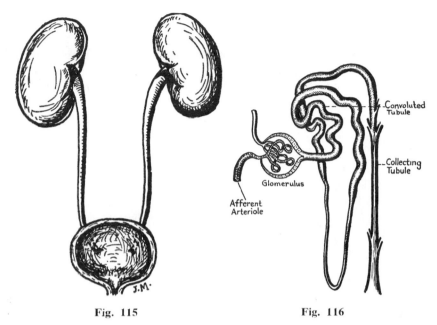

Fig. 115   Fig. 116

Fig. 115. Kidneys, ureters, bladder, and commencement of urethra.
Fig. 116. One of the kidney nephrons.

itself to a marked degree, and one of the early signs of renal disease is loss of this concentrating power.

The filtering mechanism is a very beautiful one. Each kidney, with an average weight of around 150 grams, is composed of over 1,000,000 units or *nephrons,* all of which are minute filters (Fig. 116). The nephron is a complex tube, partly coiled (convoluted tubule) and partly straight (collecting tubule), the upper end of which is formed by a spherical structure, the *glomerulus,* while the lower end opens into the chamber or *pelvis* of the kidney from which the water passes to the bladder. In the glomerulus, which is the actual filter, a small artery, the *afferent arteriole* of the glomerulus, breaks up into a little cluster of capillary loops that project like a bunch of grapes into the dilated upper end of the tubule. As the blood passes through the loops, water and solids in solution escape through the walls of the capillaries into the *convoluted tubule*, where much of the water is reabsorbed so that the urine becomes concentrated. It then passes into the *collecting tubules* and finally into the pelvis of the kidney.

The process of filtration or secretion of urine depends on the pressure under which the blood is forced through the glomerular capillaries. If the blood pressure falls markedly the secretion of urine diminishes or stops. If a large number of glomeruli are eliminated as the result of diffuse renal disease such as nephritis, the remainder have to do the extra work, and this is accomplished by means of a rise in the blood pressure, so that *high blood pressure or hypertension is one of the important signs of advanced nephritis.* There is a close reciprocal relationship between these two conditions, for not only may nephritis cause hypertension, but hypertension may cause one form of nephritis. This will be made clear a little later. Although water, urea, and salts pass from the blood through the walls of the glomerular capillaries into the tubules, the albumin and sugar of the blood plasma are not allowed to escape. The presence of albumin in the urine indicates inflammation of the glomeruli; the presence of sugar is nearly always, though not invariably, due to the raised blood sugar characteristic of diabetes.

It is evident that in the formation of the urine there are two opposite factors at work, *glomerular filtration* and *tubular reabsorption.* Were it not for the reabsorption in the tubules, the body would soon be drained of its fluid, for only one-eightieth part of the fluid that passes through the glomeruli appears as urine. The normal amount passed is about 1000 cc. a day, but this will vary with the amount of water drunk, the amount lost in perspiration or other ways.

Although we have spoken of the kidneys as excretory organs, it is now recognized that the **regulation of the acid-base balance of the body fluids and the maintenance of the normal concentrations of electrolytes** are functions of equal importance. This, as readers of Chapter 1 will recognize, represents the preservation of the internal environment (page 18). The acid-base balance is preserved by the formation of carbonic acid by the epithelium of the convoluted tubules and the reversal of the proportion of acid and alkaline phosphates with the exchange of hydrogen for sodium ions. As the result of these interchanges, the alkaline serum of the blood that is excreted by the glomeruli becomes the acid urine that enters the bladder. All this work is done by the *tubular enzymes*, one of the most important of which is *alkaline phosphatase,* readily demonstrated under the microscope in the tubular epithelium by special stains.

One of the most important features of the urine is its **specific gravity** or density, which depends on the amount of solids in solution and indicates the concentration of the urine. In health this varies between 1.015 and 1.025, the specific gravity of distilled water being taken as 1.000. The gravity is high in diabetes because the urine contains so much sugar in solution; it is low in advanced renal disease because the kidney has lost its concentrating power owing to degeneration of great numbers of the tubules. In the latter disease it is fixed as well as low, and the normal variation of about nine points in 24 hours is lost.

It is helpful to our thinking if we classify the diseases of the kidney according to the four main units of structure of which the organ is composed. These are the glomeruli (glomerulonephritis), the tubules (tubular nephrosis), the interstitial tissue (pyelonephritis), and the blood vessels (the hypertensive kidney).

Glomerulonephritis

Well over a hundred years ago Richard Bright, of Guy's Hospital, London, recognized that the combination of edema of the face and ankles with albumin in the urine was usually associated with a lesion of the kidneys which from that day to this has been known as *Bright's disease*. It is an inflammatory disease of the kidney, a nephritis, involving, as we now know, particularly the glomeruli of the renal filter and, as the filtration of the urine is dependent on blood pressure, disturbance of the blood pressure is one of the major symptoms. As a matter of fact Bright recognized the presence of hypertension in the late stages of the disease, because, although he had no blood pressure apparatus, he observed the frequent hypertrophy of the left ventricle at autopsy.

The name Bright's disease used to be confined to the condition which Bright originally described, namely glomerulonephritis, either acute or chronic. Gradually the scope of the concept became widened to include any diffuse inflammatory or degenerative process in the kidneys involving albuminuria, hypoproteinemia, and renal failure, whether or not associated with hypertension. Some writers use the term to denote the original concept, some the more modern and wider one. In order to prevent confusion I shall avoid the name as much as possible, and shall consider Bright's disease here as a clinical concept, a collection of symptoms and laboratory findings which may be due to a variety of diffuse lesions resulting in renal failure, rather than a disease entity with a uniform etiology and set of symptoms.

ETIOLOGY. Acute diffuse glomerulonephritis is an acute, nonsuppurative, proliferative inflammation *in which no bacteria can be demonstrated*. It is like acute rheumatic fever and the acute collagen diseases in this respect. The disease occurs as a sequel of acute infection with certain strains of hemolytic streptococci in the upper respiratory tract or the middle ear and following scarlet fever after an interval of two weeks or more. This latent period, together with the absence of bacteria and the peculiar proliferative rather than exudative type of lesion, strongly suggests that **sensitization of the tissue is an essential feature and that the inflammation is allergic in character owing to an antigen-antibody reaction in the glomeruli,** perhaps the most vulnerable part of the whole vascular system. The structural element of the glomerulus that is involved in the antigen-antibody reaction is the *basement mem-*

brane of the capillary loops, which forms the only continuous barrier between the vascular and urinary spaces. Not only is the basement membrane involved in this reaction; it is also involved in the all-important loss of protein from the blood into the urine.

The **lesions** vary much with the stage of the disease. Both kidneys are always affected. At first the kidneys are swollen and congested owing to the acute inflammation, but as time goes on they become small, shrunken, and present a characteristically granular surface. The kidney of chronic or advanced glomerulonephritis is therefore known as the *granular contracted kidney* (Fig. 117).

The *microscopic appearance* provides the key both to the gross change and to many of the symptoms. The brunt of the attack falls on the glomeruli, so that the condition is known as glomerulonephritis. Very large numbers of glomeruli are involved. The capillary loops are inflamed, many of them are permanently blocked, and the permeability of the remainder is so much increased that the albumin of the blood plasma is able to pass through the capillary walls into the tubules and thus appear in the urine.

As the tubule is of little use without its glomerulus, the entire nephron atrophies and finally disappears. It is on account of this wholesale destruction that the kidney diminishes so greatly in size. The remaining nephrons have to carry on as best they can, and they hypertrophy in response to the added burden, this increase in size accounting for the little granules that project on the surface between the depressed atrophic areas. Finally, the strain becomes too great and the kidneys are forced to give up their losing fight.

BASIS OF SYMPTOMS. The symptoms of glomerulonephritis are so multiform and their interpretation so difficult that large treatises have

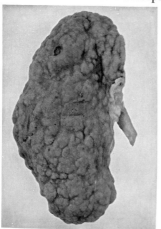

Fig. 117. Granular contracted kidney.

been written on this disease alone. In the space at our disposal we shall merely focus attention on the glomerular lesion and on the symptoms that may be attributed to it. The disease may be acute or chronic. An *acute* attack, especially that which follows scarlet fever, usually clears up completely and never progresses to the chronic stage. On the other hand, repeated attacks so mild as hardly to be noticeable by the patient may lead to the inexorable and relentless downfall of the kidney, which characterizes the chronic stage of the disease. Before this is reached the patient may or may not show symptoms of a subacute stage. The *subacute* stage is characterized by marked edema and is therefore known as *wet nephritis*. It is also called the nephrotic stage, *nephrosis* being the term that the clinician applies to a combination of massive edema and albuminuria. When the fluid collects in the abdomen it is called *ascites* (Fig. 118). In the *chronic* stage the edema disappears so that it is called *dry nephritis*. The end picture is dry nephritis with little or no albumin in the urine, a very different affair from the conception of Bright's disease as a condition marked by albuminuria and edema with which we started. Some of the principal clinical features will now be considered in brief detail.

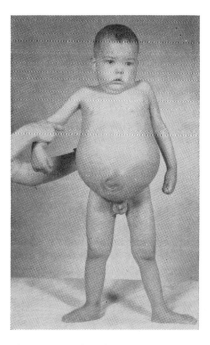

Fig. 118. Massive ascites in a child with nephrosis. (Leopold, *Principles and Methods of Physical Diagnosis;* W. B. Saunders Co.)

The main **urinary changes** are the presence of albumin, casts, and blood, and alteration in the specific gravity: (1) *Albuminuria* is due to the increased permeability of the glomerular capillaries caused by the acute inflammation. It is therefore marked in the acute stage, which is a matter of a few weeks' duration. In the subacute or nephrotic stage the damaged glomeruli still allow a certain amount of blood to pass through them, so that albumin still pours out from the blood into the urine. In the dry chronic stage the affected glomeruli have become completely closed off, no blood can traverse them, and only a trace of albumin may appear in the urine. (2) *Casts* are molds of the tubules, which may be present in the urine in large numbers (Fig. 119). They consist of coagulated albumin and blood cells. (3) *Red blood corpuscles* in the urine indicate glomerular inflammation so acute that the capillaries give way or at least allow the escape of blood cells through their walls. They are therefore characteristic of the early or acute stage and of exacerbations. (4) In the late chronic stage the *specific gravity* of the urine is *low* and *fixed, i.e.,* it does not show the normal variation of 9 to 10 points in the course of 24 hours. This is the result of loss of the concentrating power of the kidney, which in turn is due to the wholesale disappearance of the renal tubules. *Loss of concentrating power* as indicated by low fixed specific gravity is one of the most important signs of failure of renal function. This fact should emphasize to the nurse, on whom the duty of estimating the specific gravity of the urine often falls, the great necessity of accuracy in the performance of this simple test.

Edema may present in both the acute and subacute stage of nephritis, but the explanation is different in the two cases. In the *acute stage* there are streptococcal toxins circulating in the blood which act on the capillaries in general as well as on those of the kidney. There is, therefore, a widespread increase in capillary permeability with resulting general edema, especially in the face and ankles, indicated by puffiness under the eyes and swelling of the ankles. General edema is also marked in the *subacute stage* as indicated by the name *wet nephritis*. Not only are the face and legs affected, but large amounts of watery fluid may

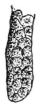 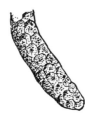

Fig. 119.   Urinary casts.

accumulate in the pleural and peritoneal cavities, so that the patient becomes in truth waterlogged. Here the explanation is quite different. The fault lies not in the walls of the vessels but in the blood itself. Two more or less equal but opposite forces are always at work in the fine capillaries: (1) *Blood pressure,* which tries to force the fluid part of the blood out through the vessel wall into the tissues. (2) The *osmotic pressure of the blood proteins,* which holds the fluid back within the vessels. The amount of blood proteins is seriously diminished by the great outpouring of albumin in the urine, which characterizes wet nephritis; the osmotic pressure falls; and edema develops. In the dry or chronic stage, as the name indicates, the edema disappears because albumin is no longer poured in large amount into the urine.

Hypertension, moderate in degree, occurs in about one-third of the acute cases. It becomes much less and sometimes disappears in the second or subacute stage. In the third or chronic stage it forms one of the dominating features, but seldom attains the extreme degree seen in essential hypertension, and usually remains under 200 mm. of mercury. The relation of the kidney to hypertension is discussed on page 385.

Blood chemistry changes indicate the gradual failure of the kidneys to function, known to the physician as *renal insufficiency.* They are of great value in the difficult task of making a prognosis, of forecasting the probable length of time that the patient has to live. Two of the important waste products that pass from the blood into the urine are *urea* and *creatinine.* These are *nonprotein nitrogenous substances,* known briefly as NPN. As the kidneys cease to function these substances accumulate in the blood in ever-increasing amount, and chemical examination of the blood shows the exact degree of retention of these nitrogenous substances. The blood nonprotein nitrogen is moderate in the acute stage, disappears in the subacute stage, and may become extreme in the third stage.

Uremia is the condition that results from renal insufficiency, and is the usual cause of death in the chronic stage of Bright's disease. It is of interest to know that it was Bright himself, well over 100 years ago, who introduced the term uremia, because he found the blood urea to be raised. Uremia is due to an accumulation of poisonous substances in the blood, although the exact nature of these poisons has not yet been determined. The blood urea and creatinine are very high, but the poisoning is not due to the presence of these nitrogenous substances. The *symptoms are mainly cerebral,* first headache, restlessness, and vomiting, then muscular twitching, convulsions, and drowsiness and finally coma and death. The patient may be *short of breath,* and the respirations develop the peculiar and ominous Cheyne-Stokes character, *i.e.,* the breathing increases in depth up to a certain point and then decreases until finally all respiration ceases for half a minute or so, when it begins again as before.

Anemia is one of the most characteristic features of the disease, and is evidenced by the increasing pallor of the patient. It is a good indication of the progress of the case. It may be due to interference with the building up of hemoglobin in the liver or to toxic arrest of the maturation of red blood cells.

It will be observed that no mention has been made of *backache* as a symptom of Bright's disease. In the acute stage, which is seldom seen, there may be some aching in the loins, but in chronic nephritis, which forms the great bulk of the cases, pain in the back is *not* a symptom. The numerous patent medicines advertised in the daily press as a sure cure for the backache which is supposed to spell Bright's disease are of no more value than a glass of water from the tap.

Tubular Nephrosis

The term nephrosis is a singularly confusing one, for it is used in two very different senses. To the clinician nephrosis, or, better, the *nephrotic syndrome,* means a *combination of albuminuria and massive edema.* It is characteristic of the second or subacute stage of glomerulonephritis. To the pathologist, on the other hand, it connotes a *tubular degeneration.* We have already seen that one of the most important functions of the kidney is to maintain a normal and constant internal environment. In performing this function selective absorption by the tubules is as essential as excretion by the glomeruli. Damage to the tubules must interfere with this function, but the most striking result is *oliguria,* a great diminution in the amount of urine passed, or *anuria,* which means complete suppression. This may be brought about as the result of two very different causes: (1) a large and important group known as *anoxic tubular necrosis* due to ischemia or loss of blood supply to the tubules; (2) *toxic tubular necrosis* due to the action of external poisons on the tubules.

ANOXIC NECROSIS. Tubular damage due to loss of oxygen supply may be caused by a bewildering variety of extrarenal conditions. Examples of such conditions are shock, burns, trauma, severe hemorrhage, intestinal obstruction, and incompatible blood transfusion. Traumatic tubular necrosis is the commonest cause of acute oliguric renal failure.

The *clinical picture* is characteristic and alarming. The primary injury is followed by a brief initial period during which all seems to be well. There is then a rapid decrease in the excretion of urine, leading to *extreme oliguria* or even complete *anuria.* The kidneys have gone on strike. Within a week the full-fledged picture of *uremia* is evident, usually terminating in death. Loss of function of the proximal tubules is indicated by inability to concentrate urea and creatinine. *Electrolyte imbalance* is also constantly associated with acute tubular degeneration. This upset may be reversible or irreversible. A *rise in serum potassium* is of particular significance, because it may poison the myocardium and be responsible for death.

The essential *lesion* is necrosis of the convoluted tubules. It used to be thought that the chief damage was to the lower or distal part of the tubule, so that the label *lower nephron necrosis* was attached to the condition. It is now realized that the proximal convoluted tubules suffer to an equal or greater degree. Disruption and rupture of the necrotic tubules may be associated with hemorrhage from the surrounding vessels, so that blood appears in the urine, a condition of *hematuria*. *Casts* are a prominent feature in the tubules, and these become colored by the blood pigment. In contrast to the devastation of the tubules, the glomeruli appear normal.

TOXIC NECROSIS. Here the problem is much simpler. An exogenous poison such as mercuric chloride, often used in attempted suicide, is excreted by the kidney, concentrated in the tubules owing to reabsorption of water, and causes massive necrosis, most marked in the proximal convoluted tubules. Anuria rapidly develops, the non-protein nitrogen in the blood rises, and death may occur from uremia.

Pyelonephritis

The word pyelonephritis means inflammation of the kidney and the renal pelvis, the emphasis on the pelvis indicating that the infection is often an ascending one. The inflammation is quite different from that of glomerulonephritis, for it is primarily an inflammation of the interstitial tissue rather than the parenchyma (glomeruli and tubules) of the kidney; it is patchy in distribution and is often suppurative in character.

It is therefore caused by pyogenic bacteria, particularly *E. coli* streptococci, and staphylococci. The colon bacilli ascend from the bladder in inflammatory conditions of the bladder, which are especially apt to occur in women and children. In men it is a common complication of enlarged prostate. The infecting organisms may also reach the kidney by the blood stream.

The kidneys are seldom equally affected, and often only one is involved. Numerous small abscesses are scattered throughout the kidney (Fig. 120). These abscesses may open into the renal pelvis, so that one of the most characteristic symptoms is the presence of a large amount of pus in the urine, a condition called *pyuria*. The progress of the disease varies, and it may end in two very different ways:

1. The suppuration may extend; more and more renal tissue is de-

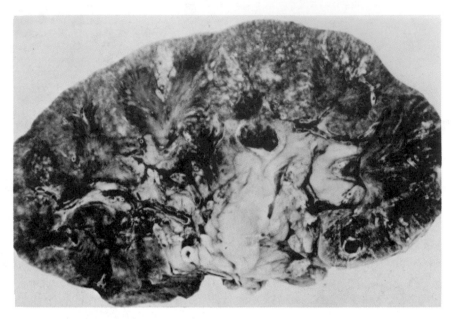

Fig. 120. Acute pyelonephritis. (Boyd's *Textbook of Pathology*.)

stroyed; and the small abscesses fuse and form large ones which communicate with the renal pelvis. The clinical picture is one of septic infection, and if the patient lives long enough one or both kidneys may become converted into *large bags of pus*. As so much kidney tissue is destroyed the patient will show symptoms of renal failure and will die of uremia, if he has not already died of septic infection.

2. In another group of cases the inflammatory process is much less violent, and in many of the inflamed areas healing occurs followed by scar formation. The infection continues in other areas, until these also become scarred. In this way the kidney is gradually destroyed, but it is now a *mass of scar tissue* instead of a bag of pus. The scar tissue contracts, so that the kidney becomes shrunken in size with a granular surface. In other words, it presents a picture of *granular contracted kidney* very similar to that of chronic glomerulonephritis. If both kidneys are involved the patient shows evidence of *renal failure* and dies of *uremia*.

Hypertension may develop in the chronic stage of pyelonephritis. Even though only one kidney is involved there may still be hypertension. This suggested the possibility of curing the hypertension by removing the diseased kidney. This has been done on a number of occasions, but the results have been disappointing. Although there is temporary benefit, sooner or later, and usually sooner, there is a return of the hypertension. There is also the danger that the remaining kidney may be affected, and then the last state of the patient will be worse than the first.

Pyelonephritis is the commonest form of renal disease, but it usually passes unrecognized. Less than one in five cases are diagnosed correctly before death. One of the reasons for this is that the disease is one of the great imitators, and it may manifest itself in different ways. It is the most frequent cause of death from uremia. A long history of renal disease should at once suggest the possibility of chronic pyelonephritis. *Microscopic examination of the urine is all-important.* In the acute stage it is loaded with pus cells, so that the diagnosis is easy. In the chronic stage there may be only an occasional pus cell, and the bacteriological examination becomes particularly important. True bacterial infection must not be confused with contamination due to the use of a catheter for obtaining a specimen of urine. The distal one or two centimeters of the urethra, both male and female, contain numbers of bacteria, so that the tip of the catheter inevitably becomes infected, and the bacteria thus collected grow readily in the urine. It is far better to use a midstream specimen, rejecting the first and the last parts. This is followed by high dilution with sterile saline, prompt inoculation of culture plates, and counting the resulting colonies. Significant bacteriuria is present when there are 100,000 bacteria or more per milliliter of urine.

Kidney and Hypertension

The general subject of arterial hypertension has been discussed in a previous chapter.

Hypertension is one of the important manifestations of the later stages of Bright's disease, for it rather than the disease in the kidneys may be the cause of death. High blood pressure may be the result of glomerulonephritis or pyelonephritis; this form is called *secondary* hypertension. Or it may have no apparent cause, and is then called *primary* or *essential* hypertension. This is the form that is associated with the hypertensive contracted kidney; the hypertension appears to be the cause of the renal condition, but this is not certain, and the reverse may prove to be the case. Experimental work on animals has shown that when the blood supply to the kidneys is gradually reduced (ischemia) by narrowing the renal arteries, hypertension results. It is evident, therefore, that the kidney is able under certain conditions to produce a substance, which has been named *renin*, that has the power of raising the blood pressure permanently. This is probably the mechanism of the hypertension of glomerulonephritis and pyelonephritis. It

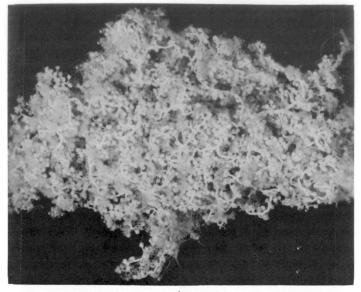

A

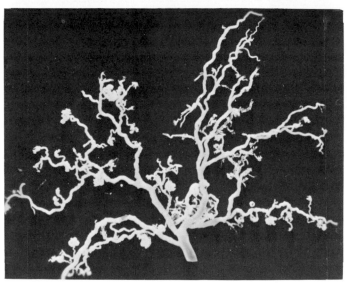

B

Fig. 121. *A*, Neoprene cast of kidney of a man 20 years of age with normal blood pressure. The blood flows through a jungle of normal arterioles and glomeruli. *B*, Neoprene cast of kidney of a man 52 years of age, with marked hypertension and a heart of 450 grams. Very few arterioles remain and still fewer glomeruli.

is not yet certain whether essential hypertension is also renal in origin. The high blood pressure is dangerous to the patient in two ways. (1) It may throw such a strain on the heart that the patient dies of heart failure rather than renal failure. (2) A blood vessel may burst in the brain as a result of the high pressure causing death from cerebral hemorrhage.

The *hypertensive kidney, i.e.,* the condition of the kidney that may develop in the course of arterial hypertension, is so similar in appearance to the kidney in the end stage of glomerulonephritis that it may be impossible to distinguish between the two at postmortem examination. The reason for this is that essential hypertension is accompanied by a great thickening of the walls of the small arteries with narrowing of the lumen, so that so little blood can reach the glomeruli through the afferent arterioles that they become ischemic and collapse (Fig. 121, A and B). The entire nephron atrophies, and as this is taking place everywhere throughout the kidney, the result is a granular contracted kidney. Various names are given to the kidney of hypertension, such as the *arteriolosclerotic kidney* (because the change in the blood vessels is a form of arteriosclerosis) and *nephrosclerosis* (because the kidney becomes scarred or sclerotic).

Renal Transplantation

There is no organ (except the heart) in which greater interest has been aroused in relation to transplantation than the kidney. This is particularly true with regard to bilateral renal disease. The kidney is an ideal organ to transplant, because it is paired; its function can be easily assessed, and its vascular supply is uncomplicated. Unfortunately the host may not approve of the graft on genetic grounds. Identical twins are ideal for transplantation, but most patients with renal failure are not fortunate enough to have an identical twin. In such cases the clinician turns to immunosuppressive drugs to combat rejection.

Tuberculosis

Tuberculosis of the kidney is always secondary to tuberculosis elsewhere, usually the lung or the pulmonary lymph nodes. The primary focus may be small and quiet, giving rise to no symptoms. The tubercle bacilli are carried by the blood to the kidney, where they are arrested. At first and often for a long time only one kidney is involved. The lesions are similar to those of tuberculosis of the lung, *i.e.,* gradual breaking down of tissue, discharge of the debris into the ureter, and formation of a series of cavities, which finally coalesce and destroy the kidney (Fig. 122).

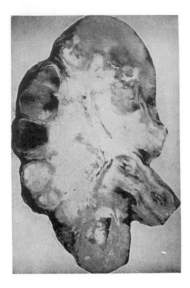

Fig. 122. Tuberculous kidney, showing cavity formation.

The **spread** of the disease is of great importance. The infection involves the ureter, producing thickening of the wall and narrowing of the lumen which may be so great that the lumen becomes completely blocked and the kidney is cut off from the bladder. The bacilli are carried by the urine down into the bladder, so that tuberculous ulcers are formed in that organ. The infection in the male may spread to the prostate gland situated in the floor of the bladder. Finally, the other kidney may be involved either by upward spread from the bladder or from the original source in the lung.

BASIS OF SYMPTOMS.　It is a curious fact that the early symptoms of tuberculosis of the kidney are referable not to that organ but to the bladder. These symptoms are *painful* and *frequent urination,* and are explained by the tuberculous lesions in the bladder. The ulcers can be seen by means of a cystoscope passed into the bladder. In this way an early diagnosis can be made of which kidney is affected, because the urine from each ureter can be collected separately by means of the cystoscope. **The urine contains pus, blood, and tubercle bacilli.** The *pus* and *blood* come from the breaking-down area in the kidney. In exceptional cases they may disappear after a time; this is due to the ureter's becoming so completely blocked that the only urine that enters the bladder is from the sound kidney. The *tubercle bacilli* may be so scanty that they cannot be detected by the microscope. In such a case the urine is cultured or injected into a guinea pig; if bacilli are present the animal will develop tuberculosis in the course of a few weeks. When the other kidney becomes seriously involved, symptoms of renal insufficiency will

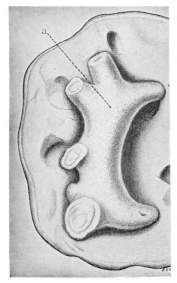 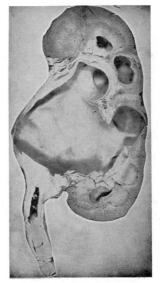

Fig. 123   Fig. 124

Fig. 123. Stone in the kidney (*a*).
Fig. 124. Hydronephrosis showing stone at upper end of ureter.

begin to make their appearance, and the development of uremia will finally bring down the curtain.

Urinary Calculus

A urinary calculus is a stone that forms in the urinary tract. The common site of formation of the stone is the kidney, but it may form in the bladder. Stone in the kidney originates in the renal pelvis (Fig. 123), the chamber into which the urine is poured and from which the ureter collects it and conducts it to the bladder. Stone in the bladder may begin in the bladder, but more frequently it starts as a kidney stone and passes down into the bladder where it continues to grow.

The **causes** of stone can be guessed at, but not with certainty. *Infection* is an important factor, probably the most important in the case of stone in the bladder. In the kidney in addition to infection a *high concentration of crystalline salts* in the urine probably plays a part, for a urinary stone is composed of such inorganic materials as uric acid, oxalates, and calcium phosphate. Some stones consist entirely of one or another of these materials, but usually there is a mixture of two or more. *Diet* may be a factor in some cases, for stone is very common in some parts of India where a large proportion of the population lives on a vitamin-poor diet. Vitamin A is perhaps the most important of the vitamins in this respect. A small *tumor of the parathyroid glands* may be the cause of stone formation. These glands, which are four in number and lie in contact with the thyroid gland in the neck, are important regulators of calcium metabolism. When they become overactive, owing to the development of an innocent tumor, too much calcium phosphate is removed from the bones, carried by the blood to the kidneys, and deposited there.

The **effect on the kidney** is partly due to pressure, partly to blockage of the ureter. Pressure on the kidney due to a stone in the renal pelvis causes gradual destruction of that organ. Infection is always superadded and intensifies the destruction. The stone tends to block the upper opening of the ureter. Sometimes it passes down the ureter and blocks the lower end. In either case the urine accumulates behind the obstruction and produces great dilatation of the renal pelvis, a condition known as *hydronephrosis* (Fig. 124).

It is obvious that hydronephrosis may be due to *causes of obstruction other* than calculus. Among such causes may be mentioned *inflammatory stricture,* particularly of the urethra, *tumor of the bladder,* and *hypertrophy of the prostate.*

If severe infection with pyogenic organisms occurs, the fluid in the dilated pelvis will be pus instead of watery urine, and the condition is then called *pyonephrosis.* Pyonephrosis may also occur without the presence of a stone. The gradual accumulation of pus or watery urine leads to pressure on and destruction of the kidney. In time the kidney will cease to function and becomes useless to the patient. The *effect on the bladder* is similar. The combined irritation of a *stone in the bladder* and the infection that accompanies it causes inflammation of the bladder wall or *cystitis.* In addition the stone blocks the exit from the bladder (the urethra), and leads to dilatation not only of the bladder but also of both ureters and the pelvis of both kidneys, a condition of double hydronephrosis. This is much more dangerous than stone in the kidney, because the patient is threatened by renal failure owing to involvement of *both kidneys.*

BASIS OF SYMPTOMS. The symptoms of urinary calculus are pain, the passage of pus and blood in the urine, and evidence of renal failure. The *pain* will be felt in the region of the kidney when the stone is in the renal pelvis. When it is in the bladder the chief pain is felt on urination owing to contraction of the bladder on the stone. If the stone in the kidney is small it may pass down the ureter causing *renal colic.* This is an agonizing pain felt along the line of the ureter, similar in nature and cause to the extreme pain of biliary colic. The *pus* and *blood* in the urine are due to the irritation of the stone in the kidney and bladder, and the inflammation that results from that irritation. *Renal failure* may develop if there is a stone in both kidneys or if the outlet from the bladder is obstructed. It is due to extensive destruction of renal tissue, which may be caused as much by the accompanying inflammation as by the back-pressure of the accumulating urine.

Tumors of the Urinary Tract

HYPERNEPHROMA.   The only relatively common tumor of the kidney is hypernephroma. It derives its name from an old and mistaken idea that the tumor originated from an adrenal "rest" or fragment of embryonic adrenal retained within the kidney, hypernephros (above the kidney) being a former name for the adrenal. It is now known to be a *renal carcinoma*, which gradually destroys the kidney and causes great enlargement of the organ (Fig. 125). The tumor invades the blood vessels, so that secondary tumors are formed in the lungs, bones, and other organs. Sometimes the first indication of the presence of a hypernephroma is the occurrence of a fracture due to weakening of the bone caused by the metastasis.

The *chief symptom* of hypernephroma is *blood in the urine*. In the early and sometimes in the late stages there is no pain in the region of the kidney. The presence of blood in the urine should always send the patient to his doctor.

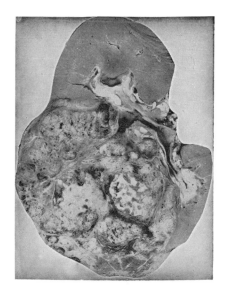

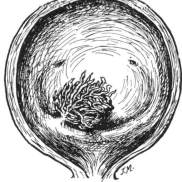

Fig. 125   Fig. 126

Fig. 125. Hypernephroma.
Fig. 126. Carcinoma of bladder, villous type.

Long-continued *fever* is a remarkable feature in some cases; it is probably a protein fever due to breaking down of tumor tissue, and is not related to infection. Removal of the kidney containing the tumor is often successful, provided that secondary growths have not occurred.

WILMS' TUMOR.   This neoplasm, first described by Wilms and also called *embryoma, is the commonest abdominal malignant tumor of early childhood.* It usually occurs during the first three years of life, and may attain an enormous size, nearly filling the child's abdomen. It is a developmental tumor; hence the name embryoma. *The diagnosis cannot be made until a tumor appears, for there is no hematuria and no pain.* Distant metastases by the blood stream are fortunately uncommon. Fever occurs in 50 per cent of the cases.

CARCINOMA OF THE BLADDER.   Carcinoma is the chief tumor of the bladder and is often of a low grade of malignancy, but it may be highly malignant. The tumor usually projects into the bladder in a papillary form. Sometimes it assumes a villous type, the growth consisting of delicate fern-like processes which unfold like a piece of seaweed when the bladder is filled with water and viewed with the cystoscope (Fig. 126). Each of these processes contains a thin-walled blood vessel, which is readily injured when the bladder contracts during urination, so that hemorrhage is common. The outstanding symptom is therefore *blood in the urine* usually unaccompanied by pain (*painless hematuria*).

ETIOLOGY.   A number of factors are known to be carcinogenic for the bladder. Workers in aniline dye factories are liable to develop the disease, the factor gaining entrance to the lung via inhaled air, and being then carried to the bladder by the blood. The sharp-pointed ova of Schistosoma hematobium or bilharzia (p. 208) can stimulate the development of cancer of the bladder, that condition having its highest incidence in Egypt, where bilharzia infection is prevalent. The latest discovery is that cigarette smoking (in excess) is associated with the disease, the carcinogenic metabolites being excreted in the urine.

TREATMENT.   The treatment consists in opening the bladder and treating the tumor either by radium or by surgical removal. If an early diagnosis is made with the aid of the cystoscope, an instrument passed into the bladder by means of which a view of the interior can be obtained, the prognosis is good in many cases.

Congenital Cystic Kidney

This condition, known also as *polycystic kidney,* is a congenital defect of the kidney, an error in development. About 30 per cent of cases occur in infants, the majority stillborn. The remaining cases present symptoms in early adult and middle life. The condition is nearly always *bilateral.* The kidneys are converted into a series of cysts, and may be

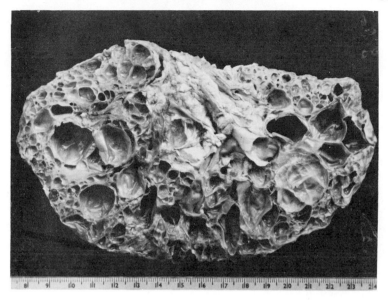

Fig. 127. Polycystic kidney. The kidney is large and converted into a series of cysts. (Kindness of Dr. N. K. Patoria, Nagpur, India.)

enormously enlarged (Fig. 127). The contents of the cysts are watery, but hemorrhage may occur from intervening vessels, so that, should the cyst rupture into the renal pelvis, there will be hematuria. Hardly any renal tissue may be left, so that the occurrence of *hypertension, renal insufficiency,* and *uremia* is easily understood. There is a strong hereditary tendency. Small *cysts in other organs,* more particularly the liver and pancreas, are an indication of a general disturbance in development.

Examination of the Urine

Examination of the urine or urinalysis serves to show the presence of disease in the kidneys and bladder. It will also indicate the presence of diabetes, although this disease is not connected in any way with disorder of renal function. In a complete urinalysis the following points are noted: color, reaction, specific gravity, a chemical examination for albumin and sugar, and a microscopic examination for blood, pus, and casts.

COLOR. The normal color of the urine is yellow or amber. The intensity of the color depends on the amount of water the urine contains. If the patient is drinking a large amount of water, the urine is dilute and pale. On the other hand if much water is lost by perspiration in hot weather or as the result of fever, the urine becomes highly colored.

In diabetes there is a marked increase in the output of water, so that the urine is correspondingly pale. The same is true of chronic nephritis, where the kidneys lose their normal power of concentrating the urine. A smoky red or brown color is usually due to the presence of large amounts of blood.

REACTION.   Although the blood is alkaline in reaction, the normal reaction of the urine is acid. In infections of the bladder the reaction tends to be alkaline owing to the action of bacteria. It is important for the nurse to remember that if the specimen of urine is forgotten and allowed to stand for many hours in a warm room, the normal acid reaction may be changed to alkaline owing to the action of contaminating bacteria. *The urine should therefore be fresh and sent at once to the laboratory.* Decomposing urine has a characteristic ammoniacal smell (to be noticed in some urinals) owing to the production of ammonia from the urea in the urine.

SPECIFIC GRAVITY.   The specific gravity or concentration of the urine depends on the amount of solids (waste products of the tissues) held in solution. When the urine is secreted by the glomeruli it is of low concentration, but during its passage along the convoluted tubules a large amount of water is absorbed; this normal process is known as *the concentrating power of the kidney.* Extensive kidney disease, particularly chronic nephritis, results in destruction of large numbers of the renal tubules, with corresponding interference with the concentrating power. This loss of the normal concentrating power of the kidneys is one of the most valuable pieces of evidence of the presence of chronic diffuse renal disease. For this reason the estimation of the specific gravity of the urine is a procedure of the greatest importance.

The specfic gravity of pure water is 1.000. The specific gravity of normal urine varies from 1.010 to 1.025, but it may be even higher as the result of loss of water through profuse perspiration, diarrhea, or other means. In health there should be a variation of at least 10 points in the course of 24 hours, the first specimen in the morning being always the most concentrated. A low *fixed* specific gravity indicates chronic nephritis. A high gravity (1.030 to 1.040) suggests the presence of sugar, *i.e.,* diabetes.

ALBUMIN.   When albumin is present in the urine (albuminuria) it comes from the blood, and is an indication of inflammation in the urinary tract as a result of which the permeability of the blood vessels is increased.

SUGAR.   In nearly all cases the presence of sugar in the urine (glycosuria) indicates diabetes mellitus. The rare exceptions need not be discussed here. The kidneys are perfectly normal, but the blood sugar is so high that some of it leaks out into the urine. As the sugar is dissolved in the urine, the specific gravity is considerably above normal, *i.e.,* 1.040 or higher.

DIACETIC ACID AND ACETONE. In the discussion of diabetes reference was made to the presence in the urine of diacetic acid and acetone, known as ketone bodies and indicative of acidosis, that grave complication of diabetes. When sugar is found in the urine it is therefore essential to test for the presence of ketone bodies.

BLOOD. If there is much blood in the urine it imparts to it a dark brown or smoky character. If the quantity is small there may be no naked eye change and microscopic examination of a centrifuged specimen for red cells is necessary. Blood in the urine (*hematuria*) with rare exceptions indicates disease of the kidney, ureter, or bladder. The disease may be inflammation (acute or chronic nephritis), tuberculosis, stone, or tumor. *Painless hematuria* without any other symptoms suggests a malignant tumor of the kidney or bladder. When associated with pain it suggests a stone in the kidney or bladder, or tuberculosis of these organs.

PUS. Pus in the urine (*pyuria*) gives a cloudy or turbid appearance. Microscopically large numbers of pus cells (polymorphonuclear leukocytes) are readily recognized. Pus in the urine may be caused by suppuration in the kidney, inflammation of the bladder (cystitis), and tuberculosis or stone in the kidney or bladder. In the male, pus may come from the urethra, and in the female from the vagina. If pus is found in female urine, a second specimen should be obtained from the bladder by means of a catheter.

When tuberculosis of the kidney is suspected a search must be made for *tubercle bacilli.* These may be found in the centrifuged deposit. If not, a guinea pig may be inoculated with a small quantity of urine or a culture made on special media. In both cases, unfortunately, several weeks may elapse before a definite result can be obtained.

CASTS. A urinary cast is a cast or mold of the renal tubules formed by a collection of precipitated albumin. Red and white blood cells and epithelial cells from the lining of the kidney are often incorporated with the cast. Casts, which are oblong in shape, tend to disappear when the urine has been kept for some time; the specimen should therefore be fresh. The importance of casts is that they form an important feature of the urinary findings in the various forms of nephritis. A few casts, spoken of in the report as "an occasional cast," may however be present in the absence of definite disease. When the urine is found to contain albumin it must always be examined for casts.

Crystals of various kinds are often found in the urine, but as they are of no special pathological significance they will not be described here.

MALE GENITAL TRACT

Prostate

HYPERTROPHY OF THE PROSTATE.   The prostate is a gland about
the size of a horse chestnut situated at the neck of the bladder in the
male and surrounding the urethra. It really belongs to the male reproductive system, but when diseased it produces symptoms associated with
the urinary system on account of its position at the outlet of the bladder.
Enlargement of the prostate is very common in men over 60 years of
age, but fortunately it only produces symptoms in about 8 per cent of
these cases. The disease is hardly ever seen in early life. The cause of
the enlargement is probably some disturbance of the hormones from
the sex glands, which is likely to occur as the period of reproductive
activity declines. It is really a hyperplasia or overgrowth rather than
a mere hypertrophy or enlargement. It is comparable to the condition

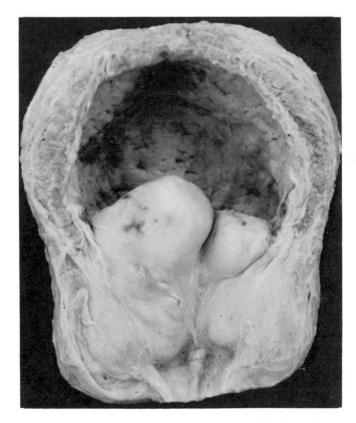

Fig. 128. Marked enlargement of prostate causing obstruction of urethra and
hypertrophy of bladder wall.

of the breast known as chronic mastitis or cystic hyperplasia which is described in Chapter 24.

The *effects* of the prostatic enlargement are *obstruction* to the outflow of urine and an inability to empty the bladder completely (Fig. 128). The *residual urine* retained in the bladder tends to undergo decomposition and becomes infected. The two great dangers that threaten the man suffering from enlargement of the prostate are (1) *urinary retention* with back-pressure on the ureters and kidneys, and (2) *infection* that ascends from the bladder to the kidneys. The results will be distention of the bladder, cystitis, dilatation of the ureters, hydronephrosis, and pyonephrosis (Fig. 129). Death is due either to sepsis or to renal failure.

Treatment has entirely changed the outlook for the man in declining years whose last days used to be made pitiable by prostatic enlargement. The enlarged gland can be removed by various surgical measures. One of these days it may be possible to control the enlargement by the use of hormones and thus render operation unnecessary.

CANCER OF THE PROSTATE. Carcinoma of the prostate is unfortunately quite common. The prostate becomes enlarged and very firm, causing symptoms of urinary obstruction. The tumor infiltrates the surrounding structures early and extensively, and on that account surgical treatment is far from satisfactory. The blood vessels are also invaded at an early date, and *secondary growths* are formed in various organs, particularly the bones. *When an elderly man is found to be suffering from a tumor of bone, the prostate should always be examined.* From what has been said it is evident that the prognosis in cancer of the prostate is very unfavorable with surgical removal.

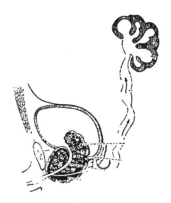

Fig. 129. Enlargement of prostate, the enlarged part projecting into the bladder and obstructing the urethra. The ureter and renal pelvis are dilated. (Joll and Leadley, *Aids to Surgery;* Baillière, Tyndall & Cox.)

New light and new hope have been shed on the subject of carcinoma of the prostate by the demonstration that the male hormone of the testicle exerts an important influence on the growth of the prostate. *Castration* (removal of both testicles) before puberty prevents development of the prostate, and castration in adult life causes regression of the normal gland. These facts have been applied to the problem of the control of cancer of the prostate with remarkable results, for castration leads to marked shrinking of the tumor and great relief of the severe bone pains caused by metastases in the skeleton, particularly the spine. The administration of *stilbestrol,* the synthetic form of the female sex hormone, also affords marked relief, probably because of interference with the male hormone. This form of therapy has largely replaced castration. Sometimes the two are combined.

A valuable means of determining the improvement produced by these methods of treatment is afforded by estimating the *acid phosphatase* in the blood. Phosphatase is an enzyme produced by the prostate, and the amount is greatly increased when cancer of the prostate develops, and especially when secondary tumors are formed in the bones. Under these circumstances there is a marked rise in the level of the blood acid phosphatase, a rise that disappears if the treatment is successful. The word success is used in only a relative sense, for it is not claimed that cancer of the prostate can be cured by these means.

Testis and Epididymis

The epididymis is the convoluted excretory duct of the testis and, although it lies separate from though attached to the testis, it may be considered with the latter in connection with disease.

EPIDIDYMITIS.   By far the commonest cause of inflammation of the epididymis is the gonococcus, which extends from the male urethra during an acute attack of *gonorrhea*. The epididymis becomes enlarged, hard, and tender. Minute abscesses are formed, but there is no extensive breaking down of tissue such as might be expected. The inflammation is acute and subsides quickly, but often leaves fibrous scars that obliterate the seminiferous tubules. When the condition is bilateral, complete sterility may result.

ORCHITIS.   The two common causes of inflammation of the testis (orchitis) are injury and mumps. *Traumatic orchitis* is caused by a blow, which is followed by an acute inflammatory edema of the organ. *Mumps orchitis* is usually unilateral, and is rarely seen before the age of puberty, being commonest in young men. It may follow or may precede the enlargement of the parotid gland which is characteristic of mumps.

TUBERCULOSIS.   Tuberculosis usually starts in the *lower pole of the epididymis.* Tuberculous nodules are formed throughout that organ, and caseation may occur later with ulceration through the skin. Infection may spread to the testis and along the spermatic cord which is felt to be thickened and nodular. If the disease is progressive there may be successive involvement of the prostate, the other epididymis, the bladder, and finally the kidneys.

TUMORS. Tumors of the testis are fairly common. There are two principal groups named seminoma and teratoma. The *seminoma* appears to arise from the seminiferous tubules of the testis, whereas the *teratoma* is believed to arise from a primitive germ cell, and consists of a variety of structures. Both of these tumors are highly malignant and tend to spread both by the lymphatics and along the blood stream. Other rare tumors are found in the testis, but these do not need to be considered here.

FURTHER READING

ALLEN, A. C.: *The Kidney: Medical and Surgical Diseases,* 2nd ed., New York, 1962.

DEWARDENER, II. E.: *The Kidney: An Outline of Normal and Abnormal Structure and Function,* London, 1958.

ELLIS, A.: Lancet, 1942, *1,* 34, 72. (Natural history of glomerulonephritis.)

HEPTINSTALL, R. H.: *Pathology of the Kidney,* Boston, 1966.

KERR, W. K., *et al.:* Can. Med. Ass. J., 1965, *93,* 1. (Cigarette smoking and cancer of the bladder.)

Chapter 23

Female Reproductive System

UTERUS

STRUCTURE AND FUNCTION. The reproductive system in woman consists of four major parts (Fig. 130): (1) the *ovaries* where the ova or eggs are produced; (2) the *fallopian tubes* by which they are conducted to the uterus and in which impregnation by the male element or spermatozoon occurs; (3) the *uterus* or womb in which the impregnated ovum develops into an embryo and then into a fetus; (4) the *vagina* or birth canal. The uterus is divided into an upper part or *body* and a lower part or *cervix*. This distinction is important because the two parts are quite different in function and in pathological behavior. The wall of the uterus is composed of involuntary muscle intermingled with fibrous tissue, and its cavity is lined by a mucous membrane called the *endometrium*. The *placenta* is the organ of communication between the mother and fetus, being derived partly from the maternal endometrium, partly from the chorion, a membrane that covers the developing fetus (Fig. 131).

Menstruation. Every month the endometrium undergoes a change of the greatest importance known as menstruation (*mensis,* a month), for every month an ovum is discharged from one of the ovaries, and the endometrium shows changes similar to those at the beginning of pregnancy in the expectation that the ovum may be impregnated. When impregnation fails to occur the prepared endometrium undergoes

400

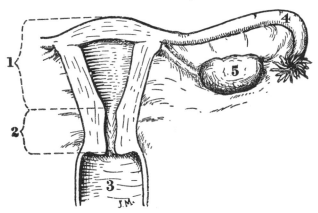

Fig. 130. Female reproductive organs. 1, Body of uterus; 2, cervix; 3, vagina; 4, fallopian tube; 5, ovary.

necrosis and is cast off, accompanied by a discharge of blood lasting for several days. When the menstrual flow is excessive, it is known as *menorrhagia;* when there is bleeding between the menstrual periods it is known as *metrorrhagia.* Absence of menstrual bleeding is called *amenorrhea.* After menstruation has ceased the endometrium is re-

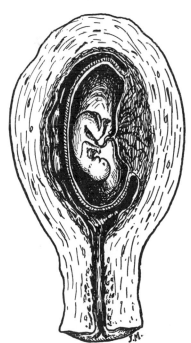

Fig. 131. Pregnant uterus showing placenta and fetus.

formed from the fragments that are left, only to be cast off again at the end of another month.

This strange cycle is directly dependent on a similar monthly cycle in the ovaries, the communication between the two organs being by chemical messengers or *hormones*. There are two of these hormones, each of which produces a different effect on the endometrium. In order to understand the origin of these hormones we must look a little more closely at what is going on in the ovary. Each ovary contains thousands of ova, but only one is discharged from the ovary every month. The chosen ovum undergoes a process of ripening. It lies in a little cavity, the *graafian follicle,* containing a watery fluid and lined by specialized cells. The follicular fluid is the source of the first of the ovarian hormones, which is carried by the blood to the uterus where it acts on the endometrium and also to the kidneys by which it is excreted in the urine. It is known as **estrogen** or *the female sex hormone.* The follicle approaches the surface of the ovary, and at the very middle of the month, about the fourteenth day, the ovum is discharged into the end of the fallopian tube (ovulation). The follicle at once undergoes a peculiar series of changes, as a result of which it is converted into a solid yellow body, the *corpus luteum,* which in turn produces a hormone of its own. This hormone is responsible for the changes in the endometrium designed to nourish the impregnated ovum when it reaches the uterus, so that in the absence of the corpus luteum pregnancy is impossible, for the fertilized ovum cannot be retained. When pregnancy occurs the corpus luteum becomes greatly enlarged (corpus luteum of pregnancy) and produces a correspondingly increased amount of hormone. The reason for this increase in size will be apparent presently. The corpus luteum hormone is called **progesterone,** because *it prepares the uterus for pregnancy* (*gestation*). It will be seen presently that failure of the corpus luteum to develop will give rise to serious pathological changes.

Progesterone has been called "nature's contraceptive," for it serves to prevent the ripening of another ovum until the next cycle starts. Chemists can now make chemically related substances known as *progestins* which are far more potent than natural progesterone in preventing ovulation. This is the basis of oral contraceptives, known popularly as *"The Pill."* Like other good things the Pill has its bad side, which we need not enter into here.

Just as the endometrium is under the influence of the ovary, so the ovary is under the influence of the pituitary gland. The periodicity of the ovary is not inherent in itself, but is dependent on the anterior lobe of the pituitary which regulates it. Injections of pituitary extract will cause an immature female animal rapidly to become mature with development of graafian follicles and production of the female sex hormone. The starting motor of the complex monthly menstrual cycle is undoubtedly the tiny pituitary gland lying on the floor of the skull and covered by the brain. The pituitary hormone that produces these effects is known as the *pituitary gonadotropic hormone.*

Functional Uterine Hemorrhage

At the time of the menopause or change of life a woman may begin to suffer from irregular uterine hemorrhage, which may take the form either of periodic bleeding or of prolonged and continuous bleeding. This irregular hemorrhage may occur at earlier age periods, and sometimes even in young women. The endometrium is markedly thickened. It used to be thought that this bleeding condition was due to some disease of the uterus, but we now know that the essential trouble lies not in the uterus but in the ovaries. For this reason the condition is called *functional uterine hemorrhage,* the associated thickening of the endometrium being *endometrial hyperplasia.*

We have already seen that two ovarian hormones act on the endometrium to produce normal menstruation, the one, estrogen, from the ripening follicles, the other, progesterone, from the corpus luteum. Menstruation is brought about by regression of the corpus luteum, a fall in progesterone production, and then desquamation of the superficial layers of the endometrium. In functional uterine hemorrhage there is an entire absence of lutein tissue, but the ovary does contain one or more ripening follicles. Apparently something prevents ovulation from occurring, there is a continued overproduction of estrogen by the persisting ripening follicles, and the endometrium shows the effect of this overstimulation by manifesting in pathological form the first or hyperplastic phase of the menstrual cycle with resulting functional hemorrhage.

Puerperal Sepsis

The normal uterus is remarkably resistant to infection, but in the *puerperium,* the period after childbirth, it is extremely liable to infection on account of the raw surface of the interior and the presence of blood clots and fragments of placenta. The danger of infection is much greater after an abortion than after delivery at full term, owing to the greater likelihood of fragments of placenta being retained and acting as a suitable culture medium for any bacteria that may be introduced. *Secondary factors* that predispose to infection are instrumental interference, exhaustion, and hemorrhage. **In the vast majority of cases infection is introduced either by the examining hand or by an unsterilized instrument used to produce abortion.** The less manual examination a woman receives during labor, the less likely is she to develop puerperal infection, for the gloved hand is apt to carry microorganisms from the vagina up into the uterus. The commonest cause of fatal puerperal infection is *Streptococcus haemolyticus*. This may come from the throat of the attending physician or nurse, so that the wearing of a mask is a valuable protective measure. In a small proportion of cases the hemolytic streptococci apparently come from the throat of the patient, being carried to the uterus by the blood stream.

In the fatal cases the cavity of the uterus is lined by dirty, necrotic, breaking-down material swarming with streptococci which have also widely invaded the uterine wall and may in this way set up general peritonitis. *Infection may reach the peritoneal cavity from the uterus by passing along the fallopian tubes, with resulting fatal peritonitis.* An equally great danger is infection of the large blood clots that occupy the gaping and torn vessels. These infected clots become broken down, converted into septic emboli, and carried by the blood stream throughout the body causing septicemia and pyemia. In such cases the streptococci will readily be found in blood culture, and the clinical picture is that of acute blood poisoning. The patient is thus exposed to the double threat of septicemia and general peritonitis.

The above account is now largely of historic interest, because with modern chemotherapy the infection can be nipped in the bud. It is well, however, for the student to know something of the risks from infection which women used to run in giving birth to a child. And they still do when they resort to illegal abortion.

Penicillin and other antibiotics are so effective against puerperal sepsis that the fear of this complication of pregnancy no longer exists. This condition was one of the first infections in which the efficacy of sulfonamide therapy was demonstrated, but the sulfonamide drugs have now largely been replaced by penicillin and other antibiotics.

Endocervicitis

The uterus, as we have already seen, is divided into an upper part, the body, and a lower part, the neck or cervix. The changes characteristic of menstruation and pregnancy are confined to the endometrium of the body. As it is on this part of the uterus that the ovarian hormones act, this is naturally the part affected by such disorders as functional hemorrhage. Up to the present in our discussion the cervix has seemed remarkably immune from disease. We have now to learn that it is the site of two common pathological conditions, namely, chronic inflammation and cancer.

Inflammation of the cervix, or rather the lining of the cervix, is known as endocervicitis. Its frequency is due partly to the structure of the mucous membrane of the cervix, partly to the fact that the lining of the cervix is not swept away every month as in the case of the uterine body, so that infection can lodge in it for long periods. The glands in the lining of the body of the uterus are comparatively simple and tubular, but those in the cervix are highly complex and branching like the streets in the native quarter of an oriental city, so that infecting organisms may lurk there for long periods, not only causing local inflammation but sallying forth and causing trouble at a distance. Two sets of organisms may give rise to chronic endocervicitis: (1) the ordinary pyogenic bacteria such as staphylococcus, streptococcus, and *E. coli,* which tend to invade the tissue as the result of a tear during childbirth; (2) the gonococcus, the infection of the cervix occurring during an attack of gonorrhea.

Cervical erosion is the name given to the inflammatory lesion that follows injury to the cervix during delivery. When the cervix is examined by means of a speculum in the vaginal canal a red patch is observed which has an appearance of rawness or erosion. The underlying tissue is filled with inflammatory cells, and the bacteria responsible for the inflammation may keep it going for months or years.

The *chief symptom* of inflammation of the cervix is *leukorrhea,* a word which means white discharge. This discharge is a sticky glairy fluid which is poured out by the irritated cervical glands. Leukorrhea is one of the commonest of female disorders. The *chief danger* of cervical erosion is the possibility that cancer may develop later, *i.e.,* that the inflammatory lesion may prove to be a pre-cancerous one. This matter will be referred to again in connection with cancer of the cervix.

Tumors of the Uterus

FIBROIDS.   A fibroid of the uterus is an innocent tumor consisting essentially of involuntary muscle, but containing a varying amount of fibrous tissue. Pathologically, therefore, it is a myoma or, more accurately, a *leiomyoma* which consists of plain unstriated muscle, but the old name of fibroid is universally used. It is an extremely common tumor, but very often it gives rise to no symptoms. One of its most striking characteristics is that it only develops during the period of reproductive activity. *It never appears before puberty or after the menopause,* although naturally fibroids that are already present will persist after the change of life. *This suggests very strongly that ovarian hormones play some part in stimulating the growth of the tumor.* The tumors are frequently multiple. In size they vary from a pea to a child's head. They somewhat resemble the surrounding uterine muscle, from which they are separated by a definite capsule, but they are whiter and more dense. The tumor may grow toward the cavity of the uterus, pushing the mucous membrane in front of it, and is then known as a

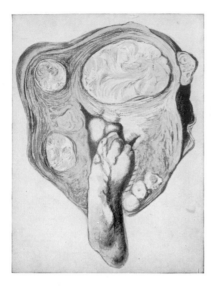

Fig. 132. Fibroids of uterus; some tumors are in the muscular wall, and one submucous fibroid hangs down in the cavity.

submucous fibroid (Fig. 132). Or it may grow outward, projecting from the surface of the uterus and pushing the peritoneum in front of it; it is then called a *subperitoneal fibroid,* and may only be attached to the uterus by a narrow stalk or pedicle.

The **symptoms** are variable. Often there are none. A submucous fibroid is likely to cause *uterine hemorrhage.* This may take the form of excessive menstrual bleeding (*menorrhagia*) or bleeding between the periods (*metrorrhagia*). A large fibroid may cause *pelvic pain,* pressure on the rectum with *constipation,* or pressure on the veins from the leg with resulting *edema.* Occasionally the narrow pedicle of a subperitoneal fibroid may become twisted, causing a sudden attack of severe pain.

CARCINOMA. Cancer of the uterus is one of the commonest forms of cancer and *this tumor grows from the cervix in 90 per cent of cases* (Fig. 133). The great susceptibility of the cervix compared with the body of the uterus is possibly related to *the frequency with which the cervix is injured during childbirth,* for at least 96 per cent of the cases are in women who have borne children.

It is equally possible that *stimulation of the cervix by the hormones of pregnancy* may be the factor that is responsible for the development of carcinoma. There is no corresponding relationship between cancer of the body of the uterus and the bearing of children. Cancer of the cervix is a disease of middle age, but may appear before the thirtieth year. Cancer of the body develops on an average about ten years later than cancer of the cervix.

A third factor may be *smegma,* which is believed to act as a carcin-

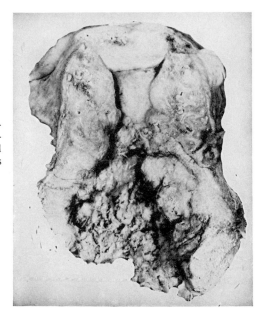

Fig. 133. Carcinoma of cervix. The cervix is converted into a ragged fungating mass. (Boyd's *Textbook of Pathology*.)

ogen in cancer of the penis. The rate of cancer of the cervix is only one-quarter as high in Jewish as in non-Jewish white women both in Israel and in New York City. The incidence is also much lower in Moslems, a group in which circumcision is practiced.

Carcinoma of the cervix arises from the epithelium of the cervix at the point where it joins the vaginal canal. It may form a cauliflower-like mass projecting into the vaginal canal, or it may grow away from the lumen, destroying the cervix and becoming ulcerated so as to form a gaping cavity where the cervix once was. **Carcinoma of the body** may project into the uterine cavity (Fig. 134), or it may infiltrate the wall

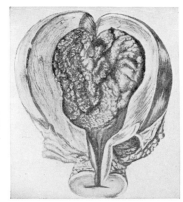

Fig. 134. Carcinoma of body of uterus. The tumor projects into the uterine cavity, but does not involve the cervix.

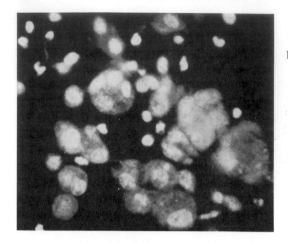

Fig. 135. Smear from patient with carcinoma-in-situ of cervix, showing marked pleomorphism of cells. Fluorescence microscopy. × 280. In the original slide the cells were flaming red-orange in color. (Bertalanffy *et al.,* courtesy of Cancer.)

of the uterus. *Smears made from the cervix or even from the vaginal fluid show the presence of exfoliated cancer cells.* The *cytological features* are: (1) great variety in form and size of the cells; (2) atypical structure of their nuclei; and (3) vacuolization of the cytoplasm. This is the method associated with the name of Papanicolaou and popularly known as the Pap smear (p. 231). *Fluorescent microscopy* may prove to be a more rapid method of identifying malignant cells in vaginal smears, and one not requiring the services of a highly trained observer. With the fluorescent dye, acridine orange, malignant cells show an intense red-orange fluorescence owing to their high DNA content (Fig. 135). This method of **exfoliative cytology** is a very valuable aid in the detection of carcinoma of the cervix in the earliest stage. It must always be checked, however, by biopsy, *i.e.,* surgical excision of small portion of tumor and subsequent examination by the pathologist under the microscope.

The **spread** of the tumor is of great importance. *Cancer of the cervix* is a highly infiltrative growth, so that it tends to invade the surrounding structures, including the bladder in front and the rectum behind. It is this quality which has made the operative treatment in the past so highly unsatisfactory. There is also spread along the lymph vessels to the lymphatic glands of the pelvis. Blood spread is of little importance and only occurs late in the disease. *Cancer of the body of the uterus is* not nearly so invasive, so that the results of operative removal are better. Spread is more likely to take place by the blood stream than by the lymphatics, and secondary growths may be formed in distant organs.

The **chief symptom** of cancer of the uterus is *hemorrhage.* As cancer of the cervix commonly occurs about the time of the menopause, the irregular bleeding from the ulcerated tumor surface may be mistaken by the patient for the irregular menstrual flow which is common at the change of life. The occurrence of uterine bleeding at a period of life when menstrual bleeding has ceased should at once arouse the alarm of the patient and send her immediately to a doctor. Unfortunately *pain is not an early symptom of cancer,* here or elsewhere, and as pain is the only certain means of sending the patient to the practitioner, much priceless time is often lost.

Cancer of the uterus, particularly cancer of the cervix, used to be regarded as a peculiarly malignant form of tumor, because operative removal of the uterus was so frequently followed by local recurrence of the tumor, owing to the tendency to invasion already referred to. It is true that the tumor is highly malignant, but at the same time it is highly radiosensitive, a fact which has entirely altered the prognosis (Fig. 136). *Radiation therapy often succeeds in destroying every one of the tumor cells,* and the patient may be restored to perfect health and strength. Everything depends on whether the case is seen sufficiently early before distant spread has occurred. Cancer of the body is not so radiosensitive as cancer of the cervix, but radiation followed by removal of the uterus has materially improved the prognosis in this form also.

CHORIONEPITHELIOMA. This is an uncommon tumor of the uterus, but deserves mention on account of its unique character. It is the only tumor that arises in the tissues of another individual. The chorion is the fetal part of the placenta, and as the tumor arises from the epithelial covering of the chorion it is a fetal tumor invading the tissues of the mother. The tumor must, of course, be preceded by pregnancy, but the pregnancy usually terminates in an abortion and does not go on to full term. Moreover the tumor is preceded in about 30 per cent of cases by the development of the peculiar condition known as hydatidiform mole, which is described in the next section.

The tumor, also called *choriocarcinoma,* is a highly malignant one,

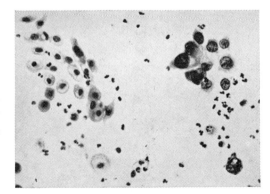

Fig. 136. Carcinoma of cervix. Group at right typical, unradiated, undifferentiated, malignant cells. Group at left shows pyknosis of basal cells. (Graham, courtesy of Surg. Gynec. and Obst.)

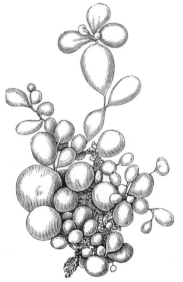

Fig. 137. Hydatidiform mole.

very soft and red like blood clot, and it invades not only the uterine wall but the large veins. As a result of this early invasion the tumor cells are carried by the blood to distant organs, particularly the lungs, where they set up secondary growths.

The only *early symptom* is *uterine hemorrhage*. The onset of hemorrhage weeks or months after an abortion should arouse suspicion of a chorionepithelioma. This suspicion will be confirmed by positive results of a pregnancy test.

HYDATIDIFORM MOLE. Mole means "mass" and hydatidiform means "like hydatid cysts" (the cystic stage of a tapeworm). A hydatidiform mole is a mass of grape-like cysts into which the placenta becomes converted in about 1 in 3000 cases (Fig. 137). In addition to the formation of cysts there is marked proliferation of the chorionic epithelium, but of an innocent, not a malignant nature. It is the chorionic epithelium that produces the chorionic gonadotropic hormone and is responsible for the reaction in the urine so characteristic of pregnancy. Even when the fetus dies the test remains markedly positive, but no sooner is the cystic mole expelled from the uterus than the test becomes negative. In the event of the mole developing into a chorionepithelioma the test will remain positive even after the mole is discharged, for the malignant chorionic epithelium continues to form gonadotropic hormone in large amounts.

The practical application of all this now becomes evident. Hydatidiform mole is an essentially innocent condition, which requires no more drastic treatment than clearing out the uterus. It always holds the threat, however, that it may develop into a chorionepithelioma. This tumor, although highly malignant, can be cured if the uterus is removed sufficiently early. The change from the benign mole to the malignant tumor is indicated by the continuance of the pregnancy reaction in the urine after the mole has been removed.

FALLOPIAN TUBES

The fallopian tubes are ducts, one on each side, which lead from the ovaries to the uterus, along which the ovum passes, and in which fertilization of the ovum takes place. The inner end of the tube opens into the uterus and the outer end into the peritoneal cavity. Both ends are readily closed by inflammation, which is by far the commonest pathological condition to affect the tubes and is called salpingitis.

SALPINGITIS. By far the most important cause of salpingitis is gonorrhea, which is responsible for at least 80 per cent of the cases. Pyogenic cocci, especially streptococci, cause 15 per cent. The remaining 5 per cent are tuberculous in nature. The effect on the tube depends largely on the virulence of the infection. The outer end usually becomes closed early, so that the peritoneal cavity is shielded from infection. If the inner end still remains open the condition is called a *pus tube.* When both ends are closed the tube becomes markedly distended with fluid. If the infection is virulent the inflammation is purulent in type, the tube is filled with pus, and the condition is known as **pyosalpinx.** If the infection is mild the inflammation is more in the nature of a catarrh and the fluid is watery in type, a condition of **hydrosalpinx.**

The infection usually reaches the tubes from the uterus, so that salpingitis is generally bilateral. The distention of the tubes may be enormous, and they may resemble bananas. Adhesions to surrounding structures may be very dense, so that operative removal may be a matter of great difficulty. *Sterility* is an inevitable result if both tubes are closed, as the ovum is unable to pass along the obstructed tubes. In addition there is often pelvic pain, menstrual disturbances, and general invalidism.

Tuberculous salpingitis is very similar to the salpingitis produced by gonococci and other organisms except that the inflammation is not purulent. The tubes are thickened, and may be greatly distended with caseous tuberculous material. The infection reaches the tubes by the blood stream from some tuberculous focus elsewhere.

TUBAL PREGNANCY. Impregnation of the ovum takes place during its passage along the fallopian tube, not in the uterus itself. If the fertilized ovum should be entrapped in the folds and crevices of the mucous membrane of the tube, it will develop into an embryo in the tube instead

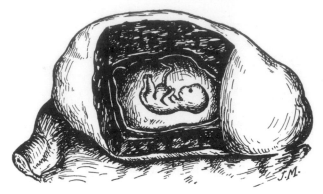

Fig. 138. Tubal pregnancy.

of in the uterus, a condition known as tubal or **ectopic pregnancy** (Fig. 138). Chronic salpingitis causes thickening of the folds and deepening of the pockets between them, so that it acts as a strong predisposing cause of tubal pregnancy.

As the embryo grows in size it burrows deeper into the wall of the tube and causes increasing distention of the lumen. An accident is almost certain to happen by the end of the second month. The pregnancy may terminate in one of two ways, by tubal abortion or by tubal rupture. *Tubal abortion* is the usual course. There is hemorrhage into the placenta which has formed in the tube, with destruction of the embryo and distention of the tube with blood clot, a condition called *hematosalpinx*. This is accompanied by severe pain in the right or left groin, and a flow of blood from the uterus. These symptoms together with amenorrhea for two months will usually allow a correct diagnosis to be made.

The great danger of ectopic pregnancy is *tubal rupture,* which occurs in about 25 per cent of cases. The wall of the tube ruptures, severe bleeding occurs into the abdominal cavity, and the patient may die of internal hemorrhage. It is on account of the danger of tubal rupture that the correct treatment of ectopic pregnancy is surgical removal of the tube.

OVARIES

The ovaries are two small flat organs, rather larger than a bean, which lie one on either side of the uterus, and are connected with it by the fallopian tubes. Each ovary contains more than 100,000 graafian follicles in which ova are formed, but only a small number of these may come to maturity. The chief pathological conditions affecting the ovaries are cysts and tumors.

Cysts and Tumors

Cysts and tumors of the ovary are so intermingled that it is convenient to consider them together, although this will be done under separate headings.

OVARIAN CYSTS. Ovarian cysts may be of two kinds, retention cysts and tumor cysts or cystadenomas. *Retention cysts* are of very common occurrence. They arise from graafian follicles, which have never matured and discharged their ova on the surface, and are usually multiple but small in size, so that the ovary is only slightly enlarged. On account of their origin they are called *follicular cysts.* It used to be a common practice to remove such cystic ovaries under the belief that they were responsible for pelvic pain and other common female complaints, but this practice has been largely given up.

Cystadenomas. These lesions are of very different character. Although they take the form of cysts, *i.e.,* cavities filled with fluid, they are really benign tumors, and may accordingly grow to an enormous size. Before the days of modern surgery it was not unusual to see the entire abdomen filled with one of these great bags of fluid. The contents are sometimes watery (*serous cystadenoma*), sometimes jelly-like (*mucinous cystadenoma*). The cavity is often multiloculated so that the main cyst contains many smaller cysts. The lining is usually smooth, but may be covered by papillary processes; in the latter case there is a distinct danger that the tumor may become malignant. The papillary processes perforate the wall of the cyst, become scattered over the peritoneal cavity, and form there large secondary malignant masses. The irritation to the peritoneum leads to an outpouring of watery fluid, a condition of ascites.

As long as the cystadenoma is benign, removal of the tumor will bring about cure. Even when it becomes malignant, removal may be successful if secondary growths have not been formed.

Dermoid Cyst. This is a common form of ovarian tumor which takes a cystic form. It is a *teratoma,* a developmental tumor arising from an ovum and representing an attempt to form a new individual. It may, therefore, contain a variety of structures such as skin, hair, teeth, bone, brain tissue, etc. It is filled with yellow buttery material produced by the glands in the skin that it contains, and hair is a constant ingredient, hence the name dermoid. Although this cystic tumor may attain a large size, it is essentially innocent in character.

OVARIAN TUMORS. Tumors of the ovary may be cystic or solid. The cystic tumors are the cystadenomas which have just been described. The solid tumors are nearly all malignant, for the most part carcinoma. Carcinoma of the ovary may be primary or secondary. **Secondary cancer** is much commoner than primary, being usually secondary to cancer of the stomach or large bowel. The tumor cells are carried from the stomach through the peritoneal cavity and are implanted on both ovaries so that the tumor is bilateral. **Primary cancer** is comparatively uncommon. It forms a large solid mass which replaces the ovary; tumor cells are often implanted on the second ovary, so that both ovaries must be removed, although only one may appear to be affected.

In addition to the tumors that have been mentioned there is a group of rare tumors referred to as **special ovarian tumors.** They all have a common origin from embryonic remnants, but what marks them out from ordinary ovarian tumors is that several of them produce sex hormone disturbances, which may be *masculinizing* or *feminizing*. The term "feminization" has its drawbacks when applied to a woman. It denotes a prolonged estrogen effect, which in infancy and early childhood produces precocious puberty, with development of the breasts and uterine bleeding. In postmenopausal women the major symptom is bleeding from the uterus.

FURTHER READING

GARDNER, W. U., *et al.:* J.A.M.A., 1938, *110,* 1182. (Hormonal stimulation in cancer of cervix.)

GRAHAM, R. M.: Surg., Gyn. and Obst., 1951, *93,* 767. (Vaginal smears in radiation of cervical cancer.)

MORRIS, J. M., and SCULLY, R. E.: *Endocrine Pathology of the Ovary,* St. Louis, 1958.

NOVAK, E. B., and WOODRUFF, J. D.: *Gynecologic and Obstetric Pathology,* Philadelphia, 1967.

WAY, S.: *The Diagnosis of Early Carcinoma of the Cervix,* London, 1963.

Chapter 24

The Breast

Structure and Function **Cystic Hyperplasia**	**Fibroadenoma** **Carcinoma**

STRUCTURE AND FUNCTION. The breast resembles the uterine endometrium in many respects, for it changes markedly in structure in response to the needs of reproduction, it is played upon by influences from the ovary and pituitary, some of its commonest disorders are connected with disturbance of these influences, and it is a very common site of cancer. It varies markedly in microscopic appearance as well as in size at varying periods of life. At all periods, however, it consists partly of glandular tissue, for the breast is essentially a gland, and partly of fat. It is worth recalling that the Latin name of the breast is mamma, with all the psychological connotation which that name suggests.

In the *newborn*, both male and female, the breasts may be slightly swollen and contain milk (witch's milk), owing to stimulation by the female sex hormone in the mother's blood. Up to puberty there is almost no glandular tissue in the breast, but at *puberty* under the influence of *ovarian hormones* there is rapid growth of glandular tissue in the female breasts, the outlines of which become rounded and full. It is, of course, during *pregnancy* and *lactation* that the glandular overgrowth is most marked, the stimulus being again due to ovarian and now also to *placental hormones*. The mother's pituitary secretes *prolactin* which starts milk production. At the *menopause* there is great atrophy of the glandular tissue.

The production of milk from the blood that flows through the breast is indeed a chemical miracle, an achievement that leaves the greatest of our chemists speechless. The glucose of the blood has to be converted to the lactose of milk, the amino acids of the blood are very different from the complex proteins of milk, and so are the fatty acids of the blood from the rich fats of milk. All this is done by the enzymes in the cells lining the glands of the breast under the stimulus of the tiny

415

pituitary gland at the base of the brain. We take these things for granted without considering their wonder.

It is evident that the breast is capable of great hypertrophy, and of correspondingly great involution in which there is an attempt to return to the former state. A similar but much smaller swing of the pendulum takes place during each menstrual cycle, the glandular tissue enlarging and then regressing. As a result of pathological conditions, *e.g.,* abnormal ovarian stimuli, there may be deviations from the normal. In the first place the hyperplasia and involution may be more localized to one part of the breast than another. In the second place, involution may be less complete than hyperplasia, as a result of which some of the gland spaces may remain dilated and become converted into cysts. These two results are often combined, so that localized areas of overgrowth are produced, which may be well or poorly demarcated from the surrounding breast and contain cysts of varying size. There are *only three common diseases of the breast, cystic hyperplasia, fibroadenoma, and carcinoma;* the first two appear to be a direct outcome of the cyclic changes that have just been described.

CYSTIC HYPERPLASIA

This, which is the commonest lesion of the female breast, is called *chronic mastitis,* but this name was given when it was supposed to be a chronic inflammation of the breast and when the true nature of the condition was not known. It usually occurs about the time of the menopause, but is by no means confined to that period of life, and a group of cases are seen in young unmarried women with menstrual evidence of disturbed ovarian function. Both in the young and in the elderly the hyperplasia is due to irregular and abnormal stimuli coming from the ovaries. As a result of these irregular stimuli a *hyperplasia* of the breast occurs which is *patchy in character,* affecting groups of the lobules into which the breast is divided, so that it is often called *lobular hyperplasia. Cyst formation* is a prominent feature. Each month the process is repeated, so that the lesion is gradually intensified.

The *clinical features* are characteristic. The woman, usually between the ages of 40 and 50 years, has commonly borne a number of children, and now complains either of *pain* or of a *lump in the breast.* The pain as a rule is worse at the menstrual period, and there is tenderness of the breast as well as pain. Both breasts are often involved and there may be several lumps in each breast. The lump may feel exactly like a tumor, especially if it contains one or more large cysts; these are so tense that they give the feeling of a solid mass.

Cystic hyperplasia is an innocent lesion, which can be treated by local removal. But it must be treated with respect for two reasons: in the first place, the doctor can never be certain before operation whether a lump in the breast is innocent or malignant, and in the second place cystic hyperplasia may act as a precancerous lesion, *i.e.,* it may develop later into cancer. The area affected may be very small and localized, so that the operation does not need to be a mutilating one. On the other hand it is advisable in an elderly woman, in whom the danger of cancer is greater and the importance of the breast less, to remove the entire breast.

It is important to distinguish between possibility and probability. No one would deny the *possibility* of certain forms of cystic hyperplasia passing into carcinoma, but the question is, how often? If it is frequent, removal of the breast, often both breasts, must become a common prophylactic procedure; if but seldom, the risk of cancer developing may be too small to justify an operation entailing physical mutilation and psychic trauma. If the majority of surgeons were women rather than men the outlook on the best practical procedure might possibly be different!

FIBROADENOMA

This is a benign tumor of the breast, occurring chiefly in young women, often originating at puberty and growing during the years of developing sexual activity. It forms a firm, circumscribed, peculiarly movable mass with no attachments to the overlying skin or the underlying tissue. It is easily removed, and carries no threat of developing into cancer. As its name implies, it is formed by an overgrowth both of fibrous and glandular tissue. Although we have spoken of the lesion as a tumor, it is really more a localized and encapsulated form of lobular hyperplasia, although without cyst formation, and may be attributed to abnormal ovarian stimuli at the beginning of the reproductive period.

It is not wise to draw too close a parallel between lesions of the breast and those of the uterus, but it is allowable to compare cystic hyperplasia of the breast with endometrial hyperplasia and fibroadenoma of the breast with fibroids of the uterus.

CARCINOMA

Carcinoma of the breast is one of the commonest forms of malignant disease, and it is the commonest cancer in women. It usually occurs in the years before the menopause, but may develop at the age of 80 or 90 years; it is rare before the age of 35. It is rather commoner in those who have not borne children. Injury to the breast bears no relation to the development of cancer. Cystic hyperplasia may act as a predisposing cause in some cases, although this is a contentious subject which we had better avoid. Cancer of the breast is often called *scirrhous can-*

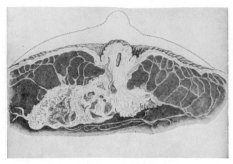

Fig. 139. Cancer of the breast. The white mass is the tumor. The nipple is retracted. Dotted line shows normal outline of breast.

cer. The term means hard, and describes a common characteristic of breast cancer. Other forms of cancer also occur, but for convenience in this brief outline only the characteristics of scirrhous carcinoma will be described.

It usually begins in the upper and outer segment of the breast, and forms a hard nodule which can be best appreciated by the palm of the hand rather than the fingers. It may not be nearly so readily felt as a fibroadenoma. It is important to realize that no matter how small a lump in the breast may be, it may still be cancer. I have seen a nodule of the breast no larger than a pea, but when it was removed it was found to be a carcinoma. It is wise to regard every lump in the breast as malignant until it has been proved to be innocent. If the advanced signs are waited for, it is then too late. These advanced signs are fixation of the tumor to the overlying skin and to the chest wall, indrawing of the nipple (Fig. 139), dimpling of the skin, and enlargement of the lymph nodes in the axilla (armpit) and in the neck.

The tumor in the patient may seem to be a circumscribed lump, but when it has been removed it will be found to blend with the surrounding breast. It cuts with the peculiar hard grittiness of an unripe pear, and the cut surface is concave instead of convex, as in the fibroadenoma.

Spread of the tumor occurs by infiltration, by the lymph stream, and by the blood stream. By *infiltration* the tumor cells spread throughout the breast, to the overlying skin, and to the underlying muscle (Fig. 140). This microscopic spread is very much wider than the tumor that can be seen with the naked eye, so that the surgeon has to remove a wide area of skin and muscle as well as the entire breast itself. *Lymph spread* carries the tumor cells to the lymph nodes in the axilla, so that the contents of the axilla have also to be dissected away lest any cancer be left from which a recurrence of the tumor may occur. Unfortunately lymph vessels may also carry tumor cells to lymph nodes in the chest

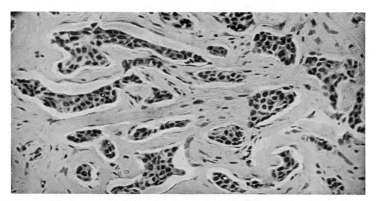

Fig. 140. Microscopic picture of cancer cells infiltrating the breast. The tumor cells are lying in lymph channels.

and in the neck. *Blood spread* carries the tumor to distant organs such as the brain, lungs, and bones.

The **prognosis** or outlook for the patient depends partly on the earliness of the diagnosis, partly on the thoroughness of the treatment. Statistics vary much in different clinics and in different countries, but it has been estimated that of patients treated efficiently and thoroughly, 50 per cent are alive and well after three years and 30 per cent after ten years. Of patients in whom the disease is confined to the breast without involvement of the lymph nodes, over 85 per cent are alive and well at the end of ten years. These figures apply to groups of patients who have received the best surgical treatment, with or without radiotherapy. As regards the individual patient the spread of carcinoma of the breast varies enormously for reasons that are beyond our comprehension. In some instances a tiny tumor is removed the moment it is observed, yet the patient is dead from generalized metastases within six months, whereas another tumor grows slowly and remains localized for many years without any treatment. Such facts as these indicate in unmistakable fashion the need for further basic research into the problems of neoplasia.

FURTHER READING

CURRIE, A. R. (Edit.): *Endocrine Aspects of Breast Cancer,* Edinburgh, 1958.

HAAGENSEN, C. D.: *Diseases of the Breast,* Philadelphia, 1956.

JANES, R. M.: Can. J. Surg., 1959, 2, 252. (Prognosis of breast cancer.)

LENDRUM, A. C.: J. Path. and Bact., 1945, 57, 267. (Cystic hyperplasia.)

LEWISON, E. F.: *Breast Cancer and Its Diagnosis and Treatment,* Baltimore, 1959.

Endocrine System

The *ductless* or *endocrine glands* form the most interesting group of organs in the body. Ordinary glands, such as those concerned with digestion, pour their secretion into the mouth, stomach, or intestine where they act upon the foodstuffs. The endocrine glands have no ducts, so that their secretions, instead of passing into one of the cavities of the body such as the mouth or the intestine, are absorbed directly into the blood. But the difference between the two sets of glands is much greater than this, for the secretions of the endocrine glands, known as *hormones,* govern some of the most fundamental metabolic processes of the body, and exert a far-reaching influence on the personality itself. This becomes evident when we remember that the sex glands belong to this group. Moreover, it is now known that subtle and but dimly understood relationships exist between the various endocrines. They may be compared to an orchestra in which, when one instrument is out of tune, a perfect ensemble is impossible. As has been remarked in a previous chapter, the leader of the glandular orchestra is the pituitary. It is not only the conductor of the orchestra, but it itself plays several important instruments in the ensemble, as well as acting as a link or mediator between soma and psyche. It is constantly monitoring the internal environment, and it is ideally situated to function in response to psychic stimuli.

Large treatises have been written on the ductless glands, but in this place it will be possible to give brief consideration to only five members of the group, disturbance of the function of which is reflected in the symptoms of disease. These are the pituitary, adrenals, thyroid, parathyroids, and islets of Langerhans. Reference has already been made to disorders of the female sex glands. Speaking generally, the endocrine glands may show evidence of disorder in one of two ways: there may be *hyperactivity* associated with the production of an excess of hormone, or there may be *hypoactivity* associated with an insufficient production of hormone. Overproduction of hormone may be caused by the presence of a tumor, usually benign in character, but this is not necessarily the case. Hypoactivity is usually the result of destruction of the gland produced by disease.

PITUITARY

STRUCTURE AND FUNCTION. It is no exaggeration to say that in the light of modern knowledge the pituitary gland, also known as the *hypophysis,* is the most remarkable organ in the human body. In size it is insignificant, being only slightly larger than a cherry stone, but its importance is indicated by the care with which it is protected from injury, for it lies in a little roofed-in chamber on the floor of the skull with the entire mass of the brain above it and the nasal cavity below. Its name indicates the relation it bears to the nose, for the ancients, who were well aware of its existence, imagined that its function was to produce the "pituita" or nasal secretion. Others, more idealistic, considered it to be the seat of the soul. Modern materialistic medicine regards it as the master gland of the body, regulating and coordinating the action of the other endocrine glands, and exercising a profound influence on the growth of the body, on the development of sex, on the subsequent functioning of the sex organs, and on the mind of the individual.

Like the adrenals, the pituitary consists of two parts, which may be regarded as two separate organs that happen to be united in one. These parts are the *anterior lobe,* which is formed by an upgrowth from the pharynx and is glandular in nature, and the *posterior lobe,* which is

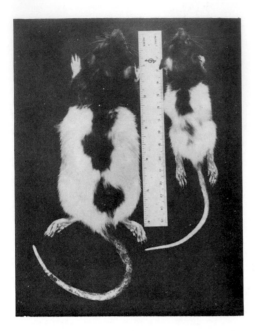

Fig. 141. The effect of hypophysectomy and of replacement therapy on growth. Litter mate rats were hypophysectomized at the age of 30 days. The animal on the left was injected daily thereafter for 3 months with the growth hormone of the adenohypophysis. The rat on the right received no treatment. (Reproduced from Grollman, A.: *Clinical Endocrinology,* courtesy of J. B. Lippincott Co.)

derived from a downgrowth from the base of the brain, remains connected with the brain by a narrow stalk, and is composed of nervous tissue.

Anterior Lobe. The anterior lobe is the part that produces the various hormones that play such an important part in the development and functioning of the body. The principal hormones are as follows:

1. *Growth hormone.* If the anterior pituitary is removed in an animal, growth is retarded to an extreme degree and the animal remains a dwarf (Fig. 141). The human dwarf is usually an individual in whom the growth hormone of the pituitary has been lacking. When the dwarfed animal is given the growth hormone, it catches up with its normal brother and may even surpass it in size, provided that the period of growth is not ended. Removal of the anterior lobe in a tadpole prevents its metamorphosis into a frog, but if an extract of the lobe is injected, normal development takes place.

2. *Gonadotropic hormone, i.e., the gonad-stimulating hormone.* This is necessary for the proper development of the reproductive organs, both male and female. It is on this hormone that the menstrual cycle in the female depends, for it stimulates the ovaries to monthly activity, and these in turn produce hormones that are responsible for the changes in the uterus that result in menstruation. One of the first signs of pituitary disease in the female is cessation of the menstrual function.

3. *Thyrotropic hormone.* Injection of this hormone in an animal stimulates the thyroid to great activity, and produces both the symptoms and the thyroid lesions of exophthalmic goiter.

4. *Lactogenic hormone.* When this is injected, it stimulates the production of milk in the female animal, and it is probably through the pituitary that the changes of pregnancy finally lead to lactation.

5. *Adrenocorticotropic hormone.* There exists the closest relationship between the pituitary and the adrenal cortex. Removal of the anterior pituitary reduces the adrenal cortex to a mere shell, and the administration of this hormone, now known by the abbreviation ACTH, restores it again to normal and stimulates it to produce cortisone.

6. *Diabetogenic hormone.* If experimental diabetes is produced in an animal by removal of the pancreas, the condition is relieved by removal of the pituitary. It would, therefore, appear that the anterior pituitary exercises an antagonistic effect on the islets of Langerhans in the pancreas.

Posterior Lobe. The posterior lobe, also called the *neurohypophysis* because of its intimate connection with the brain in both structure and function, produces three hormones: vasopressin, oxytocin, and the antidiuretic hormone. (1) *Vasopressin* is so-called because it can produce a marked rise in the blood pressure by causing vasoconstriction. (2) *Oxytocin* derives its name from its ability to cause contraction of smooth muscle, notably the uterus (*oxus,* swift; *tokos,* birth). The hormone is of value in inducing uterine contractions during labor. (3) *Antidiuretic hormone* or ADH increases the rate of reabsorption of water and electrolytes by the renal tubules, so that it reduces the output of urine or diuresis, and thus performs the extremely important function of guarding the organism against excessive water loss. Lack of the hormone results in the development of *diabetes insipidus.*

Like the other endocrine glands, disturbance of the pituitary may manifest itself either by overactivity, *i.e.,* hyperpituitarism, or by underactivity, *i.e.,* hypopituitarism. The former is associated with and dependent on the presence of an adenoma or benign tumor of the anterior lobe. The latter is caused by destruction of the anterior lobe by disease.

Hyperpituitarism

This manifests itself by excessive growth, particularly of the skeleton, but the results depend on whether the disturbance develops during the period of skeletal growth or after it is completed. In the former case the result is *gigantism* (Fig. 142). Every giant has an overactive pituitary, and at autopsy an *adenoma of the anterior pituitary* will be found. If the adenoma develops after growth is completed the result is *acromegaly,* a name that signifies enlargement of the hands and feet (Fig.

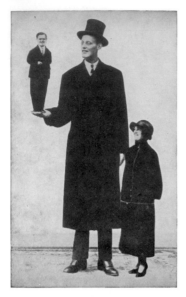

Fig. 142. Effects of pituitary disease, showing a pituitary giant and dwarf; the
woman is of normal height.

143). The acromegalic is unable to increase his stature, but his face
becomes very large with a markedly projecting lower jaw, which serves
to match the huge hands and feet. Curvature of the spine develops, and
the patient with his bent back, enormous hands reaching to the knees,
and protruding lower jaw may present a gorilla-like picture in extreme
cases. The overgrowth affects the connective tissue as well as the bones,
and the skin becomes thick, coarse, and furrowed. The disease does
not necessarily shorten life, for it is self-limited, and the tumor responsible for the condition not only stops growing but tends to undergo
degeneration.

Hypopituitarism

This is a much commoner condition than hyperpituitarism, but the
clinical pictures produced are more varied and confusing, and a detailed
consideration of their complexities would be out of place here. The most
common form is **Fröhlich's syndrome,** which is a disturbance of genital
development and fat (Fig. 144). It commonly develops about the time
of puberty. *Depression of the sexual function* is the earliest and most
constant symptom. In the female there is absence of menstruation, and
lack of libido in the male. The sexual organs remain undeveloped. The
connective tissue of the skin atrophies, so that the skin is smooth and
delicate like a child's, the reverse of the condition seen in acromegaly.
Adiposity may be very marked or may be absent. When the condition
develops in an adult male, deposits of fat in the breasts, hips, and buttocks give the figure a distinctly feminine cast. *Mental dullness* and

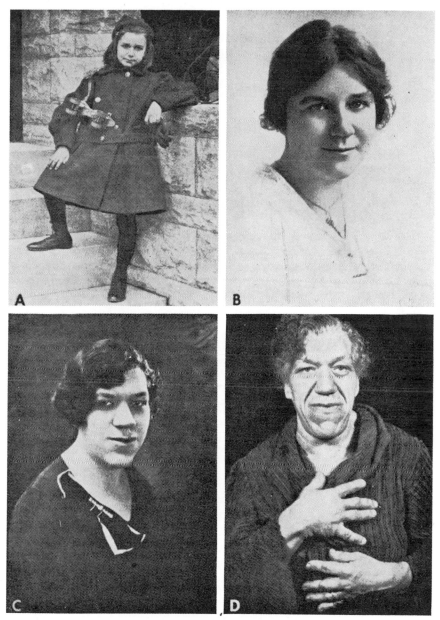

Fig. 143. The progression of acromegaly is illustrated in these photographs: *A,* normal, age 9 years; *B,* age 16 years with possible early coarsening of features; *C,* age 33 years, well-established acromegaly; *D,* age 52 years, end-stage acromegaly with gross disfigurement. (Clinical Pathological Conference, *Am. J. Med., 20:*133, 1956.)

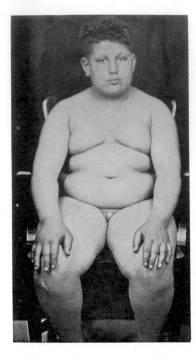

Fig. 144. Frohlich's syndrome showing adiposity and sexual underdevelopment. (Bell, *Textbook of Pathology.*)

lethargy are common. The syndrome or collection of clinical features is perfectly illustrated by the Fat Boy in Pickwick, with his round, chubby face, his fat body fairly bursting through his buttons, his slow mind, and his ability to drop asleep at a moment's notice.

A different form of hypopituitarism is *pituitary dwarfism* (Fig. 142). The patient is bright mentally, but remains small and undeveloped sexually. When he grows up he remains like a graceful and attractive child, a Peter Pan who never really grows up.

Still another form of hypopituitarism is **Simmonds' syndrome,** which is an example of *progeria* or premature senility. When the condition develops in childhood, growth ceases and the patient may present a pathetic picture of a child with the aspect of a decrepit old man or woman (Fig. 145). When Simmond's syndrome develops in an adult it is likely to be the result of necrosis of the anterior pituitary in women during delivery, owing to thrombosis of the pituitary vessels caused by collapse after severe hemorrhage.

The common *cause* of hypopituitarism is an adenoma of the pituitary composed of undifferentiated cells which apparently have not the power of producing pituitary hormones. The cells do not stain well with the dyes used in microscopic work, so that the tumor is known as a *chromophobe adenoma*. The chromophobe adenoma is not only nonfunction-

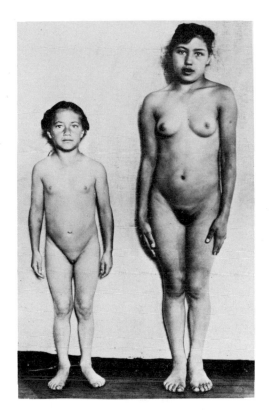

Fig. 145. Hypophyseal infantilism. Girl on left, age 15, sexually infantile, next to normal sister on right, two years younger and fully matured. Striking example of pituitary dwarfism plus sexual infantilism. (Lisser and Escamilla, *Atlas of Clinical Endocrinology*. 2nd Ed., St. Louis, The C. V Mosby Company, 1962.)

ing, but it destroys the functioning cells that produce the hormones and thus leads to pituitary insufficiency. Other lesions may destroy the pituitary, but these are much rarer.

Tumors

The only tumor of the pituitary that we need to consider is the adenoma. Two types of adenoma are recognized, the chromophobe and the acidophil. The **chromophobe adenoma** is composed of cells that contain few or no granules, so that they are colorless (chromophobe) in a stained section. When endocrine symptoms are present they are those of pituitary insufficiency. This is the usual type of adenoma. The **acidophil adenoma** is composed of cells containing granules that stain with acid dyes. As it is these cells that are concerned with skeletal growth, the tumor is associated with gigantism in early life or acromegaly in the adult.

In addition to endocrine symptoms a pituitary adenoma may produce the general symptoms of cerebral tumor such as increased intracranial pressure. If the tumor remains small there will be no general symptoms, but *neighborhood symptoms* caused by pressure on neighboring structures may develop and indicate the correct diagnosis. The pituitary lies between the two optic nerves, so that an adenoma may press on the inner fibers of these nerves causing a peculiar form of blindness involving only half of the visual field on each side. This half blindness is known as **hemianopia.** The tumor also presses on the surrounding bone, causing **enlargement of the sella turcica,** the little bony pocket that contains the pituitary. This enlargement is very evident in the roentgenogram, so it is the radiologist who may make the final diagnosis.

ADRENALS

STRUCTURE AND FUNCTION. The adrenals are two little glands shaped like a cocked hat, one on either side of the spinal column situated just above the kidney. Each adrenal consists of two parts, an outer portion or *cortex* and an inner portion or *medulla*. These are not merely two parts; *they are two different organs joined together as one, different in origin, in structure, in function, and in pathology.*

The **cortex** is essential to life, for when removed on both sides in the animal, death occurs in a few days. For over a hundred years it has been known that patients with adrenal insufficiency often die from minor infections and stresses. We now know that it is the adrenal that enables the body to withstand the large variety of environmental stresses and strains to which it is subjected. The adrenal plays perhaps the largest single role in determining whether a person is sick or well. It is, however, the pituitary that controls the adrenal cortex, through the hormone ACTH, so that the pituitary still remains the master gland. More than 20 distinct steroids with varying degrees of physiological action have been isolated from the adrenal cortex. These may be divided into three groups, which regulate three broad types of body activity, namely, salt or electrolyte balance, carbohydrate metabolism, and sex function. For those of weak memory or mentality, the three functions may be represented as the letter S: salt, sugar and sex. To the more sophisticated they are the mineralocorticoids, the glucocorticoids, and the androgens (masculinizing hormones).

(1) *Mineralocorticoids.* The *salt* or *electrolyte group* of hormones are represented by **aldosterone,** produced by the cells of the first or most superficial layer of the cortex, and the synthetic **deoxycorticosterone.** As the name implies, the hormone governs *sodium* and *chloride retention* and *potassium excretion,* and therefore the amount of fluid in the body. Administration of the hormone leads to edema and increase of body weight due to retention of sodium and chloride, and also fatigue and electrocardiographic changes due to depletion of potassium. **It is**

essential to life. Deficiency of this group of hormones results in the picture of *Addison's disease* and leads to death.

(2) *Glucocorticoids.* The *sugar* or *carbohydrate metabolism group* convert amino acids into sugar instead of into protein, thus increasing blood sugar and the amount of glycogen in the liver. The principal members of this group are **cortisone** and **hydrocortisone,** produced by the second or intermediate layer of the cortex, a production stimulated by ACTH, the adrenocorticotropic hormone of the pituitary. These hormones cause the eosinophils of the blood to disappear and have a destructive action on lymphocytes. In excess they produce the picture of *Cushing's disease,* while deficiency is associated with the lesions seen in Selye's alarm reaction in experimental animals, and possibly with the collagen diseases in man.

In addition to its influence on protein and carbohydrate metabolism, **cortisone suppresses the inflammatory response of the tissues to practically all forms of irritation.** This anti-inflammatory action relieves the pain and discomfort of inflammation, and is of particular value in non-bacterial inflammations such as rheumatoid arthritis and the other collagen diseases, particularly when the inflammation is short-lived, as in acute rheumatic fever. Unfortunately cortisone relieves the symptoms of disease without influencing the cause. It does not put out the fire nor does it repair the damage after the fire, but it does seem to provide the tissues with an asbestos suit, although the suit may be only temporary. We must remember that the object of inflammation is protection and the limitation of infection. In experimental infections treated with cortisone the microorganisms grow unrestrained, a fulminating bacteremia develops, and the animals remain active and happy until they die. It is evident that cortisone is a two-edged sword, which must be used with respect and understanding.

(3) *Androgens.* The *sex* or *nitrogen group* of hormones tend to masculinize the body (*andro,* male) and to build up amino acids and protein from nitrogen. When this hormone is metabolized the substances known as 17-*ketosteroids* are formed and excreted in the urine. The urine is examined for these steroids in cases of virilism where some disorder of the adrenal is suspected. They are extremely low in Addison's disease.

Medulla. The medulla is derived from the sympathetic nervous system, and an extract made from the medulla, known as **Adrenalin** or **epinephrine,** has a remarkable stimulating effect on that system. *Noradrenalin* (norepinephrine), a recently arrived first cousin of epinephrine, is even more potent. When injected into an animal or person it causes a marked rise in the blood pressure owing to contraction of the involuntary muscle in the walls of the arterioles, this contraction in turn being due to stimulation of the sympathetic nerves which supply this muscle. Epinephrine also converts the glycogen in the liver into sugar, which is poured into the blood and at once carried to the voluntary muscles, allowing these to perform a markedly increased amount of work. It appears that under *severe emotional stress* such as rage or fear a marked excess of epinephrine is poured into the blood, thereby enabling the animal or person to perform feats of muscular exertion (attack, flight, etc.) of which he would not ordinarily be capable. This has been called the *emergency function of the adrenals*. It is much more difficult to say what the function of the adrenal medulla is under conditions of ordinary life.

Hypoadrenalism

ACUTE ADRENAL INSUFFICIENCY. Failure of adrenal function may be acute or chronic. The chronic form or Addison's disease was recognized long before the acute form was even thought of. Acute failure is increasing in importance, partly because of the development of adrenalectomy (surgical removal of both adrenals), partly on account of the great popularity of steroid therapy with its organic and functional effects on the adrenal cortex.

An **acute adrenal crisis** may be precipitated in three ways. (1) *Bilateral adrenalectomy* unless accompanied by adequate replacement steroid therapy. At the present time the adrenals are removed principally for carcinoma of the breast and intractable arterial hypertension. (2) *Sudden stress* (trauma, surgical operation, acute illness) superimposed on adrenals gravely damaged by chronic disease or atrophied as the result of prolonged administration of cortisone. (3) *Massive adrenal hemorrhage,* which may occur in the *newborn* and in massive *meningococcal infection,* and nearly always in childhood. This combination of meningococcemia and massive bilateral adrenal hemorrhage is known as the *Waterhouse-Friderichsen syndrome* and marked by acute and fatal peripheral circulatory collapse.

The *clinical picture* of acute adrenal crisis comprises abdominal pain, headache and lassitude, which may be accompanied by nausea, vomiting, and diarrhea. Unless treatment is prompt, acute circulatory collapse develops, terminating in death. The condition is due to loss of sodium and corticosteroids.

ADDISON'S DISEASE. This is a condition of *chronic adrenal insufficiency,* which was described over a hundred years ago by Thomas Addison, of Guy's Hospital, London, who was a colleague of Richard Bright, of Bright's disease fame. It is of great historic interest, because Addison's description was the means of directing attention for the first time to the ductless glands, which had previously been structures of complete mystery. In the years that have intervened since this epoch-making contribution we have come to regard the endocrine glands as among the most important in the entire body.

The *lesions* responsible for the condition are those that destroy both adrenals. Of these, the commonest used to be chronic *tuberculosis,* the infection being carried by the blood from some focus in the lung or elsewhere. More frequent now is *atrophy of the adrenals* for some unknown reason, possibly due to one of the countless new drugs poured into the bodies of patients. In very rare cases there are *tumors* of both glands, either primary or secondary.

Symptoms. The symptoms are multiform. The two most characteristic are a gradually *progressive weakness* and a remarkable *pigmentation of the skin.* This pigmentation varies from a light yellow to a deep brown, and in severe cases the patient may resemble a Hindu in appearance. It is most marked on the nipples, the genital region, and other places which are normally pigmented, as well as on exposed parts such as the face and hands. The *blood pressure* is very low. There may be *gastrointestinal symptoms,* such as nausea, vomiting, and diarrhea. Sometimes these occur in the acute and alarming form known as *crises,* in which abdominal pain is a prominent feature. Hypoglycemia is apt to develop, and death may be due to hypoglycemic shock.

The *biochemical disturbances* produced by the hormonal insufficiency may be summarized as (1) salt and water imbalance, and (2) changes in general metabolism. *Loss of salt and water balance* includes *depletion of sodium and chloride together with a rise in the plasma potassium.* This involves a flow of water from the extracellular compartment into the cells, with an accompanying decrease in plasma volume, fall of blood pressure, and circulatory failure (Fig. 146). A high blood potassium leads to muscular weakness. Interference with salt and water balance may be traced to a deficiency in mineralocorticoids produced by the superficial layer of the cortex. *Changes in general metabolism* affect principally the carbohydrates, and are due to deficiency in the glucocorticoids produced by the intermediate layer of the cortex. Sugar is not formed from the proteins, so that hypoglycemia develops.

Pigmentation is under the influence of a pituitary hormone, the release of which is normally inhibited by cortisone and hydrocortisone from the adrenals. When these are no longer available, the pituitary hormone is produced in excess, and stimulates the pigment-forming cells in the skin, with results that we have already seen.

Mild cases of Addison's disease may be *treated* by the addition of salt to the daily intake. However, in the more severe cases the use of deoxycorticosterone, a synthetic compound that controls the salt and water metabolic disturbances of Addison's disease, will restore the pa-

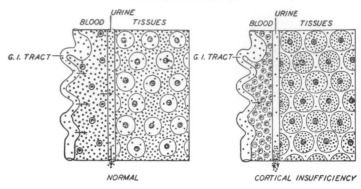

Fig. 146. Distribution of water in a normal animal compared with one with adrenal insufficiency. The stipples represent water molecules. The diagram shows the shift of water from the extracellular compartment (blood and interstitial fluid) into the intracellular compartment with resulting hemoconcentration, vascular collapse, and oliguria. (Turner, *General Endocrinology;* W. B. Saunders Co.)

tient to a normal state in many cases. This may be given by injection or by the implantation of pellets under the skin, from which the drug is slowly absorbed. Cortisone has been found to be satisfactory in the maintenance treatment of these cases. It has to be emphasized that these treatments are by no means a cure for the disease, but merely act as a replacement of the missing hormones.

Hyperadrenalism

Hyperfunction of the adrenals may be either cortical or medullary. Overfunction of the first or superficial layer of the cortex will involve the mineralocorticoids and lead to *aldosteronism;* overfunction of the second layer will involve the glucocorticoids with the clinical picture of the *Cushing syndrome;* overfunction of the deep layer leads to overproduction of sex hormones with resulting *adrenal virilism,* the *adrenogenital* syndrome; overfunction of the medulla leads to *noradrenalism.* The lesion responsible in the case of the cortex is usually bilateral hyperplasia, sometimes adenoma, and rarely carcinoma.

CUSHING'S SYNDROME. In this condition there is a confusing array of symptoms, the only ones that we shall mention being *painful adiposity* confined to the face, neck, and trunk; *hirsutism* in females and preadolescent males; *sexual atrophy;* and *muscular weakness.* The adiposity gives the face a peculiar round appearance to which the name of "full moon face" has been given (Fig. 147C). Although adrenal tumors are rare, Cushing's syndrome has suddenly become of importance, because when patients are given ACTH or cortisone for too long a period, as in rheumatoid arthritis, they tend to develop this peculiar appearance.

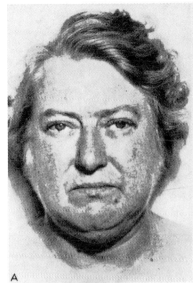
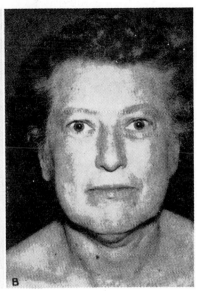

A

B

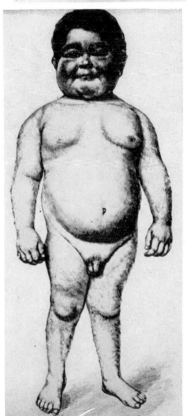

C

Fig. 147. *A*, Face of a patient with Cushing's syndrome due to bilateral hyperplasia of the adrenals. This 45-year-old patient underwent a two-stage bilateral total adrenalectomy. *B*, Disappearance of all signs and symptoms eight months after the second adrenalectomy, during which period patient received complete substitution therapy. (A and B from Williams, *Textbook of Endocrinology*. 4th Ed. Philadelphia, W. B., Saunders Company 1968.) *C*, Adrenal virilism in boy 4½ years of age.

ADRENAL VIRILISM. This condition, known also as the *adreno-genital syndrome,* is due to an excess of masculinizing hormones (androgens), and is marked by premature sexual development in children with an intensification of maleness, a condition known as *virilism.* In boys, even when quite young, there is precocious development of the sex organs, growth of hair on the face (hirsutism), and great muscularity, so that the boy may present the picture vividly termed *the infant Hercules.* In girls and women the uterus and ovaries atrophy, but the clitoris hypertrophies, hair appears on the face and upper lip, the voice becomes deep, and normal healthy interest in the opposite sex is lost. A puzzling feature is the frequent occurrence of *high blood pressure,* which is usually paroxysmal rather than constant. Removal of the tumor in women has been followed by a dramatic return to a normal sexual condition, the change including the voice, the abnormal hair, the blood pressure, and the sex instincts.

ALDOSTERONISM. This is an overproduction of aldosterone, the astonishingly powerful mineralocorticoid produced by the most superficial layer of the cortex, which serves to regulate fluid balance and the excretion of electrolytes, causing *retention of sodium* and *increased loss of potassium.* The biochemical picture is thus the opposite of that of Addison's disease. The *adrenal lesion* is much more likely to be adenoma than cortical hyperplasia or carcinoma.

The *clinical picture* is known as *Conn's syndrome.* It is characterized by *periodic severe muscular weakness amounting to paralysis, arterial hypertension,* and *renal dysfunction.* The serum potassium is very low, thus accounting for the muscular weakness, while the sodium level in the blood is raised. The urinary aldosterone level is extremely high. Surgical removal of the cortical tumor is followed by a dramatic and complete disappearance of the clinical signs and symptoms, including the hypertension.

NORADRENALISM. This term signifies hypersecretion of the hormones of the adrenal medulla. The lesion responsible is *pheochromocytoma,* a *tumor of the medulla* usually benign and unilateral. The classic *clinical picture* is characterized by *symptoms of hypertension, often paroxysmal* rather than continuous. The paroxysms, marked by headache, dyspnea, dizziness, vomiting, and convulsive twitching are often precipitated by stooping or abdominal palpation.

THYROID GLAND

STRUCTURE AND FUNCTION. The thyroid gland is an organ of some size, shaped like a shield, which lies on either side of the neck in the region of the larynx. It is composed entirely of a large number of spaces or *acini,* lined by low epithelial cells, and filled with jelly-like material

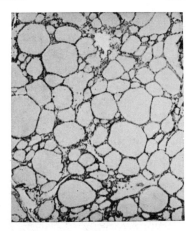

Fig. 148. Microscopic picture of normal thyroid gland.

known as *colloid,* which is richer in iodine than any other substance in the body (Fig. 148). Between the acini run thin-walled capillaries, into which the secretion of the epithelial cells is poured. But part of this secretion, when not actively needed by the body, passes into the acini and is stored as colloid, which may be regarded as an emergency ration to be given up to the body on demand.

The chief **function** of the thyroid is to maintain a certain rate of metabolism, as evidenced by oxygen consumption and heat production, and to regulate this rate according to the needs of the body. This is done by means of its iodine-containing hormone, *thyroxin.* The effect of feeding thyroid gland or injecting thyroxin is to raise the rate of metabolism. Removal of the thyroid is followed not only by a loss of heat production, but also by poor physical, mental, and sexual development, most marked, of course, in the young. It would appear, therefore, that an adequate supply of thyroid secretion is necessary for the development of the young animal. Similarly an excess of secretion will accelerate development, as can be shown by the rapidity with which thyroxin brings about the change from a tadpole into a frog. *Thyroid secretion appears to act as a general and necessary stimulant without which there can be no health or vigor of the body, no flash and speed of the mind.* Someone with a turn for the picturesque has remarked that thyroxin converts the sluggish toad into the lively frog. The bearing of these observations will become very evident when diseases of the thyroid are considered.

The iodides consumed in food and water are absorbed and carried to the iodide pool in the extracellular fluid, from which they pass into the blood. The thyroid has been called the *iodide trap,* the only one in the body. It functions to the iodide in the blood flowing through its vessels as a flypaper does to the flies in its neighborhood. The iodide trap can be paralyzed by so-called antithyroid drugs such as thiouracil. Thyroxin cannot now be formed on account of lack of iodine, so that these drugs can be used in the treatment of hyperthyroidism.

The activity of the thyroid can also be gauged by estimating the **basal metabolic rate** (BMR), the amount of metabolism in a person at complete physical and mental rest. This is actually done by determining the amount of oxygen consumed when a person is under these basal conditions. If during the test the person makes the slightest physical or mental exertion, the metabolic rate at once goes up, and the test is invalidated. Even the effort required to digest a meal is sufficient to spoil the test.

Iodine is found in the blood in two forms: (1) *inorganic iodide,* and (2) *organic* or *protein-bound iodine.* The level of protein-bound iodine, abbreviated to PBI, is a reliable index of thyroid secretory activity, and is therefore used as a laboratory test for thyroid function. The normal PBI level is 4 to 8 μg. per cent. In hypothyroidism (myxedema) it is about 2 μg. per cent, whereas in hyperthyroidism it is usually around 15 μg., but may go up as high as 30 μg. per cent.

The introduction of *radioactive iodine* or I^{131} has advanced our knowledge of thyroid physiology in health and disease, for the labeled iodine can be followed by means of a Geiger counter from the source of the raw material to the factory, thence to the warehouse (the thyroid), and finally to the users (the tissues). The *radioactive iodine uptake* (RAIU) provides a valuable laboratory test, together with the PBI, for the state of thyroid activity. It indicates the degree of *avidity* of the thyroid for the iodine in the iodide pool. Thus iodine-deficient goiters, to which group most endemic goiters belong, will be associated with a high RAIU, as the gland hungrily soaks up what iodine is available.

The thyroid takes iodine from the blood that flows through it and converts it into thyroxin, and gives it back to the blood or stores it as the case may be. If there is an insufficiency of iodine (as iodide) in the food or water, the thyroid finds itself in the same position as the Children of Israel when they were ordered by the Egyptians to make bricks without straw. But as the Israelites rose to the occasion by redoubling their efforts, so the thyroid responds by working overtime, and in doing so it becomes larger. This enlargement is known as *goiter.* It is evident that this enlargement is compensatory in character, being analogous to the enlargement of the heart when that organ is given too much work to do. It is not associated with symptoms of hyperthyroidism or overactivity of the thyroid. Other forms of goiter, as we shall see, are of a different nature, and are accompanied by marked symptoms of hyperthyroidism.

The **pituitary-thyroid axis** is a term that indicates that an intimate relationship exists between the thyroid and the anterior pituitary. The thyroid-stimulating or *thyrotropic hormone* (TSH) of the pituitary is the most powerful known stimulant of thyroid activity. The TSH probably acts mainly by increasing the collection or trapping of iodide, but it may also have some effect on the synthesis of thyroxin. As the term axis suggests, there is a two-way activity, for the thyroid hormone inhibits the production of TSH in the pituitary, so that a balance is maintained in health. Theoretically this balance may be upset at either end.

Goiter

The term goiter simply indicates enlargement of the thyroid. This enlargement may be due to more than one cause, such as iodine deficiency or overstimulation by the pituitary, and the clinical picture will vary accordingly. It is customary to recognize three forms of goiter: (1) simple or diffuse colloid goiter, (2) nodular or adenomatous goiter, and (3) exophthalmic goiter or Graves' disease. The last-named is essentially a manifestation of hyperthyroidism and will be considered under that heading.

SIMPLE COLLOID GOITER. This is by far the commonest form of goiter. It is known by a variety of names: *adolescent goiter,* because it so frequently occurs during the years of adolescence; *endemic goiter,* because it is prevalent in certain regions and peoples (*demos,* people); and *colloid goiter,* because it is characterized by an accumulation of colloid in the acini with corresponding dilatation of these spaces and consequent enlargement of the gland. The regions where goiter is endemic are the Alpine districts of Switzerland and the Himalayas where almost every thyroid gland is more or less enlarged, the region of the Great Lakes in North America, and the valley of the St. Lawrence River. These areas have one thing in common: the soil is poor in iodine, so that the enlargement of the thyroid is compensatory in character, a work hypertrophy in order to perform the necessary amount of work with an inadequate supply of raw material. Animals as well as men living in these regions tend to suffer from this deficiency form of goiter. The occurrence of goiter during adolescence is due to a relative deficiency in iodine. The demands on the thyroid made by the girl at puberty blossoming out into womanhood are greater than those in later life, and it is for this reason that the enlargement is usually only temporary, the gland returning to its normal size when the period of stress is past.

The incidence of this form of goiter has been greatly diminished in certain endemic districts by the judicious use of iodine in the form of iodized salt. In one part of Ohio a mass experiment was performed by giving the school children a small amount of iodized salt for one or two weeks twice a year (spring and fall), and this simple expedient was followed by an astonishing reduction in the incidence of goiter in the school community, a striking demonstration of the value of the application of the results of scientific research in the laboratory to the needs of the people.

Lesions.   The lesions of simple goiter depend on the stage of the disease. During the early and more active stage, the chief microscopic change is hyperplasia, an overgrowth of the glandular epithelium which will be more fully described in connection with exophthalmic goiter. When the demand for increased work is no longer felt the gland tends to return to its former state. Should the supply of iodine be much below normal, a stage of exhaustion follows the overactivity, and although the epithelial hyperplasia disappears, the acini become distended with colloid, and the thyroid may remain permanently enlarged. Such colloid goiters are met with at any period of adult life, and these are the goiters that are so prevalent in Switzerland and the hill districts of India.

Symptoms.   The symptoms of simple goiter, apparent from enlargement of the neck, are naturally few or absent, for the needs of the body are attended to by the work hypertrophy. Occasionally the hyperplasia may be carried too far, so that the girl may suffer from nervous irritability and other signs of hyperthyroidism. On the other hand, the return of the gland to a colloid state may be attended by symptoms of thyroid insufficiency. In the great majority of cases, however, the only evidence of disease (if it can be called such) is the enlargement of the neck (Fig. 149).

The *treatment* of simple goiter consists of providing an adequate supply of iodine, and regulating the life of the patient so that no undue strain is thrown on the organism during the critical period at which the goiter is likely to develop. From what has already been said it is evident that operation is the worst thing that could be done for such a patient.

NODULAR OR ADENOMATOUS GOITER.   In adult life a rather different form of goiter may develop, again more common in goitrous districts. The thyroid is not only enlarged, but is also nodular, the nodules being called adenomas. These may be regarded as the result of repeated hyperplasia followed by involution, the process affecting some parts of the gland more than others so that a series of nodules tend to develop, some of considerable size. Microscopically, these nodules may show either hyperplasia or a resting colloid condition. With the passage of years they tend gradually to become larger.

Symptoms.   The symptoms of adenomatous goiter may be of two different varieties. The chief symptom is *pressure* of an adenoma upon surrounding structures, especially the trachea, causing difficulty in breathing. Or there may be so-called *toxic symptoms,* indications of hyperthyroidism, such as rapid pulse, tremors, nervousness, sweating,

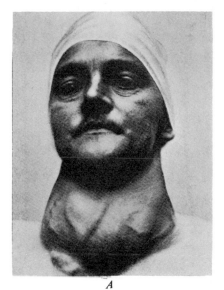 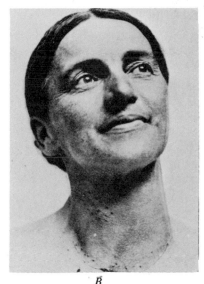

A *B*

Fig. 149. *A,* Diffuse multinodular colloid goiter, showing the compressed veins and congested appearance of the face. *B,* Same patient 15 days after removal of the goiter. Note rapid relief of congestion of the veins of the face. (From de Quervain: Goitre and Thyroid Diseases. New York, William Wood & Co., 1924.)

and an increased basal metabolic rate. In these cases there is evidently an overproduction of thyroxin by the adenomas, for these are the very symptoms produced by an injection of thyroxin or by an overdose of thyroid extract. Such a clinical condition is known as *toxic adenoma,* and is similar in many ways to that of exophthalmic goiter except that there is no exophthalmos. The main danger is the effect on the circulatory system. The blood pressure is raised, and the constant acceleration of the heart's action, which may last for years, gradually leads to cardiac exhaustion.

Treatment consists in removal of the part of the thyroid containing the adenomas. It is evident that this must not be delayed too long, else the heart may suffer irreparable damage.

Hyperthyroidism

Hyperthyroidism is overactivity of the thyroid with overproduction of thyroxin. We have already seen that it may occur in so-called toxic adenoma when localized hyperplasia is marked. The most striking manifestation of hyperthyroidism is afforded by exophthalmic goiter or Graves' disease, which will be considered now.

GRAVES' DISEASE. Graves' disease or *exophthalmic goiter* is marked clinically by the classic triad of: (1) *hyperthyroidism,* the picture produced by an excess of thyroxin, (2) *exophthalmos* or protrusion of the eyeballs, and (3) *goiter.* Unfortunately one or another of these may be absent, at least for a time. That is why Graves' disease is a more satisfying name than exophthalmic goiter. The condition is characterized by hyperplasia of the gland and great overactivity of its function, but without any corresponding call on the part of the body for such overactivity. There is often a very definite history of nervous or psychic shock, or some terrifying experience, which is sometimes followed in the course of a few days by the development of the symptoms. This suggests that the disease is in some way connected with the nervous system. It seems probable that overstimulation of the thyroid by the TSH of the pituitary gland is the basis of the disease. This idea may ultimately lead to some satisfactory form of treatment.

Lesions. The lesions are due to diffuse epithelial hyperplasia. The thyroid is diffusely enlarged, but not necessarily to a great degree, and presents no nodules. The cut surface has a dense, meaty appearance, in marked contrast to the translucency of the normal thyroid or the colloid goiter. The microscopic appearance presents a great change in structure; for the normal colloid in the acini has disappeared and is replaced by numerous projections of epithelium from the lining of the acini (Fig. 150). (Compare Fig. 150 with Fig. 148.) It is, therefore, a picture of great glandular activity. The thyroxin that is normally stored in the colloid has gone, having been poured into the blood stream. The blood vessels in the walls of the acini are widely dilated.

Symptoms. Graves' disease is much commoner in women than in men in the proportion of 5 to 1. It usually begins in early adult life, and the onset is often sudden and acute. The symptoms are those of extreme overactivity of the thyroid. The patient has a strained tense expression and is in a highly *nervous excitable condition.* The outstretched hands show a fine *tremor.* The pulse is very rapid (*tachycardia*) and *palpitation* is common, the *skin* is *moist,* and the patient is peculiarly *insensitive to cold* owing to the heat produced by the excessive metabolism, which is indicated by the *high metabolic rate.* It is as if some blast were blowing on the furnace of the body, fanning it to furious activity. The nitrogen of the tissues is consumed by this fire, so that the patient wastes away. A peculiar symptom, which gives its name to the disease, is *exophthalmos* or protrusion of the eyeballs. The staring eyes, the strained expression, and the enlargement of the neck give the patient so striking an appearance that in a severe case the diagnosis can be made at a glance (Fig. 151). The exophthalmos is peculiarly difficult to explain, because it bears no direct relation to the degree of hyper-

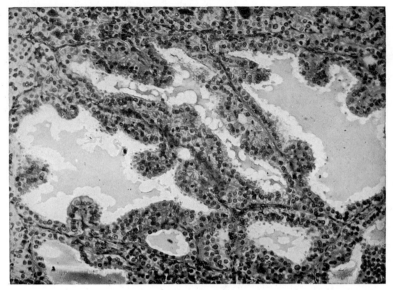

Fig. 150. Thyroid of Graves' disease undergoing involution under iodine treatment. The papillary processes are being withdrawn from the enlarged acini, and the colloid is reappearing. Above and below there is still dense hyperplastic tissue. × 150. This picture should be compared with Fig. 148. (Boyd, *Textbook of Pathology;* Lea & Febiger).

thyroidism, nor can it be produced by the administration of thyroxin to laboratory animals. It is now believed that it is related to overactivity of the anterior pituitary which elaborates some exophthalmos-producing substance. The actual displacement of the eyes is due to edema of the fat tissue at the back of the orbit.

The *course* of the disease varies. In some cases it is acute and fulminating, the patient being consumed by the inward fire and dying of exhaustion. More frequently the course is marked by exacerbations and remissions without any apparent cause; gradually the fire burns itself out, the thyroid becomes incapable of hyperplasia, and the final picture may be one of thyroid insufficiency or myxedema.

There are *several methods of treatment* of hyperthyroidism now available and the choice of treatment in an individual case depends on several factors and must be selected in light of the severity of the disease, the patient's age, heart complications, and other situations. *Propylthiouracil* or methylthiouracil will control the disease in many cases by reducing the amount of thyroxin liberated from the gland. Some cases may be controlled in this manner for periods of six to twelve months or longer, and subsequently they remain normal after one or more courses of such treatment. Or alternatively, after such preparation with

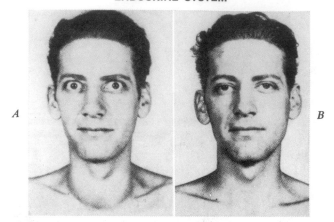

Fig. 151. *A,* Exophthalmic goiter in man, age 27; duration, 16 months. BMR, plus 85%; sleeping pulse rate, 110; radioiodine uptake, 72% in 24 hours. Note staring expression and uniform enlargement of thyroid; thrill and bruit present. *B,* Same patient four months after treatment with 6.4 millicuries of I^{131}. Marked improvement one month after administration. Note calmer expression, recession of exophthalmos, and disappearance of goiter. Pulse normal; BMR, minus 10%. Had slight hypothyroidism for one year; did not require thyroid medication; was well and active eight years later. (Lisser and Escamilla, *Atlas of Clinical Endocrinology.* 2nd Ed., St. Louis, The C. V. Mosby Company, 1962.)

this drug, *removal of the thyroid gland* may be performed which will result in a cure of the condition in a large majority of patients. The introduction of *radioactive iodine* as a treatment measure in this condition offers another possibility. Here radioactive iodine is deposited in the active thyroid gland and emits radiation in diminishing amounts over a period of two weeks, during which time the active tissue is either destroyed or returned to a normal functional state. This method of treatment requires the provision of very careful laboratory control of the administration of this potentially dangerous method of treatment.

Hypothyroidism

So far we have discussed overactivity of the thyroid as evidenced by symptoms of hyperthyroidism. An exactly opposite picture results from hypothyroidism, but the effect differs greatly, depending on whether the deficiency of thyroid secretion is due to absence of development of the gland during fetal life or to atrophy of an already developed thyroid in adult life. The former condition, which is congenital, is known as *cretinism;* the latter condition, which is acquired, is called *myxedema.*

CRETINISM. A cretin is an individual in whom the thyroid has failed to develop, so that a study of the disease serves to throw light on the functions of the gland. We have already seen that normal thyroid func-

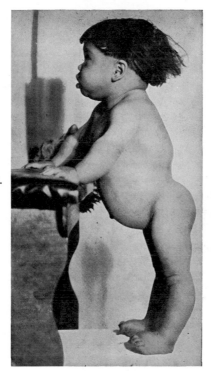

Fig. 152. A cretin.

tion is necessary for the proper development of the body and the mind. The cretin is a dwarf physically and mentally (Fig. 152). The mind, the skeleton, and the sexual organs do not develop. Like Peter Pan, the cretin never grows up, but he has none of Peter's vivacity, for the vitalizing influence of the thyroid is lacking. He is a sad, old child. Sir William Osler's pen picture of the cretin is a masterpiece: "No type of human transformation is more distressing to look at than an aggravated case of cretinism. The stunted stature, the semi-bestial aspect, the blubber lips, retroussé nose sunken at the root, the wide-open mouth, the lolling tongue, the small eyes half closed with swollen lids, the stolid expressionless face, the squat figure, the muddy dry skin, combine to make the picture of what has been termed, the pariah of Nature."

Cretinism occurs in two forms, endemic and sporadic. *Endemic cretinism* is very common in the great regions of endemic goiter, the Alps and the Himalayas. The mother suffers from simple goiter, and the tragedy of cretinism can be prevented by giving the pregnant woman a sufficient supply of iodine. The *sporadic form* develops in nonendemic regions, and is fortunately a rare disease. The mother is not goitrous,

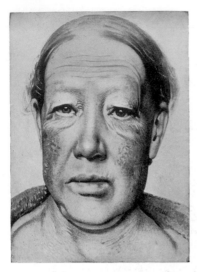

Fig. 153. Myxedema. (Bramwell's *Atlas of Clinical Medicine.*)

but apparently something interferes with the development of the thyroid during fetal life.

If *treatment* with thyroid extract is not commenced until a few years have passed it is useless to hope that the child may be restored to normal, for the critical period of brain development has been lost; "the moving finger writes, and, having writ, moves on."

MYXEDEMA. This is thyroid deficiency in the adult. Like other diseases of the thyroid, it is commoner in women, usually appearing about the age of 40 years. The thyroid atrophies until only a remnant is left, but the cause of the atrophy is unknown. It is not commoner in the regions of endemic goiter than elsewhere.

The *clinical picture* in an advanced case can be recognized at a glance, for it is the reverse of that of Graves' disease (Fig. 153). All the processes, both mental and physical, are slower, the fire burns low, the basal metabolism is much below normal. The patient is heavy, obese, intensely phlegmatic, and will sit for hours without moving. The face is broad, the features coarse like those of an Eskimo. The skin is rough, dry, and wrinkled, and the patient is very sensitive to cold. Premature baldness is common and the hair falls out of the outer third of the eyebrow. There is an infiltration of the skin with a mucus-like substance, giving an appearance of edema but not pitting on pressure. It is this infiltration which gives the disease its name, and which is responsible for the ironing away of all lines of expression in the face, so that most myxedema patients look more or less alike. A comparison of Figures 153 and 151 will serve to demonstrate some of the differences between myxedema and Graves' disease.

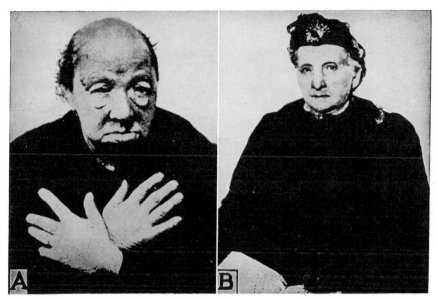

Fig. 154. *A,* Myxedema of 20 years' duration; patient bedridden and imbecile. *B,* After treatment with thyroid extract; the same patient 30 years later, aged 94 years. (Harrington, *The Thyroid Gland—Its Chemistry and Physiology;* Oxford University Press.)

The above description applies to the full-blown case. Milder degrees of thyroid insufficiency are very much commoner, and are much more difficult to recognize. Increased sensitiveness to cold is always suggestive of the condition, and the diagnosis can be confirmed by testing the basal metabolic rate.

Treatment consists in giving thyroid extract (thyroxin) by mouth. Few therapeutic results are more dramatic. The metabolic fire begins to burn again, the infiltration of the skin disappears, the normal lines and expression of the face return, the mind reawakens, the patient becomes indeed a new man, or rather a new woman (Fig. 154).

Tumors

There are two main types of tumors of the thyroid, adenoma and carcinoma. Each of these has been endlessly subdivided, but we shall not concern ourselves with these minutiae.

ADENOMA. From what has already been said it is evident that it may be very difficult to determine when a lump in the thyroid is really adenoma, *i.e.* a neoplasm, or when it is merely a nodular hyperplasia. The chief characteristics of a true adenoma are the pressure of a single nodule compared with the multiple nodules of nodular goiter, good encapsulation, and a different growth pattern from that of the surrounding gland. One of the most contentious matters in relation to thyroid adenoma is the possibility that it may develop into carcinoma. Certain it is that the occasional case may do so. The difficulty is to say how frequent is this occurrence. This is not the place to engage in such a debate.

CARCINOMA. Cancer of the thyroid varies enormously in microscopic structure, in rate of growth, and in the danger of spread. Some of these tumors are very indolent in growth, extending slowly. Others are highly anaplastic and disseminate rapidly and widely by the blood stream. The *microscopic appearance* agrees to some extent with the speed of spread, but seeing that in this book we have tried to avoid the question of microscopic appearance, it would be well if we did not pursue this subject.

Secondary carcinoma of the thyroid is uncommon, with the exception of bronchogenic carcinoma and malignant melanoma.

PARATHYROID GLANDS

STRUCTURE AND FUNCTION. In the wonderful volume of endocrine romance there are few more thrilling chapters than that dealing with the story of the parathyroids. For more than seventy years the presence of these four tiny glands, each no larger than a pea, had been known. They are situated in the neck, two on each side behind the thyroid, but their function was not even guessed at. Gradually it came to be suspected that they had something to do with the regulation of calcium metabolism, but it was not until Collip, in 1925, succeeded in preparing an extract of their active principle, which he called *parathormone,* that a flood of light was cast upon the subject.

By injecting the extract into animals it was found that an amazing *mobilization of the calcium in the body* was brought about. Normally the calcium in the food is absorbed from the bowel, carried by the blood to the bones, and stored in the skeleton which acts as the great reservoir of calcium in the body, just as the thyroid is the reservoir of iodine. The normal average is 10 mg. per 100 cc., with a range of 9 to 11 mg. Calcium is essential for tissue health and activity, but it must be supplied in minute and exactly correct amounts. In health this small amount is given up by the bones to the blood, and carried to the body in general and to the muscles in particular. When parathyroid extract is injected into an animal, the mobilization of calcium is enormously augmented, and the blood is flooded with calcium, which pours through the kidneys into the urine and is lost to the body. As a result of this loss the bones become decalcified, they lose their rigidity and are easily bent, they no longer cast a dense shadow in the roentgenogram, and cystic spaces develop in their substance.

The plasma calcium level has to be regulated with great accuracy, because at levels under 4 to 5 mg. per cent the patient may have tetanic convulsions and die, whereas at high calcium levels fatal nephrocalcinosis and cardiac disturbances may occur. It used to be thought that the remarkable constancy of the plasma calcium level, what may be termed **calcium homeostasis,** was entirely due to parathormone; when the calcium level fell more parathormone was produced, and when the level became too high the hormone production was decreased. In 1962 Copp showed by an ingenious and elegant series of experiments that this is not so. The lowering of calcium to the normal level depends on a second hormone, a hypocalcemic factor, called by Copp **calcitonin,** because it is involved in regulating the level or "tone" of calcium in body fluids. There is thus a highly efficient "calciostat" with dual hormonal feed-back mechanism that accounts for the precise control of the level of plasma calcium in the normal animal. This may be compared with the production of two hormones by the islets of the pancreas, insulin and glucagon, both involved in the regulation of the level of blood glucose.

At first the parathyroids were thought to be the site of production of calcitonin, but now it is known that it is formed by the cells of the ultimobranchial glands situated just below the parathyroids in the lower vertebrates such as the salmon, but which become fused with the thyroid and to a lesser extent with the parathyroids in mammals. For this reason the hormone is sometimes called *thyrocalcitonin.*

It becomes evident that the maintenance of a constant serum calcium level is mediated by the action of the hypercalcemic hormone, parathormone, and the hypocalcemic hormone, calcitonin. Fortunately calcitonin has now been synthesized, as it may possibly have considerable therapeutic value in osteoporosis and similar diseases such as Paget's disease of bone (see p. 526), in which there is early rarefaction, followed later by overproduction of bone.

Like the thyroid and other ductless glands the parathyroids may show disturbance in the direction either of underactivity or overactivity. In underactivity or *hypoparathyroidism* there is insufficient mobilization of calcium, and the tissues are starved of that element; in overactivity or *hyperparathyroidism* there is undue mobilization of calcium; the blood is flooded but the bones are depleted.

Hyperparathyroidism

Hyperparathyroidism can be produced experimentally by the administration of parathyroid extract, but in human pathology it is the result of the growth of a parathyroid tumor. This is an innocent tumor, an adenoma, but the effect it produces on the body may be far from inno-

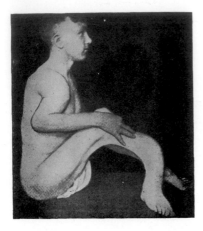

Fig. 155. Osteitis fibrosa cystica. Showing marked bending of the arms and legs.

cent. The adenoma may be no larger than a bean or it may be the size of a plum, but even a large tumor may not be detected by the physician because it is tucked away behind the thyroid. It is readily recognized, however, by the remarkable effects that it produces.

In 1891 the Viennese pathologist, von Recklinghausen, described a peculiar disorder of bones which is known as *osteitis fibrosa cystica* or *von Recklinghausen's disease*. In this condition the bones are softened as the result of decalcification, and the softened bones, having lost their rigidity, become greatly deformed. The arms and legs are bent (Fig. 155), the pelvis is wedge-shaped, there is spinal curvature, and there is a loss of weight. With the passage of the years it has come to be recognized that such a picture may be given by fibrous dysplasia of bone, and it is possible that the patient shown in Figure 155 may have suffered from this condition. Severe pains in the bones are a distressing feature. It is now known that this long-recognized disease of bones is due to the presence of a previously unsuspected tumor of one of the parathyroids. A striking feature in many cases is the formation of cysts in the bones, readily seen in roentgenogram; these cysts may so weaken the bones that *spontaneous fractures* occur.

Two other points of importance are the condition of the blood and the condition of the kidneys. The *blood is flooded with calcium* from the bones, so that the normal blood calcium of 10 mg. per 100 cc. is raised, sometimes to 18 or even 20 mg. Other conditions associated with decalcification, such as secondary tumors of bone, may cause the blood calcium to be raised, but there is an additional blood change which is even more characteristic of hyperparathyroidism, *i.e., lowered blood phosphorus.* Calcium in bone is combined with phosphorus in the form of calcium phosphate, so that it might be supposed that the blood phosphorus would also be raised in the decalcification of hyperparathyroidism. But in this condition the permeability of the kidney for phosphorus is markedly lowered, so that more escapes into the urine than is poured into the blood from the bones, and the level of the blood phosphorus is accordingly lowered.

The *kidneys* may show a change of very great importance, namely, *deposits of calcium*. The calcium pouring from the blood into the urine may be partly arrested in the kidney, giving a shadow in the roentgenogram. Sometimes these deposits of calcium form a *stone in the kidney,* even though the changes in the bones may be comparatively slight. It is, therefore, desirable in every case of stone in the kidney to estimate the blood calcium and phosphorus in order to determine if a parathyroid tumor may be the underlying cause of the stone.

Treatment by removal of the tumor in the neck, even though this be so small that it cannot be felt, is followed by dramatic consequences. The blood calcium at once falls and the phosphorus rises to normal, the pains in the bones are relieved; in a remarkably short space of time the bones become recalcified, and the patient is converted from a chronic invalid to a robust individual.

Hypoparathyroidism

The chief clinical manifestation of hypoparathyroidism is *tetany*. This is a disorder marked by intermittent muscular contractions affecting particularly the hands and feet which are drawn into peculiar attitudes that are highly characteristic. These spasms are due to *increased irritability of the muscles,* which in turn is *due to the low calcium content of the blood.* The condition used to be common in the early days of the surgical treatment of goiter, when the great importance of leaving the parathyroids behind when the thyroid was removed was not properly recognized. Tetany may also occur in other disturbances of calcium metabolism such as rickets, but this aspect of the subject need not be entered into here. The disorder is at once relieved by the administration of parathyroid extract, which ensures an adequate supply of calcium to the starved muscles.

ISLETS OF LANGERHANS

The islets of Langerhans are small groups of cells scattered through the pancreas, which really constitute one of the endocrine glands, for they pour their secretion or hormone into the blood and not into the intestine like the pancreatic cells proper. The hormone of the islets is known as *insulin.* Like the other endocrine glands, there may be underactivity or overactivity of the islets, *i.e.,* hypoinsulinism and hyperinsulinism. *Hypoinsulinism* is the condition known as diabetes, which has already been studied in connection with the pancreas. It is relieved by the administration of insulin.

Hyperinsulinism

Hyperinsulinism is caused by the presence of a *tumor of the islets,* which may be either a benign adenoma or a carcinoma of low malignancy. The *symptoms,* which are remarkable and highly distinctive, are due to a condition of *hypoglycemia* or lowering of the blood sugar (glucose). The normal blood sugar is about 1 per cent, but when an excess of insulin is produced the blood sugar may fall to low levels. When it reaches 0.5 per cent symptoms of hypoglycemia develop, which are similar to those caused by an overdose of insulin (*insulin shock*). The patient suffers from attacks of faintness of increasing severity, convulsions, and loss of consciousness. The tell-tale feature of these attacks is that they always occur when the patient has been fasting for some hours, the sugar absorbed from his last meal being exhausted. The attacks can be prevented by eating sugar, and even when the patient is unconscious the injection of glucose solution into the blood will at once revive him. As the tumor grows in size, the attacks increase in severity, and the only adequate treatment is removal of the tumor. Such removal is usually not difficult for the skilled surgeon, and is followed by brilliant and most satisfactory results.

FURTHER READING

Copp, D. H., *et al.:* Endocrinology, 1962, *70,* 638. (Calcitonin.)

Copp, D. H.: Am. Rev. Physiol., 1970, *32,* 61. (Endocrine regulation of calcium metabolism.)

Ezrin, C.: Ciba Foundation Clinical Symposia, 1963, *15,* 71. (The pituitary gland.)

Levitt, T.: *The Thyroid, a Physiological, Clinical and Surgical Study,* Edinburgh, 1954.

Simpson, S. L.: *Major Endocrine Disorders,* 3rd ed., London, 1959.

Thorn, G. W.: *Diseases and Treatment of Adrenal Insufficiency,* Springfield, Ill., 1951.

Blood and Lymph Nodes

BLOOD

Structure and Function

The hematopoietic system consists of the bone marrow, the circulating blood, and the lymphoid tissue. The cells of the blood in extrauterine life are formed in the bone marrow, *but only in the red marrow* which is confined to the flat bones, *i.e.,* vertebrae, sternum, ribs, skull, and pelvic bones. The marrow in the interior of the long bones is called *yellow marrow,* consisting almost entirely of fat. When the marrow has to be examined during life it is taken from the upper part of the sternum with a needle and syringe. The blood should really be regarded as a tissue, for it is composed of cells, the red and white blood corpuscles,

451

and intracellular stroma, the plasma, which happens to be fluid for reasons of motility, because the red cells must move in order to function. These three tissues together constitute one of the largest organs in the body. The total volume of the blood is from 4000 to 8000 cc., depending on the size of the individual.

In this consideration of the diseases of the blood and the blood-forming organs we are concerned mainly with the blood cells. These are of two varieties, the red cells or erythrocytes (*erythros,* red), and the leukocytes or white cells (*leukos,* white). In addition there is a third element, the blood platelets, minute particles which cannot be regarded as cells. In the case of both the red and the white cells there may be too few cells or too many cells. A diminution in the number of cells is always a sign of disease. An increase in the number may be a manifestation of blood disease, or it may be a physiological response to a temporary demand from the body for more red or white cells; the leukocytosis of infection is an example of the latter condition.

THE ERYTHROCYTES. The erythrocytes are globules filled with hemoglobin, which gives them their color, but *possessing no nucleus.* The shape is that of a *biconcave disc,* because this gives the largest interface between each erythrocyte and plasma, thus ensuring not only efficient absorption and release of gases, but ready penetration of gases from the surface to the center of the cell. Under disease conditions the biconcave shape may be lost, and the cell becomes spherical (*spherocytosis*) with unfortunate results as we shall see presently.

In health the erythrocytes number from 5,000,000 to 6,000,000 per c.mm. in the male, and from 4,500,000 to 5,000,000 per c.mm. in the female. They are formed in the bone marrow. Some knowledge of this formation is necessary for an understanding of what happens in anemia, the commonest disease affecting the red blood cells. In the bone marrow, in addition to the vessels through which the blood circulates, there is a series of lagoons or sinusoids in which red cells are formed and released into the blood stream as required. The endothelial cells lining the sinusoids give rise to large nucleated cells called primitive erythroblasts (Fig. 156). These are the earliest blood cells, and they do not at first contain any hemoglobin, the coloring matter of the red cells which enables them to perform their sole function, the carrying of oxygen from the lungs to the tissues and the return of carbon dioxide from the tissues to the lungs. The primitive erythroblasts multiply, and their daughter cells develop into *normoblasts, i.e.,* smaller cells which become filled with hemoglobin but still retain a nucleus. The last stage of development is the change from a normoblast into an *erythrocyte,* which is brought about by loss of the nucleus. The adult erythrocyte is the only cell in the body that does not possess a nucleus, and as a

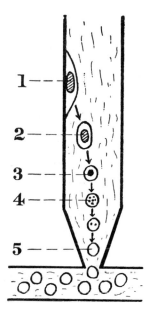

Fig. 156. Steps in the formation of red blood cells. Immature cells in marrow sinusoids maturing and entering blood stream. 1, Endothelial cell; 2, primitive erythroblast; 3, normoblast; 4, reticulocyte; 5, erythrocyte.

nucleus is essential to the life of a cell, it follows that the days of an erythrocyte are numbered. Their average duration of life is from 100 to 120 days.

The *developing red cells* show changes not only in their nucleus, but also in their cytoplasm. The cytoplasm of the early cell is basophilic, that is to say it stains blue owing to the presence of ribonucleic acid, but as hemoglobin gradually begins to make its appearance the cytoplasm presents a slaty color, a mixture of red and blue which is given the descriptive name of *polychromatophilia* (love of many colors). When a wet film is stained with brilliant cresyl blue the basophilic substance appears in the form of a fine reticulum with no diffuse staining. Young erythrocytes which stain in this manner are known as *reticulocytes*. Finally, as a result of pathological processes, lead poisoning in particular, the basophilic substance may become aggregated into granules in the fixed film, a condition known as *basophilic stippling* or *punctate basophilia* of the red cells. I have introduced these three terms because when detected in the laboratory their presence points to the entry of immature red cells from the marrow into the circulating blood, and indicates the possibility of some serious blood condition such as hemolytic anemia.

Hemoglobin. Hemoglobin is the essence of the erythrocyte, whose function it is to carry oxygen from the lungs to the tissues. In the normal adult the quantity of hemoglobin is about 16 gm. per cent in males and

14 gm. in females. Perhaps the simplest and most accurate method of determining the *hemoglobin content* is to expel a measured amount of blood into a fixed volume of diluting fluid and read the mixture with the aid of a photoelectric colorimeter.

Packed Cell Volume. This is measured by the hematocrit. Blood is drawn into a *hematocrit tube* 10 cm. long, which is centrifuged until the cells are completely packed, and the result read on the graduated tube. The volume of packed cells is normally about 47 cc. for males and 42 cc. for females per 100 cc. of blood. When the cells are smaller than normal the hematocrit reading will be lower, and when the cells are larger, as in macrocytic anemia, the reading will be higher.

The *color index* used to be the important method of determining the mean corpuscular hemoglobin, but it has been largely replaced by the methods outlined above. The color index is determined by dividing the percentage of hemoglobin by the percentage of erythrocytes compared with the normal.

It must be emphasized that a *well-stained blood smear* studied by an educated eye and brain still affords one of the best means of arriving at an accurate diagnosis. It provides the observer with information as to the size and shape of the red cells, the concentration of hemoglobin in these cells, and the presence of nucleated cells and reticulocytes. The size and shape of the red cells demand special attention. *Anisocytosis* or variation in size and *poikilocytosis* or variation in shape are indications of disease. Anisocytosis is seen very early in pernicious anemia, while poikilocytosis develops at a later stage and helps in the diagnosis. All of these abnormalities tell us something of the functional activity of the bone marrow.

Sedimentation Rate. The sedimentation rate of red blood cells is an indication of the suspension stability of these cells, and may be taken as a *nonspecific index of the presence and intensity of organic disease*, being comparable in this respect to fever and leukocytosis. The rate of sedimentation is expressed as the distance in millimeters which the cells fall in one hour. The rate depends on the type of tube in which the test is carried out. With the Wintrobe tube the average rate for men is about 3.5 and for women 9.5. With the Westergren tube the figures are somewhat higher. There is, however, a wide normal variation. An increase is present in destructive disease of the tissues, which may persist for a long time in chronic infections such as tuberculosis and rheumatic fever, and the test is of particular value in following the progress of such diseases. The rate is also increased in acute infections, but in such conditions it quickly returns to normal.

Leukocytes. The leukocytes or white blood cells number from 6000 to 8000 per c.mm. of blood. Large numbers, however, are trapped in the unused capillaries, and as physical exertion causes great numbers of these capillaries to become opened up, the leukocyte count shows a corresponding rise after exercise. The white blood cells are not uniform in type like the erythrocytes, but are of three different kinds: the polymorphonuclear leukocyte, the lymphocyte, and the monocyte. The *polymorphonuclear* (*polys,* many, *morphe,* form, and *nucleus*) is a cell whose nucleus may have various forms, in comparison with the spherical nucleus of the lymphocyte and monocyte. It is further characterized by the presence of fine granules in the cytoplasm. In one variety the granules are large and stain bright red with eosin, a red dye used for staining blood films; this is known as the *eosinophil.* The polymorphonuclears constitute about 70 per cent of the leukocytes, but this figure varies considerably. The eosinophils form only 2 per cent of the total leukocyte count. Both types of cells are formed in the sinusoids of the bone marrow, in very much the same way as the erythrocytes are formed, *i.e.,* they go through two immature stages before the adult form is reached. These stages are the *myeloblast* and the *myelocyte.* Granules appear for the first time in the myelocyte, and these cells are present in large numbers in the marrow, but do not enter the blood stream under normal conditions. Some of the myelocytes are eosinophil myelocytes. Both forms are found in the blood in large numbers in leukemia. The *function* of the polymorphonuclears is defense of the body against bacteria by means of phagocytosis, a process that has already been studied in connection with inflammation. The number in the blood is enormously increased in acute infections, owing to the depots in the bone marrow pouring their reserve into the blood stream, and at the same time speeding up the rate of production. The function of the eosinophils is uncertain, but their number may be markedly increased in allergic conditions.

The *lymphocytes* form about 20 per cent of the total leukocyte count. They are rather small, uninteresting-looking cells, with very little cytoplasm around the spherical nucleus. Large numbers of lymphocytes appear at a focus of chronic inflammation, some being derived from the blood, others from the tissues. Though they arrive on the field of battle, they appear merely to play the part of interested spectators, for they have no phagocytic power. This appearance is deceptive, however, for the lymphocytes are an important source of the immune bodies which play so important a part in the defense of the body against bacterial infection. They are therefore *immunocompetent cells.* Unfortunately they also play a part in the rejection of foreign material introduced to help the patient, as in transplantation of the kidney or heart. The lymphocytes are produced in the lymphoid tissue, mainly the lymph nodes and spleen.

The *monocytes* or large mononuclears, on the other hand, are actively phagocytic, and play an important part in the inflammatory process. In acute inflammation they form the second line of defense, arriving later than the polymorphonuclears and serving the useful purpose of scavengers. They are formed in the bone marrow and constitute about 8 per cent of the total leukocytes.

In a blood examination the leukocytes may be examined in two ways: (1) leukocyte count and (2) differential count. The object of the *leukocyte count* is to estimate the total number of leukocytes, and to determine if there is a leukocytosis or increase in the number. This extremely useful procedure is quite simple and takes only a few minutes. In a *differential count* several hundred leukocytes are examined, note being taken whether each cell is a polymorphonuclear, eosinophil, lymphocyte, or monocyte. In this way the percentage of the various cells is determined. Such a procedure is much more laborious and time-consuming, and in most diseases gives information of little value. In selected cases, however, it may prove of great use. It is essential in the leukemias.

BLOOD PLATELETS. Blood platelets are the third formed element of the blood but the last to have their function recognized. These small round or rod-shaped bodies, from 250,000 to 300,000 per cu. mm., are capable of great good, but they may also do great harm.

This electron microscope has revolutionized our concept of the platelet. It used to be regarded as an inert particle, structureless and possibly an artifact. Now it is known to possess abundant metabolic equipment, numerous microtubules, three types of granules, and 80 enzymatic activities.

The *function* of the platelets is *hemostasis,* the arrest of hemorrhage. This is brought about partly by their extreme tendency to agglutination when they encounter any roughness (the process of thrombosis), partly by their role in coagulation, a very different and much more innocuous process. The platelet is the first element to appear at a break in the lining of a blood vessel. Within 1 to 3 seconds they start to adhere to the damaged wall, surely the promptest first aid we could imagine. And this is the element of the blood we used to consider structureless, without function, and possibly an artifact!

BLOOD GROUPS. The fact that the red cells of one individual may be clumped when mixed with blood of many others, with fatal results if transfusion is done, is old knowledge. The modern era was inaugurated in 1900 by Karl Landsteiner of the Rockefeller Institute when he showed that all persons can be divided into four groups as regards the reaction of the serum of one on the red cells of another. The red blood cells and serum of each individual are perfectly adapted to one another, but the cells of one person may not be adapted to the serum

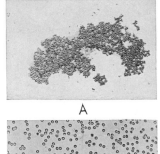

A

Fig. 157. Blood grouping. *A,* Incompatible bloods. *B,* Compatible bloods.

B

of another; they may be incompatible. The gravest accidents may follow transfusion of an incompatible blood. It is this fact that for centuries retarded the use of so obvious a procedure as blood transfusion.

When two bloods are incompatible the red cells of the injected blood from the donor are clumped together or agglutinated by the serum of the patient, the recipient, owing to the presence of agglutinins in the serum of the latter (Fig. 157). The basis of the incompatibility lies in the fact that in human blood the red cells contain either no antigens or one or both of two antigens, known as A and B, which may produce agglutination, while the serum contains corresponding antibodies or agglutinins known as beta or anti-B and alpha or anti-A. Under natural conditions an antigen and its corresponding agglutinin cannot be present simultaneously in the same blood. If, however, blood containing antigen A or B is introduced by transfusion into a person whose blood contains the corresponding antibody, agglutination occurs. Moreover, solution as well as agglutination of the transfused red cells may occur. *This solution of red cells or hemolysis is the real danger of blood transfusion.*

Depending on the presence of the two antigens the blood of all persons can be divided into four great groups known as O, A, B, and AB. Group O contains no antigen, group A contains A antigen, group B contains B antigen, and group AB contains both A and B antigens. As group O contains no antigen, it does not react with the blood of other groups, even though they contain agglutinins. Persons belonging to this group are therefore called *universal donors* because their blood is compatible with that of any of the four groups. Fortunately this is the largest group, comprising over 40 per cent of persons. A person in any one group may receive blood from anyone in the same group. The AB group, having no agglutinins in the serum, is a *universal recipient,* just as we have seen that group O, having no agglutinogens in the red cells, is, *or used to be,* regarded as a universal donor. The term "universal" unfortunately ignores the Rh factor which is discussed below.

The specific antigens and agglutinins (antibodies) are governed by hereditary factors and are transmitted from parent to child, a fact that is sometimes made use of in cases of disputed parentage. *An agglutinin in the blood of a child must also be present in at least one of the parents.* If the blood group of one parent and the child is known, in certain cases the group of the other parent can be determined.

The suitability of a donor is determined by two methods known as *grouping* (or typing) and *matching* (or cross-matching). The blood group to which an individual belongs can be decided by testing his red cells against serum from both a known group A (which contains anti-B agglutinins) and a known group B (which contains anti-A agglutinins) and noting if any agglutination occurs.

Cells agglutinated by serum from a known:		*Individual belongs*
Group A	*Group B*	*to*
No	No	Group O
No	Yes	Group A
Yes	No	Group B
Yes	Yes	Group AB

When this has been done both the cells and serum of the prospective donor should be cross-matched against the serum and cells of the patient, even though both belong to the same group, because each group contains subgroups which are not shown by the usual method of grouping. **If the same donor is to be used after an interval of time for a second transfusion, the two bloods should be matched again even though they belong to suitable groups,** for agglutinins may develop in the patient's blood as the result of the first transfusion with alarming and even fatal results.

Rh Blood Group.   Reference has just been made to the subject of what is called intragroup incompatibility. An important example of this incompatibility is afforded by the antigen known as the *Rh factor,* so-called because it was first discovered in the blood of the rhesus monkey. About 85 per cent of persons possess this factor or antigen, so that they are said to be Rh positive, whereas 15 per cent lack the factor and are Rh negative. Anti-Rh agglutinins are not normally present in human serum, but may be formed in Rh negative persons following transfusion by Rh positive blood. Such serum is the agent used for Rh typing, because it contains an antibody called anti-D, and naturally it is not too easy to obtain this serum in quantity. If a second transfusion is given, using the same donor, it is evident that there will be a transfusion reaction owing to combination of the antigen with the corresponding agglutinin.

The Rh factor may prove a menace in another and more subtle way. It has been found that a Rh positive father can transmit the factor to the fetus. If the mother is Rh negative, anti-Rh agglutinins may be formed in her blood in response to the presence of the Rh factor in the fetus. *There is now a twofold danger:* (1) If the mother is given a transfusion because of excessive blood loss at delivery, and the donor happens to be Rh positive, there will be a transfusion accident, even though the two bloods belong to the same general group (intragroup incompatibility). (2) The maternal anti-Rh agglutinins may reach the fetal blood through the placenta and cause a slow continuous hemolysis of that blood. The result of this intrauterine hemolysis of fetal blood is a severe hemolytic anemia known as *erythroblastosis fetalis* or *hemolytic disease of the newborn.* The reason for this name is that the most striking feature of the blood, apart from the anemia, is the presence of great numbers of nucleated red cells or erythroblasts. These calamities due to primary Rh immunization of the Rh negative childbearing woman can now be prevented by one injection of anti-Rh gamma globulin by the third day after delivery (Bowman and Chown). It will be evident to the reader what a major advance this represents.

BLOOD TRANSFUSION. The novelist speaks of the life blood ebbing away. The phrase is hardly an exaggeration, for, as we have seen in Chapter 1, it is the blood that carries to the innumerable cells of the body their requisites for life, namely, food and oxygen. Without sufficient blood the cells are both starved and asphyxiated. As a severe loss of blood is so injurious, it is natural that the injection of blood from another person should be correspondingly beneficial. When this injection is made into a vein it is called transfusion of blood.

The chief value of blood transfusion is replacement of blood after a severe, acute hemorrhage, when it is truly a lifesaving procedure. It is also useful for combating shock following surgical operations, especially those associated with much loss of blood, as in operations on the brain. Repeated small transfusions are sometimes used in the treatment of chronic anemias with a low red cell count and in severe infections.

Unfortunately it is not possible to use the blood of all and sundry for the purpose of transfusion.

In testing for incompatibility the criterion is the presence or absence of agglutination of the red cells in the test tube, but it is hemolysis rather than agglutination that is the great danger in **transfusion reactions.** If the bloods of the donor and recipient are incompatible there may be immediate signs of shock as evidenced by restlessness, pallor, shortness of breath, feeble rapid pulse, and fall in blood pressure. Or there may be a more delayed type of reaction, marked by chills, fever, pain in the back, jaundice, and the presence of hemoglobin in the urine. *These delayed symptoms are all due to breaking down of the red blood cells.* About 40 per cent of the patients showing these symptoms of hemolysis make a complete recovery. In the remaining 60 per cent symptoms of renal failure develop in the course of a week, there may be complete suppression of urine, and the patient dies in convulsions or coma. From a consideration of these facts it is evident how extremely important it is to prevent reactions to transfusions, and how necessary are the preliminary laboratory tests to determine the question of blood incompatibility. It is essential that blood for cross-matching be correctly and adequately labeled so that there can be no doubt about the identity of the person from whom it was collected. For many purposes, particularly in the treatment of shock, **blood plasma** can be used instead of whole blood. As the plasma contains no red cells, the question of incompatibility does not arise and the dangers of using unsuitable blood are thus avoided. Plasma has a great advantage over whole blood in that it can be dried, and can be kept in the dry form for an indefinite period, but unfortunately it may contain a virus that will cause jaundice owing to the production of viral hepatitis.

Anemias

The term anemia signifies a reduction in the amount of oxygen-carrying hemoglobin in a given volume of blood. This reduction involves the number of red cells, the quantity of hemoglobin, and the volume of packed red cells in a given unit of blood. The decrease may be more marked in the number of red cells or, more important, in the amount of hemoglobin they contain. The presence of anemia is detected by estimation of the amount of hemoglobin or measurement of the packed red cell volume in the hematocrit, not by counting the number of red cells, for in some hypochromic anemias the red cell count may be normal or even above normal.

It is obvious that there are two main ways in which anemia may develop: (1) **too much blood may be lost,** and (2) **too little blood may be formed.** *Increased loss* of red cells may be due to *hemolysis* of these cells within the body, giving us the various forms of hemolytic anemia, or due to *loss of blood from the body,* as in peptic ulcer, cancer of the colon, or excessive menstrual bleeding. *Diminished production* of red cells may be due to deficiency of iron or of vitamin B_{12}, or to hypofunction of the bone marrow.

There are endless ways of classifying the anemias. In our discussion of the subject we shall consider two forms named from the appearance of the red cells in the blood film (macrocytic and microcytic hypochromic), and two named from the method of production of the anemia (hemolytic and aplastic).

Macrocytic anemia can occur in a number of conditions. By far the most important and interesting of these is pernicious anemia.

PERNICIOUS ANEMIA. The form of anemia commonly called pernicious was first described by Addison more than a hundred years ago, so that it is sometimes known as Addison's anemia, a more appropriate term, as the disease is no longer "pernicious" and uniformly fatal as it was before the introduction of modern therapy.

Pernicious anemia is now classed among the nutritional anemias. This does not necessarily mean that it is due to some defect in the diet; the defect is rather in the mechanism that converts certain elements of the diet into substances necessary for proper blood formation. The end-result, however, is the same as if the defect was primarily in the food. We have seen that erythrocytes are formed in the bone marrow from normoblasts, and that these in turn are formed from the more primitive erythroblasts. A continuous evolution is going on in normal marrow, primitive nucleated blood cells being converted into adult non-nucleated erythrocytes, which are then liberated into the circulation It would appear that for this process to continue, building bricks are necessary. If these are missing the primitive red blood cells fail for the most part to develop into erythrocytes, and accumulate in the bone marrow where they appear unduly large and are known as megaloblast. Only a few erythrocytes reach the blood stream, so that a condition of bloodlessness or anemia develops which tends to be steadily progressive. Occasionally a few primitive megaloblast escape into the blood, but for the most part they crowd the bone marrow where, of course, they are of no use to the patient. In biology as well as in economics it is evident that there may be the paradox of poverty in the midst of plenty.

Two factors are involved in the pathogenesis of pernicious anemia, an *intrinsic factor* in the gastric juice, and an *extrinsic factor* in the diet, now known to be vitamin B_{12}. The intrinsic factor used to be regarded as an enzyme, but it is now known as a "carrier" which carries B_{12} safely through the intestinal canal to the terminal ileum. It is believed that the intrinsic factor permits the passage of the very large molecules of the essential vitamin B_{12} across the intestinal mucosa, the vitamin being stored in the liver and used as required. Absence of the intrinsic factor is the basis of pernicious anemia, and this is associated with great atrophy of the gastric mucosa and loss of free hydrochloric acid.

Another member of the vitamin B group known as *folic acid* also provides a powerful stimulus for maturation. It is of even greater value in the treatment of the other macrocytic anemias such as that of pregnancy and the malabsorption states.

Blood Picture. The red blood corpuscles are greatly diminished in number, so that a condition of extreme anemia may exist. Instead of the normal 5,000,000 red cells per c.mm. the number may fall to 1,000,000 or even less. The large macrocytes naturally contain more hemoglobin than do normal erythrocytes. Owing to their greater thickness, which allows less light to pass through them, they appear dark in the stained smear (Fig. 158C), and this used to be regarded as an indication that the *relative* amount of hemoglobin was increased. For this reason the cells were called hyperchromic, and pernicious anemia was labeled as a hyperchromic anemia. We now know that this was a mistake. In several other respects the red cells are far from normal. Some are very small (*microcytes*), but the average size is larger than normal and these large cells are known as *macrocytes.* This is a highly characteristic feature of the blood picture, so that pernicious anemia is a perfect example of a *macrocytic anemia.* The average diameter of normal red cells is 7.5 microns, but in this disease it may be 8 or 8.5 microns, and individual macrocytes may be 12 microns in diameter. From the standpoint of diagnosis this is the most important single feature of the blood picture. Primitive red cells, sometimes normoblasts but usually megaloblasts, may be found in the blood. Normal erythrocytes are perfectly rounded and are all of the same size. In pernicious anemia many of the red cells are misshapen and distorted (*poikilocytosis*), and they vary much in size (*anisocytosis*).

Reference must now be made to one of the most important features of the blood picture, the presence of *reticulocytes*. These are primitive

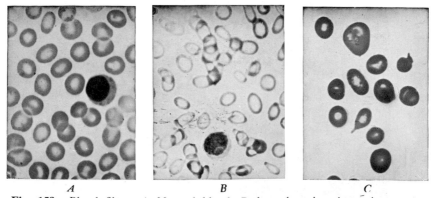

          A   *B*   *C*

Fig. 158. Blood films. *A,* Normal blood; *B,* hypochromic microcytic anemia; *C,* macrocytic pernicious anemia, showing variation in size and shape.

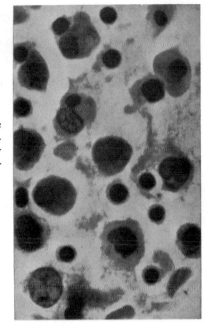

Fig. 159. Megaloblastic reaction of the bone marrow in pernicious anemia. All of the cells are either megaloblasts or normoblasts. × 1000. (Boyd's *Textbook of Pathology.*)

red cells which have lost their nucleus, but in which a fine network or reticulum is present in the cytoplasm. Normally about 1 per cent of the red cells are reticulocytes, but in pernicious anemia there may be 5 per cent. The great importance of reticulocytes, however, lies in their relation to therapy. If a patient with severe anemia is given adequate therapy there will be a marked rise in the number of reticulocytes, a sure indication that the treatment is proving of benefit. If there is no increase in the reticulocytes it is a strong indication that the case is not one of pernicious anemia.

Basis of Symptoms. The disease, which usually develops in middle life, is marked by a *progressive anemia,* and the development of a blood picture which has already been described. The basis of the anemia is the inability of the immature red cells, the megaloblasts, to develop into mature erythrocytes, so that they remain locked up in the bone marrow and are unable to enter the blood stream (Fig. 159). This lack of maturation is due to the lack of the intrinsic factor in the stomach. One of the most characteristic features of the disease is the *absence of the normal hydrochloric acid* of the stomach. Unless this is absent, a diagnosis of pernicious anemia must not be made. The alteration in the gastric juice is responsible for digestive disturbances which may be severe. There may be marked *loss of appetite,* which may amount to aversion for food, and in severe cases there may be dyspepsia, nausea, and even vomiting. The *tongue* is often characteristically *sore, smooth,* and of a *glazed appearance* (Fig. 160).

Every patient with severe anemia is *pale* and suffers from *shortness of breath and palpitation.* The shortness of breath (*dyspnea*) is due to the fact that there are not enough red blood cells to carry oxygen from the lungs to the tissues. Just as dyspnea may result from disease of the heart or the lungs, equally so it may result from disease of the red blood cells.

There is one more group of symptoms that must be mentioned, those pointing to *disease of the nervous system.* Common symptoms of pernicious anemia are *numbness, tingling,* and a *feeling of pins and needles in the arms and legs,* particularly the hands and feet. In more severe cases there may be *unsteadiness in walking* or other indications of changes in the spinal cord. Very definite degenerative lesions are often found in the cord at autopsy. The exact cause of these changes is still uncertain, but it is apparently due to some deficiency similar to, but not necessarily identical with, that which is responsible for the changes in the bone marrow. Treatment with large doses of vitamin B_{12} serves to arrest these changes, and may relieve the symptoms either partially or completely. Treatment of severe nervous symptoms, however, is much less satisfactory than treatment of the blood condition.

Other Macrocytic Anemias. A blood picture similar to that of per-

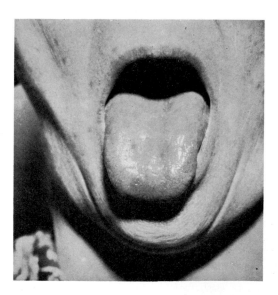

Fig. 160. Smooth tongue in a case of pernicious anemia. (Wintrobe, *Clinical Hematology.*)

nicious anemia may occasionally be seen in other conditions, more particularly sprue, fish tapeworm infection, pregnancy, and gastrectomy. *Sprue* is a tropical intestinal infection marked by the passage of pale bulky fatty stools and atrophy of the tongue and intestinal mucous membrane. The intestinal lesions seem to interfere with the absorption of the vitamins necessary for the health of the bone marrow. *Dibothriocephalus latus* (fish tapeworm) infection is occasionally associated with a macrocytic anemia identical with pernicious anemia, the reason being that the tapeworm competes very successfully for available vitamin B_{12} in the intestine, thus "stealing" it all before it can reach the absorptive area of the gut in the ileum. The macrocytic anemia of pregnancy is due to an increased requirement for folic acid—up to 10 times that required in the normal person. The same is true for the very occasional macrocytic anemia of *pregnancy*. *Gastrectomy* may be followed by a similar picture if the acid-bearing part of the stomach has been removed. This is easy to understand.

MICROCYTIC HYPOCHROMIC ANEMIA. In pernicious anemia each red cell contains the normal amount of hemoglobin, although the cells appear darker in a blood film because of their greater volume. *In hypochromic anemia the hemoglobin is diminished to a greater degree than the red cells,* so that each erythrocyte has a pale, washed-out appearance. In contrast to pernicious anemia, this is a microcytic anemia, the average diameter of the red cells being smaller than normal.

In spite of these facts, the *clinical picture* resembles in many respects that of pernicious anemia. There are the same digestive disturbances, loss of appetite, absence of hydrochloric acid, glazed tongue, and numbness and tingling in the arms and legs. One important difference is that the *fingernails* are *brittle* and easily broken, and are turned up at the edges so that they become "spoonshaped." The disease is much commoner than pernicious anemia, being mainly a disease of middle-aged women, often following pregnancy. Iron deficiency is also common in young women, especially shortly after puberty, in the period of rapid growth combined with the onset of menstruation.

Like pernicious anemia this form of anemia is a deficiency disease, but in this case it is a **deficiency in iron,** which is an essential ingredient of hemoglobin. Several factors combine to produce this deficiency. During pregnancy there is a great depletion in the store of maternal iron which is needed for the formation of the red blood cells of the baby. The absence of hydrochloric acid and the gastric disturbance probably interfere with the digestion and absorption of the iron in the food. Finally, the marked distaste for food is apt to lead the patient to adopt a diet of slops which is greatly deficient in iron. *An exact determination by examination of the blood of the type of anemia is of* *the highest importance, because the administration of large amounts of iron in hypochromic anemia is followed by as dramatic an improvement as is produced in pernicious anemia by modern therapy.*

HEMOLYTIC ANEMIAS. The hemolytic anemias form a large and heterogeneous group, but the basis of each member of the group is *a shortened life span of the red blood cells with resulting hemolysis,* that is to say, lysis or solution of the red cells with liberation of the hemoglobin into the plasma. The mechanism by which this is brought about may be one of two profoundly different types. In the first the defect is *hereditary,* being transmitted by a gene, and the resulting disease is *congenital* in type. In the second form the defect is *acquired,* being commonly caused by *circulating antibodies* which become adherent to the red cells with resulting hemolysis. These antibodies are frequently the product of autoimmune reactions. Thus the red cell may either be *born* vulnerable or it may *become* so owing to acquired external factors. In the congenital (hereditary) form the fault lies in the red cells, whereas in the acquired form it lies in the environment. For this reason removal of the spleen, the graveyard of the erythrocytes, may be markedly beneficial in the congenital type, particularly in the variety known as congenital spherocytic anemia, whereas ACTH or cortisone, with their antihypersensitivity action, may be equally beneficial in the acquired form. The two types are differentiated in the laboratory by means of the *Coombs test,* which is designed to show the presence of *antibodies (agglutinins) adsorbed to the surface of the red cells in the acquired but not in the congenital form.*

We must recognize the fact that increased hemolysis does not necessarily result in anemia. Bone marrow activity may compensate for destruction of the erythrocytes. Under these circumstances a person is said to have hemolytic disease but not to suffer from hemolytic anemia, which only occurs when the bone marrow is unable to compensate for the shortened life span of the erythrocytes. *The best single signpost of hemolytic anemia is a persistent increase to 5 per cent or more in the number of reticulocytes.* Other evidence of bone marrow overactivity is leukocytosis, nucleated red cells, and increased platelets.

The hereditary defect may involve abnormal red cells or abnormal hemoglobin. The outstanding example of a red cell defect is spherocytic anemia; a corresponding example of a hemoglobin defect is sickle cell anemia.

Congenital Spherocytic Anemia. The obvious blood anomaly in this condition is the spheroidal shape of the erythrocytes in place of the normal biconcave discs. Their shape is responsible for their increased fragility, which in turn is responsible for the excessive red cell destruction or hemolysis. The basic genetic defect, however, involves a defect in the red cell envelope and, as a result, a change in shape from biconcave to spherical.

The *blood* shows anemia, usually mild, but severe in crises (see below). The two chief characteristics of the film are microspherulocytes and reticulocytes. A *spherocyte* is smaller than normal and spherical instead of biconcave. *Reticulocytes* are more numerous than in any other disease. In place of the usual 1 per cent there may be 20 per cent. As biconcave cells become globular when placed in hypotonic saline, it is evident that the more spherical cells will rupture more readily. Thus there is an *increased fragility* of the red cells when placed in a salt solution of a strength that leaves normal cells untouched. This is the basis of the laboratory test for spherocytic anemia.

The disease may remain latent for many years, although the fragility is there, hanging like the sword of Damocles over the head of the person carrying the defective gene. For some reason which I do not understand there may be occasional *crises,* in which there is increased blood destruction with attacks of pain in the region of the liver and the spleen. It has been suggested that the crises may really be due to an acute aplastic condition in the bone marrow with complete cessation of formation of red cells. This sounds good, but it explains nothing, for we are ignorant as to the cause of the aplasia of the marrow.

Jaundice is the characteristic feature of the crises, although a mild degree of jaundice, often unrecognized, may be present all the time. It is, of course, the result of the increased fragility of the red cells, the actual destruction taking place in the spleen, which appears to assume a function of overactivity to which the name of *hypersplenism* is given. On this basis splenectomy has become the recognized treatment for congenital spherocytic anemia, often with dramatic and satisfying results. The jaundice is peculiar and distinctive in character, being known as *acholuric jaundice.* As the name indicates, there is no (*a*) bile (*chol*) in the urine (*uric*), whereas in ordinary obstructive jaundice the increased supply of bile in the blood pours into the urine. (The reasons for this difference have been discussed in Chapter 20.) The blood gives an *indirect van den Bergh reaction. Gallstones* of the pure bilirubin type are frequent for an obvious reason, and enlargement of the spleen (*splenomegaly*) is a constant feature.

Sickle Cell Anemia. Although this disease is dependent on an *anomaly in the formation of the hemoglobin molecule,* it has much in common with spherocytosis in which there is an *enzyme deficiency in the structure of the erythrocyte.* Both are familial and hereditary, in both there may be active disease (anemia) or merely the hereditary fingerprints (spherocytes or sickle cells as the case may be), both are characterized by a *hemolytic type of anemia, acholuric jaundice,* and

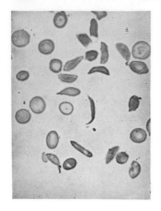

Fig. 161. Sickle cell anemia. Many erythrocytes are sickle shaped. × 500. (Boyd, *Textbook of Pathology*.)

the appearance of *large numbers of reticulocytes* in the peripheral blood. A major difference is that the genetic defect in sickle cell anemia is largely confined to the Negro race, and the disease is very prevalent in the colored population of the deep South of the United States. It is transmitted as a dominant Mendelian characteristic by either sex. It would appear that *sickle cell anemia is homozygous,* the defective gene being inherited from both parents, while the *sickle cell trait* represents a heterozygous state.

The *blood* presents a striking picture in the *active phase* of the disease. There is marked anemia as well as leukocytosis, and the blood film shows an extraordinary change in the shape of the red cells, for large numbers of these are crescentic or sickle in form (Fig. 161). As in spherocytic anemia, reticulocytosis forms a prominent feature owing to the pressure put on the bone marrow to compensate for the anemia. The serum is deep yellow owing to the great increase in bilirubin produced by hemolysis of the sickle cells.

In the *latent phase* sickle cells are not present in the circulating blood, but they can be readily demonstrated in the presence of a diminution in the oxygen tension. When a *wet* film of the blood is made, covered with a cover glass, and sealed so as to exclude air, large numbers of the red cells will be found to have assumed the sickle form in the course of 18 to 24 hours.

The state of health of the patient varies greatly. At times he feels well, at other times he presents the symptoms of severe anemia, in addition to the acute crises mentioned below. The patient, although outwardly well, has to bear the burden of a blood dyscrasia whose outstanding feature is an abnormally high rate of destruction of red blood cells. At the same time he manages to live on good terms with his disease. He is apt, however, to break down under stress, and his normal life span, like that of his red blood cells, is considerably shortened.

Acute crises may occur in sickle cell anemia, just as we have seen to occur in spherulocytic anemia. Not only is the anemia intensified, but the patient suffers from attacks of acute abdominal pain, which may be confused with acute appendicitis or ruptured peptic ulcer. Infarcts of the spleen are common owing to thrombosis in the splenic vessels.

Thalassemia. This is another of the hereditary group of hemolytic anemias. The gene responsible for the defect in hemoglobin formation is distributed among the peoples of the eastern Mediterranean basin. For this reason it has long been known as Mediterranean anemia or thalassemia from the Greek word, *thalasse,* meaning sea, for in olden times there was only one sea, the Mediterranean. The trait has now been carried far and wide throughout the world by the migration of peoples. The hemoglobin defect results in a decreased life span of the circulating red cells.

The characteristic features of the *blood film* are: (1) the great numbers of erythroblasts and (2) the presence of *leptocytes* or thin cells (*leptos,* thin), oval cells, and *target cells.* The leptocytes are comparable to sickle cells, both being a departure from the normal form of the red cell. Target cells have a central rounded area of pigment, surrounded by a clear zone, with further out a thick pigmented capsule, an appearance responsible for the names target cells and *Mexican hat cells.* The most suggestive feature of the film is the presence of great numbers of nucleated red cells, both normoblasts and megaloblasts.

The *clinical features* are: (1) a constant familial and racial incidence (most often in Greeks but also in Italians and Armenians, and even more common in Africa than in the United States), (2) a typical facial appearance, and (3) enlargement of the spleen. Thalassemia usually appears in the first two years of life and sometimes in the newborn. The skin is yellow, the face mongoloid, the head enlarged, the abdomen prominent owing to the large spleen, and the stature stunted. There is a moderate or marked anemia, and a pronounced leukocytosis.

Acquired Hemolytic Anemias. Many hemolytic anemias are caused by extraneous agents. Among these may be mentioned chemical agents and drugs, bacterial toxins such as those of hemolytic streptococci, and the malaria parasite which we have already seen to specialize in destroying the red cells in which it resides. Here we are more interested in immune antibody anemias, and in particular hemolytic disease of the newborn, to which reference has already been made in connection with the subject of blood groups.

Hemolytic Disease of the Newborn. Here the hemolysis with resulting anemia is caused by incompatible antibodies transferred across the placenta during pregnancy. The incompatibility can only occur when there is a difference between the blood groups of a mother and her fetus,

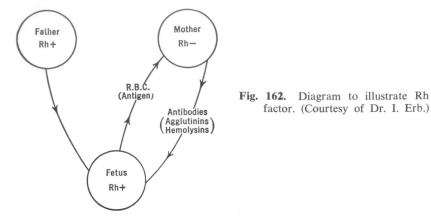

Fig. 162. Diagram to illustrate Rh factor. (Courtesy of Dr. I. Erb.)

more particularly the Rh blood group system. It is an interaction of Rh fetal antigens inherited from the father and maternal antibodies. If the father is Rh positive and the mother Rh negative, anti-Rh agglutinins may be formed in her blood as the result of sensitization by the Rh factor of the fetus (Fig. 162). If the maternal anti-Rh antibodies reach the fetal blood through the placenta, a slow continuous hemolysis of the red cell takes place. It should be pointed out that a pregnant woman may be sensitized not only by paternal Rh antigens via the fetus but also by blood transfusion. The simplest and best method of detecting the passive transfer of maternal antibody to the infant's circulation is to determine whether the infant's erythrocytes have been coated with antibody. This is demonstrated by the *Coombs antiglobulin test.* Hemolytic disease of the newborn occurs once in every 200 pregnancies, and accounts for 2 to 3 per cent of all neonatal deaths.

The *clinical picture* varies. The child may be born dead in a condition of extreme general edema or hydrops. About 7 per cent of those that survive are mental defectives. *Jaundice* may or may not be present. The blood picture is one of *congenital anemia* and *erythroblastosis fetalis,* that is to say great numbers of nucleated red cells (erythroblasts) owing to compensatory activity of the bone marrow. The mortality formerly was 70 to 80 per cent, but with modern treatment the recovery rate is now over 80 per cent. *Exchange transfusion* given at birth when there is evidence of disease or when there is a history of disease in a previous baby is the treatment of choice. If this is not possible, repeated simple transfusions can be given.

OTHER ANEMIAS. Anemia may be produced in a number of ways other than those just described. **Aplastic anemia,** as the name indicates, is due to aplasia or atrophy of the bone marrow. This may be caused by *industrial poisons, drugs, and ionizing radiation.* The blood picture is aplastic in type, with reduction in the number of red cells, leukocytes, and blood platelets.

Secondary anemia is a conveniently vague term to describe a rather heterogeneous group in which the blood is of the hypochromic type. The hemoglobin is diminished to a greater degree than the number of red cells, so that each erythrocyte is correspondingly poor in coloring matter. The cause of the anemia is defective formation of hemoglobin, and this occurs as the result of all sorts of *acute* and *chronic infection, chronic renal disease,* or *cancer.* Secondary anemia is, therefore, a complication or accompaniment of many other diseases. The same type of anemia develops as the result of hemorrhage, which may be acute and profuse, as in the vomiting of blood due to gastric ulcer, or chronic and almost unnoticed, as in the continued bleeding from piles. In the treatment of secondary anemia, iron is the most valuable therapeutic agent.

Polycythemia

The term polycythemia means an increase in the number of the cells of the blood, but in practice this increase applies only to the red cells, so that a more accurate although less popular name is *erythremia.* The condition may be primary or secondary.

POLYCYTHEMIA VERA. As the name indicates, this is true or primary erythremia. The red cells are greatly increased, usually from 7,000,000 to 10,000,000 per c.mm. The blood volume is also increased, and the blood becomes viscid owing to the burden of cells it carries. There is a moderate leukocytosis, and occasional primitive red and white cells. As might be expected, the bone marrow is markedly hyperplastic, so that the condition may be regarded as neoplastic in type, being comparable with leukemia in this respect. It is perhaps significant that occasional cases have changed from erythremia into leukemia of myelogenous type.

The *clinical picture* is striking, for the skin and mucous membrane of the mouth are red and the conjunctiva is blood-shot. The color is due to the increased number of red cells. The spleen is always enlarged. At autopsy the visceral vessels are greatly distended and often thrombosed. The blood volume may be effectively reduced by repeated venesection.

Erythrocytosis. This is *secondary* polycythemia, a compensating increase of red cells in conditions of *insufficient oxygenation* such as congenital heart disease, congestive heart failure, emphysema, and residence at high altitudes. It will be obvious that the condition is in no sense one of disease, but rather corresponds to leukocytosis. There is *no increase in leukocytes,* a diagnostic point of great value in distinguishing erythrocytosis from polycythemia vera.

Bleeding Diseases

The bleeding diseases are those in which the normal mechanism for the control of hemorrhage is deficient or deranged. The two important tests in the study of these diseases are: (1) the *bleeding time, i.e.,* the time blood continues to flow from a minute puncture of the skin, the platelets acting as a plug for such a puncture; (2) the *coagulation time, i.e.,* the time that blood continues to flow from a cut before clotting or coagulation takes place. The two tests form a useful basis for the classification of the bleeding diseases into three main classes: (1) bleeding and coagulation times normal; (2) bleeding time prolonged and coagulation time normal; (3) coagulation time prolonged and bleeding time normal. A discussion of the general subject of the arrest of hemorrhage will be found in Chapter 4. There are many diseases in which bleeding is a prominent feature, but we shall only consider two in this place, namely hemophilia and purpura.

HEMOPHILIA. Hemophilia, "the bleeding disease," is characterized by prolonged bleeding following a cut or trauma, although not from a needle puncture. *It is the most hereditary of all hereditary diseases, and repeats itself in generation after generation.* Famous examples that occurred in the Royal families of Europe are known to anyone interested in history, for the tragic gene weaved itself across the tapestry of modern Europe like a scarlet thread, probably originating as a mutation in one of the parents of Queen Victoria. It is almost invariably confined to males, but the gene is transmitted by females of the family. It is therefore *a perfect example of sex-linked heredity*. The hemorrhagic tendency appears in early childhood. A simple injury such as the extraction of a tooth or circumcision may give rise to a fatal hemorrhage. Hemorrhage into the large joints after slight trauma is common, and results in grave disability.

The striking *blood change* is the very *prolonged coagulation time* combined with a *normal bleeding time*. The reason for the difference is that **hemorrhage from a cut is arrested primarily by the formation of a clot, whereas hemorrhage from a puncture is stopped by a plug of platelets. The essential deficiency is that of a plasma factor necessary for coagulation.** This *anti-hemophilic factor* (AHF) is associated with the globulin or fibrinogen fractions of the plasma proteins, so that it is also known as *anti-hemophilic globulin* (AHG). Other defects in the clotting mechanism are responsible for other bleeding diseases.

PURPURA. Purpura is a condition in which there are spontaneous hemorrhages in the skin and mucous membranes. **The tendency to bleeding is connected with a marked fall in the number of blood platelets, so that the bleeding time is prolonged although the clotting time is normal.**

Two forms of the disease can be recognized, a *primary* form in which no cause for the fall in blood platelets can be discovered, and a *secondary* form in which it is possible to demonstrate some definite cause for the fall.

The primary form is known as *thrombocytopenic purpura hemorrhagica*. The *platelets* fall from 250,000 (normal) to below 60,000, and may indeed disappear completely (thrombocytopenia). *There are small and large hemorrhages in the skin, and bleeding from the mucous membranes of the nose, mouth, stomach, intestines, and uterus;* blood appears in the urine. When a tourniquet is applied to the arm petechial hemorrhages develop below the tourniquet. Acute cases may end fatally in a few weeks. In chronic cases removal of the spleen (splenectomy) may produce great benefit.

Secondary purpura may be caused by replacement of the bone marrow by secondary carcinoma. The reason for this is that the cells that produce the platelets in the marrow are destroyed by the cancer. In septicemia and in infectious fevers there may be purpuric hemorrhages, owing to damage to the capillary walls by the bacterial toxins. Secondary purpura is seldom so severe as the primary form.

Vascular purpura is an increased permeability of the small blood vessels, as a result of which both plasma and red cells can pass out into the tissues. *The platelets are normal.* The condition is an *exudative diathesis* rather than a tendency to true hemorrhage, and it may have an allergic basis. When the transudation is into the wall of the stomach and bowel causing abdominal pain, vomiting, and diarrhea, the condition is called *Henoch's purpura;* when it occurs into a large joint giving symptoms of acute arthritis, it is known as *Schönlein's purpura.* These old names die hard.

Leukemias

The essential feature of leukemia is *a neoplastic proliferation of the leukoblastic tissues,* as a result of which there is usually a great increase in the white cells of the blood. It is important to realize that in spite of its name *leukemia is essentially a disease of tissue, not of the blood.* The increase may involve the myeloid cells (*myelogenous leukemia*), the lymphoid cells (*lymphatic leukemia*), and in rare cases the monocytes (*monocytic leukemia*). To these must be added a fourth, *acute leukemia,* a disease of childhood and rapidly fatal, lasting from a few days to a few months, and associated with hemorrhage from the gums and other mucous membranes. Leukemia in childhood is always a more devastating disease than in adult life. Occasionally there is a proliferation of white cells in the tissues, but they fail to appear in the blood stream. To this condition the confusing name of *aleukemic leukemia* is given. In the two common forms, chronic myelogenous and lymphatic

leukemia, there is a progressive anemia, owing to infiltration and replacement of the bone marrow by enormous numbers of proliferating
white cells. **It will be realized that leukemia is essentially cancer of the
bone marrow.** We are ignorant as to its cause, apart from the fact that
ionizing radiation is definitely leukemogenic. It is (or used to be) 8
to 10 times as common in radiologists as in nonradiologists. Many cases
of leukemia developed after the explosion of atomic bombs at Hiroshima and Nagasaki. There is also much to suggest a viral origin.

MYELOGENOUS LEUKEMIA. In myelogenous leukemia there is a
great increase in the granular series of cells, both primitive (myelocytic)
and adult (polymorphonuclear) in type. The cells in either of these
groups may be neutrophil, eosinophil, or basophil. The *myelocyte* usually forms the prominent feature of the film (Fig. 163). It is a large
cell about double the size of the polymorphonuclear, with an indented
or lobed nucleus and abundant cytoplasm containing granules which
may be fine and neutrophil, or coarse and eosinophil, or basophil. The
total white cell count averages 200,000 per c.mm., but it may go as
high as 500,000 or even 1,000,000. As a result of irradiation, drug
treatment, or even an acute infection such as pneumonia, there may
be a great drop in the cell count, sometimes to normal, but *abnormal*
white cells (stem cells) are still in evidence. Primitive red cells also

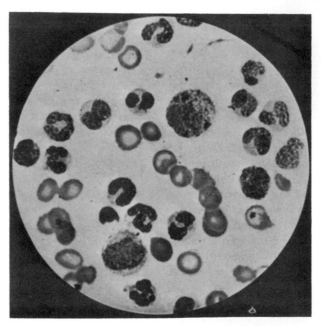

Fig. 163. Myelogenous leukemia. Several myelocytes and very many polymorphonuclear leukocytes. × 800. (Boyd's *Textbook of Pathology.*)

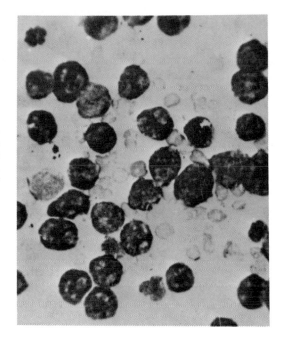

Fig. 164. Lymphatic leukemia. Enormous in-
crease in the number
of lymphocytes × 850.
(Boyd's *Pathology for
the Physician.*)

appear in the blood, and *normoblasts* are more numerous than in any
other disease. Finally there is a great increase in *blood platelets,* owing
to proliferation of megakaryocytes, which make the platelets in the bone
marrow. We have already seen that the *red blood cells* are greatly reduced in number. *If it is remembered that there may be 1,000,000 white
cells, 1,000,000 red cells, and 1,000,000 platelets, some of the principal
features of the blood picture may be recalled.*

LYMPHATIC LEUKEMIA. In the lymphatic form of leukemia only
the lymphoid cells are increased in number, and they may form as much
as 99 per cent of the total white cell count, although 90 per cent is
a commoner figure (Fig. 164). The average count is 50,000 to 100,000
per c.mm., distinctly lower than in the myelogenous form. The lymphocytes contain less cytoplasm than the normal small lymphocytes, so that
they may appear as naked nuclei. The *bone marrow* becomes infiltrated
and replaced by lymphoid tissue, but there is none of the erythroblastic
activity characteristic of myelogenous leukemia, so that although some
degree of anemia develops there are no normoblasts in the peripheral
blood and the platelets are greatly reduced, with resulting hemorrhage
in the skin and mucous membranes. A consideration of the red cells
and the platelets is of more use for differentiating myelogenous from
lymphatic leukemia in difficult cases than is a study of the primitive
white cells.

Basis of Symptoms.   A patient suffering from leukemia presents two entirely different groups of symptoms: The first are those of *anemia, e.g.,* weakness, dyspnea, palpitation; the second are due to *infiltration and enlargement of the organs.* In addition there is often *a marked tendency to hemorrhage,* as shown by bleeding from the gums and the uterus. Extraction of a tooth may be followed by prolonged bleeding. In *myelogenous leukemia* the *spleen* is usually much *enlarged,* and sometimes it may be so huge that it fills the greater part of the abdominal cavity, producing a feeling of dragging and great weight. The *liver* and other organs may be enlarged to a lesser degree owing to accumulation of white cells within their substance. In the *lymphatic form* the chief organs enlarged are the *lymph nodes,* in which the lymphocytes are formed, although the spleen is also often increased in size. Not only the superficial nodes are enlarged such as those in the neck, axilla, and groin, but also the deep nodes in the thorax and abdomen, and these may produce symptoms by pressure on neighboring structures.

Radiation may lead to some prolongation of life, and in most cases of chronic leukemia it will produce abatement of symptoms. Several drugs are known to be of value in the treatment of chronic myeloid leukemia, but none produces permanent cure.

Agranulocytosis

As the name suggests, this is a remarkable disappearance of the granulocytic series of leukocytes from the blood with an accompanying drop in the total white cell count. The change in the blood picture is accompanied by *necrotizing gangrenous lesions of the mouth* involving the gums, the tonsils, and even the bone of the jaw. The association of leukopenia with gangrenous lesions of the mouth is known as *agranulocytic angina,* the word "angina" in this sense meaning an acute inflammation of the throat.

Two groups of cases can be distinguished: (1) those occurring in persons who have been *taking too much of some of the pain-killing drugs,* particularly amidopyrine and the barbiturate series, *i.e.,* chemicals containing the benzene ring; (2) cases in which *no obvious cause can be discovered,* although a huge variety of industrial and household agents have been incriminated. The two factors, diminished leukocyte count and severe mouth infections, probably assist one another. Disappearance of the leukocytes, which are the natural defenders of the body against infection, facilitates the spread of infection in the mouth. On the other hand a severe mouth infection with production of bacterial toxins is known in some cases to depress the production of leukocytes. Certain persons are peculiarly susceptible to the action of amidopyrine and other drugs, and respond by a marked lowering of the leukocyte count. Unfortunately the victim, on account of the pain of the mouth lesions, may continue to take even larger doses of the drug, and such cases cannot fail to go on to a fatal termination, as the leukocytes fall almost to the vanishing point.

The disease often begins with the extraction of teeth. It is marked by fever, increasing weakness and fatigue, sore mouth, and sore throat. There may be extensive destruction of the gums and even the jaw, so that the teeth may fall out. Some cases are very acute, death occurring in a week or two.

It is important to discontinue the use of any dangerous drugs that the patient may have been taking. The use of antibiotics has prevented the occurrence of serious infections in these cases, so that the patient's bone marrow will have a better chance of recovery from the damage done by the toxic drug. Repeated transfusions of fresh blood may be of help also in the treatment.

Infectious Mononucleosis

This condition with the descriptive name is apparently due to an infection, most probably viral in nature, through the tonsils or the upper respiratory tract, as a result of which the lymphoid tissue is unduly stimulated, many of the newly formed mononuclear cells appearing in the blood stream. Although sporadic cases occur, the disease is most readily recognized in epidemic form.

The *clinical features* are a mild degree of *fever* lasting for two or three weeks in young persons, frequently medical students, nurses, or laboratory technologists (perhaps because the diagnosis is more likely to be made by reason of the likelihood of a blood examination in this group), a very *sore throat,* enlarged and tender cervical *lymph nodes* and sometimes the axillary and inguinal groups, moderate *enlargement of the spleen,* and a constant increase of the *mononuclear cells* of the blood. The total leukocyte count rarely exceeds 20,000 or 30,000, but the percentage of mononuclears may be 50 to 95 per cent of the total count, so that at first a distinction from lymphatic leukemia may be extremely difficult, but the absence of anemia and the normal platelet count are differential features of value. The blood contains *heterophile antibodies, i.e.,* the serum will clump sheep's red cells in high dilution. This is the *Paul-Bunnell test,* a useful one in doubtful cases, but by no means specific.

The *lesions* are seldom seen by the pathologist, because recovery is the almost invariable rule unless one of the rare complications such as rupture of the spleen proves fatal. There is a widespread proliferation of a characteristic mononuclear cell in the lymphoid tissue throughout the body, most marked in the spleen. Very occasionally there may be *spontaneous rupture of the enlarged spleen.* Still more rarely the nerve roots and meninges become infiltrated by the proliferating cells with slowly ascending motor paralysis and severe root pains, the picture known as the *Guillain-Barré syndrome.*

In concluding this brief outline of diseases of the blood it is obvious that anyone whose task it is to examine blood films in the laboratory must familiarize himself with the appearance of blood and bone marrow cells, both red and white, when stained appropriately. This can be done by studying the color plates in such textbooks as Wintrobe's *Clinical Hematology* and Miale's *Laboratory Medicine—Hematology,* as well as the special color atlases devoted to the subject.

LYMPH NODES

The lymphatic tissue forms one of the most all-pervasive indispensable parts of our anatomy, although it is very little in evidence in a state of health. It consists of lymphatic vessels and lymphoid tissue, the latter being collected in two groups, namely lymph nodes situated in the lymph stream and lymphatic tissue in mucous membranes. The lymph nodes, with which we are concerned here, consist of: (1) *lymphocytes,* which are free cells in a framework or (2) *reticulum cells,* which are part of the reticuloendothelial system and are both supporting and phagocytic.

The *function* of lymphoid tissue is twofold: (1) *filtration* and (2) *production of lymphocytes.* All the lymph passes through one or more nodes, which act as filters not only for bacteria and dust particles but also for cancer cells. The reticuloendothelial cells arrest and destroy immense numbers of invading bacteria by phagocytosis and dust particles of varying kinds are prevented from entering the blood stream, but whether cancer cells are injured or destroyed when arrested is open to question. The life span of the lymphocytes is only a few days, so they must be produced in overwhelming numbers, yet their precise function remains in doubt. There can be no question that they are involved in immunological processes, but at the present time they seem to be carriers of antibodies made by the plasma cells, rather than the maker of those antibodies as used to be thought.

Lymph node biopsy is a frequent and valuable procedure. Usually it is done to determine whether or not an enlarged node is malignant. The neoplasm may be *primary* (lymphosarcoma) or much more often *secondary* (carcinoma). Usually the pathologist has no difficulty in arriving at a correct answer from the microscopic picture, but in some cases the diagnosis is very difficult because the reaction of the reticuloendothelial cells to a bacterial irritant may closely resemble a neoplasm.

When a bacterial infection is suspected, part of the specimen must be placed in a sterile container for subsequent culture, while the other part is placed in a fixative for microscopic section.

Many of the diseases in which the lymph nodes are involved have already been considered, including two discussed in the present chapter, namely lymphatic leukemia and infectious mononucleosis. Brief mention will be made of only one or two pathological processes.

Lymphosarcoma

This is a malignant tumor of the lymphoid tissue, and so it is characterized by enlargement of the lymph nodes, both superficial and deep (Fig. 65, page 229), the lymphoid tissue in the throat and intestine, and sometimes the spleen. It presents a clinical picture similar to that of lymphatic leukemia, but the lymphoid cells that multiply and cause such great enlargement of the lymph nodes do not escape into the blood. Treatment with roentgen rays and the newer drugs is remarkably effective for a time, the masses of enlarged nodes melting away like snow before the sun, but eventually this power is lost, and the patient is killed by the pressure of huge masses in the chest and abdomen (Fig. 165).

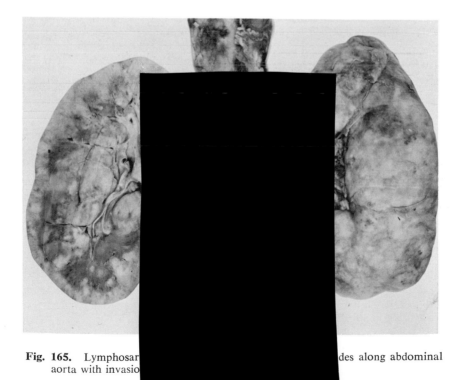

Fig. 165. Lymphosar[...]des along abdominal aorta with invasio[...]

From the foregoing brief summary it might be thought that the subject of primary malignant tumors of lymphoid tissue, lymphomas or *lymphoblastomas* as they are called, was a simple one. The reverse is the case. In addition to the neoplasm of lymphocytes just described there are tumors of reticuloendothelial cells (*reticulum cell sarcoma*), which are more rapid and malignant in their course, as well as one type of low malignancy (*macrofollicular lymphoma*). Mere mention of these possibilities must suffice. Nor need anything more be said here about the subject of lymph nodes involved in secondary carcinoma.

Hodgkin's Disease

The clinical picture of Hodgkin's disease is similar to that of lymphosarcoma, being marked by the development of large glandular masses in the neck (Fig. 166), axilla, groin, thorax, and abdomen. Enlargement of the spleen is more frequent and more marked than in lymphosarcoma. The microscopic picture is quite different from that of lymphosarcoma. In lymphosarcoma the cells are all of the same type, all lymphocytes. In Hodgkin's disease, on the other hand, the cells are extremely varied, resembling the picture seen in a chronic granuloma, although the condition is without doubt a true neoplasm. In spite of this fact the disease has the same progressively fatal character as lymphosarcoma, although the progress may be arrested for a time by means of radiation.

Fig. 166. Hodgkin's e neck.

Fig. 167. Tuberculous lymph nodes of the neck, showing sinuses and scars.

Tuberculosis

Tuberculosis used to be one of the commonest causes of glandular enlargement in the neck, but improvement in the milk supply has greatly diminished the number of these cases. The lymph nodes in the neck are infected from the mouth and throat, the bronchial nodes are infected from the lungs, the abdominal nodes from the bowel. The enlarged nodes are at first firm, but when caseation occurs they undergo softening and break down, and the softened material is discharged on the surface if the glands are in a superficial position. Sinuses are formed which connect the softened glands with the skin of the neck. These persist for a long time, but eventually they heal, leaving deep scars that cause considerable deformity (Fig. 167). In many cases the nodes heal without undergoing softening and sinus formation, especially if the patient is placed under the best hygienic conditions. Perhaps I should omit Figure 167. The only reason it is still included from earlier editions of this book is because of its historic interest to me, for when I was a medical student in Edinburgh this was one of the commonest surgical conditions. Its present rarity is a striking example of the changing incidence of disease.

Sarcoidosis

It is difficult to know where the subject of sarcoidosis should best be discussed. It was first described almost 100 years ago, and yet we are still completely ignorant as to its cause. The microscopic lesions are granulomatous in character, closely resembling those of tuberculosis, yet the nature of the condition remains obscure. The disease is endemic in regions of pine forests such as the Scandinavian countries and the New England region of the United States, so that it has been suggested

that pine pollen may be at least one etiological agent which can excite
arcoidosis.

e for the diversity of their distribution, the
he lymph nodes, both superficial and deep,
lungs, and many other organs may be
r months or years, with a tendency to fibro-
re is an astonishing absence of symptoms.
is that of circumscribed masses resembling
istaken for these lesions.

elevation in the total plasma protein, more
on. The *Kveim test* for sarcoidosis is an
antigen being made from cutaneous sar-
expressed either as a gross nodule at the
croscopic sarcoid lesion when it is excised.
t is a worthwhile diagnostic procedure in
patients who do not have skin lesions or palpable lymph nodes accessi-
ble for biopsy.

FURTHER READING

BOWMAN, J. M., and CHOWN, B.: Can. Med. Ass. J., 1968, *99,* 385. (Pre-
    vention of Rh immunization after massive Rh-positive transfusion.)
DAMESHEK, W., and GUNZ, F.: *Leukemia,* New York, 1958.
QUICK, A. J.: *Hemorrhagic Diseases and Thrombosis,* Philadelphia, 2nd ed.,
    1966.
RACE, R. R., and SANGER, R.: *Blood Groups in Man,* 5th ed., Oxford, 1968.
WINTROBE, M. M.: *Clinical Hematology,* Philadelphia, 6th ed., 1967.

Chapter 27

Nervous System

STRUCTURE AND FUNCTION

The nervous system is divided into a central part consisting of the brain and spinal cord, and a peripheral part consisting of the nerves carrying motor messages from the brain and cord to the muscles and those carrying sensory messages from the skin and other parts of the body to the cord and brain. In this place only the central nervous system will be considered, although passing reference will be made to the peripheral nerves.

The brain is made up of the cerebrum consisting of the right and left cerebral hemispheres, the brain stem which connects the cerebrum with the spinal cord, and the cerebellum or little brain (Fig. 168). The **cerebrum** initiates motor impulses which pass to the muscles, receives sensory impulses from the periphery, and is the seat of thought and reason. The **brain stem** is composed from above downward of the midbrain, the pons, and the medulla, which is continued into the spinal

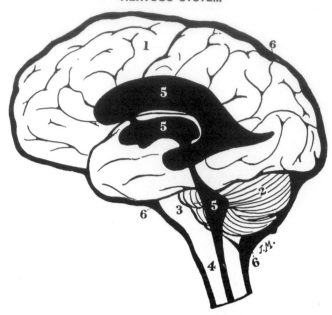

Fig. 168. Brain and cerebrospinal fluid. 1, Cerebrum; 2, cerebellum; 3, pons; 4, medulla; 5, ventricles; 6, subarachnoid space.

cord. Through the brain stem pass the innumerable motor and sensory nerves, and it also houses the groups of nerve cells from which arise the cranial nerves that pass to the eye, ear, face, and mouth. The **cerebellum** is concerned principally with coordination and equilibrium, so that cerebellar disease is marked by incoordination and loss of equilibrium (ataxia).

The **spinal cord** is traversed by all the nerves going to and coming from the body. Those passing to the arm leave the cord in the upper or cervical region; those passing to the leg leave in the lower or lumbar region. The motor fibers from the brain terminate around nerve cells in the *gray matter,* which occupies the center of the cord, and from these motor cells a second set of fibers carries the motor messages to the muscles. The upper relay is called the *upper motor neuron* and is injured in cerebral hemorrhage; the lower relay is called the *lower motor neuron* and is injured in infantile paralysis. *Complete paralysis may be produced by destruction of either neuron, and by injury to the nerve cell or the nerve fiber which arises from it.*

NEURONS. The *central nervous system* is composed of neurons and neuroglia (Fig. 169). The *neurons* consist of nerve cells and the nerve fibers that arise from them and pass sometimes for a long distance through the brain and spinal cord. The *motor efferent nerve fibers* arise

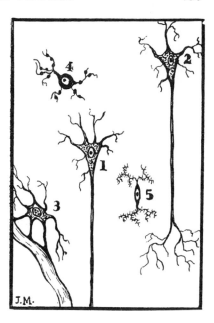

Fig. 169. Nerve cells and neuroglia. 1
and 2, nerve cells; 3, 4, and 5,
various types of neuroglial cells.

from nerve cells in the gray matter of the spinal cord and leave the
cord by the anterior nerve roots to become the motor peripheral nerves.
These nerve cells and their fibers constitute the *lower motor neurons,*
which receive and respond to impulses coming from the *upper motor
neurons, i.e.* the motor cells in the brain and their descending fibers.
Paralysis will result from injury either to upper motor neurons, as from
a cerebral hemorrhage, or to the lower motor neurons, as from poliomyelitis. Sensory impulses of various kinds are carried by the *afferent
sensory nerve fibers,* which enter the cord in the posterior nerve roots
and pass up to the appropriate centers in the brain. Here the messages
upon reaching our consciousness give information concerning the outside world.

The **nerve cells,** of which there are some 10 billion, have certain
peculiarities which distinguish them from all other cells. Two of their
most striking characteristics are their longevity and their unfortunately
great susceptibility to environmental and metabolic disturbances. The
nerve cells can live for 100 years (compare this with the short life of
the lymphocyte), but they pay a heavy price for their relative immortal-
ity because they cannot be replaced when they are destroyed, so that
the paralysis of poliomyelitis is permanent, as repair is impossible. They
have great metabolic activity, but on that account they require a constant large supply of oxygen and glucose, so that the cells of the cerebral
cortex cannot survive five minutes of anoxia due to complete arrest of

the circulation *at normal body temperature,* and a marked fall in blood sugar level results in loss of consciousness.

The **nerve fibers** in the central nervous system consist of two elements; the *axis cylinder,* which conducts the nervous impulses, and the *myelin sheath* that surrounds it. In the peripheral nerves a nucleated sheath, the *neurilemma,* is added. The myelin sheath consists of lipid or fatty material. When a peripheral nerve is cut the myelin breaks up into fine droplets which eventually disappear. This process is called *demyelination* and it is of particular significance in the central nervous system where it constitutes the principal feature of a group of so-called demyelinating diseases, of which multiple sclerosis is of special importance.

The nerve cells that send out motor impulses along nerve fibers and those that receive sensory impulses along corresponding fibers are situated in the *gray matter* of the brain, which is spread for the most part as a thin layer over the surface to form the cerebral cortex. These cells are collected in groups known as *centers* or *nuclei.* The various centers are linked by bundles of fibers known as association fibers. In the performance of an action many centers are associated, and when this is repeated many times the nervous impulse appears to flow along the corresponding *association paths* with increasing ease; the resistance to their passage seems to be diminished. Some such mechanism may form the physical basis of *habit.* Every act, indeed every thought, serves to make these paths more open and easily traversed. Every smallest stroke of virtue or of vice leaves its little scar. Nothing we ever do is, in strict scientific literalness, wiped out.

NEUROGLIA. The interstitial tissue of the central nervous system has long been known as the neuroglia. Glia means glue, and the neuroglia was regarded as a kind of putty which served the humble purpose of holding together the more noble neurons. We now know this to be nonsense. With ordinary stains the interstitial elements appear for the most part as naked nuclei, but with gold and silver impregnation the cells are seen to be provided with a forest of fibers. By the aid of these methods it is possible to distinguish three elements in the interstitial tissue: (1) astroglia, (2) oligodendroglia, and (3) microglia.

(1) The *astrocytes,* the cells of the astroglia, have peculiar processes called *sucker feet,* which are attached to the capillaries (Fig. 169, 3). For this reason the astroglia is believed to be involved in the transport of water and electrolytes between the capillaries and the nerve cells. The repair of wounds in the brain is due entirely to the activity of the astrocytes, and the *gliosis* seen in general paresis and other chronic inflammations of the brain consists of astrocytes and their fibers. Finally, it is from the astroglia that the glioma, the common brain tumor, takes its

origin. (2) The *oligodendroglia* is the largest group of the interstitial cells, but their function is still unknown, perhaps to the relief of the reader. The cells are smaller than the astrocytes and they possess a small number of processes (*oligos,* few) (Fig. 169, 4). (3) The *microglia* cells are very small (hence the name) and are provided with numerous fine branching processes (Fig. 169, 5). These cells are the phagocytes or scavengers of the central nervous system and when called on to perform this function they become greatly swollen, their processes are withdrawn into the cell, and the cytoplasm is filled with droplets of disintegrating myelin which they carry away and discharge into the nearest vessels.

PATHOLOGICAL PHYSIOLOGY. The normal physiology of the brain may be changed into dysfunction involving the motor or sensory fields or those of intellect or behavior. It is customary to speak of (1) "*organic*" disorders in which gross or microscopic lesions can be demonstrated, associated with interference with the supply of oxygen or carbohydrate to the brain or with abnormalities of cerebral enzyme activity, and of (2) "*functional*" disorders in which no such changes can be shown. It is becoming more and more probable that this failure is due to inadequacy in our technique. **What in the past we have called mental disease and stigmatized as insanity or madness is probably in most cases merely a biochemical disturbance of nerve cells which will be corrected in the future by biochemical means.** It seems likely that most of the popular tranquilizers and "psychic energizers" act upon the mechanism concerned with biochemical interactions in the nerve cells, that is to say the action of enzymes on carbohydrate in the presence of oxygen, and thus change the utilization of cerebral energy. It should be added that these ideas come from a pathologist who was once a psychiatrist. The weight of current psychiatric opinion runs counter to these assumptions. This also applies to the discussion of schizophrenia which follows. We must bear in mind that so much neurotic illness is related to personal difficulties and emotional disturbances.

Memory is the ability to receive a sensory impression, to retain it, and to recall it at the appropriate moment. Learning and memory are intertwined, and both may be lost because of disease and age. RNA (ribonucleic acid) is now known to play a part in learning and memory processes. It has been shown that RNA tablets can improve remembering in senile patients with impaired memory, although this procedure cannot be recommended to a student preparing for an examination.

Schizophrenia. It would be obviously absurd to think of considering the all-important subject of *mental disease* in this place, but a word may be devoted to schizophrenia in this discussion of the pathological physiology of the brain, for it is the principal cause of chronic mental illness, and is said to be responsible for more grave disability than any other illness in the whole of medicine. More than one-half of the beds for chronic disease in our hospitals are devoted to mental disorder, although the segregation of these beds in separate institutions conceals this fact from us. The frontier of the mind and its diseases remains one of the last frontiers to be pushed back in this day of incredible medical advances.

The word schizophrenia is derived from the Greek meaning *a divided mind,* and it connotes a disconnection between thoughts and feeling on the one hand and actions on the other. It manifests itself most often between the ages of 15 and 25 years (hence the older name of *dementia praecox*), first by a gradual social withdrawal, followed by the development of all sorts of bizarre hallucinations. It involves a fragmentation, a breaking-up, of all the processes of thought and feeling which enable a healthy person to remain in touch with his world; it might be regarded as a cancer of the mind gnawing into the very soul of the patient. What interests us in the present discussion is that similar hallucinations can be induced in a normal person by means of the so-called *hallucinogenic drugs,* as a result of which the volunteer subject may experience marked distortions of reality. The significance of these observations is that they indicate that *a chemical abnormality in a brain that is structurally normal may result in a condition of temporary insanity.*

Finally, there is the possibility that a *defective gene* may be at fault, for we know the genes control enzyme activity in the brain as elsewhere. In at least one of the inborn errors of metabolism, a subject already referred to in Chapter 14, there is a low level of serotonin in the serum, associated with severe mental deficiency in children. The condition is known as *oligophrenia,* which is simply Greek for feeblemindedness. The metabolic disturbance is reflected in the excretion of abnormal metabolites (phenylpyruvic acid) in the urine, thus allowing a laboratory diagnosis to be made. We may look forward to the day when a chemical test on the urine will be used to diagnose schizophrenia and when appropriate means will be available for correcting the metabolic defect while the condition is still in an early stage.

Even with the drugs now available many victims of mental illness need not be sent to public (mental) hospitals. Psychotherapy in the shape of psychoanalysis has proved its great value, but we should not let this exclude therapy with the aid of chemical agents. In our consideration of mental disease it would appear that we must bring back the soma as well as the psyche, just as in Chapter 1 we saw that in our study of physical disease we must not concentrate too much on the soma to the exclusion of the psyche.

CEREBROSPINAL FLUID. The brain and spinal cord are enclosed in two bony cases which are continuous with one another, namely, the skull and the spinal column. They are, therefore, unable to expand when they become swollen with blood or as the result of inflammation, and the increased tension causes headache, that commonest of symptoms. And yet there is an ingenious mechanism which serves to take up some of the temporary increases of pressure which may occur inside the skull. This mechanism is the *cerebrospinal fluid,* which bathes the brain and in which it is suspended as in a water-bath. This fluid not only covers the brain but also passes down the spinal canal outside the spinal cord. There is far more spare space in the canal than in the cranial cavity, so that when the brain becomes swollen the fluid flows out into the spinal canal and thus provides a much needed safety valve. The fluid is produced in a series of cavities in the interior of the brain which are known as the *cerebral ventricles* (Fig. 168).

From one of these (the fourth ventricle) it escapes by one or two tiny openings in the roof of the ventricle to reach the exterior of the brain, or rather the subarachnoid space through the walls of which it is absorbed into the blood stream. The **subarachnoid space** with its contained fluid passes down outside the spinal cord to the third piece of the sacrum, while the cord ends at the level of the first lumbar vertebra, so that in its lowest portion the sac contains only fluid. As production of fluid is more rapid than absorption, there is a constant flow out of the ventricles into the subarachnoid space. Should the openings in the root of the fourth ventricle become blocked the fluid accumulates and distends the ventricles, pressing the brain against the skull with serious results, a condition of *hydrocephalus* or water on the brain (Fig. 170).

The spinal fluid can be withdrawn by the simple procedure of **lumbar puncture;** a hollow needle is passed into the spinal canal between two contiguous vertebrae in the lumbar region, below the point where the spinal cord ends, and the fluid that escapes is collected. This procedure is of great value in two ways: (1) It is a simple means of lowering a dangerously high intracranial pressure, which may be threatening the life of the patient by injuring the vital centers; (2) it is a valuable means of diagnosis in diseases of the nervous system, for the fluid is a mirror in which are reflected many of the changes which may be affecting the brain and spinal cord.

The changes that the cerebrospinal fluid undergoes in conditions of disease, and the diagnostic value of such changes as revealed by laboratory examination will be better appreciated after these disease conditions have been discussed (p. 513).

One structure still remains to be described, the membrane or rather membranes that cover the brain and cord, just as the pleura covers the lungs and the peritoneum the abdominal organs. These membranes are known as the **meninges,** of which there are three, the dura mater, the

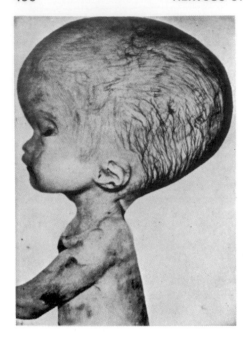

Fig. 170. Hydrocephalus showing huge sac of fluid. (Anderson, W.: Boyd's *Pathology for the Surgeon.* W. B. Saunders Co., 1967.)

arachnoid mater, and the pia mater. The *dura* is a tough membrane which lies in the cranial cavity and the spinal canal. The *pia* clothes the brain and cord like a glove, and the *arachnoid* like a mitt; there is, therefore, a space between these membranes, and that space, known as the *subarachnoid space,* is occupied by the cerebrospinal fluid. Fortunately this space extends a good deal lower than the termination of the spinal cord, so that in lumbar puncture a needle can be inserted into the space without danger of damaging the cord.

It may be of interest to know that dura mater is derived from the Latin *durus,* hard, and *mater,* mother, while *pia* means soft. To the ancients the meninges were the "mother" membranes. Hence Shakespeare's phrase, "nourished in the womb of pia mater." The ancients were not aware of the existence of the arachnoid, which means a spider's web.

STROKES

The most frequent organic lesions of the brain are the result of vascular disturbances. The word *apoplexy* comes from the Greek meaning a striking down, *i.e.,* a seizure or stroke. It is a very old term, for the condition was described by Hippocrates. To Galen it was "a sudden loss of feeling and of movement of the whole body, with the exception of respiration." The victim was believed to be struck down by some external force, as by the act of one of the gods. It is now restricted to a condition caused by acute vascular lesions in the brain which result in a sudden loss of consciousness, often accompanied by loss of sensation and motor power. What are known as **minor strokes,** "little strokes" or "strokelets," are characterized by *fleeting attacks of faintness, localized paralysis, aphasia* (loss of speech), and *visual disturbances.* The attacks are so temporary that they are accompanied by no structural damage, and are apparently a manifestation of temporary cerebral anoxia due to a combination of cardiac failure and cerebrovascular narrowing.

A great change has taken place in our thinking regarding **major strokes.** Not so long ago a stroke used to be synonymous with cerebral hemorrhage, and certainly a massive hemorrhage gives a classic picture of apoplexy. It is now realized, however, that the local ischemia responsible for a stroke may be due to (1) thrombosis, (2) embolism, or (3) hemorrhage, and that **the site of occlusion is more likely to be extracranial than intracranial.** The main arteries carrying the blood to the cranial cavity are (1) the *internal carotids* in the neck, and (2) the *vertebral arteries* which arise from the subclavian at the root of the neck and pass upward in the vertebral canal. *Revolutionary changes in the medical and surgical treatment of strokes demand accurate localization of the cause of the ischemia by means of cerebral angiography using radiopaque material and radiographic technique.*

The **clinical picture** of a stroke varies within the widest limits. It may take the form of a violent assault, in which the patient falls as if felled by an axe, deprived of sense and motion. This is the only variety that used to be recognized and it earned the condition its title of stroke or apoplexy. Far the most frequent type is that in which there is only a slight defect of speech, thought, motion, sensation, or vision; consciousness is not lost, and some degree of recovery is nearly invariable. It is obvious that the former type is likely to be caused by massive cerebral hemorrhage, the latter type by thrombosis.

CEREBRAL HEMORRHAGE. With advancing years the arteries in the brain tend to degenerate and become brittle. If at the same time the blood pressure is raised, there is danger of one of the brittle arteries bursting. When this happens the person is said to have an **apoplexy.** Even in the absence of hypertension, massive hemorrhage may occur in an area of softening produced by vascular occlusion (Fig. 171). The effect will naturally depend on the site of the hemorrhage and also on the extent. The most common position is unfortunately that part of the brain where the motor nerves to the body are gathered together into a comparatively small space before passing down the spinal cord. The hemorrhage destroys these nerves, the motor impulses are cut off from the muscles, and the side of the body (face, arm, and leg) supplied by the side of the brain affected is paralyzed, a condition known as **hemiplegia.** Should the patient survive, the paralyzed arm and leg gradually become flexed and assume the characteristic appearance shown in Figure 172. As the motor nerves from one side of the brain cross to the opposite side before passing down the cord, it follows that hemorrhage on the right side of the brain will be followed by a left-sided hemiplegia, and *vice versa.* The speech center in right-handed persons is on the left side of the brain, so that hemorrhage on the left side will destroy the nerve fibers that go to the organs of speech, producing a condition of speechlessness or *aphasia* in addition to a right-sided hemiplegia.

Apoplexy almost never produces sudden death, because the part of the brain in which it occurs contains no vital centers. Sudden death is nearly always due to sudden heart failure. But if the hemorrhage is large and close to the ventricles it may rupture into those cavities in the course of a day or two, a complication that is sure to prove fatal. On the other hand, if the hemorrhage is small the amount of damage to the brain is correspondingly limited, and only the arm or the leg may

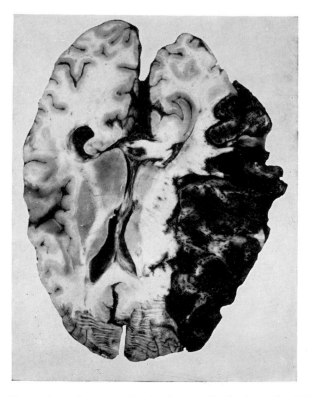

Fig. 171. Hemorrhage in area of softening in distribution of middle cerebral artery. (Boyd, *Textbook of Pathology.*)

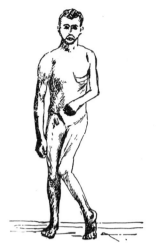

Fig. 172. Old hemiplegia due to cerebral hemorrhage.

be affected. The blood is gradually absorbed, and the patient may make a good recovery, with only a slight disability in the affected limb. Of course, there is always the danger of another hemorrhage later, a danger that hangs suspended over his head like the sword of Damocles but may never fall. The cerebral faculties are not necessarily interfered with. Pasteur did some of his best work after a stroke of apoplexy.

THROMBOSIS. *This is the most common cause of strokes, comprising probably 50 percent of all cases.* Atherosclerosis is the primary lesion with narrowing of the lumen, the occluding thrombus being added at a late stage to produce an *ischemic* stroke. The main site of obstruction is not in the brain but in the *extracerebral vessels,* often in extracranial vessels, more particularly the internal carotid in the neck (Fig. 173) and the vertebral artery. *Diagnosis of occlusion,* and in particular the exact site of the occlusion, can be established with certainty by cerebral angiography, to which reference has already been made. Excision of the occluded segment of the artery and anastomosis or insertion of an arterial or plastic graft may yield highly gratifying results in selected cases. This is a development impossible to imagine only a few years ago. The *lesions* are infarcts followed by cerebral softening with eventual liquefaction and the formation of a cyst. The myelin sheath of the nerve fibers breaks down into droplets of fat, which are taken up by the phagocytic microglia and carried away, while the astrocytes lay down a layer of gliosis around the cavity which may eventually be obliterated.

The *clinical picture* will vary so much with the site of the vessel occluded and the size of the area of brain affected that it would be fruitless to give a detailed description here. The neurological symptoms may take

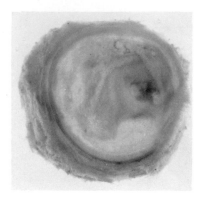

Fig. 173. Occlusion of internal carotid artery at site of carotid sinus. (Kindness of Dr. C. Miller Fisher.)

several days to develop. Compare this with the stroke of a cerebral hemorrhage in which the period is measured in minutes or at most in hours, or cerebral embolism in which the period is so short that it cannot be measured. There is a tendency for the stroke to develop while the patient is asleep or within an hour of arising, compared with a stroke due to hemorrhage which is likely to develop during waking hours of activity, while that due to embolism may of course occur at any time.

CEREBRAL EMBOLISM. The third great cause of strokes is embolism of the smaller cerebral vessels within the brain. The embolus most often arises in the left side of the heart, either as a vegetation on the mitral or aortic valve, or as a clot in the appendix of the left atrium, or a mural thrombus that has formed in the left ventricle at the site of a myocardial infarct. The embolus usually passes into the left carotid artery and is most likely to lodge in the middle cerebral. The accompanying paralysis may be very extensive, and is distinguished from other forms of strokes by the extreme suddenness of the onset of symptoms, with complete development in from ten to thirty seconds and a total absence of warning.

MENINGEAL HEMORRHAGE

Hemorrhage in relation to the meninges may be *extradural, subdural,* or *subarachnoid.*

EXTRADURAL HEMORRHAGE. Extradural hemorrhage (Fig. 174) is a condition in which blood is poured out between the skull and the dura mater. It is commonly called *middle meningeal hemorrhage,* because the bleeding occurs from the middle meningeal artery. This artery lies in contact with the inside surface of the skull in the region of the temple, and is liable to be torn by a fracture of the skull in this region. The condition is readily diagnosed because the patient is first stunned

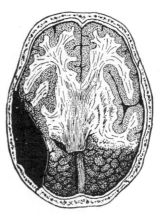

Fig. 174. Extradural hemorrhage. A dark blood clot lies between the skull and the brain.

by the blow to the skull; he then recovers consciousness and appears to be all right for a few hours—this is known as the *"lucid interval";* at the end of that time he becomes dull, drowsy, and finally loses consciousness again owing to the increasing pressure of the blood which is accumulating between the skull and the brain outside the dura mater. The condition *must* be diagnosed, for by immediate operation the collection of blood can be removed, the bleeding vessel tied, and the life of the patient saved. There is *no blood in the cerebrospinal fluid* at lumbar puncture, because the thick dura mater intervenes between the bleeding vessel and the cerebrospinal fluid.

SUBDURAL HEMORRHAGE. Subdural hemorrhage is **venous in origin,** not arterial, and in this respect it differs fundamentally from extradural and subarachnoid hemorrhage. The condition is at least four times as common as extradural hemorrhage, and it is of great importance because *the life of the patient depends on a correct diagnosis and this is easily missed.* The cause is a blow in the frontal or occipital region (*e.g.,* knocking the head against a shelf or door in the dark) which injures the cerebral veins passing into the subdural longitudinal sinus. The extravasated blood spreads slowly throughout the subdural space. The blood clot so formed is converted into a kind of cyst in which cerebrospinal fluid continues to collect. There is thus a continually increasing pressure on the underlying brain with the production of symptoms similar to those of a brain tumor. The confusing feature is the fact that many weeks may intervene between the relatively slight injury to the head and the development of cerebral symptoms, so that all memory of the injury may have been forgotten.

Intracranial hemorrhage of the newborn, a common cause of death, is a variety of subdural hemorrhage. The hemorrhage is due to injury during delivery producing tears in the cerebral veins crossing the subdural space to enter the longitudinal sinus. Death may occur in a few hours or in the course of a day or two. If the child survives, paralytic and mental symptoms may develop later.

SUBARACHNOID HEMORRHAGE.   Subarachnoid hemorrhage is hemorrhage into the subarachnoid space between the arachnoid and the pia mater. As the cerebrospinal fluid is contained in this space, *blood in large amount will be found in the fluid* at lumbar puncture. Such hemorrhage occurs when the surface of the brain is torn by a fracture of the skull, or it may be due to rupture of an aneurysm of one of the arteries that lie beneath the arachnoid at the base of the brain (Fig. 175). The latter variety is known as *spontaneous* subarachnoid hemorrhage, and produces a clinical picture that is easily mistaken for ordinary cerebral hemorrhage. The condition, which is not uncommon in young people, was usually fatal in the past, but modern neurosurgery has made it possible to deal with the aneurysm and arrest the hemorrhage.

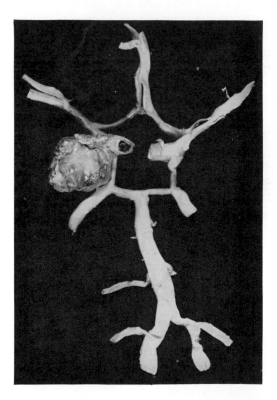

Fig. 175.   Aneurysm of circle of Willis. The aneurysm, which is of unusually large size and still unruptured, arises from the internal carotid artery. The location adjacent to a bifurcation is characteristic. (University of Alabama Medical School.)

FRACTURE OF THE SKULL

This may be considered in connection with cerebral hemorrhage, because the essential danger of this condition is laceration of the surface of the brain with accompanying hemorrhage. The fracture may involve the upper part of the skull or *vault,* or the *base* of the skull. The latter is by far the more serious, and is apt to prove fatal if not properly treated. The fracture itself is of little moment, although it may open into the ear or nose, causing bleeding from those organs. There is nearly always an accompanying laceration of the base of the brain with rapidly developing edema of that structure. Some of the most important vital nerve centers essential for life, those for the heart and for respiration, are situated in this part of the brain, and the increasing pressure on these centers caused by the edema may prove fatal. At the same time there is an accumulation of cerebrospinal fluid in this region which still further increases the pressure. It is evident that the most urgent need is to reduce the pressure inside the skull before the vital centers become paralyzed, and this is done most rapidly and effectively by repeated lumbar puncture and withdrawal of large amounts of spinal fluid. Since this method of treatment has been introduced, the mortality in cases of fracture of the base of the skull has been greatly reduced. Lumbar puncture also serves as a means of diagnosis, for the fluid is found to contain blood when the skull has been fractured and the brain torn.

ABSCESS OF THE BRAIN

The microorganisms that cause abscess of the brain may come from a focus of infection in the skull or may be carried by the blood stream from a distance. By far the commonest local source used to be the middle ear or mastoid, which is so often the site of suppuration, but antibiotic therapy has now given us control of this condition. The infection spreads inward and causes abscess formation in the adjacent part of the brain. Another source of danger is infection in the frontal and other air sinuses which communicate with the nose. Here the abscess is likely to be in the frontal part of the brain. If the infecting organisms come from a distance, the most common source is an abscess or other septic process in the lung. Indeed, *one of the dangers of abscess of the lung is the formation of a secondary abscess in the brain.*

SYMPTOMS. The symptoms of abscess of the brain are apt to be very misleading. It might be imagined that a collection of pus in so delicate a piece of mechanism as the brain would cause a violent disturbance, but the reverse is the case. Many parts of the brain are what are called *silent areas,* that is to say, a lesion of that part produces no characteristic symptoms, and this is particularly true of those parts in which an abscess is likely to occur. Moreover, the inflammation is usually of a quiet rather than a violent character. For these reasons the abscess may give rise neither to "localizing symptoms" nor even to those indicating infection. The clinical picture will rather be that of gradually increasing intracranial pressure, which may suggest a tumor instead of an abscess. Suspicion, however, will be aroused by the coexistence of middle-ear and mastoid infection, inflammation in the frontal sinus, or lung abscess.

Remarkably good results may follow the opening of a brain abscess, provided the operation is performed by a surgeon who knows what he is doing, but there is always danger of the infection's reaching the meninges with the production of a fatal meningitis. This complication may now be avoided by the use of antibiotics.

MENINGITIS

We have already seen that the brain and spinal cord are covered by membranes or meninges, inflammation of which constitutes the condition known as meningitis. This inflammation is confined to the pia and arachnoid, which are in intimate contact with the brain, and which contain between them the cerebrospinal fluid. Many organisms may cause meningitis, but the common ones are the meningococcus, streptococcus, pneumococcus, and tubercle bacillus. These cause, respectively, *meningococcal meningitis, streptococcal meningitis, pneumococcal meningitis,* and *tuberculous meningitis,* of which the first and the last are the most frequent. The first three organisms are pyogenic or pus-forming bacteria, so that the diseases they produce are acute and violent in type; the tubercle bacillus is less violent in action, yet it used to be the most fatal of the four types.

The *streptococcus* and *pneumococcus* reach the meninges from the middle ear or the frontal sinus, but they may be carried by the blood stream from distant parts, especially the lung. The *meningococcus* comes from the cavity of the nose or throat. It is an intracellular organism, usually found inside polymorphonuclear leukocytes (see Fig. 33). Meningitis may assume an epidemic form, with many cases developing in one locality or in many places throughout the country. Such epidemic meningitis is always due to the meningococcus. The infection is spread by *carriers,* who harbor the organisms in their throat, but do not themselves develop infection of the meninges. The term *cerebrospinal meningitis* is often applied to the meningococcal type, but the other forms are also cerebrospinal in the sense that the meninges of both the brain and the spinal cord are inflamed.

Tuberculous meningitis is in a class by itself. It has none of the acuteness of the other forms of meningitis and yet it used to be the most uniformly fatal, with a mortality of 100 per cent. The hopeless outlook has been dramatically changed in recent years by the use of streptomycin and still more by a combination of streptomycin, isoniazid, and para-aminosalicylic acid, which has given a survival rate of over 80 per cent. The infection is carried by the blood stream from some other tuberculous lesion, often a quiescent and unsuspected one.

At *autopsy* the subarachnoid space is filled with an acute inflammatory exudate in the meningococcal, streptococcal, and pneumococcal forms, so that the brain and cord are covered with yellow pus. In tuberculous meningitis, however, there is only a thin milky white layer in which tubercles may be distinguished with difficulty. As the subarachnoid space over the brain is continuous with that of the cord, lumbar puncture serves to show what is going on inside the skull in cases of meningitis.

Examination of the cerebrospinal fluid obtained by lumbar puncture gives the final diagnosis, including the type of bacterial infection. When normal cerebrospinal fluid is removed by this means it is as clear as water, and the pressure is so low that it flows out drop by drop. In *meningitis due to the pyogenic bacteria* the fluid is turbid, because in reality it is thin pus, and the pressure is raised to such a degree that it may spurt from the needle. When the fluid is examined under the microscope it is found to be crowded with polymorphonuclear leukocytes (pus cells), and to contain varying numbers of the bacteria responsible for the infection. In *tuberculous meningitis* the spinal fluid is only slightly milky or may be almost clear, for, as the inflammation is less acute, the cells are much fewer in number and are for the most part lymphocytes. The pressure is raised, as in the other forms of meningitis. When the fluid is allowed to stand, a fine *web of fibrin* forms. The *protein* is increased, the *sugar* is decreased and sometimes disappears, and the *chlorides* are very low. This is the most valuable of all the chemical tests, for no other condition gives a really low chloride reading. The demonstration of *tubercle bacilli* is the conclusive proof. Both the web and the centrifuged deposit should be examined for bacilli.

VIRAL DISEASES

A large number of known viruses can attack the central nervous system, sometimes setting up an inapparent infection, not infrequently meningitis or nonparalytic poliomyelitis, less often encephalitis. Viruses with a special affinity for the nervous system are called *neurotropic* and cause some of the most serious diseases of that system, such as poliomyelitis and rabies. There is another group of very common febrile viral diseases (measles, chickenpox, smallpox, vaccinia) in which injury of the nervous system occurs on rare occasions. Neurotropic viruses are peculiar in that they may reach the central nervous system *via* peripheral nerves, traveling actually in the axis cylinder of the nerve fiber, an excellent example being rabies. Neurotropic viruses diffuse throughout the entire nervous system, both central and peripheral.

Two great classes of lesions produced by neurotropic viruses may be distinguished: (1) nonsuppurative encephalitis (brain) or myelitis (spinal cord), in which an infecting agent enters and **destroys certain groups of nerve cells,** with poliomyelitis, rabies, and herpes as characteristic examples; (2) encephalomyelitis, in which the essential lesion is a primary **demyelination of nerve fibers.** The evidence that this second group is caused by viruses is not absolute. An acute disseminated demyelinating encephalomyelitis may follow specific viral fevers. The question which naturally suggests itself is whether a demyelinating disease such as multiple sclerosis, on which so much popular interest is focused, should be included in this group. Only a few of the viral diseases that affect the nervous system of man and still more of domestic animals will be mentioned in the discussion that follows.

ACUTE ANTERIOR POLIOMYELITIS. Poliomyelitis or *infantile paralysis* is an acute infectious disease of the spinal cord and brain caused by a filterable virus (poliovirus) and chiefly affecting children, although now also adults with increasing frequency. The name signifies an inflammation of the gray matter or marrow of the spinal cord (*polios,* gray; *myelos,* marrow). It is the anterior part of the gray matter of the cord containing the motor nerve cells which is chiefly affected, thus explaining the term anterior in the full title (Fig. 176). The disease may occur in sporadic, *i.e.,* occasional, form, or it may become epidemic. An epidemic usually begins about the end of June and for some unknown reason disappears with the onset of cold weather.

The virus is carried from one person to another in the throat or the intestine where it can live without producing any symptoms and without invading the nervous system. Such individuals are called carriers. They are immune to the disease, but they can carry the infection. During an epidemic there are far more carriers than patients suffering from the disease, that is to say, there is a much larger carrier epidemic than dis-

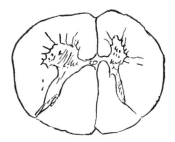

Fig. 176. Late effects of poliomyelitis: atrophy of right anterior (motor) horn of the spinal cord.

ease epidemic. The virus has also been found in the feces of patients convalescing from the disease, and even in sewage.

The general virology of the poliovirus has already been outlined in Chapter 10, including the cytopathogenic effect when grown in tissue culture, and immunization against the infection by either attenuated or dead vaccines. It was the crowning triumph of tissue culture which made possible the large-scale commercial production of polio vaccine.

The infection is primarily one of the alimentary canal rather than the respiratory tract as we used to believe. Nor is the route by which the virus spreads from the original site of infection to the central nervous system along the axis cylinders of nerves, as in the case of rabies. While this can occur, serving to explain the spread up and down the cord, it has been displaced by the concept of *viremia.* Invasion of the blood stream probably develops in every case, only to be quenched as a rule by circulating antibodies. It is only when these are not forthcoming in sufficient quantity that the central nervous system becomes involved. Or overexertion, fatigue, or trauma may tip the balance against the defense even when the antibodies are adequate. Invasion of the spinal cord and brain may never develop if the immunological barrier in the blood is sufficiently strong. Once invasion of the nervous system has occurred the progress of the virus cannot be influenced in any way. *The immunity that follows an attack is life-long, immune bodies being demonstrable in the blood during the remainder of the patient's life.*

The **lesions** are most evident in the *motor cells of the anterior horn of the gray matter of the spinal cord*. The motor nerve cells of the lower part of the brain (pons and medulla) may also be attacked, so that respiration may be severely impaired, and if death occurs it is due to destruction of these cells. The destruction produced by the virus in the nerve cells is devastating. All the fine structure of the cells is lost, together with their enzymes, as can be seen in Figure 177. Finally, there may be complete disappearance of all the motor cells. Small wonder that the result is complete paralysis of the part or parts involved. The process of cell death and disintegration may be incredibly rapid, as can be seen in the experimental animal. The *meninges* are also involved, so that the cerebrospinal fluid may be expected to show changes.

Basis of Symptoms.   The child or adult shows *general symptoms* of infection, such as fever, malaise, irritability, and loss of appetite. After a day or two of these symptoms the *paralysis,* which is so characteristic and tragic a feature of the disease, suddenly makes its appearance. Only one arm or one leg may be paralyzed, or both legs, and occasionally both arms as well.

Nerve cells differ from most cells of the body in being unable to proliferate, so that no repair or replacement of the injured cells is possible.

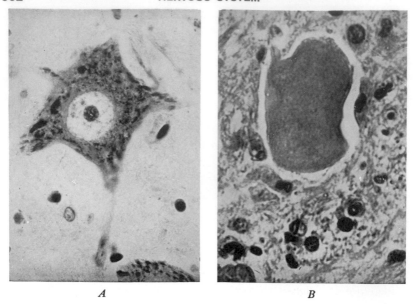

A B

Fig. 177. *A,* Normal nerve cell showing processes, concave borders, Nissl granules, nucleus, and nucleolus. × 600. *B,* Degenerated nerve cell; borders convex, loss of processes, Nissl granules, and nucleus. × 600.

For this reason the paralysis is permanent. The paralyzed muscles atrophy from disuse, so that the limb becomes wasted and shriveled (Fig. 178). If the vital centers in the lower part of the brain are also affected there may be *paralysis of swallowing and respiration,* which may result in death. The symptoms are not purely motor, for there is usually *pain* in the back and the affected limbs. *Stiffness of the neck* and *rigidity of the back* are constant and early symptoms. The explanation of these sensory symptoms is not certain, but they are supposed to be due to irritation of the meninges and the sensory nerves. During an epidemic many children manifest only the sensory disturbances and never develop paralysis, owing probably to their motor nerve cells possessing a certain degree of immunity against the virus.

The *cerebrospinal fluid* in the paralytic form shows a moderate increase of lymphocytes of not more than 200 or 300 per c.mm. The protein is normal or slightly elevated at first, rising later, as the cell count falls, to 300 mg. per 100 cc. In the nonparalytic form or the pre-paralytic stage the cell count is much higher, with polymorphonuclears predominating. The spinal fluid of tuberculous meningitis can be distinguished from that of poliomyelitis by the presence of a fibrin web, the decrease of sugar and particularly of chlorides, and the much greater increase of protein, as well as the occasional finding of tubercle bacilli.

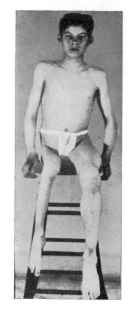

Fig. 178. End-result of poliomyelitis; marked atrophy of right leg.

RABIES. There is no more dramatic and deadly example of viral infection than rabies. It has already been discussed in Chapter 10, but one or two points of distinction from poliomyelitis may be noted. In poliomyelitis infection comes from a human carrier, whereas in rabies it comes from the saliva of an animal. In poliomyelitis the virus is carried to the central nervous system by the blood, whereas in rabies it passes along the axis cylinders of the afferent sensory nerves from the point of inoculation. The characteristic Negri inclusion body of rabies has already been illustrated (p. 174). Its practical significance is that when a person has been bitten by a dog suspected of being rabid, microscopic examination of the animal's brain will show whether or not the fingerprint of rabies, the Negri body, is present in the nerve cells, and preventive lifesaving inoculation can be commenced at once if necessary. Finally, in poliomyelitis we are now beginning to practice preventive vaccination, yet this practice was introduced by Pasteur with complete success for the prevention of rabies nearly 100 years ago.

ENCEPHALITIS. *Viral encephalitis* constitutes a group of diseases, some of which are epidemic. Any detailed consideration of this group is beyond the scope of this *Introduction,* but one or two members may be mentioned. *Lethargic encephalitis,* also called "sleeping sickness," appears in epidemic form at long intervals and sweeps across the world. In an epidemic that I studied in Winnipeg in 1919 the patient was dull, lethargic, and somnolent. He would lie like a log in bed with drooping lids or closed eyes, sunk in a stupor that no external stimuli could penetrate, the dim rushlight of reason hardly flickering. About 20 per cent of these cases subsequently developed some degree of *post-encephalitic paralysis agitans* or *Parkinsonism,* a condition of generalized rigidity of the face and body which is described later in relation to Parkinson's disease (p. 509). *Equine encephalitis,* as its name indicates, is a viral disease of horses which appears in epidemic form. Farm workers may also fall victim to it. Human infection is probably due to mosquitoes, which convey the infection from horse to man, although this has not been proved. Wild birds may act as the reservoir hosts of the virus. *Secondary encephalitis* may occur as a complication following one of the common viral fevers, usually *measles,* more rarely mumps and chickenpox. Finally, *post-vaccinal encephalitis* must be mentioned, in which in rare instances a severe form of encephalitis follows vaccination for smallpox.

HERPES. Herpes is a viral disease characterized by the formation of small vesicles. The name is derived from the Greek word meaning to creep. There are two distinct forms: (1) herpes zoster or *shingles,* in which the vesicles follow or creep along the distribution of a sensory nerve, and (2) herpes simplex, in which there is no such distribution. An attack of the former is followed by lasting immunity, but in the case of the latter there is no immunity. They are caused by entirely different viruses. *Herpes zoster* is the sensory analogue of poliomyelitis, with lesions in the posterior root ganglia. A puzzling feature is that the eruption is always unilateral, running in a zone (zoster) as far as the middle line, being preceded by neuralgic pains, which *in old people* may be very persistent and severe. The virus appears to be identical with that causing chickenpox, the spread in the latter case being by the blood stream whereas in zoster it is along the nerves. *Herpes simplex* is the common form of herpes, usually on the lips as a complication of infective fevers, pneumonia, and even the common cold, so that it is best known as a "cold sore." Again the lesion is in a sensory nerve ganglion and spread is along the nerve.

ASEPTIC MENINGITIS. This should really be called **viral meningitis,** in contrast to the usual bacterial or septic meningitis. It is not strictly a disease entity, because it can be caused by a variety of viruses. Particular mention should be made of *Coxsackie virus* infection, so named from the village in New York State where the virus was first isolated. Its distinguishing feature is that it is pathogenic for the suckling mouse in whom immunity has not yet developed, but not in older animals, thus differing sharply from the virus of poliomyelitis. Other viruses which may be responsible for aseptic meningitis are those of *poliomyelitis, herpes simplex* and *mumps.* The *clinical features* are an acute onset, fever, headache, stiffness of the neck, and in particular a very high lymphocyte count, many hundreds in number, in the cerebrospinal fluid.

SYPHILIS OF THE NERVOUS SYSTEM

Among the most tragic manifestations of syphilis are those due to infection of the central nervous system in cases untreated by modern antibiotic methods, particularly by penicillin. A peculiarity of these lesions is that they do not develop for many years after the original infection; it may be 10, 15, or even 20 years later. The patient may have been without symptoms for years, may have almost forgotten that he ever had syphilis, when suddenly, without warning the sword of Damocles may fall. Various parts of the nervous system may be attacked, so that the symptoms may be very varied, but there are two clearly cut clinical pictures or diseases which alone will be described here. The first and most terrible of these is general paresis or general paralysis of the insane, the second is tabes dorsalis or locomotor ataxia.

GENERAL PARESIS.   The name is descriptive, for it implies not only a weakness of the muscles but a general weakening of all the faculties of the mind. The even more sinister "general paralysis of the insane" describes the final state of the patient. The spirochetes of syphilis are scattered widely throughout the brain, and produce multiple areas of inflammation together with destruction of the nerve cells and nerve fibers. As a result of this destruction the brain atrophies and wastes away, becoming much smaller than normal. This wasting affects particularly the cerebral cortex in the frontal region, that is to say the part of the brain concerned with the highest functions of the mind. The areas concerned with muscular movements and with sensation are also involved.

Basis of Symptoms.   The symptoms of the disease are as diverse as the lesions are widely disseminated. The first indication that all is not well is a painful *deterioration in the higher life of the mind and the soul.* The moral sense is impaired, and there is a weakening of the faculties of judgment, reason, and self-control. *Delusions of grandeur* lead to domestic and financial difficulties, for if a man believes that he is worth millions and orders motor cars and grand pianos in corresponding amount, it is not conducive to domestic happiness. The structure of the mind crumbles, and the final stage is one of childishness and *complete dementia.* All of these changes are due to destruction of the nerve cells in the cerebral cortex. *Tremors* are highly characteristic; they involve the face, lips, and tongue so that the speech becomes thick and indistinct, and the hands are tremulous. These tremors are due to lesions in the motor centers. The sensory centers are also involved, so that sensibility is dulled and pain may hardly be felt. The pupil of the eye no

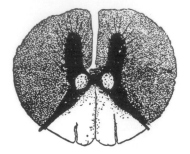

Fig. 179. Spinal cord in tabes dorsalis; marked degeneration (white) of posterior columns.

longer contracts when exposed to bright light, although it still does so when the eye looks at a near object, a condition known as the *Argyll-Robertson pupil. Convulsive seizures* followed by unconsciousness are common. The *weakness of the muscles* implied in the name of the disease becomes extreme. In the end the patient is not only mindless but helpless. To describe his existence as that of an animal is unjust to even the lowest member of the animal kingdom.

The *cerebrospinal fluid* shows changes that are of great importance, because they allow the physician to make an early diagnosis at a time when treatment may arrest the progress of the disease. The cells of the fluid, particularly lymphocytes, are markedly increased, especially at the beginning of the malady. The protein is increased, but far more significant is the fact that the Wassermann test on the fluid is positive, showing that the patient is suffering from syphilis of the central nervous system. The colloidal gold reaction gives a significant paretic curve.

TABES DORSALIS. The word tabes means a wasting away, and as the lesion in this syphilitic disease of the spinal cord is a wasting of the posterior or dorsal part of the cord, the condition is called tabes dorsalis (Fig. 179). In the dorsal columns of the cord run the nerves that carry the sensation of position, what is called muscle sense and joint sense. When these are lost the patient is no longer certain of the position of his legs, so that he becomes unsteady or *ataxic* in his locomotion. For this reason the disease is also known as **locomotor ataxia.** The first name is a pathological term indicating the lesion, the second is a clinical term indicating one of the principal symptoms.

Anyone wishing to read a description of the onset of the *symptoms of tabes* by a master of literature should look up Kipling's wonderful little story, "Love o' Women." There is no muscular weakness, for the lesion is confined to the sensory nerves, but the power of muscular co-ordination is gradually lost, so that the patient is unable to make his legs do what he wants them to. Things are not so bad as long as he has the assistance of sight, but in the dark he is completely at sea. The ordinary person walks by faith (without watching the ground), but the tabetic walks by sight. He walks with his legs wide apart to increase his stability, and is unable to stand with his feet together and his eyes closed without swaying or falling (*Romberg's sign*). To the trained eye the tabetic can be recognized at once as he walks down the street by his peculiar wide-based gait and the way he throws his feet out and brings them down with a stamp.

Other sensory disturbances are sudden, severe shooting pains passing down the legs known as *lightning pains,* and occasional attacks of abdominal pain and vomiting, called *gastric crises,* which may be mistaken for acute appendicitis. There is *loss of the knee-jerks, i.e.,* lack of response when the tendon below the knee cap is tapped, loss of the normal contraction of the pupil to light (*Argyll Robertson pupil*) as in general paresis, and gradual wasting of the optic nerve, *optic atrophy,* with corresponding impairment of vision. The disease may last many years, because it involves no vital centers. The *cerebrospinal fluid* shows the same changes as in general paresis so that its examination is of the greatest help in diagnosis. Again, in this form of central nervous system syphilitic infection, penicillin is the best *method of treatment* and may often serve to arrest the progress of the condition and relieve many of the symptoms.

If the reader should ask why the *Treponema pallidum* attacks the brain in one patient and the spinal cord in another, there is at the present time no answer.

DEMYELINATING DISEASES

A glance at the Outline of Contents at the beginning of this chapter will show that it is easy to group many of the diseases of the central nervous system under such headings as strokes, meningitis, viral infections, and syphilis. In these instances we have a fairly good idea of the etiological agent involved and the meaning of the pathological changes. Unfortunately there remains a large and heterogeneous collection of conditions of unknown etiology, which are referred to vaguely as degenerative diseases of the nervous system. From this large collection it seems justifiable to separate off at least one group known as the demyelinating diseases.

We have already considered some of the characteristics of the myelin sheath of the nerve fibers both in the central nervous system and in the peripheral nerves. The essential feature of a demyelinating disease is destruction of the myelin sheaths and relative sparing of the axis cylinders as well as other elements such as nerve cells and neuroglia.

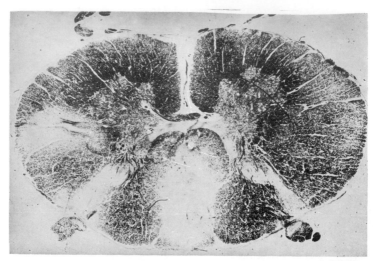

Fig. 180. Multiple sclerosis. There are irregular asymmetrical patches of degeneration in the posterior and lateral columns. (Weigert's myelin stain.) × 8.

By far the most important member of this group is multiple sclerosis, with which may be included Schilder's disease, as well as others which will not even be mentioned. Although we are ignorant as to the etiology and pathogenesis of the demyelinating diseases it would appear at the present time that an allergic process, perhaps autoimmune in character, is the best working hypothesis for this baffling group.

MULTIPLE SCLEROSIS.   This condition, also known as disseminated sclerosis, is a chronic disease of the nervous system, characterized by curious remissions and relapses, and by the presence of multiple patches of demyelination associated with sclerosis or hardening scattered diffusely throughout the gray and white matter of the brain stem and spinal cord. The nerve fibers in the white matter degenerate and are replaced by glial (neuroglial) scar tissue (Fig. 180). The cause is unknown but may be related to a condition of allergy or autoimmunity.

The **clinical picture** is extremely varied. The patient, usually a young man, suffers from an assortment of sensory and motor symptoms, some of which may be quite fleeting. The *sensory disturbances* take the form of *numbness* and *tingling* in the hands and feet, or definite loss of sensation. *Motor disturbances* are seen in the *gait,* which is *peculiarly* stiff, in *fleeting paralyses,* in tremor of the hands when they are used (*intention tremor*), a jerky movement of the eyes (*nystagmus*), and a characteristic *staccato speech.* The patient is absurdly cheerful, considering the progressive and incurable nature of his ailment.

There is no satisfactory treatment, but on account of the remissions the patient may live for many years.

The *cerebrospinal fluid* with one exception shows little change, although in the early cases there is a mild lymphocytosis and a slight increase in protein, but in the advanced sclerotic stage these changes are absent. The exception is the *colloidal gold reaction,* which in about one-half of the cases *gives a paretic curve,* though the Wassermann reaction is uniformly negative.

SCHILDER'S DISEASE.   This fortunately rare condition, which affects children and young adults, closely resembles multiple sclerosis in its pathology, but it involves the cerebral hemispheres, not the brain stem and spinal cord. The onset is acute and the course rapidly progressive, in these respects differing completely from multiple sclerosis. There is early blindness, deafness, sensory disturbance, motor paralysis, and mental deterioration.

PARKINSON'S DISEASE

Parkinson's disease, also known as *paralysis agitans* or, more colloquially, "the shaking palsy," is a chronic, nonkilling, but profoundly disabling degeneration of the brain, perhaps the best known member of the group known as degenerative diseases of the central nervous system. The *clinical picture* was drawn in 1817 by Parkinson with the hand of a master. The classic triad of symptoms are rigidity, tremor, and an attitude of flexion. The *rigidity* involves all the voluntary muscles, until in an extreme case the unhappy sufferer becomes as rigid as a block of marble. This rigidity gives the face the familiar "Parkinsonian mask." The *tremor* affects the fingers and hands, giving a cigarette-rolling movement. Curiously enough it is present when the part is at rest, disappearing for a few minutes with movement, thus justifying the term "shaking palsy," and differing from the "intention tremor" of multiple sclerosis. The whole attitude is one of flexion. The head is flexed on the chest, the body is bowed, the arms and wrists are flexed, the knees are bent, and the forward-leaning posture enforces steps that are short and almost running, so that an advanced case of the disease can be diagnosed at a glance (Fig. 181).

Parkinsonism is seen in two forms. The first is the rare *primary* form of unknown etiology described long ago by Parkinson. The other is a form *secondary* to the great epidemic of *encephalitis lethargica* just before and after 1920, due almost certainly to a virus. In both cases the lesion is a degeneration of the nerve cells of the corpus striatum consisting of the globus pallidus and substantia nigra in the midbrain. In the primary form there is marked disappearance of the large pale motor cells of the globus pallidus, whereas in the secondary form the degenera-

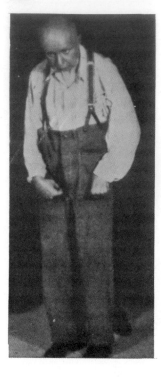

Fig. 181. Parkinsonism. (Grinker's *Neurology,* Charles C Thomas.)

tive changes are in the substantia nigra with loss of melanin in the pigmented cells and also of the neurohormonal transmitter *dopamine,* of which *dopa* is a precursor. The dopamine stores in the basal ganglia are markedly depleted. There is a correspondingly low content of dopa in the urine. The essence of the condition is an enzyme defect. The most recent method of treatment is the daily intramuscular injection of dopa in the form of L-dopa, a derivative. This results in a dramatic improvement in both the appearance and the behavior of the patient through reversal of the crippling effects of the disease. The disease used to be a rarity, but during the last 40 or 50 years, that is to say since around 1920, it has become much commoner. This may be because the causal agent of the encephalitis epidemic damaged the subthalamic cells, but not to a sufficient degree to produce clinical symptoms. The passage of the years or possibly some kind of delayed-fuse action brought the submerged disturbance to the surface. If this idea is correct, Parkinson's disease will happily soon once more become a rarity.

Many other uncommon or rare degenerative diseases of unknown etiology and therefore classified as *idiopathic* (from the Greek meaning individual, thus originating in one's self) involving the central nervous system will be found described in textbooks of medicine and pathology, but I feel that it would be out of place to consider or even mention them here.

INTRACRANIAL TUMORS

We have already seen that the brain is composed of two types of cells, the nerve cells and the neuroglial cells. Tumors of the brain only arise from and are composed of neuroglial cells and therefore are called *gliomas*. Not uncommonly a tumor grows from the meninges which cover the brain, and is therefore called a *meningioma*. There is a fundamental difference between these two types of tumor, for the meningioma is a benign tumor, which is encapsulated and merely presses upon the brain, whereas the glioma is a malignant tumor which infiltrates the brain and is not demarcated from it in any way.

Two points might be added to the above brief summary. (1) It is evident that intracranial tumor may be intracerebral or extracerebral. The *intracerebral tumors* are the gliomas and metastatic carcinoma, as well as a few rarities which will not be mentioned. The *extracerebral tumors* are the meningiomas, tumors of the acoustic nerve, pituitary tumors, and craniopharyngiomas which arise from the remnants of the epithelial tract from which the pituitary is formed. (2) The reason that intracerebral tumors are gliomas rather than nerve cell tumors is that glial cells, particularly astrocytes, are capable of unlimited mitotic division, whereas the adult nerve cells live on but are incapable of multiplying. Cells that are not capable of division are not likely to give rise to neoplasms.

GLIOMA. Although gliomas are malignant by virtue of their infiltrative power, they vary greatly in their degree of malignancy, and while some are rapidly growing and kill the patient in a few months, others grow very slowly and the patient may live for many years, especially if he receives skillful surgical treatment. Moreover, gliomas do not form metastases or secondary growths in other parts of the body as most malignant tumors do, probably because the tumor cells fail to escape from the interior of the skull.

There are many different kinds of glioma, but only four of these will be described. Of these four, two occur principally in the adult, namely, glioblastoma multiforme and astrocytoma; two occur in children, namely, medulloblastoma and ependymoma. The *glioblastoma multiforme* is a highly malignant tumor occurring in middle life and is usually found in one or other of the cerebral hemispheres. The margin is ill-defined so that the surgeon may have great difficulty in knowing where the tumor ends and the normal brain begins (Fig. 182). It is highly invasive and is likely to kill the patient in the course of a few months. The *astrocytoma* is much less malignant, and the average time of survival after operation is six years. It may occur in any part of the brain,

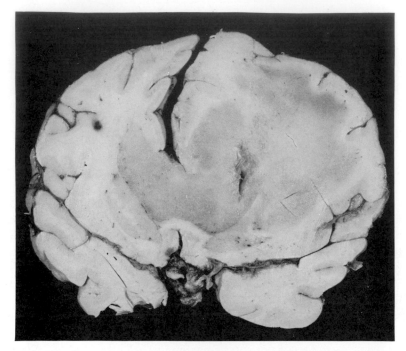

Fig. 182. Glioblastoma multiforme, showing massive infiltration of right and left frontal lobes. (University of Alabama Medical School.)

but in children the common site is the cerebellum. The cerebellar tumor in children is usually completely benign. The *medulloblastoma* is a highly malignant and rapidly growing tumor in the roof the fourth ventricle in the midline of the cerebellum. The prognosis of this tumor of children is therefore the very opposite to that of astrocytoma. The *ependymoma* is the rarest of the four. It usually occurs in children and in the same location as the medulloblastoma. It is, however, much less malignant than that tumor.

MENINGIOMA. This nearly always benign tumor arising from the meninges covering the brain is one of the common forms of intracranial neoplasm. Although benign it will obviously kill the patient in due time by virtue of its intracranial position and the pressure it exerts on the brain *unless it is removed*. The meningioma is usually much firmer than the glioma, and it is adherent externally to the dura. As it presses on the brain from the outside, it forms a deep bed for itself, from which on the autopsy table it can readily be lifted out (Fig. 183). In the operating room things are much less simple, for there is danger of severe or even fatal hemorrhage from large vessels that pass between the highly vascular overlying bone and the tumor. *Local changes in the skull* may

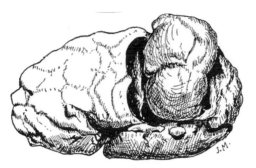

Fig. 183. Meningioma lifted out of cavity which it has produced in brain by pressure.

be of great help in diagnosis. In about 25 per cent of cases there is bony thickening of the skull over the tumor which can be detected radiographically and sometimes even by physical examination.

Acoustic nerve tumor is another intracranial tumor which is much more closely related to meningioma than to the gliomas. It grows from the eighth cranial nerve at the angle between the pons and the cerebellum and forms a firm, round, well-encapsulated tumor. It presses upon the nerve supplying the muscles of the face as well as upon the acoustic or auditory nerve. The principal symptoms are therefore facial paralysis and deafness on one side. It is important to realize that the tumor is perfectly benign, so that when removed surgically there is no chance of its return.

METASTATIC TUMORS. When a diagnosis is made of tumor of the brain the doctor has to bear in mind the possibility that the tumor may be a secondary carcinoma. In such cases *by far the commonest primary tumor is bronchogenic carcinoma, next in frequency being carcinoma of the breast*. The tumors are usually multiple rather than single, and on this account the clinical picture may be perplexingly confused. To add to the confusion the signs and symptoms may be entirely cerebral, with the primary tumor remaining completely silent. This is particularly likely to happen in the case of bronchogenic carcinoma.

BASIS OF SYMPTOMS. The symptoms of a brain tumor may be divided into two groups, the first general and the second localizing. The **general symptoms** are due to the increased intracranial pressure produced by the mass of new tissue inside the skull, and are more or less the same in whichever part of the brain the tumor is situated. The chief of these is *headache,* which may become excruciating in intensity. The *cerebrospinal fluid pressure* is greatly increased, as shown by lumbar puncture. *Vomiting* may be marked in the later stages, but is often absent. The pressure on the optic nerves produces swelling of the termination of these nerves in the eye, a condition called *optic neuritis* followed by *optic atrophy,* which can be recognized when the retina of the eye is viewed with the ophthalmoscope. X-ray examination may show *thinning of the skull.*

The **localizing symptoms** are naturally very varied, because they depend on the site of the tumor in the brain. If the *motor centers* are involved there will be weakness of the muscles of the face, arm, or leg. If the *sensory centers* are affected there will be corresponding disturbance of sensation. Involvement of the *special senses,* such as sight or hearing, will point to the areas concerned with these functions. It is for this reason that these symptoms are known as localizing, because by a careful analysis of these disturbances the physician is able to arrive at a conclusion as to the exact location of the tumor, and the surgeon is then able to open the skull at the correct spot where he will have access to the lesion. Unfortunately, there are fairly extensive regions of the brain known as *silent areas,* so-called because lesions of these areas do not give rise to any localizing symptoms. If the tumor is situated in one of the silent areas, it may be impossible to determine its exact location, impossible even to decide on which side of the brain to operate.

The *radiologist* may provide invaluable information in the diagnosis and localization of intracranial tumors. Gases that are radiolucent when introduced into the subarachnoid space and thus into the cerebral ventricles serve to outline the ventricles and indicate the site of a tumor which may distort that outline. Of particular value is *angiography,* which consists of injecting a radiopaque oil into the cerebral circulation. By this means, the outline of the tumor may be indicated even in those lesions that do not distort the ventricles. The procedure is of special importance in the case of intracranial aneurysms and other vascular anomalies.

If the reader would like to get a vivid idea of what it is like to be a patient with a brain tumor, he should read "A Journey Round My Skull," by the distinguished Hungarian novelist, Frigyes Karinthy, who himself was the patient. The rather terrifying description of the operation under a local anesthetic is perhaps somewhat highly colored.

The *treatment* of brain tumors is discouraging but by no means hopeless. If the tumor can be located, much or the whole of it may be removed. In the case of a meningioma a complete cure may be expected. With the gliomas it is very much more difficult for the surgeon to know if he has removed all the tumor, so that there is great danger that some of it may be left behind and that the growth will recur. But even if a cure cannot be assured, several years of comfort and comparative health may be added to the patient's life. Perhaps the most important point for the patient with a brain tumor to decide is to choose the right surgeon.

CEREBROSPINAL FLUID IN DISEASE

The normal spinal fluid is as clear as water, contains sugar and chlorides, no protein, less than 5 lymphocytes per c.mm., and no polymorphonuclears. In *acute meningitis* the vessels in the inflamed meninges allow the constituents of the blood to pour into the fluid, so that it contains much protein and great numbers of polymorphonuclears. The fluid is therefore purulent and turbid. The bacteria feed on and destroy the sugar, so that this substance is reduced in amount or disappears entirely. Bacteria are found in smears of the pus and in culture. *Tuberculous meningitis,* which is much less acute, gives rather different spinal fluid findings. The fluid is clear or only slightly milky, as it usually contains less than 100 cells per c.mm., most of which are lymphocytes. The protein (globulin) is only moderately increased, and the sugar correspondingly diminished. The most characteristic findings are a marked diminution in the chlorides and the presence of tubercle bacilli in the smears. In poliomyelitis the picture is identical with that of tuberculous meningitis, except that the chlorides are normal and there are, of course, no tubercle bacilli.

In suspected *brain tumor* the spinal fluid must be examined for *tumor cells.* These are much more likely to be found in secondary carcinoma than in glioma, although in the latter condition there may be a marked increase in the lymphocyte count. The use of the millipore membrane filter gives considerably better results than the conventional sedimentation methods. In *spinal cord tumors,* which resemble intracranial tumors and are not considered here, the spinal fluid may show the "compression syndrome" if the canal is blocked. Below the obstruction the characters of the fluid are as follows: (1) massive spontaneous coagulation, (2) xanthochromia or yellow coloration of the fluid, (3) marked increase in the protein, (4) no corresponding increase in the cells. This is known as the *Froin syndrome,* of which only the last two features may be present. The exact site of a spinal cord tumor may sometimes be determined by the intraspinal injection of *Lipiodol* followed by radiography. It is evident that lumbar puncture can be of great value in the diagnosis of suspected spinal cord tumors.

FURTHER READING

BOGOOCH, S.: *The Biochemistry of Memory,* New York, 1968.
CONSTANTINIDES, P.: Arch. Path., 1967, *83,* 422. (Pathogenesis of cerebral artery thrombosis.)
ENESCO, H. E.: Can. Psychiat. Ass. J.: 1967, *12,* 29. (RNA and memory.)
FISHER, C. M.: Can. Med. Ass. J., 1953, *69,* 257. (Strokes.)
HUGHES, J. T.: *Pathology of the Spinal Cord,* London, 1966.

Chapter **28**

Locomotor System

Human locomotion depends on a number of structures and functions. Bones, joints between the bones, and muscles, the contraction of which results in movement, are the three obvious structures that will be discussed in this chapter. It is equally obvious, of course, that without motor nerves, the cells in the spinal cord from which these nerve fibers arise, and the impulses from the motor areas in the cerebral cortex, locomotion is impossible, as we have seen in the previous chapter.

BONES
Structure and Function

A bone is not a dead thing. It is true that it is impregnated with a nonliving material which gives it its rigidity, but the bone itself is just

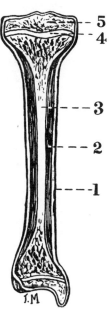

Fig. 184. Long bone. 1, Periosteum; 2, shaft; 3, medullary cavity; 4, epiphyseal cartilage; 5, epiphysis.

as much alive as the heart or the brain. It consists of bone cells surrounded by a modified fibrous tissue saturated with salts of calcium, in which there are spaces or interstices which are particularly numerous at the ends of the bone. In the center of the shaft of the bone there is a cavity, the *medullary cavity,* filled with the *bone marrow* which manufactures the red blood cells and the leukocytes (Fig. 184). The marrow also extends into the interstices of the bone, and is therefore particularly abundant at the ends of the bone. Lining the medullary cavity and the interstices are primitive bone cells called *osteoblasts,* which are the precursors of the adult bone cells, and whose function it is to form new bone. It is from these cells that the commonest form of malignant bone tumor, the osteogenic sarcoma, is formed. In the same situations there are much larger cells, giant cells containing several nuclei, called *osteoclasts.* They are concerned with removal instead of formation of bone, and from them also a tumor, the giant-cell tumor, is believed by many to arise, but unlike the osteogenic sarcoma it is essentially benign.

During childhood and adolescence the bones grow in length. This they do entirely by virtue of a layer of cartilage at each end of the bone known as the *epiphyseal cartilage.* When the child grows up this cartilage becomes calcified and converted into bone, after which no more growth is possible. The growth of the cartilage is under the control of the pituitary gland. When this gland becomes overactive in early life as the result of a pituitary tumor, the growth of the epiphyseal cartilage is speeded up and the individual becomes a giant. It is evident that *gigantism* is not possible once the cartilage has become converted into bone. Conversely, if the pituitary is insufficiently active, growth ceases and the person remains a dwarf. But while there is only one cause of gigantism, there are many causes of dwarfism. Indeed the study of dwarfism is a subject in itself, a subject so extensive that to discuss it here is out of the question.

A bone must grow in thickness as well as in length. This increase of thickness is brought about by the *periosteum,* a fibrous membrane that closely covers the bone and contains osteoblasts on its deep surface. It is through the periosteum that the superficial part of the bone receives its blood supply, so that anything that injures or removes the periosteum threatens the health and even the life of the bone.

We have said that the epiphyseal cartilage is at the end of the bone, but this is not strictly true. It is separated from the actual end of the bone, *i.e.,* the joint surface, by a small piece of bone known as the *epiphysis.* The epiphyseal cartilage therefore intervenes between the shaft of the bone and the epiphysis. Many of the most important diseases of bone (inflammation, tuberculosis, sarcoma) commence in this region of the bone on one or other side of the epiphyseal cartilage.

Calcium is stored overwhelmingly in the bones, which contain 99 per cent of the total body calcium as well as 90 per cent of the *phosphorus* combined with calcium in the form of *calcium phosphate.* Yet the very small amount of calcium that is not in the bones plays a vital role in body function, for it affects enzyme activity, cell membrane permeability, cardiac rhythm, and neuromuscular excitability. A fall in the level of serum calcium may produce tetany and death. The serum calcium and phosphorus maintain a delicate inverse equilibrium with one another: when one goes up the other goes down. A minor change in calcium results in a major disturbance of health, but a marked change in phosphorus causes only a slight disturbance.

The metabolism of calcium and phosphorus in relation to bone must be considered as a whole. When we speak of *calcification* we mean of course the deposition of calcium phosphate and not merely calcium. The metabolism of calcium and phosphorus is influenced by many different factors, chief among which are the **hormone of the parathyroid glands and vitamin D,** the latter controlling absorption of calcium from the small intestine, but such hormones as estrogens, androgens, adrenal corticoids, thyroxin, and those of the anterior pituitary may all play a part. When the complexity of the entire mechanism is considered it becomes almost a matter of surprise that anyone has normal bones.

Osteoblasts, when multiplying rapidly, produce the enzyme *alkaline phosphatase* which splits organic phosphate compounds, thus upsetting the local calcium-phosphate balance and causing the precipitation of calcium salts in the soft tissues. The phosphatase level of the serum may be raised either in excessive bone formation or in bone destruction, for in both of these increased osteoblastic activity comes into play.

OSTEOPOROSIS. Bone consists of an organic protein matrix laid down by osteoblasts, and an inorganic calcium-phosphate complex deposited in the matrix from the serum. Generalized bone deficiency may take one of *three different forms.* (1) **Generalized osteitis fibrosa,** in which there is excessive bone resorption (p. 448). This condition may be due to (a) *hyperparathyroidism* or (b) *renal glomerular failure with phosphate retention.* (2) **Osteomalacia,** in which the calcium complex is not deposited in the protein matrix owing to calcium deficiency (p. 529). The condition may be due to (a) *deficient calcium absorption from the intestine,* or (b) *various renal tubular deficiencies* resulting in excessive loss of calcium in the urine. (3) **Osteoporosis,** in which there is poor formation of the protein matrix of bone, but normal calcium deposition and bone resorption.

Osteoporosis may occur in a variety of *clinical conditions,* of which three deserve special mention. (a) **Atrophy of disuse,** seen in paralysis or immobilization of a limb, especially in paraplegics (paralysis of the legs). Bone formation is diminished, and calcium is drained from the bone and excreted in the urine, where it may give rise to the formation of stones in the kidney or bladder, thus explaining the frequent association of poliomyelitis and urinary calculi. (b) **Gonadal deficiency,** whether male or female, leads to osteoporosis. It is much commoner in the female owing to the occurrence of the menopause. *Senile osteoporosis,* with its brittle bones and tendency to fractures, is for the most part due to loss of gonadal (sex) hormones. (c) **Adrenocortical hormone hyperactivity,** as is best seen in Cushing's disease (p. 432).

The *end results* of osteoporosis demand serious consideration because of the disabling effects on the aging and old. There is deficient bone formation, that is to say *too little bone,* although what is formed is completely calcified. This is the reverse of osteomalacia, in which there is insufficient calcification rather than deficient bone formation, with bending of the softened bones and deformities of the legs and pelvis (p. 529). In osteoporosis we may expect fracture of the brittle bones, especially *fracture of the neck of the femur* from a minimal degree of trauma, a frequent and tragic occurrence in elderly females, and *compression fracture of the vertebrae* with loss of height.

Inflammations

ACUTE OSTEOMYELITIS. The word osteomyelitis means inflammation of the bone (osteitis) and of the bone marrow (myelitis). The inflammation actually involves only the soft parts of the bone, *i.e.,* the marrow in the medullary cavity and the interstices of the bone, but the calcium is dissolved away from the hard structures as the result of the inflammation, so that the bone becomes softened.

The inflammation is usually caused by staphylococci, which generally gain access to the body through the skin causing a boil, and are then carried to the bone by the blood stream. The disease is essentially one of children and adolescents in whom the bone is still growing, and it is three times as common in boys as in girls, probably because the former are liable to trauma. As growth takes place only in the region of the epiphyseal cartilage, and as this is therefore the part most abundantly supplied with blood vessels, it follows that the disease affects the end of the bone, usually on the side of the epiphyseal cartilage next to the shaft. Injury to the bone is a common accessory factor, because this is apt to cause rupture of a small vessel, and the circulating staphylococci are enabled to settle down in the blood clot and grow rapidly. The injury may be a twist or a direct blow. I once saw a boy develop acute osteomyelitis twelve hours after he had been struck on the knee by a golf ball. The bones most frequently affected are the femur, tibia, and humerus.

The **lesion** begins as an *abscess of the bone*. As the result of acute inflammation pus is produced, and this tends to spread down the medullary cavity and outward to the surface. When it reaches the surface it raises the periosteum from the bone, and may spread along the surface for a considerable distance. As it is from the periosteum that the bone receives a considerable proportion of its blood supply, it follows that a fairly large area of the shaft may become devitalized and die. Such a piece of dead bone is called a *sequestrum,* and in the course of time this becomes separated from the living bone by the action of the osteoclasts. The inflamed periosteum is stimulated to form a thick layer of new bone, called the *new case,* which surrounds the sequestrum. In the new case there are a number of openings, *cloacae,* through which purulent discharge escapes from the interior (Fig. 185). *One of the most serious results of the inflammation is thrombosis of the vessels in the marrow*. The thrombi become heavily infected with staphylococci, and they may break down and be carried by the blood to the lungs and other organs, where they set up multiple abscesses, a condition of *pyemia.*

Basis of Symptoms. From what has been said it is apparent that osteomyelitis tends to be both a local and a general infection, and the symptoms are therefore both local and general. The *local symptoms* are *pain* and *tenderness* at the end of one of the long bones, usually in the region of the knee, together with *heat, redness,* and *swelling:* the classic signs, in short, of acute inflammation.

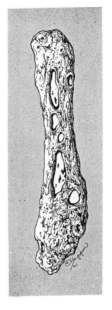

Fig. 185. Extensive osteomyelitis showing the rough new bone, cloacae, and sequestra (white).

The *general symptoms* are those of any severe acute infection, *i.e.,* high fever, chills, rapid pulse, marked leukocytosis, and the presence of staphylococci in blood culture. Although it is the local lesions which cause the patient the pain that is his chief complaint, it is the general infection which threatens his life.

The entire picture of osteomyelitis has been changed since the introduction of antibiotic therapy. The disease used to be a surgical one, the only treatment being opening up the bone so as to allow the pus and the infecting organisms to escape. The condition is now treated by medical means and if the diagnosis is made early and correct treatment started at once, the widespread bacterial infection described in the preceding paragraphs will be prevented. It is evident also that if the case is properly treated there will be no development of a sequestrum or of sinuses.

TUBERCULOSIS. Tuberculosis of bone is like osteomyelitis, except that it is a chronic disease from the beginning. Like the acute disease, it affects the ends of the bones, but begins in the epiphysis much more frequently than does osteomyelitis. The bones most often attacked are the long bones of the arms and legs, the bones of the wrist and ankle, and the vertebrae. As in the case of acute osteomyelitis, the region of the knee (lower end of femur and upper end of tibia) is a common site.

The lesion consists of a slow destruction of the end of the bone, not a wholesale destruction but a nibbling here and there, giving the bone

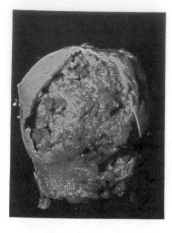

Fig. 186. Tuberculosis of head of femur. Only a small part of smooth articular cartilage remains at the left. (Boyd, *Pathology for the Surgeon;* W. B. Saunders Company.)

a worm-eaten appearance known as *caries,* a word that means dry rot. If the disease begins in the shaft, the epiphyseal cartilage is gradually eaten away and the epiphysis is invaded. From the epiphysis, whether it is infected primarily or secondarily, the disease spreads to the articular cartilage, which is eroded bit by bit until the articular surface comes to be formed by the diseased and roughened bone (Fig. 186).

Tuberculosis of the spine, also known as *Pott's disease,* is of frequent occurrence in children, although it may also occur in the adult. The disease affects one or more vertebrae, which it slowly destroys, just as the ends of the long bones are destroyed. The pressure from above causes the softened vertebrae to collapse, with resulting deformity of the spine, so that the child develops a "humpback" (Fig. 187). A more

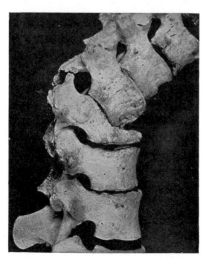

Fig. 187. Pott's disease, showing destruction of the middle vertebra.

serious result is pressure on the spinal cord, with the gradual production of paralysis of the legs (Fig. 188). A tuberculous or *cold abscess* may develop, the peculiarity of which is that it tends to spread along the psoas muscle, which passes from the lumbar part of the spine to the upper end of the femur. This *psoas abscess,* as it is called, will therefore tend to appear in the groin as a soft swelling, which may easily be mistaken for a hernia.

Basis of Symptoms.   Whichever joint is affected, be it the wrist, the knee, or the joints of the spine, the first symptom will be *limitation of movement.* This is natural, because no one moves a diseased joint more than is absolutely necessary. If the disease starts in the bone, symptoms do not appear until the joint also is involved. The joint is *swollen* owing to tuberculous swelling of the synovial membrane. The *affected limb tends to be shorter than the normal one,* partly because of the bone destruction, but mainly because the epiphyseal cartilage, which is responsible for the growth in the length of the bone, is killed. When the articular cartilage is destroyed and the roughened ends of the bones come in contact, *pain* develops. There may be no pain during the day, because the muscles around the joint contract and prevent movement from occurring. But when the child falls asleep the muscle

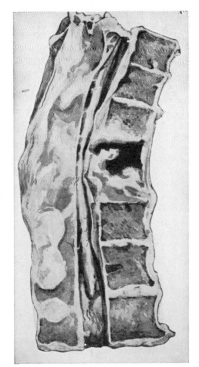

Fig. 188.   Pott's disease of spine. A vertebra is destroyed (right) and the spinal cord is compressed.

watch-dogs are no longer on guard, and the joint may be moved, causing intense pain, the child waking up with a start and a cry, so that these pains are known as "starting pains" or "night pains." For a long time the patient may show none of the general symptoms of tuberculosis such as fever or loss of weight.

It is hardly necessary to add that modern antibiotic therapy with streptomycin and isoniazid has completely altered the picture painted above.

Perthes' Disease. This condition, also known as *Legg-Perthes disease,* is merely the commonest of a group of lesions known as *aseptic* or *ischemic necrosis of bone.* In Perthes' disease the lesion is confined to the head of the femur, but in other members of the group known by other men's names the epiphyses in a variety of bones are involved. The lesions are of clinical importance not because of any marked disability that they produce, but because they are so easily mistaken for bone tuberculosis. In all cases the lesions represent a quiet necrosis of bone, aseptic and nonbacterial in character and apparently due to ischemia, which develops for some unknown reason.

Perthes' disease usually occurs in boys between the age of five and ten years. There is often a history of recent injury. The bone in the center of the epiphysis is fragmented, so that it may resemble fragments of mortar. As a result the head of the femur becomes flattened and

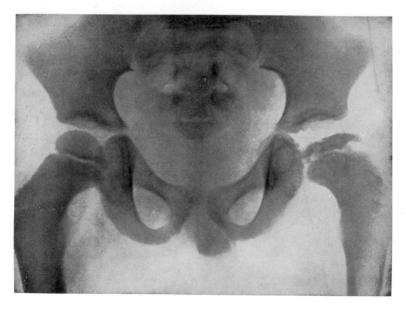

Fig. 189. Perthes' disease: extreme flattening of the head of the femur. (Boyd, *Pathology for the Surgeon,* W. B. Saunders Co.)

splayed out. When healing occurs the fragments coalesce, and the bone regains some of its structure, but the flattening is permanent. The roentgenogram is absolutely characteristic, and it is by means of it that a final diagnosis is made (Fig. 189). The *earliest symptom* is a limp, accompanied by little or no discomfort. The condition *must be distinguished from early tuberculosis in a child.*

SYPHILIS. Syphilis of bone used to be a disease of great importance, but modern chemotherapy has changed a common type of lesion into a rarity, so that we may dispose of the subject with welcome brevity. It differs from tuberculosis in the following respects: (1) it affects the shaft of the long bones rather than their ends, (2) the joint is seldom involved, and (3) osteosclerosis with new bone formation is much more prominent than osteoporosis or rarefaction. The tension produced by this new tissue within the bony canals is responsible for the nocturnal boring pains alluded to by the Psalmist. Destruction of the bones of the nose and hard palate used to be common, so that the bridge of the nose fell in at the root (*saddle-nose*), and there might be a large *perforation of the palate.* It may avoid embarrassment to remember that not every saddle-nose is caused by syphilis.

Osteodystrophies

The osteodystrophies, as their name implies, are *disturbances in the growth of bone.* Some are due to lack of vitamins, others to overproduction of hormones, but in the case of the majority the cause is quite unknown. The disturbance may be in the direction of *too little* or *too much,* and naturally the effect on the bone in the former will be the opposite to that in the latter. *The radiologist occupies a commanding position in determining the location and nature of bone lesions, and it is he who can determine whether the basic pathology is one of too little or too much undue absorption or undue formation of bone substance.*

OSTEITIS FIBROSA. This condition, also known as *osteitis fibrosa cystica* and *von Recklinghausen's disease,* is characterized by highly porous and decalcified bones which may be much deformed and curved, sometimes with the formation of bone cysts and spontaneous fractures of the rarefied bone. The decalcification is a manifestation of *hyperparathyroidism,* usually due to an adenoma but occasionally to hyperplasia of the parathyroid glands, a condition that has already been described on page 448. The calcium removed from the bones appears in the blood, so that the serum calcium rises from 10 mg./100 cc. to 15 or 20 mg., and the serum phosphorus is correspondingly low. The calcium may be deposited from the blood in the kidneys, giving a shadow in the x-ray film, or it may form a stone in the kidney.

FIBROUS DYSPLASIA.　Fibrous dysplasia of bone is readily confused clinically with osteitis fibrosa, indeed the case illustrated in Figure 155 on page 448 may well have been a case of fibrous dysplasia, but the pathogenesis of the two conditions is entirely different. Fibrous dysplasia is not related to hyperparathyroidism, but, as the name implies, is a congenital anomaly in the development of bone, with the formation of fibrous swellings that replace the bone and give rise to deformities like those of osteitis fibrosa. There is no disturbance in the serum calcium and phosphorus.

PAGET'S DISEASE.　Paget's disease of bone is an example of overproduction, not rarefaction, of bone. The cause is unknown, but it is associated with a greatly increased blood flow to the affected bones, which are principally the skull, the vertebrae, and the bones of the leg. At first there is softening and later overgrowth and hardening of bone; during the period of softening characteristic deformities develop. The disease usually begins in persons past the age of 40 years, and it may be familial. The softened bones of the legs are bent, the femur outward, the tibia forward. They become hardened again in this position and look as if they had been bent by the hands of a giant (Fig. 190). The head enlarges owing to the great thickening of the skull (Fig. 191), and the patient's history reveals that he has to buy hats of ever-increasing size. A posterior curvature of the softened spine is very common and reduces the height of the patient, so that the final clinical picture can be recog-

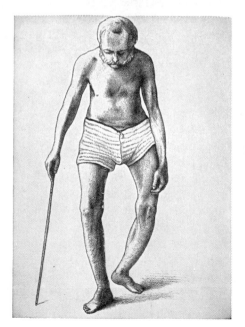

Fig. 190.　Paget's disease. A picture of one of Paget's original cases. (Sir James Paget, *Medicochirurgical Transactions,* 1877.)

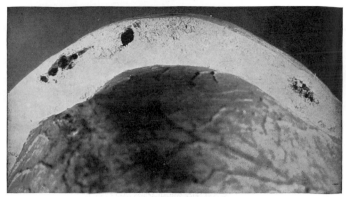

Fig. 191. Paget's disease of the skull; great thickening of the bone (white) and cyst formation. Water ran readily through the thick skull cap.

nized at a glance. The roentgenogram is characteristic even before any deformity is evident. The affected bones are thick and dense, and the vault of the skull presents a peculiar serrated (cock's comb) appearance which is pathognomonic. The disease is progressive, but does not usually shorten life, nor are the mental powers impaired in spite of the thickening of the skull. **The serum alkaline phosphatase is very high,** and may be over 100 units, a sure indication of the overactivity of osteoblasts.

RICKETS. Rickets is a form of osteodystrophy completely different from those already considered, because it is a manifestation of a vitamin deficiency. We have already seen that the chief mineral constituents that impart rigidity to the bones are **calcium** and **phosphorus,** combined in the form of *calcium phosphate.* These substances are absorbed from the food and deposited in the bones. If they are not present in the food in sufficient amount, the bones remain soft and are easily bent. A deficiency in phosphorus is much more serious than a deficiency in calcium.

But there is another factor in deficiency which is even more fatal to proper calcification. This factor is **vitamin D.** The ordinary food of a child usually contains a reasonable amount of calcium and phosphorus, but may be gravely lacking in vitamin D. This vitamin is *necessary for the proper absorption of calcium and phosphorus from the intestine,* and in its absence, no matter how abundant the minerals may be in the food, the body is unable to utilize them and rickets will result. Vitamin D is a fat-soluble vitamin, in contrast with some of the other vitamins which are water-soluble. It is therefore contained principally in fatty foods, although also found in certain vegetables.

A third factor is **light** (ultraviolet light). The relation between ultraviolet light and vitamin D has already been discussed on page 61.

The *cause* of rickets is therefore a deficiency in some of the factors necessary for the proper calcification of bone. The most important of these is vitamin D. A marked deficiency in phosphorus and, to a lesser degree, in calcium is a predisposing factor. *The fault lies in the quality, not the quantity, of the food.* A child may be starved and emaciated but show no signs of rickets, while a plump baby may show marked rickets. The disease is much commoner in artificially-fed infants than in those that are breast-fed. Owing to the absence of light it is commoner in large smoky cities and during the winter months. Negro children are especially susceptible, as their dark skin prevents the light from acting on the ergosterol. All the factors are included in the statement that *rickets is a disease of the slums of large cities in countries that get little sunshine.*

Clinical Picture. The symptoms are partly connected with bones, partly constitutional. The disease is one of infancy and early childhood (six months to two years), and a period at which there is the greatest demand for calcium and phosphorus by the rapidly growing bones. The softened bones become deformed, especially those that bear the weight of the body (Fig. 192 and Fig. 193), and backward *curvature of the*

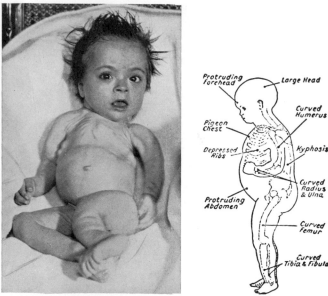

Fig. 192   Fig. 193

Fig. 192. Rickets, showing large forehead, deformed chest, curvature of arms and legs, and pot belly.

Fig. 193. Clinical features of severe rickets. (Harris, *Vitamins in Theory and Practice;* Cambridge University Press.)

spine develops (kyphosis). The *head* is large and square. The sternum is pushed forward (*pigeon-breast*), and a series of nodules develop at the anterior ends of the ribs called the *rickety rosary. Nodular swellings* are formed at the *wrists, knees,* and *ankles.* The most serious deformity is a *narrowing of the inlet of the pelvis,* which in the female may make normal delivery impossible in later life. Among the constitutional disturbances are sweating, restlessness, flabbiness of the muscles giving the child a "pot belly," and enlargement of the spleen. The *blood phosphorus is markedly decreased.*

Treatment consists in making good the deficiencies that may have been present. Cod-liver oil is an old and well-proved remedy. Halibut (haliver) oil is also rich in vitamin D, and is more palatable than cod-liver oil. The most potent form of vitamin D is viosterol, *i.e.,* ergosterol which has been irradiated by ultraviolet light. An abundance of sunlight is desirable. Sunlight loses its ultraviolet rays when passed through window glass, for the short-wave rays are screened out by the lead in the glass. Special lead-free glass may be used in the nursery, or the child may be exposed to the light of a lamp capable of producing ultraviolet rays, such as the mercury vapor lamp or the carbon arc lamp.

OSTEOMALACIA. Osteomalacia may be regarded as adult rickets, and is also due to vitamin D deficiency. As the name implies, it is a softening of bone (Greek *malakia,* soft), but only after growth is completed. It is a rare disease in North America, fairly common in Europe, particularly during wartime, and is extremely common in North China with its absence of sun. Osteomalacia often comes on during pregnancy owing to the great drain on the calcium of the woman's bones which occurs at that period. It is interesting to compare the pathogenesis of osteomalacia and rickets with that of osteitis fibrosa cystica. In the two former not enough calcium is deposited in the bones, whereas in osteitis fibrosa, which in essence is an osteoporosis, too much calcium is removed from the bones as a result of hyperparathyroidism. In both, the bones become decalcified and soft.

Tumors of Bone

We have already seen that bone is a complex structure into the composition of which a number of tissues enter, *e.g.,* bone cells, marrow, periosteum, and cartilage. Tumors of various kinds may arise from any of these elements. For the purpose of this brief outline, however, bone tumors may be divided into primary and secondary, while the primary tumors may again be divided into benign and malignant.

PRIMARY TUMORS. Primary tumors of bone may be benign or malignant. The three chief *benign* tumors are osteoma, chondroma, and giant cell tumor. The *osteoma* and *chondroma* are very similar tumors, the former consisting of bone cells and the latter of cartilage. Both are hard tumors which usually arise at the end of a long bone, although they may occur in practically any bone in the body. Being benign they are localized and usually remain small, but occasionally they grow to a great size. When removed they show no tendency to recur.

Giant cell tumor develops in children and young adults, usually before the age of 30. It occurs principally at the ends of long bones, and the common location is the knee. It is highly destructive locally, but does not cause metastases or kill the patient. It consists of a soft red hemorrhagic mass which greatly distends the bone and almost completely destroys it. This gives the highly characteristic roentgenographic picture of large bubbles separated by thin strips of bone. The tumor gets its name from the large number of giant cells that are seen in the microscopic section.

The *three chief primary malignant tumors of bone* are osteogenic sarcoma, Ewing's tumor, and multiple myeloma.

Osteogenic Sarcoma. This is the commonest of the three tumors. It is a disease of young persons between the ages of 10 and 30 and is very rarely seen after the age of 50. The location is similar to that of giant-cell tumor, namely, at the ends of the long bones, usually in the region of the knee joint. The tumor expands the end of the bone, so as to give it a "leg of mutton" appearance (Fig. 194). The perios-

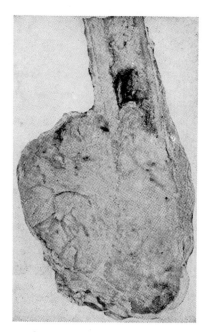

Fig. 194. Osteogenic sarcoma of the lower end of the femur. The tumor has destroyed the shaft. (Boyd, *Textbook of Pathology*.)

teum is lifted from the bone by the tumor, and spicules of new bone are laid down which radiate outward from the central mass giving a characteristic *"sunray" effect* in the roentgenogram. Spread takes place by the blood stream, and secondary growths are formed first in the lungs. Secondary growths in other bones are very rare; multiple bone tumors suggest Ewing's tumor in the young and multiple myeloma in the middle aged.

Ewing's Tumor. This tumor occurs at an earlier age period than osteogenic sarcoma, usually between the ages of 5 and 15. It is rarely seen after the age of 30. It involves the bone much more diffusely than does osteogenic sarcoma, giving rise to a uniform thickening. The tumor does not begin at the end of a bone. One of the more striking features of the disease is that *as the tumor progresses other growths become apparent in many widely distant bones, particularly those bones known as the flat bones, such as the scapula, sternum, vertebrae, and skull.* The *roentgenogram* shows diffuse involvement of the greater part of the shaft. There is a combination of bone formation and bone destruction; formation in the early stage, destruction later. The new bone on the surface may present a laminated appearance in the film like the layers of an onion. One of the most striking characteristics of the tumor is its *response to radiation;* it may melt away like a lymphosarcoma, but only to return again later.

Multiple Myeloma. This neoplasm is also known as *plasma cell myeloma,* for not only is it composed of plasma cells, but these cells are responsible for one of the most important characteristics of the tumor. As the name myeloma suggests, this is a tumor of bone marrow rather than of bone. It is multiple, and by the time the patient comes to the doctor a large number of the flat bones may be involved. The *age incidence* is in striking contrast to that of Ewing's tumor, 80 per cent of the cases occurring after the age of 40 years. Huge amounts of calcium may be freed from the bones, with resulting high serum calcium and deposits of calcium in the kidneys, so that pathological fractures are common. Marrow aspiration shows tumor cells in the sternal marrow, even though there is no other evidence of a tumor. The tumor is highly malignant and invariably fatal.

Plasma cells normally produce gamma globulins, so it is only natural that a neoplasm of plasma cells should produce these and related globulins in excess quantity. *The total serum proteins are raised to 10 mg. or higher, and there is a marked inversion of the normal albumin-globulin ratio* owing to the great overproduction of gamma globulin by the tumor cells. In addition there is a copious excretion in the urine of a unique protein, the *Bence Jones protein,* which was recognized in the urine over 100 years ago by Bence Jones. It appears as a cloud when the urine is heated to 55°C., disappears at 85° or on boiling, but re-appears on cooling. The reason it is found in the urine and not in the serum is that its molecular weight is only half that of albumin, so that it can readily escape from the blood into the urine through the glomerular filter. It must be noted that Bence Jones protein is present in the urine in less than 50 per cent of cases of myeloma, so that its absence does not mean that the patient is not suffering from the disease. Renal failure occurs in the later stages, and may be so severe as to lead to uremia and death. This may be due to the fact that large numbers of renal tubules may be blocked by casts of abnormal protein, and the calcification already alluded to cannot improve the functional capacity of the kidneys.

Treatment of malignant bone tumors consists in amputation at the earliest possible moment, in the hope that metastases may not yet have been set up. Roentgen examination of the lungs must first be made, because if secondary growths are found in these organs no treatment is of any avail. Some forms of sarcoma respond well to x-ray treatment, and the tumor may disappear for a time, but the relief is only temporary, and sooner or later the tumor will recur.

SECONDARY TUMORS. Secondary tumors of bone are carcinomas, the tumor cells coming from a cancer in some other organ. The most common forms of cancer which are likely to metastasize to bone are *cancer of the breast, lung, prostate,* and *kidney.* The metastatic tumor destroys the bone, and the first indication of its presence may be the occurrence of a fracture from a very trivial injury. The bones commonly affected are the ribs, vertebrae, sternum, and skull (the flat bones), and the upper end of the femur and humerus. In all of these bones the marrow is of the red variety and therefore well vascularized, so it is natural that the blood-borne tumor cells will be arrested at these sites. It is evident from the nature of the condition that nothing in the way of treatment is of any avail.

JOINTS

Structure and Function

A joint is a structure of peculiar delicacy, and one that responds only too readily to injurious stimuli. When we consider the amount of stress and strain, not to mention abuse in sports, to which the joints are subjected in a long life, it is little wonder that disease of the joints is among the commonest of clinical disorders. Man was not originally designed to stand upright, so it is but natural that the weight-bearing joints, in particular those of the lower limbs and vertebral column, should be among the principal sufferers.

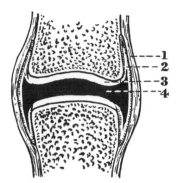

Fig. 195. Normal joint. 1, Capsule; 2, synovial membrane; 3, articular cartilage; 4, joint cavity.

A *joint* or articulation consists of **two articular surfaces,** a **capsule** or strong fibrous structure, which joins the two ends of the bone together, and a **synovial membrane,** which lines the capsule and produces an oily fluid that lubricates the articular surfaces and ensures the smooth working of the mechanism (Fig. 195). **Any or all of these structures may be damaged by disease.**

Acute Arthritis

Suppurative arthritis used to be the most important form of acute arthritis, pyogenic cocci being introduced through a wound or spreading to the joint from a bone that is the seat of acute osteomyelitis. Antibiotic therapy has now pushed this complication into the background. *Gonorrheal arthritis,* formerly an occasional complication of acute gonorrhea affecting many joints, has also passed into the realm of the forgotten as the result of the present adequate treatment of the infection with penicillin in the acute stage of the disease. *Rheumatic arthritis* is the acute nonsuppurative arthritis of rheumatic fever, which has been considered on page 138. There is an acute synovitis with excess of turbid fluid in the joint. Extreme tenderness is characteristic of the swollen and acutely inflamed joint. *The inflammation usually undergoes complete resolution,* but some permanent stiffness occasionally may persist. *Traumatic synovitis* is a good example of acute nonsuppurative arthritis, the inflammation being confined to the synovial membrane (acute synovitis), with no destruction of tissue and therefore no permanent stiffness. The synovial membrane is swollen, juicy, and congested, while the synovial fluid is increased in amount and cloudy.

Tuberculous Arthritis

Tuberculosis of the joints is a disease of children, and is usually secondary to tuberculosis of the adjacent bone, a subject that has already been considered (p. 521). When it occurs in an adult it is more likely to be primary in the synovial membrane, infection being carried by the blood stream from some distant focus. The *synovial membrane* may be even thicker and more voluminous than that of rheumatoid arthritis, so that it may fill the entire cavity. The *fluid* is usually scanty but highly fibrinous, so that it contains flakes of fibrin which may develop into foreign bodies known as *melon-seed bodies* or *rice bodies*. The destruction of the articular surfaces that may develop and the resulting clinical picture already have been described in connection with tuberculosis of bone, and will not be discussed here.

Rheumatoid Arthritis

This very common, tragic, and crippling disease, known also as chronic arthritis, is a chronic inflammatory condition affecting particularly the small joints of the hands and feet, although the larger joints may be affected later. The condition usually occurs in women between twenty and forty years of age. *It is the oldest of all known diseases,* having been observed in many of the Egyptian mummies. Rheumatoid arthritis is one of the greatest causes of disability, and it has been estimated that it is responsible for an annual loss of $200,000,000 in the United States. This is perhaps not remarkable when we consider that there are an estimated 4,500,000 persons who suffer from the disease in this country, and that 200,000 are totally disabled. The English figures are very similar.

Etiology. An enormous amount has been written about the causation of rheumatoid arthritis, a sure indication that little is known about the subject. The most reasonable view appears to be that the arthritis is the result of a **combination of minimal hematogenous bacterial infection with tissue hypersensitivity.** The sensitization may be the result of a series of minor infections or a chronic focus which periodically discharges a few bacteria into the blood. At no time do the bacteria reach the joint in sufficient numbers to produce conventional lesions, but all the time the tissues are becoming sensitized, until finally one bacteremic episode culminates in a definite arthritis. Psychological factors such as *stress,* operating perhaps through the adrenal cortex, seem to play a part. Marked and sometimes startling relief of the arthritic symptoms is common during the early months of pregnancy.

Laboratory tests support the idea of an immunological pathogenesis. A *specific agglutination reaction* occurs when the serum of the arthritic is added to a suspension of a variety of particles. At first sheep red cells coated with tannic acid and sensitized with human gamma globulin were used, but more recently a suspension of latex particles mixed with gamma globulin. Only a drop of serum is needed, a positive *latex fixation test* being indicated by an agglutination of the particles visible to the naked eye. The latex particles simply act as inert carriers of gamma globulin, and the same is true of the coated red blood cells. The reaction seems to be due to the presence of a **rheumatoid factor** in the blood, which has now been isolated and shown to be a macroglobulin antibody or *antigen-antibody complex. By fluorescence microscopy it has been demonstrated that the rheumatoid factor originates in the lymphocytes and plasma cells of the lymph nodes and the hypertrophied synovial membrane.*

Lesions. The synovial membrane is primarily affected, so that the disease might be called synovioarthritis in contrast to osteoarthritis, the other great form of chronic arthritis. The pathological changes resemble in certain respects those of joint tuberculosis, although it attacks many joints instead of a single one, and does not lead to destruction of the bone. There is the same swelling of the synovial membrane with the formation of pulpy masses or fringes and tags, which cause the joints to be enlarged, the same gradual destruction of the articular cartilage, the same interference with the function of the joint resulting finally in complete disability and fusion of the joint surfaces. The most significant feature is the superabundance of lymphocytes and plasma cells, indicating the immunological character of the process. The periarticular soft parts share in the inflammatory swelling and edema. The ligaments become softened and absorbed, thus contributing to the deformities that form so distressing a feature of the end picture of the disease. Subcutaneous inflammatory nodules may be found in the neighborhood of the affected joints, particularly in the arms (Fig. 196). The course of the disease is marked by curious remissions and exacerbations, and at any stage the progress may be arrested, but as in tuberculosis the injury to the joint is permanent, and the hands and feet are twisted, gnarled, and crippled for life (Fig. 197). On this account, and because of its commonness, the disease is of great industrial importance.

Symptoms. The symptoms are *pain* and *swelling* of the joints, together with increasing *stiffness* and *disability*. In the later stages the joints become distorted and deformed. During the exacerbations the patient often suffers from mild fever, malaise, anemia, and sweating, all pointing to a chronic infection.

Treatment. During the acute phase of the rheumatoid disease *rest* is of great importance together with methods of physiotherapy that help to restore function and particularly to prevent crippling deformities. The *maintenance of correct posture* of the joints involved provides for the maximum of function when the acute process subsides. *Relief of pain* with heat and mild analgesics is necessary in most cases. The *use of cortisone and ACTH* in rheumatoid arthritis has provided marked benefit in many cases. This treatment is accompanied by relief of pain, decrease in swelling, and increase in movement of affected joints. Unfortu-

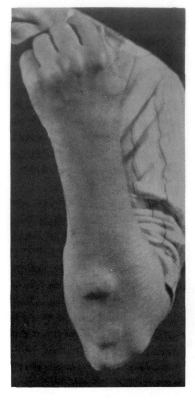

Fig. 196. Subcutaneous nodules in rheumatoid arthritis. (Kindness of Dr. A. J. Blanchard.)

nately, in many instances this improvement is not maintained after the drug is stopped.

ANKYLOSING SPONDYLITIS. The name of this unusual variant of rheumatoid arthritis means *stiffness of vertebral joints.* Although rheumatoid in character, it differs from rheumatoid arthritis in having a high male sex incidence and a negative serological reaction for the rheumatoid factor. The articular cartilage is destroyed, fibrous adhesions develop, and eventually bony fusion with calcification of the intervertebral discs. The condition begins in the sacroiliac joints and spreads slowly upward, ending with extreme rigidity which may justify the term *poker back.* In early cases the roentgenogram shows a fuzziness of the opposed surfaces of the bones, followed by calcification and later ossification of the vertebral ligaments. In exceptional cases there are *lesions of the aortic valve and ascending aorta* resembling those produced by syphilis.

Osteoarthritis

Osteoarthritis is a *degeneration of articular cartilage and bone,* so that it might well be called degenerative arthritis; in this it differs from

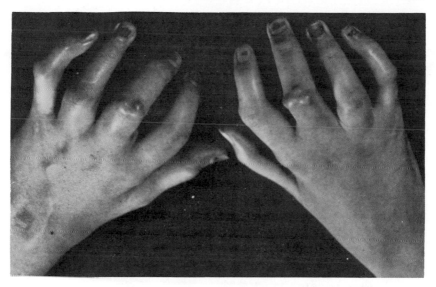

Fig. 197. Hands of a 17-year-old girl with juvenile onset at age 12, with typical rheumatoid changes, including subcutaneous nodules over middle proximal interphalangeal joints, except for radial (rather than ulnar) deviation. (Hollander, *Arthritis and Allied Conditions.*)

rheumatoid arthritis, which is primarily an inflammation of synovial membrane, and indeed it differs from that condition in almost every respect. Thus it is as common in men as in women, it is a disease of the later period of life, there are no general symptoms, the large joints are commonly involved, often only one joint, particularly the hip, and there is no true ankylosis or fusion between the articular surfaces. The small joints of the hands and feet may also be involved, the knuckles becoming greatly swollen and knobby.

The *lesions* are primarily atrophic, followed later by localized hypertrophy. The articular cartilage undergoes degeneration and softening, so that it is gradually worn away until the underlying bone is exposed. There is atrophy of the central part of the bone, so that much of the head and neck of the femur may disappear. The peripheral part of the cartilage has a much better blood supply than the central area, and overgrowths of cartilage, which resemble candle drippings, develop at the edge of the articular cartilage, a condition known as *lipping* of the joint. These cartilaginous excrescences tend to become ossified, so that the atrophied head of the bone is surrounded by a ring of bony excrescences which may gravely limit movement and form a striking feature in the roentgenogram. *Thinning of the intervertebral discs* is also a feature of diagnostic importance in the film.

The *etiology* of osteoarthritis is obscure. It is a degenerative condition
in which the ageing process, probably associated with local ischemia,
plays a leading part. If a joint is continually exposed to trauma, as in
a trade or in professional athletes, it may show the characteristic
changes. The condition may indeed be described as "wear and tear"
arthritis.

Charcot's Joint

The peculiar and puzzling condition known as Charcot's disease of
joints may be regarded as acute osteoarthritis, although not related in
any way to the usual form of osteoarthritis. It is marked by the rapid
destruction and disintegration of the articular surfaces as well as the
soft structures of the joint, so that a hinge-joint like the knee or the
elbow can be moved passively in any direction, sometimes with a horrible crunching sound, *yet with a remarkable absence of pain or even
discomfort.* At a later stage, new cartilaginous and bony processes develop at the periphery, a point to be noted in the roentgenogram. The
condition is neuropathic in origin, that is to say it is a complication
of a disease of the nervous system. One of the large joints of the leg
(hip, knee, ankle) may be involved in *tabes dorsalis,* and the same is
true of the arm in *syringomyelia,* a destructive disease of the upper part
of the spinal cord which is not described in this book. In both diseases
there is an absence of pain sensation in the parts involved, so that the
joint is unduly exposed to trauma and attrition. The reader will perceive
that these words really explain nothing. In exceptional cases the spine
may be involved.

Villo-Nodular Synovitis

This is a rather rare benign proliferative lesion of the synovial membrane of the knee and only very occasionally other joints. The greater
part or the whole of the synovial membrane is covered by villous projections, which may fuse into grape-like nodular masses. The *clinical picture* is one of chronic arthritis with painful exacerbations followed by
long remissions. The painful attack is due to hemorrhage, sometimes
profuse, from the villi into the joint cavity. The blood gives the synovial
lesions a characteristic pigmented appearance.

Gout

Gout is the most intriguing of all the diseases that involve the joints.
It has been known since the earliest of times, although under the name
of *podagra,* a Greek deviation from *pous,* foot and *agra,* attack. Colchicine, the most effective and specific drug in its treatment, was used
1500 years ago, yet lost its popularity in the fifteenth century. The
disease is known to be a hereditary disorder of uric acid metabolism

with a great increase in the uric acid of the blood, yet it remains a mystery wrapped in an enigma.

Gout is an inborn error of metabolism, with an overproduction of uric acid, which may be regarded as a partial reversion to the normal situation in birds and reptiles. In man the end product of nitrogenous metabolism is highly soluble urea, which is excreted in the urine. Birds, on the other hand, excrete nearly all their nitrogenous wastes as uric acid, and the same is true of reptiles.

But our knowledge of the metabolic defect does not serve to explain the mechanism of the acute attack or of the curious periodicity of such attacks. For this it is customary to blame precipitating factors such as rich foods, beer, and red wines. We are left wondering why the big toe should be picked out. Equally confusing is the fact that colchicine has no effect on the synthesis or excretion of uric acid.

Gout may present itself in one of three phases. (1) The **acute attack** is the classic form described by writers of genius and drawn by cartoonists. The joints chiefly affected are those of the big toe, and less frequently those of the fingers and knee. The suddenness of onset is one of the mysteries of the disease. The joint is acutely swollen, exquisitely painful and tender, and the overlying skin tense and shiny. At the same time there is a systemic reaction with fever, chills, malaise, and a leukocytosis up to 20,000. (2) The **intercritical period** is the interval of months or years between acute crises. The patient appears well, but the blood uric acid remains as high as before. (3) The stage of **chronic gout** is one of joint deformities and subcutaneous nodules called tophi.

The **lesions** with which we are familiar are confined to chronic gout, for no one has ever looked into the interior of the acutely inflamed joint. *Chronic gout* is due to the formation of masses of urate crystals in the joint and the surrounding soft tissues. The crystals are laid down in the superficial layers of the articular cartilage as white chalky deposits rather like drops of paint, an appearance from which the name gout is derived (Latin *gutta,* a drop). The cartilage disintegrates, so that a variety of osteoarthritis is produced. Deposits also occur in the synovial membrane and capsule. *Tophi* are masses of crystals that accumulate in the soft tissues around the joints, causing marked deformities of the fingers and toes (Fig. 198). Tophi are also formed in the cartilage of the ear. A useful diagnostic procedure in a doubtful case is to prick a suspected tophus with a needle and look for the characteristic crystals under the microscope. The *kidneys* suffer from deposits of urate crystals in the pyramids. Gross hematuria may be the first thing to draw attention to the kidneys, and *renal failure is the commonest cause of death in gout.*

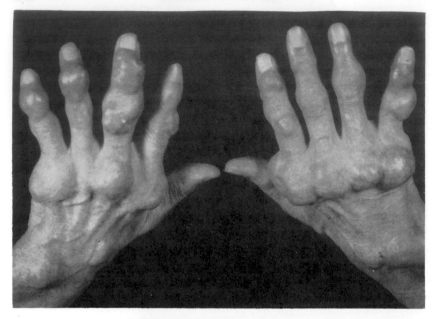

Fig. 198. Marked formation of gouty tophi in the hands of a man who was supposed for years to have rheumatoid arthritis, and was treated as such. (Boyd, *Pathology for the Physician*).

Lesions of the Intervertebral Discs

When we consider the important joints of the body we are apt to forget the intervertebral discs. And yet there is perhaps no part of the body where strain and movement are so constant, and where impairment of movement, especially when associated with pain, so cripples the full enjoyment of life. Owing to man's upright position the discs are subjected to constant strain for which they were not originally intended, so that degeneration in later life is commoner than in any other organ, with corresponding loss of the normal cushioning function.

The *nucleus pulposus* is the essential part of the disc, and plays the chief role in pathological changes. It is a highly elastic semi-fluid mass compressed like a spring between the vertebral surfaces. In youth it presents a very marked elastic turgor, depending on the fluid content of the tissue. With age this turgor gradually diminishes, and is completely lost in various degenerations. A frequent lesion is *herniation of the nucleus pulposus* into the body of a vertebra, due usually to degeneration or tearing of the cartilage plate which separates the nucleus from the vertebral body. The lesion is known as a Schmorl node. The condition is of little clinical significance.

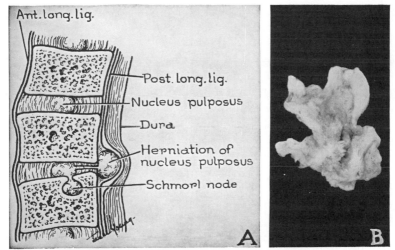

Fig. 199. *A*, Herniated nucleus pulposus and Schmorl node. *B*, Herniated disc removed at operation. (Peet and Echols, courtesy of Arch. Neurol. Psychiat.)

PROTRUSION OF DISC. An intervertebral disc may be protruded or herniated into the vertebral canal and press on the spinal cord or stretch the nerves. This is the condition known popularly as "slipped disc." Protrusions occur at the sites of the maximum anterior spinal curvature, that is to say the region between the fourth lumbar and first sacral, and between the fifth and seventh cervical vertebrae (Fig. 199). The causation of the protrusion varies. The most common cause is *trauma,* either sudden as in a fall from a height, or repitititious as in heavy labor involving lifting. The turgid nucleus pulposus is confined by a circular band of fibrous tissue, the annulus fibrosus, and when this is torn or degenerates, the disc is forced backward into the canal. In many cases no cause can be suggested.

The chief *clinical features are low back pain* and *sciatica* or pain passing down the back of the leg along the course of the sciatic nerve, symptoms that carry little threat to life but may interfere greatly with living. In addition to the sensory disturbances there may be severe spasm of the muscles of the back causing marked disability. It is possible to localize the lesion accurately by clinical findings in over 75 per cent of cases. Excision of the protruded disc is required in only a small proportion of cases.

MUSCLES

Structure and Function

Muscle forms the largest mass of tissue in the body, what we refer to as "the flesh," yet we know less about the pathological changes in this tissue than in any other. Much of this ignorance is due to the mass of tissue involved. It is easier to make a searching microscopic examination of the kidney or the pituitary than of the muscles of the back.

Each muscle is composed of innumerable *fibers,* and each of these so-called fibers is really an elongated multinucleated cell boiling with enzymes, for muscle is a unique organ in that it is capable of converting stored chemical energy into the mechanical energy needed to make the fibers contract. Moreover the chemical charge, *adenosine triphosphate* (ATP), is fired by a spark from a motor neuron. For this reason **disorders of the muscle may have their origin:** (1) *in motor nerve cells* (poliomyelitis), (2) *in nerve fibers* (neuritis), (3) *in the myoneural junction between muscle and nerve* (myasthenia gravis), and (4) *in the muscles themselves* (primary muscular dystrophy).

Two chemical points may be mentioned. **Potassium** plays an important part in muscle metabolism. Both too little potassium (potassium loss) and too much potassium (potassium intoxication) will cause paralysis of muscle. **Transaminase** (glutamic oxaloacetic transaminase) is an enzyme present in greatest concentration in cardiac and skeletal muscle. Destruction of this tissue results in a liberation of the enzyme into the serum, and an estimation of the transaminase serum level is a valuable test for determining the presence and extent of such injury, more particularly in myocardial infarction. It would be absurd for us to consider more than one or two of the large number of obscure diseases that may involve the muscles and tax the resources of the physiotherapist.

Ischemic Necrosis

When a young adult without previous training engages in strenuous athletic exercises such as running, jumping or kicking a football, or in long marches, he may rapidly develop firm swelling, aching pain, and paralysis of the muscles in front of the tibia. In its milder form this is known to athletes and their coaches as "shin splints." A more severe form in which the affected muscles actually become necrotic carries the more academic title of the *anterior tibial syndrome.* It is believed that the strenuous exercise of an untrained muscle liberates excess quantities of metabolites which lead to swelling of the muscle, and that this in turn causes pressure first on the veins and later on the arteries, resulting in ischemic necrosis. *Volkmann's contracture* usually occurs in young people and affects the muscles of the forearm. It is commonly associated with the pressure of splints or a tourniquet or with hemorrhage resulting from a fracture. Within a few hours of the receipt of injury burning pain develops in the hand or forearm. This is followed by contracture of the fingers which become fixed in the flexed position. Once again this is an example of ischemic necrosis or infarction of the muscle, the ischemia being caused by arterial spasm resulting from injury to the vessel wall.

Myositis Ossificans

There are two kinds of ossifying myositis in which new bone is formed in the muscle. *Traumatic myositis ossificans* is a not uncommon condition which may be the result of repeated injury to a muscle or a single severe injury, especially when accompanied by hemorrhage. There is a danger that the lesion may be mistaken for an osteogenic sarcoma of bone invading the muscle. *Progressive myositis ossificans* is fortunately a very rare progressive disease, which commences in child-hood and slowly kills the patient. Soft swellings develop in the muscles which are gradually converted into bone, until finally the body is en-closed in a bony sheath which makes breathing impossible.

Myasthenia Gravis

This disease with the ominously descriptive name is characterized by great weakness or rather fatigability, most marked in the muscles of the face, which is blank and expressionless, but shared to a lesser extent by all the voluntary muscles. After the muscle has been used a few times it rapidly loses its power of contraction, only to regain it as rapidly with rest. In extreme cases the limbs are so weak and easily fatigued (myasthenia) that they can hardly be lifted. This is not the same as paralysis.

The *cause* of the condition remains unknown, despite the enormous amount of work that has been devoted to the problem. **No lesions to explain the astonishing weakness can be found in the motor nerve cells, the nerves, or the muscles they supply.** It is presumed that there is some defect at the myoneural junction where the nerve enters the muscle fiber, perhaps a biochemical abnormality, which blocks the transmission of the nerve impulse to the muscle. Normally, the chemical substance acetylcholine is released at the myoneural junction when im-pulses are passed across it, and this is believed to stimulate the muscle fiber to contract. The enzyme cholinesterase is normally present and destroys whatever acetylcholine remains after the contraction is effected. It has been suggested that in myasthenia gravis there is either an over-abundance of cholinesterase or too little acetylcholine. Although there is no proof of this theory, treatment consists of the use of drugs antago-nistic to cholinesterase. Neostigmine is by far the most useful drug dur-ing acute attacks. In many cases there is hyperplasia or a neoplasm of the thymus gland in the neck. What this means is unknown, but in occa-sional cases surgical removal of the thymus has been attended by dra-matic improvement.

Passing reference may be made to the *myotonias* in spite of their rarity, because the condition is the reverse of myasthenia. As the name indicates, there is an increase of muscle tone, with the result that there is prolonged contraction of a muscle after cessation of the stimulus, the fibers being unable to relax. When a movement is repeated a number of times the muscles warm up, and normal contraction and relaxation may then occur.

Muscular Dystrophies

This is a group of rare diseases of muscle that represent *a genetic disorder of muscle metabolism*. The disease generally begins in childhood, shows a very marked familial tendency, attacks only the males, but is transmitted only by the females. The large muscles of the hip and later the shoulder are chiefly affected. In striking contrast to the myasthenias and myotonias, the dystrophies show marked changes in muscle structure, as again indicated by the name. The affected muscles are enlarged and bulging, as is well seen in the calves of the legs, but this is not a true hypertrophy of muscle fibers, but merely a marked replacement by fat, so that the academic name of the usual variety is *pseudohypertrophic muscular dystrophy*. The *biochemical lesion* of the muscular dystrophies is *loss of storage of creatine* by the affected muscle, with excessive loss in the urine. In health over 95 per cent of the body's supply of this nitrogenous substance is stored in the skeletal muscles, and none of it appears in the urine. The *serum transaminase* (glutamic oxaloacetic transaminase) is raised, the increase being most marked when there is much pseudohypertrophy of the muscles.

TENDONS

TENOSYNOVITIS.　The tendons in which the muscles terminate are nonvascular and therefore immune to inflammation, but the tendon sheath in which they move, especially those at the wrist and ankle, are often infected. *Suppurative tenosynovitis* may result from spread of infection from a septic process in the fingers. *Tuberculous tenosynovitis* is marked by the formation of tuberculous granulation tissue causing a "white swelling" like that seen in tuberculosis of a joint. *Traumatic tenosynovitis* is the commonest form, occurring in piano players, typists, and others whose tendons are subjected to excessive use. Fibrin is laid down on the surface of the tendon and the wall of the sheath, so that crackling is felt when the tendon is used.

GANGLION.　This is a cystic swelling that develops in connection with a tendon sheath. The common site is the back of the wrist. It is attached to the outer surface of the tendon sheath. It appears to commence as a proliferation of the connective tissue of the sheath, which undergoes mucoid degeneration with the formation of numerous small cysts that eventually fuse to form one large cyst filled with soft mucoid material.

BURSITIS. A bursa is a sac lined by synovial membrane, containing viscid fluid and situated at points where friction would otherwise develop, usually close to a joint. Those with an interest in words may care to know that bursa is derived from the Latin word meaning a purse, from which comes our bursar, the man who holds the purse. *Traumatic bursitis* is usually caused by chronic and repeated irritation ("housemaid's knee," "student's elbow"), but occasionally it is due to a blow. A common site is the region of the shoulder involving the subdeltoid and subacromial bursae (*subacromial bursitis*), with pain most marked on motion, so that the arm is not moved and a "frozen shoulder" results. The bursa is distended with serous fluid (hydrops). *Tuberculous bursitis* usually takes the form of hydrops with melon-seed bodies, or the bursa may be filled with granulation tissue.

FURTHER READING

ADAMS, R. D., DENNY-BROWN, D., and PEARSON, C. M.: *Diseases of Muscle,* 2nd ed., New York, 1962.

AEGERTER, E., and KIRKPATRICK, J. A., JR.: *Orthopedic Diseases,* 3rd ed., Philadelphia, 1968.

COLLINS, D. H.: *Pathology of Bone,* London, 1966.

HOLLANDER, J. L. (Ed.): *Arthritis and Allied Conditions. A Textbook of Rheumatology,* 7th ed., Philadelphia, 1966.

JAFFE, H. L.: *Tumors and Tumorous Conditions of Bones and Joints,* Philadelphia, 1958.

WALTON, J. N. (Ed.): *Disorders of Voluntary Muscle,* London, 1964.

Chapter 29

The Care of the Patient

INTRODUCTION

In the opening paragraph of Tinsley Harrison's *Principles of Internal Medicine* there occurs this sentence: "He who cares for the sick needs technical skill, scientific knowledge, and human understanding." In bygone days it was the last of these that was the physician's chief asset. This can be seen in Luke Fildes' famous picture, *The Doctor* (Fig. 200). The family doctor bends over the sick child with loving care, but we know that he is probably powerless to cut short by any specific means the infection (diphtheria) that threatens the life of his little patient. The doctor had far more to offer by way of compassion than by way of skill. In spite of this the father regards him with a complete and touching faith and trust which, sad to say, has somewhat declined in an age when the doctor can work miracles in his treatment of the disease.

The picture of the relationship of doctor to patient has not always been so sweet. In Turner's *Serial History of Medical Men,* we read the following pieces of advice given by some leading London doctors of Chaucer's day, such as John of Gaddesden, the first Englishman to be Court Physician. "When called to a patient, find out from the messenger

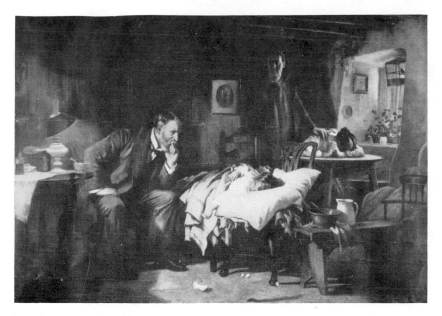

Fig. 200. The Doctor. (Luke Fildes.)

as much about him as you can before you arrive. Then, if his pulse and urine tell you nothing, you can still surprise him with your knowledge of his condition" . . . . "Whenever possible, ensure that the patient has confessed before you examine him. If you wait until after your examination before asking him to confess, he will suspect the worst" . . . . "Tell the patient that, with God's help, you hope to cure him, but inform the relatives that the case is grave. Then, if he dies, you will have safeguarded yourself. If he recovers, it will be a testimony to your skill and wisdom" . . . . "Do not look lecherously on the patient's wife, daughters, or maidservants, or kiss them, or fondle their breasts, or whisper to them in corners. Such conduct distracts the physician's mind from his work. It may also disturb the patient and fill him with suspicions and worries which will negative any good that may be wrought by the medicine."

Times change. In recent years there has been a terrific upsurge of total medical knowledge which has made specialization inevitable, so that the individual doctor's share of the knowledge must be either narrow, knowing more and more about less and less, or superficial. But it must never be forgotten that general practice (family care) is not what is left when the specialists get through, but the practice of medicine that uses the specialist only when he is needed.

In this modern age medicine has become a science as well as an art, a science demanding the cooperation of a team of experts, doctors, laboratory scientists, medical technologists, radiologists, nurses, dietetic experts, physiotherapists, specialists in rehabilitation, and still others. With the exception of the doctor, this is the team for whom the book is written. No one member of the team is better than any other, but the captain of the team must still be the doctor who is responsible for the care of the patient. It is hardly necessary to say that only a few members of the team may be needed in any given case.

We should not forget that the prevention of disease has been even more miraculous than modern advances in treatment. To quote the opening sentence of the Preface to Wain's intriguing book: "Once upon a time and not so long ago, the world was a very unsafe place in which to live. Periodically plague, pestilence, pandemics and epidemics swept across the world like great disastrous tidal waves, leaving behind them a terrible toll of death, disease and human misery." Freedom from the fearful epidemics of the past and the control of contagion are relatively recent accomplishments. Now we can concentrate on the care of the sick person. We must realize, however, that the present alarming explosion in population is essentially due to the success of preventive medicine, especially among children.

Until the early part of the nineteenth century medical advance depended on deduction from clinical (bedside) observation. Then laboratory research took over, and now there are between 14,000 and 20,000 scientific journals published, some of them once a week. As Stephen Leacock, the Canadian humorist and professor of Political Science, puts it in Laugh Parade: "When an up-to-date doctor looks at you, in place of a human personality he sees a collection of tubes, feed-pipes, conduits, joints, levers, and food and water tanks. But the really good doctor knows that the patient must still be dealt with as a person, not as a case or a disease, a person who is unique and different from every other human being, and who cannot be assessed by a computer."

The proper care of the patient involves correct diagnosis and skilled treatment. Various members of the team may be involved in these two activities.

DIAGNOSIS

The first step in the care of the patient is to make a correct diagnosis. Medicine is a science in that it uses scientific methods and principles, but of equal importance is the fact that it still remains an art demanding judgment and experience. In order to arrive at a correct diagnosis three very different disciplines are employed. These are: (1) history taking, (2) physical examination, and (3) laboratory investigations.

HISTORY TAKING.   The taking of a history of the illness by cross-examination of the patient may seem to the uninitiated to be the simplest of the three techniques, but in reality it is the most difficult, demanding all the skill, insight, and patience of the physician, and often it is the most valuable. Further discussion of this subject would be out of place in a book of this character.

PHYSICAL EXAMINATION. By this term we mean the employment of what used to be called the five senses, more particularly sight (inspection), touch (palpation), and hearing (auscultation). Of these *inspection* appears the easiest, yet it serves to distinguish the really skilled from the ordinary observer. *Palpation* of the abdomen, breast, and other parts reveals much to sensitive, educated fingers. *Auscultation* involves the use of the stethoscope, mention of which brings us to the use of *instrumental aids* in diagnosis.

Modern science has vastly extended the range of the unaided senses. With the *ophthalmoscope* we look into the eye and form an opinion as to the vessels of the retina, with the *bronchoscope* we see into the trachea and bronchi, with the *gastroscope* into the stomach, with the *proctoscope* into the bowel, with the *cystoscope* into the bladder, and so on. The development of *x-rays* is a special extension of vision by means of which the radiologist can see into the interior of the body. The *microscope* represents another extension of vision, allowing the pathologist to determine whether the specimen removed from a lump in the breast is or is not cancer. Even the *electrocardiograph* is merely a highly refined method for enabling us to picture the electric currents involved in every beat of the heart, thus adding a visual record to the clinical impression gained from feeling the pulse and listening to the heart. The physician of a bygone age would determine the presence of fever by laying his hand on the patient's brow; now we answer the question more accurately by placing a *clinical thermometer* in the mouth or the rectum. Richard Bright decided that patients with chronic nephritis had an elevated blood pressure merely by compressing the radial artery at the wrist with his finger; now we apply a *blood pressure apparatus* to the arm. *In all of these instances the principle is the same, and merely represents an extension and amplification of our special senses by exaggerating the sounds or the sights, or by translating one sense into another.*

LABORATORY EXAMINATIONS. It is in the field of laboratory investigation of material from the patient that modern medicine has made its greatest leap forward, involving an incredible development of new methods, particularly those that are chemical in character. Laboratory methods, which were first developed in connection with research, are now applicable to the patient. For this reason the pathology laboratory, which used to be mainly concerned with the investigation of the dead, has now become vital for the diagnosis and care of the living. A patholo-

gist who is medically qualified should be the director of such a laboratory, but he can no longer expect to carry out all the highly specialized
chemical, biological, and bacteriological procedures involved. These are
performed by trained laboratory technologists, while even more complex
operations may be entrusted to those whom we may call medical laboratory scientists, science graduates of a university who do not necessarily
hold a degree in medicine.

The explosive development of new methods of laboratory investigation during recent years is responsible for a natural tendency to place
undue reliance on these techniques as opposed to the more old fash-
ioned clinical methods outlined above. It is well to recognize the limitations of laboratory procedures as well as their extreme value. The data
are compiled by fallible human beings who are as liable to errors of
technique and interpretation as are the clinicians. Mistakes may be made
by those responsible for the collection and labeling of the material to
be tested. Finally, it must be remembered that the normal figure for
any given chemical value is variable from one person to another, just
as are the height, weight, and color of the hair. Moreover we must
recognize the fact that emotions can influence biochemical processes,
even though these are controlled by enzyme systems, themselves under
the direction of the genes. The patient is no mere collection of symptoms, signs, damaged organs, and disordered functions, but a whole person related to his environment.

From this brief outline it becomes evident that the art of diagnosis
depends on the skillful combining of two sets of facts, the one procured
from the patient at the bedside, the other obtained indirectly through
the microscopic or the chemical study of blood, excretions, secretions,
and tissues. These two disciplines, although seemingly so disparate, are
in reality interwoven. The patient is interrogated and observed, first with
the unaided senses, then with the stethoscope and thermometer, and
finally, for reasons of convenience, in the laboratory with the microscope, the test tube, and the automatic mechanisms of modern science.
It is foolish to argue whether one of these disciplines or methods is
more scientific than the other merely because one is carried out in the
laboratory and the other at the bedside. The bedside can be a laboratory
for accurate observation and deduction, but the facts are locked up in
the patient, and it is none too easy to find the key. The scientist (so-
called) constructs a hypothesis or theory, which he then tests by applying it to the observed facts. Exactly the same process is followed by
the clinician, whose working hypothesis is the clinical diagnosis. Both
alike observe, reflect, verify, and then generalize. Finally it must be remembered, as has already been suggested, that the skilled use of the
five senses may be far more valuable in diagnosis than a handful of

laboratory reports or radiographs. Nor must it be forgotten that there remain large areas in the realm of disease which are not susceptible of laboratory investigation, for the art of medicine is not confined to organic disease, but deals also with the mind of the patient and with his behavior as a thinking, feeling human being.

TREATMENT

Having arrived at the correct diagnosis, we may now turn our attention to the question of treatment. But before becoming immersed in details we must ask ourselves the question, "What is it that we are trying to treat?" The word disease is sometimes used to describe the hostile agent, as in the case of tuberculosis; sometimes the bodily disturbance, as in the case of diabetes. It is the business of the physician, in conjunction with his team of helpers, to restore normal functioning by correcting disease, which is really abnormal functioning rather than damaged structure. The importance of lesions is being replaced to some extent by that of disordered enzyme systems. Indeed the change from normal to abnormal structure may be beneficent rather than evil. When the wall of the left ventricle becomes greatly hypertrophied in arterial hypertension, when one kidney becomes twice the normal size following removal or destruction of the other kidney, it is good, not bad for us, because otherwise we might be dead. **Finally it must be emphasized that the proper treatment of a disease is usually based on the physician's knowledge of its natural course without treatment so that he may depend on the healing power of nature.**

The infinite variety of measures that can be taken for the sick person may be divided into a number of main groups, in particular: (1) *supportive,* such as rest, nursing care, diet, and physiotherapy in its various forms, all designed to encourage the natural resistance of the body; (2) *specific,* directed against the causal agent; and (3) *symptomatic* or *palliative,* designed to relieve symptoms such as pain (with analgesics), fear (with sedatives), and sleeplessness (with hypnotics), when it is not possible to remove the cause.

GENERAL MEASURES

REST. This is perhaps the most important single therapeutic measure in combating disease. Rest in bed is the oldest and still the best household remedy. A sick animal does this by instinct when he crawls into the bushes and lies low. It is difficult to explain on scientific grounds the exact manner in which rest helps the sick person. All infections are benefited by rest, which may be general or local. An example of the value of local rest is afforded by immobilization of an infected hand by a splint or a sling. By this means upward spread of the invading organisms, particularly streptococci, along the lymphatics as a result of muscular movements is reduced to a minimum. Other examples of local rest to an organ are the use of light diets or predigested foods for gastric disorders, and of digitalis, which slows the rate of the heart beat in heart disease and strengthens the power of contraction.

It is important, however, to remember that rest is not simply a state of inactivity, of freedom from toil. There must be rest of the mind as well as rest of the body, relaxation, and freedom from unnecessary worry. Mental fatigue is often more harmful than physical fatigue and more difficult to relieve. Sometimes the best way of resting a tired person is by changing from mental work to recreation through physical activity. The patient who lies in bed with his mind occupied with worries is far from resting. Rest is a state of tranquillity, of quiet and repose, a freedom from all that harasses and disturbs. *The nurse may play a most important part in enabling the patient to attain this state of tranquillity.* A simple example is her function of protecting a very sick patient from importunate visitors, who are certain to exhaust him both physically and mentally. As improvement sets in, one visitor at a time may be allowed, and when two are present they should both be at the same side of the bed. A good nurse can keep a patient's mind off his troubles much better than can the doctor, and thus contribute to his state of rest.

But rest can be overdone, especially in the aged. When the octogenarian takes to bed for too long, he may never be able to get out of it again. Prolonged disuse of an organ inevitably leads to deterioration of function, to be followed sooner or later by disintegration of structure. The dangers of prolonged rest in bed, particularly for the elderly, have been summarized as follows: "Look at a patient lying in bed. What a pathetic picture he makes with the blood clotting in his veins, the lime draining from his bones, the scybala stacking up in his colon, the flesh rotting from his seat, the urine leaking from his distended bladder, and the spirit evaporating from his soul." Prolonged and complete rest in bed has been much overprescribed.

DIET.   Correct food is assuming a position of ever-increasing importance in the treatment of disease as well as in the preservation of health. This illustrates the need of an expert dietitian in a well-organized hospital. Proteins are the sole source of material for the maintenance and repair of tissues. Such maintenance and repair may be specially needed in febrile and other diseases where there is marked breakdown of tissue. The proteins of the highest biological value are contained in meat, fish, milk, and eggs, as they have the most essential amino acids. This is of special importance when the diet is restricted, as in conditions associated with albuminuria. The principal role of fats and carbohydrates is to furnish energy, a requisite of the well rather than the sick person. It is only necessary to mention here the all-important role of food, and particularly of vitamins and minerals such as iodine, calcium, and iron, in the dietary deficiency diseases. Edema is often associated with a retention of sodium, which holds fluid in the tissues, so that a low-sodium or even a salt-free diet may be advisable.

The possible relationship of fat in the diet to the development of atherosclerosis is gaining recognition. *In this respect a distinction must be drawn between saturated (with an additional H atom) and unsaturated fats.* Those fats that are liquid in an icebox or refrigerator are likely to be highly unsaturated and are not apt to cause disease of the arteries, but those that are solid in the icebox are usually highly saturated, and these are believed to favor the development of arterial degeneration. It may be remarked that fats derived from fish are different from those from land animals in the sense that fish oils are much more unsaturated. Were it otherwise the fish in the ocean would be completely stiff on account of the cold, and would not be able to swim at all.

On the nurse rests the responsibility of seeing that the patient eats the prescribed diet; she must report to the doctor if he does not do so. The regulation of fluids may be as important as the regulation of food. Thus when there is much fluid loss, which may be due to vomiting or diarrhea, that loss must be made up. Conversely, when the tissues are water-logged, as in myocardial failure, the intake of fluid must be diminished.

NURSING. This needs no more than mention in a book of this type, not because the subject is not of supreme importance, but rather because the author does not feel qualified to discuss it. With the patient safely in bed, the nurse may become the most important member of the team concerned with his care. There are endless services by which the nurse not only ministers to his comfort, but contributes to his eventual recovery. If he is to receive the rest, both physical and mental, which we have seen to be so essential, it is the nurse who is best qualified to provide it. She must exercise keen observation of the patient together with accurate recording of any changes in the symptoms and physical condition, including the functioning of the bowel and bladder. It may be added that a broad cultural education with knowledge of past and current events enabling the nurse to converse with and interest the patient is an asset of very great value. **There are many diseases for which it is better to have a good nurse than a good doctor.**

DRUGS

It has been said of drugs that they sometimes cure, often relieve, and always console. This is not only a scientific age, but also a health-conscious age, so that the old faith in a bottle of medicine (now commonly converted into a box of pills) has not weakened but rather become stronger. Man has been differentiated as "the animal with the desire to take medicine." When sick he craves the comfort of the doctor, particularly one who will prescribe drugs.

This is remarkable when one considers what the healthy person used to say about drugs. Even at the beginning of the twentieth century, with the exception of one or two drugs such as quinine for malaria, medicine was palliative and symptomatic in approach. Voltaire's cynical definition of medical treatment as the art of pouring drugs of which one knew nothing into a patient of whom one knew less, was still applicable. Oliver Wendell Holmes, in the second quarter of the nineteenth century, remarked that if most of the medicines prescribed in his day had been poured into the sea, only the fishes would have suffered.

Drugs may be divided into two main groups. (1) Members of what may be called the *empiric group* were discovered before the beginning of the present century, not by scientific investigation but mostly by happy chance in conjunction with an enquiring mind. Among the most ancient and valuable examples of this group are *opium* and *castor oil*. More modern are *digitalis* for heart disease, *quinine* for the control of malaria, and *cocaine* for the relief of pain. All of these are derived from plants, a fact of which the herbalists may be proud, and they may be regarded as a symbol of man's ancient hope to discover a magic plant that would cure all his ills. (2) A second class is represented by the *specific group,* which is based on a scientific knowledge of the etiological agent responsible for the physiological disturbance involved. This modern group includes the antibacterial agents such as the antibiotics and sulfonamides, the products of endocrine glands in glandular deficiencies, the substances lacking in deficiency diseases, and so on. The right of some of these latter examples to be considered as drugs in the classic sense of the word may of course be challenged.

It may be said without exaggeration that the two supreme scientific discoveries in relation to care of the patient are anesthesia, both general and local, and knowledge of bacterial infection, to which must be added knowledge regarding treatment and prevention of such infections. Since 1930 the mortality from gastrointestinal infections, one of the chief causes of death in infants, has fallen by over 80 per cent, and that from pulmonary infections by nearly 70 per cent. As late as 1940 there were 2,500 deaths from diphtheria in England and Wales, now the disease has disappeared. (The child in Luke Fildes picture was suffering from diphtheria.) And what has happened to cholera, plague, and smallpox?

ANTIBIOTICS.   Many microorganisms such as molds and soil bacteria secrete metabolic products which inhibit or prevent the growth of other microorganisms. These chemical substances of microbial origin are known as antibiotics, because they inhibit growth and even destroy bacteria in dilute solution.

The first antibiotic to be discovered was *penicillin.* In 1928 a British bacteriologist, Alexander Fleming, noticed that a culture of staphylococci accidentally contaminated with green mold ceased to grow and was destroyed. This mold is the common green mold, Penicillium notatum, which grows on moist bread, old cheese, and jams. Fleming, therefore, gave the name of penicillin to the active substance in the culture fluid. In 1940 Florey and his associates at Oxford worked out methods for its isolation and purification, and applied it to the treatment of human infections. So incredibly powerful is the substance thus obtained that it inhibits the growth of staphylococci in a dilution of one in eighty million. It is apparent that the green mold developed its atomic bomb a very long time before Homo sapiens invented his own. When we come to the antibiotic resistant strains (see below) it will be evident that the microorganisms have outdistanced man in self-defense. *Streptomycin* was discovered by Waksman in 1944, being obtained from a soil organism.

Although some antibiotics kill bacteria directly as do antiseptics, others merely delay or inhibit multiplication of the bacteria. This inhibiting process is known as *bacteriostasis.* As a result of bacteriostasis spread of the infection is prevented, and the natural defenses of the body, such as leukocytes and antibodies, have time to overcome the invading organisms and neutralize their toxins.

When the antibiotics were first introduced they were called the wonder drugs. It was soon discovered that some acted only against one group of microorganisms, others against other groups. Five main groups may be distinguished, depending to a large degree on whether the microorganisms are gram-positive or gram-negative, thus indicating that the distinction has a biochemical basis.

Group 1 possesses high activity against *gram-positive bacteria.* This includes the *penicillins,* of which a number have been developed, as well as *bacitracin* and the *erythromycin* group. **Group 2** has a nearly equal action against *gram-positive* and *gram-negative organisms.* This group includes the *tetracyclines*—such as *aureomycin* and *terramycin*—as well as *chloramphenicol.* As these agents are active against a wide variety of organisms they are known as *broad-spectrum antibiotics.* **Group 3** shows high activity against the *tubercle bacillus* and *gram-negative organisms.* In this group *streptomycin* is prominent, and also *neomycin.* **Group 4** shows exclusive activity against *gram-negative organisms.* The only member in this group is *polymyxin.* **Group 5** acts only against *fungi,* an outstanding example being *griseofulvin* and the *polyene antibiotics.* It is evident that the antibiotic of choice against gram-positive cocci is penicillin (which is also invaluable against the spirochete of syphilis); against gram-negative organisms, polymyxin; against both gram-positive and gram-negative organisms, the tetracyclines; and against the tubercle bacillus, streptomycin and neomycin. In actual practice the best combination against the tubercle bacillus is streptomycin, para-aminosalicyclic acid (PAS), and isoniazid. **It is self-evident that an accurate bacteriological diagnosis is of the greatest importance in deciding the choice of an antibiotic in treating an infection, for not only must the nature of the organism be determined, but also its sensitivity to the drug selected.**

We have discussed the very serious question of the development of *antibiotic-resistant strains,* more particularly of staphylococci in relation to penicillin in hospital populations, among whom they may cause what has come to be known as hospital fever (p. 134). *It is not so much a question of the individual organisms acquiring resistance as of the more resistant strains multiplying and taking command.* The transmissibility of these newly emerging strains is also greatly increased, so that a population of carriers of antibiotic-resistant organisms develops in the hospital staff as well as among the patients. Finally the indiscriminate use of antibiotics has resulted in the development of infections by yeasts and microorganisms that formerly were nonpathogenic.

Bacterial resistance may be due to: (1) ability of the microorganisms to destroy the drug, or (2) impermeability of the surface of the bacterial cell to the drug. *Penicillin-resistant strains of staphylococci owe their resistance to the fact that they elaborate an enzyme that destroys penicillin and is therefore called penicillinase.* The mechanism of resistance may develop either by exposure to the drug, stimulating the production of enzymes, or by mutation, altering the gene constitution that controls the ability to synthesize enzymes. In the case of those bacteria that are naturally resistant to an antibiotic, the bacterial cell wall probably presents an impenetrable barrier, just as does the protecting wall of animal cells.

The problem of penicillin-resistant staphylococci may have been cracked, at least in part, by the development of newer forms of penicillins. The basic penicillin nucleus, 6-amino-penicillanic acid, has now been isolated, and in 1956 it was first synthesized. This has made possible various modifications of the side chains of the nucleus, giving a wide variety of penicillins, one of which is penicillinase-resistant, and is thus effective against resistant strains of staphylococci—a most important advance. A recent synthetic penicillin is wide-spectrum in character, being effective against both gram-positive and gram-negative organisms. Unfortunately it is not resistant to penicillinase, so that it is unable to cope with penicillin-resistant staphylococci.

Penicillin and streptomycin tend to be destroyed by the gastric juice and the bacteria of the large intestine, so that they are given by *intramuscular injection,* penicillin in the form of procaine penicillin. *Oral tablets* of penicillin can be used, but a higher dosage is required and there is some danger of poor absorption. Aureomycin, chloramphenicol, and terramycin are given orally every four to six hours, because success depends on maintaining a high antibiotic level in the infected area. When collections of pus are separated by some distance from blood vessels, *local injections* of penicillin or streptomycin are made into the pus cavity. *Topical applications* of the antibiotics are used in the form of ointment in skin infections or as drops in infections of the eye.

No therapeutic roses are without their thorns. *It is well to remember that the antibiotics are potentially dangerous, although the danger is only to a small number of people who are either naturally unduly sensitive to these drugs,* or, as more commonly happens, have acquired sensitivity as the result of previous (? unnecessary) antibiotic therapy. Penicillin may be responsible for allergic reactions, sometimes quite serious, chloromycetin may inhibit bone marrow function, and so on. In view of the potential danger of these drugs it seems reasonable to state that the wonder drugs should ordinarily be used only under the following conditions: (1) when the nature of the infection has been clearly demonstrated by culture, (2) in desperately ill patients when there is not time to await the results of culture, or (3) in the rare instance of an unexplained febrile illness when the most extensive studies have failed to reveal the cause. It is only in the latter group that there is any justification for the too common practice of shooting in the dark with antibiotics simply because the patient happens to have a fever. *It may be added that the ordinary respiratory infections are usually caused by viruses, as is always the case in the common cold, and that antibiotics have no action on viruses, safely lodged as they are in the interior of the cells.*

The Sulfonamides. The sulfonamides were the first of the wonder drugs, being introduced into medical practice in 1936, and their advent marked a revolution in the treatment of infections caused by such common bacteria as the staphylococcus, streptococcus, pneumococcus, meningococcus and gonococcus. They have now been largely replaced by the antibiotics, although they still have their uses. The first member of the group was sulfanilamide, from which were derived others such as sulfapyridine, sulfathiazol, and sulfadiazine. All members of the group are potentially dangerous to a small number of hypersensitive persons. The chief toxic effects are fever, acute hemolytic anemia, leukopenia, and suppression of urine with renal failure.

IATROGENIC DISEASE.   The Greek for a physician is *iatros,* so that the rather modern term iatrogenic diseases signifies the unpleasant concept of disorders of health caused by the doctor. These disorders have increased greatly during the past decade, drugs being the worst offenders. Reference has just been made to the dangers of the overenthusiastic and indiscriminate use of *antibiotics.* These and other drugs may damage the liver. Many *synthetic drugs* may be responsible for agranulocytosis, that is to say a marked decrease in the number of circulating granulocytes (polymorphonuclear leukocytes). The abuse of *steroid therapy,* especially the prolonged use of adrenal corticosteroids, tends to lower resistance to bacterial infection and predisposes the patient to adrenal insufficiency and gastric ulcer with perforation. *Anticoagulation therapy* intended to prevent a recurrence of coronary thrombosis carries with it a threat of fatal hemorrhage if the patient should develop a very minor rupture of a myocardial infarct. *Blood transfusions,* as we have already seen, may serve to spread the infection of viral hepatitis from an immune carrier to a susceptible subject who may develop the disease and die as a result. The over-use of *intravenous fluids* sometimes causes patients to be drowned in life-giving fluid or to develop electrolyte imbalance. The prolonged use of *x-radiation* in the treatment of a benign condition such as ankylosing spondylitis may precipitate the development of malignant leukemia. The object of giving this depressing catalogue of unpleasant possibilities is to impress on us all, medical workers and laity alike, that **what is powerful for good can be potent for evil,** and that drugs and other priceless therapeutic agents should only be used when the need is real. Perhaps it is well to add that there are psychological as well as physical iatrogenic disorders, and that tactless talk by nurses and technologists as well as by physicians can often produce grave anxiety states in the patient.

IMMUNOTHERAPY

The natural means by which the body defends itself against infection is by immunity reactions, in which antibodies and leukocytes play a leading part. It is possible to assist these reactions by immunotherapy. There are two ways in which this can be done.

1. The production of antibodies may be stimulated by the injection of vaccines, which consist of the dead bodies of bacteria. In this way an *active immunity* is built up. It will be evident that the great field for active immunity is in the **prevention** of infection. Outstanding success in prevention has been attained in connection with typhoid fever, smallpox, and diphtheria. It should be noted that the technique differs

in each of these three examples. In the case of *typhoid* the vaccine consists of the dead bodies of typhoid bacilli. *Smallpox* vaccine contains a greatly attenuated living virus. The agent used in immunization against *diphtheria* is not really a vaccine, but is neutralized diphtheria toxin, known as *toxoid*. The result, however, is the same in all three, namely, active immunity.

2. An animal may be used for the production of the antibodies by means of inoculation; the blood serum containing these antibodies is then injected into the patient. The patient is given a *passive immunity,* so called because the patient himself takes no active part in producing the immune state. The serums or sera used in the treatment of disease are usually antitoxins, which are prepared by injection of gradually increasing doses of toxin into an animal. If bacteria instead of toxins are employed, the serum is an antibacterial one. One of the oldest and still the most efficient of the antitoxic sera is that used against diphtheria. The prophylactic injection of antitetanic serum has proved invaluable in war wounds as well as in civilian injuries. The antibacterial sera on the whole have been disappointing.

ORGANOTHERAPY

This form of treatment may be employed in two ways. The first is also known as substitution therapy, because it consists in the administration of the extract of an organ that has become deficient in activity. This deficiency is likely to be permanent, so that the organotherapy must be continued for the duration of the patient's life. In spite of this drawback, organotherapy has achieved some of the most brilliant results in the entire field of therapeutics. Examples of substitution therapy are provided by insulin in diabetes, liver extract in pernicious anemia, and thyroid extract in myxedema.

Organotherapy can also be used to produce a more temporary physiological effect by the administration of hormones rather than by prolonged replacement therapy. Some of the best known examples are the hormones of the adrenal cortex (corticosteroids such as cortisone and hydrocortisone), of the anterior pituitary (ACTH), of the male and female sex glands (androgens and estrogens), as well as many others.

PHYSIOTHERAPY

This form of therapy, also known as physical therapy, is probably the most ancient of all forms of treatment, and within recent years it has assumed increasing importance, particularly in the treatment of injuries. Physiotherapy is involved in two major areas. The first is physical restoration, which uses exercises and an activity program to promote the highest level of physical fitness. The second lies in the activation of the patient, for with the application of exercise programs and the demonstration of increased ability in the activities of daily living, there seems to be a concomitant raising of the level of interest in participation in normal activities. Physiotherapy may take the form of massage, exercise, heat therapy, electrotherapy, and radiation therapy.

MASSAGE. Massage is essentially manipulation of the tissues. It may be either stimulating or sedative. While in theory it can be applied by anyone, it must be realized that it demands skill and training, just as do other forms of treatment, and in the hands of an inexperienced person it may be responsible for much harm. The movements must be carried out rhythmically and smoothly. Not all persons can become masters of the art, for they may lack the necessary rhythm or the strength of hand that is needed to manipulate the great muscles of the back. **A thorough knowledge of anatomy is necessary, and also a knowledge of the physiological effects desired.** The principal types or techniques of massage are *stroking* (superficial or deep), *kneading,* and *friction.* These techniques are used for different purposes. Massage is employed both for local and general conditions. Examples of *local conditions* in which it may prove useful are organic nervous diseases associated with paralysis and wasting of the muscles, *e.g.,* poliomyelitis, chronic arthritis, fractures, sprains and strains, and atonic conditions of the alimentary canal. Among the *general conditions* in which it is used are debilitating diseases with loss of muscle tone, and neurasthenia (here used for its soothing effect). Massage is also valuable in patients who are inactive or bedridden, although not necessarily seriously ill.

It is not easy to state with certainty the exact mechanism by means of which massage produces its valuable effects. It appears to be partly mechanical and partly reflex. The flow of venous blood and lymph is mechanically assisted by stroking in the direction of that flow. The lightest touch will serve to empty the superficial veins and lymphatics. Some reflex mechanism must be presumed as the basis of the remarkable relief of muscular spasm that follows massage in cases of fracture. Skillful massage may cause rapid disappearance of the swelling after a fracture, and in such cases the mechanism is probably as much reflex as mechanical. Massage does not produce lactic acid in the muscles, but it serves to remove the lactic acid produced by violent muscular exertion. It appears to stimulate the interchange between the blood and the tissues. Finally it soothes the nervous system in a remarkable manner, as can be demonstrated in many cases of neurasthenia.

EXERCISE. The place of exercise in physiotherapy is the re-education of neuromuscular pathways and the strengthening of muscles weakened by disease or disuse. Therapeutic exercise requires the full cooperation of the patient. It may take the form of active exercise or resistance exercise. *Active exercise,* such as swimming or setting-up exercise, is that performed by the patient. In *resistance exercise* the resistance can be provided either by the patient or by the technician, and it is of special use in isolating groups of muscles and overcoming muscle spasm. Planned exercise is of particular value in the re-education of paralyzed groups of muscles in such conditions as poliomyelitis, multiple sclerosis, and hemiplegia or paraplegia caused by strokes.

HEAT. Heat may be applied to the body in a variety of forms. *Radiant heat* utilizes the infrared rays, which produce heat within the body. The source of these rays is not in contact with the body. The usual source is the ordinary electric light bulb, but an infrared baker may be used, which gives out no light but much heat. In *conducted heat* therapy the source of heat is in direct contact with the body. The source may be: (1) a hot water bag, hot packs, or a hot bath; (2) an electric pad or other dry forms of heat; (3) *diathermy,* in which heat is generated in the tissues as the result of the passage through them of an electric current. *Ultrasonic radiation* is a heat that may be created deep in the tissues by the release of energy when the direction of a sound is altered, as by hitting articular cartilage. The ultrasonic waves are produced by piezoelectric phenomena in the sound generator. The frequency of alteration is now of the order of 50,000,000 cycles per second.

Heat acts in various ways, but particularly by dilating the small blood vessels and increasing the capillary circulation in the part. This leads to muscular relaxation and reduction in the amount of pain. Radiant heat acts principally on the skin, but diathermy goes much deeper into the muscles. The commonest of all physiotherapeutic prescriptions is baking followed by massage. The baking produces dilatation of the superficial vessels, while massage helps to eliminate waste products from the part. This combination frequently provides great relief and comfort.

Cold plays a much less important part in therapy than does heat, but it has its place. It is of particular value in stopping hemorrhage after a sprain, in which a ligament, together with the surrounding vessels, is torn.

ELECTROTHERAPY. This may be applied in the form of the sinusoidal current or diathermy. The *sinusoidal current* is a galvanic current which increases from zero to a maximum in voltage, then returns to zero and to a negative voltage equal to the positive maximum. It is thus an electric current that oscillates between a given positive and negative voltage. A slow rate of oscillation is valuable for producing painless contractions of muscles that have been weakened from long disuse. *Diathermy* creates heat as the result of the passage of a high frequency alternating current. A very high rate of frequency of alternation is employed, between 500,000 and 3,000,000 cycles per second. The advantage of the high frequency is that the passage of the current is harmless and painless. The tissues act as a high resistance to the current, and heat is generated as a result. The special field of diathermy is in the application of heat to a limited, deepseated, inaccessible part of the body, as in neuritis, muscle strains, sprains, and bursitis. It is of no value for heating a large area of body surface; for this purpose radiant heat should be used.

Finally mention must be made of the role of the physiotherapist in health education. She teaches the patient to walk with his prosthesis, the patient with lumbar disc disease to live within his limitations, the patient with deforming arthritis to avoid deforming stresses, and the postcoronary patient to exercise at a reasonable level.

RADIATION THERAPY

This is a special form of radiation treatment in which x-rays and radium are employed. The gamma rays of radium produce the same effects on the tissues as do x-rays. The chief field of usefulness of radiotherapy is in the treatment of malignant tumors and allied conditions. Radiation arrests the reproduction of cancer cells, and at the same time leads to degeneration and destruction of these cells. Not all malignant tumors are equally suitable for this form of therapy. Some are very radiosensitive and melt away under the influence of radiation almost under the eye of the observer. Others are equally radioresistant. Rapid disappearance of the tumor does not necessarily indicate a good prognosis, for unless all the tumor cells are killed it will inevitably reappear. The question as to whether x-rays or radium should be used depends a good deal on the location of the tumor. A small superficial growth, such as carcinoma of the lip, is better treated with radium. In a widespread condition such as lymphosarcoma x-rays would be employed. Experience has shown that radiation is of particular value in carcinoma of the mouth, cervix, and skin, and in lymphosarcoma. It may be used alone or in conjunction with surgery. In the latter case it may be used preoperatively or postoperatively. Radiation is used as a palliative measure in leukemia and in Hodgkin's disease, but cure of these conditions cannot be expected. **In conclusion it may be pointed out that the safe use of x-rays and radium demands as great skill and as extensive a training as does the safe use of a knife by the surgeon.** Indeed, much more irreparable damage may be done by radiotherapeutic agents than by the surgeon's knife.

PSYCHOTHERAPY

In concluding this brief review of the various aspects of the care of the patient, the all-important matter of the relation of the mind to the body must not be passed over in silence. No reference will be made to that aspect of psychotherapy known as psychoanalysis, but the connotation of psychotherapy is far wider than that of the psychoanalytic techniques of Freud and his followers.

In our enthusiasm for medical science it is salutary for us to realize that the physician conducting a busy practice soon discovers that at least half the patients who walk into his office fail to show evidence of organic disease; there is apparently nothing really wrong with any one organ. And yet they are sick and need to be treated with skill, consideration, and sympathy. When a person is out of mental harmony with his environment, when he finds the stresses of life too hard to be borne, he may feel as ill as if an organ was seriously diseased, and the symptoms complained of may be similar to those of an organic disease. **The symptoms are real and not imaginary.** Moreover, much of the state of distress induced by organic disease is due to the emotional and mental disturbances resulting from a realization that disease exists. It is inherent in human nature to magnify the unknown. The manner in which the patient reacts to the disease may be more important than the disease itself. As the old French proverb puts it: "There are no diseases, but only sick people."

Medicine can never be purely a science; it contains too many immeasurables. Clinical medicine must not be regarded merely as the application of physics, chemistry, and physiology to the sick person. The patient goes to the doctor because of pain or some other discomfort from which he wishes to be relieved rather than in the pursuit of health. A human being is much more than a number of organs packaged into a minimum of space. The patient with heart disease is not just an internal combustion engine with a leaking valve, but a sensitive man or woman with a diseased heart. It may be the man or woman rather than the disease that needs to be treated. All medicine to some extent must be psychosomatic, for there is always the psyche to be considered as well as the soma.

The object of these remarks is to emphasize that from the patient's point of view the pathological lesions that we have described in the previous chapters of this book are by no means the sum total of the disease. The relief of mental distress and the promotion of contentment are just as vital as the alleviation of the physical suffering. In bringing about this relief the skilled, wise and understanding nurse may play an even more important part than the doctor who pays the patient an occasional and often too brief visit. In the wise words of a great physician: **The secret of the care of the patient is in caring for the patient.**

After going through this book I trust that the reader will agree that health is the greatest gift that anyone can receive and retain. It is this which confirms the supreme importance of the medical profession and the group of paramedical workers without whom the modern doctor would be powerless.

FURTHER READING

HARRISON, T. R. (Ed.): *Principles of Internal Medicine,* 5th ed., Ney York, 1966.

HAVARD, C. W. H.: *Fundamentals of Current Medical Treatment.* (Chapter 1: Principles of Treatment by Sir Derrick Dunlop), London, 1968.

MOSER, R. H. (Ed.): *Diseases of Medical Progress,* 3rd ed., Springfield, Ill., 1969.

PEABODY, F.: *Doctor and Patient* (The Care of the Patient), New York, 1930.

SIMPSON, J.: *An Introduction to Preventive Medicine.* London, 1970.

TURNER, E. S.: *A Serial History of Medical Men,* London, 1958.

WAIN, W.: *A History of Preventive Medicine,* Springfield, Ill., 1970.

Prefixes and Suffixes

An appreciation of the meaning of Latin and Greek prefixes and suffixes serves to make obscure and forbidding medical terms easy to understand and therefore far more interesting. Some of those more commonly used in the subjects we have been considering are given below. To make the subject more living the reader may care to put together the prefix and suffix in such words as hematemesis, pathogenesis, osteomalacia, dyspnea, and menorrhagia.

PREFIXES

a- without or not: *achlorhydria,* absence of hydrochloric acid.
acro- extremity: *acromegaly,* large extremities
adeno- gland: *adenitis,* inflammation of a gland.
an- without: *anuria,* suppression of urine.
ante- before: *antemortem,* before death.
anti- against: *antitoxin,* antagonistic to a toxin.
arthro- joint: *arthritis,* inflammation of a joint.
auto- self: *autolysis,* self-dissolution.
bio- life: *biology,* study of living things.
chol- bile: *cholecystitis,* inflammation of the gallbladder.
cyst- bladder: *cystitis,* inflammation of the bladder.
dia- through: *diarrhea,* a flowing through.
dys- difficult, bad: *dysmenorrhea,* difficult menstruation.
en- in, into: *encapsuled,* inclosed in a capsule.
endo- within: *endometrium,* lining of the uterus.
entero- intestine: *enteritis,* inflammation of the intestine.
epi- upon, outside: *epidermis,* outer layer of the true skin.
ex- out of: *exostosis,* bony growth from surface of bone.
hem-, hemo- blood: *hemoglobin,* coloring matter of red blood cells.
hetero- dissimilar: *heterophile* antibody, having affinity for antigen other than that for which it is specific.
homeo- similar: *homeostasis,* stability of normal body states.
hydro- water: *hydrothorax,* fluid in the pleural cavity.
hyper- above, excessive: *hyperacidity,* excessive acidity.
hypo- deficiency or beneath: *hypoacidity,* deficient acidity; *hypodermic,* beneath the skin.
hyster- uterus: *hysterectomy,* excision of the uterus; *hysteria,* nervous condition in women long believed to have origin in uterus.
infra- below: *infraorbital,* beneath the orbit.
inter- between: *intercellular,* between cells.

intra- within: *intracellular,* within cells.

leuko- white: *leukocyte,* a white blood cell.

macro- large:*macrocyte,* an abnormally large red blood cell.

mal- bad: *malnutrition,* poor nutrition.

mast- breast: *mastitis,* inflammation of the breast.

mega- great: *megacolon,* enlargement of the colon.

melan- black: *melanin,* a black pigment.

men- month: *menses, menstruation,* monthly blood flow from uterus.

micro- small: *microcyte,* an undersized red blood cell.

myo- muscle: *myositis,* inflammation of muscle.

myx- mucus: *myxedema,* mucinous edema.

necro- death: *necrosis,* death of cells.

neo- new: *neoplasm,* a new growth or tumor.

nephr- kidney: *nephritis,* inflammation of kidney.

oligo- few: *oliguria,* scanty urination.

osteo- bone: *osteomyelitis,* inflammation of bone.

para- beside: *paramedical,* having a secondary relation to medicine.

peri- around:*pericardium,* the membrane around the heart.

phago- to eat, devour: *phagocyte,* a cell that devours bacteria and other foreign material; *esophagus,* the gullet.

phleb- vein: *phlebitis,* inflammation of a vein.

polio- gray: *poliomyelitis,* inflammation of gray matter of spinal cord.

poly- many: *polycythemia,* excess in number of red blood cells.

post- after: *postmortem,* after death.

pro- before: *prophylaxis,* measures taken to prevent disease.

pseudo- false: *pseudopodia,* false feet of astroglia.

pyo- pus: *pyosalpinx,* fallopian tube filled with pus.

syn- together with: *syndrome,* a constant complex of symptoms.

xantho- yellow: *xanthochromia,* yellow coloration of the cerebrospinal fluid.

SUFFIXES

-angio, vessel: *lymphangiitis,* inflammation of a lymph vessel.

-algia, pain: *neuralgia,* pain involving nerves.

-ase, designating an enzyme: *amylase,* a starch-splitting enzyme of the pancreas.

-cele, a protrusion: *meningocele,* a hernial protrusion of the meninges.

-centesis, perforating or tapping: *thoracentesis,* aspirating fluid from the thorax.

-chole, bile: *acholic,* without bile.

-ectasis, dilate: *bronchiectasis,* dilatation of the bronchi.

-ectomy, excision: *tonsillectomy,* removal of a tonsil.

-emesis, vomit: *hematemesis,* vomiting blood.

-emia, blood: *anemia,* deficiency of red blood cells.

-esthesia, sensation: *anesthesia,* absence of sensation.

-genesis, generation of: *pathogenesis,* generation of disease.

-iasis, a process, especially a morbid one: *amebiasis,* state of being infected with amebae.

-itis, inflammation of the part named: *appendicitis,* inflammation of appendix.

-lith, stone: *phlebolith,* calcified body in a vein.

-lysis, to dissolve: *autolysis,* self-dissolution.

-malacia, softening: *osteomalacia,* softening of bone.

-megaly, large: *splenomegaly,* enlargement of spleen.

-odynia, pain: *pleurodynia,* pain in the region of the pleura.

-oid, like, resembling: *mucoid,* like mucus.

-oma, tumor: *osteoma,* a tumor of bone.

-osis, a morbid process: *amyloidosis,* amyloid degeneration.

-ostomy, mouth: *gastrostomy,* to make an artificial opening into the stomach.

-otomy, cut: *gastrotomy,* to cut into the stomach.

-pathy, disease: *neuropathy,* any nervous disease.

-penia, poverty: *thrombocytopenia,* decrease in the thrombocytes or blood platelets.

-phila, affinity for: *eosinophil,* leukocyte staining with eosin.

-plasia, to form: *hyperplasia,* overgrowth of tissue.

-plegia, paralysis: *hemiplegia,* paralysis of one half (side) of the body.

-pnea, breath: *dyspnea,* difficult breathing.

-ptosis, falling: *visceroptosis,* falling of abdominal viscera.

-rhagia, bursting forth: *menorrhagia,* profuse menstruation.

-rhea, flow: *diarrhea,* abnormal flow from bowel.

-sclerosis, hardening: *arteriosclerosis,* hardening of the arteries.

-stasis, standing still: *hemostasis,* arrest of circulation.

-trophy, nourish: *atrophy,* wasting.

-uria, relating to urine: *anuria,* absence of urine.

Index